The Textbook of Children's Nursing

Tina Moules
Principal Lecturer
Head of Division
Childhood Studies
Anglia Polytechnic University
UK

and

Joan Ramsay
Clinical Nurse Manager
Paediatric Unit
Luton and Dunstable Hospital
UK

with contributions from

Judith Hendrick
Law Department
Oxford Brookes University
Headington
Oxford
UK

Stanley Thornes (Publishers) Ltd

First published by Stanley Thornes (Publishers) Ltd in 1998
Ellenborough House
Wellington Street
CHELTENHAM
GL50 1YW
United Kingdom

98 99 00 01 02 / 10 9 8 7 6 5 4 3 2 1

A catalogue record for this book is available from The British Library.

ISBN 0 7487 3340 X

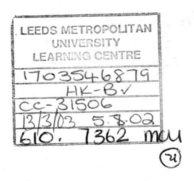

Typeset by Columns Design Ltd, Reading, Berkshire
Printed and bound in Italy by STIGE, Turin

This book is dedicated to our own children,
all the children that we have nursed,
and all the students we have taught.

CONTENTS

PREFACE

Give a man a fish and you feed him for a day
Teach a man to fish and you feed him for life
Old Chinese Proverb

This book does not merely give you facts about children's nursing because it aims to teach you how to nurse children in a way that you can remember and apply to any child in your care. It has been written to enable you to explore many different aspects of children's nursing and to actually participate in the learning process by undertaking various activities within the text. We encourage you to add your own notes, either within the text or, if you prefer, in a separate notebook. This idea is based on the philosophy that learning is an active process and occurs more effectively if the learner is actively involved. Because learning is a life-long process, you are encouraged to review the content at a later stage and explore how it has changed. By adding your thoughts about these changes you will prolong the life of the content and build up a valuable resource of past and current issues.

The book does not profess to give you all the answers. In fact it should stimulate you to ask more questions and to reflect upon your experiences, past and present. The content is structured on a modular format and will provide you with a wealth of literature and resources for further study. Each module begins with an introduction and a number of learning outcomes, and is divided into parts which can be studied separately, thus allowing you to study at your own pace. You can also choose to use the book as part of a course of study, in which case the modular format could be used to structure your learning.

The book has a strong emphasis on the differing roles of the children's nurse and in particular the role as a health promoter. This is an important role of the children's nurse so that children can be helped to achieve their full potential. The caring role of the children's nurse is complex requiring you to use your skills to make reasoned judgements and decisions about the needs of children of varying ages and levels of development. This book aims to help you in this problem-solving process by encouraging reflection, critical analysis and exploration.

ACKNOWLEDGEMENTS

The idea for this book was conceived on a beach near Herstmonceux in East Sussex many years ago and signed and sealed over a bottle of good red wine. It has come to fruition through the dedication of our dear friend and editor Rosemary Morris. Rosemary has supported us with her patience, persistence, sense of humour and her continued belief in us. She continued to give us encouragement even through her own difficult times. Rosemary we thank you.

We would also like to thank Judith Hendrick for contributing to the section on legal and ethical issues. Judith's knowledge and expertise (and her ability to keep to our deadlines) was invaluable in compiling this part of the book.

Finally we would both like to show our gratitude to Bob Walker whose creative drawings have added to the text.

> Thank you
> Tina and Joan

I would like to acknowledge the support given to me by my partner Eddy who has put up with the trials and tribulations of such a long-term project. He has never ceased to have faith that I would finish but has got rather cross about the mess in the study. As I write this, he lies in a hospital bed but fortunately not because of this! My children Tom and Kate have been a great inspiration to me – they have brought me down to earth when the going has been tough. I have been able to reflect upon and use some of their experiences. I must also give grateful thanks to my colleagues at Anglia Polytechnic University for giving me time and support.

> Thank you all.
> Tina

I would like to thank my husband Alex for his continued support and his help with typing the manuscript. Like Eddy he has had to put up with chaos in the study, postpone his own work and the loss of any shared activities over the final months of preparation. I am sure that my daughter Helen, whose bedroom is next to the study, meant to give me support by playing heavy metal music at earth shattering levels. I would also like to thank all my colleagues on the children's unit at the L&D Hospital who gave me ideas and encouragement.

> Thank you all.
> Joan

HEALTH IN CHILDHOOD

UNDERSTANDING FAMILIES

Tina Moules

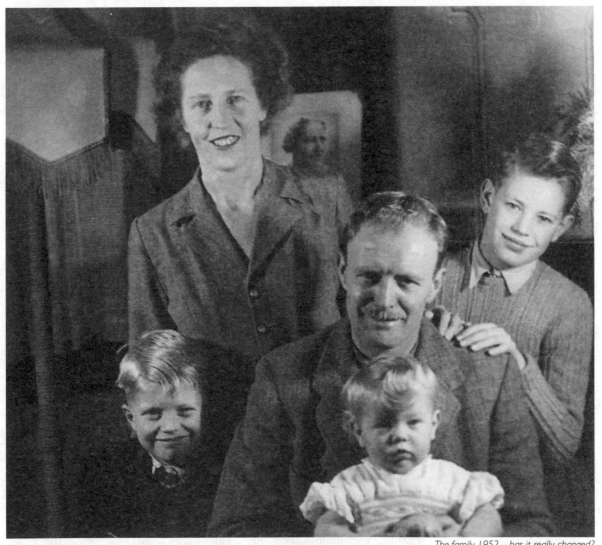

The family 1952 – has it really changed?

OBJECTIVES

The material contained within this module and the further reading/references should enable you to:

- Explore the nature of the family with special reference to the changes which have occurred in structure.
- Analyse the nature of relationships and roles within families and the factors which influence family life.
- Consider critically the role of the family in the development of children.
- Analyse different child-rearing patterns.

INTRODUCTION

For most people the family is by far the most significant institution in terms of the impact it has on the quality of their daily life and experience.

(White and Woollett, 1992)

Many different types of family structure exist in Britain today, influenced by cultural and social factors. Children are born into and grow up in these units, and, as such, develop within the context of the family and have themselves an impact on the family. Debates about the state of the family have been numerous in recent years as changing social constructs have led to changes in family structures and the social 'norm'. Thus the world of children changes as they adapt to cope with, for example, divorce, parents who work, reconstituted families, etc. It is vital that children's nurses have an understanding of the nature of the 'family' and its role in the development and lives of children, so that they can provide real family-centred care.

This module will begin by examining the nature of the family, the changes in structure which have occurred and the effect of family break-up on children. Families consist of individual members, each with a variety of roles. The way in which these roles and the relationships associated with them interact and influence family members will be explored. One of the main functions of the family is the socialisation of children. It is within the family that most infants develop the first basic social relationships and learn primary social skills. This function and the contribution that the family makes to child development will be discussed. Finally, the module will consider different styles of child rearing. Throughout the module you will be urged to consider the implications of issues for your practice.

THE FAMILY 1

INTRODUCTION

'The family' is considered by many people to be the smallest and most personal of all social institutions, and one which is a universal phenomenon varying from culture to culture. The structure of the family in the UK has changed over the last 40–50 years and continues to do so. It is not a static concept, but one which alters and adapts to the needs of a changing society. Before exploring the ways in which the nature of the family has changed it is worth considering some definitions of the family. According to various authors the family is:

- 'A group of people tied by relationships of blood, marriage or adoption' (Jorgensen, 1995).
- 'A group of people living with or near each other, who are closely related by marriage or blood' (Moore, 1996).
- 'Two or more persons who share resources and responsibilities for decisions, values and goals, and have a commitment to each other over time' (Davidson and Moore, 1996).
- 'A group of people living under one roof, commonly a set of two or more adults living together and rearing their children' (*Longman New Universal Dictionary*, 1982).
- 'A married or cohabiting couple with or without children or a lone parent with children' (CSO, 1995).
- 'A social group, characterised by common residence, economic cooperation and reproduction. It includes adults of both sexes, at least two of whom maintain a socially approved sexual relationship, and one or more children, own or adopted, of the sexually cohabiting adult' (Murdock, 1949, cited by Jorgensen, 1995).

Activity

Consider and analyse each of the definitions above. What does each really say? Do they reflect the concept of the family as you perceive it? Using the definitions try to write one which you feel reflects society today.

Since the concept of what constitutes a conventional family seems to have changed, any definition of the family must allow for all possibilities. Narrow definitions based on the conventional family may increase the social pressures on individuals to conform. When caring for children and their families, it is important to recognise the value of all forms of family unit and acknowledge the importance placed on individuality. What is considered to be the conventional family? Conventional families (White and Woollett, 1992):

- are headed by a married heterosexual couple;
- consist of two to three children genetically and biologically linked with their parents;
- consist of children born to mothers between the ages of 20 and 35;
- live together in a nuclear household unit;
- have fathers who are breadwinners and mothers who are full-time housewives.

Activity

To what extent do you believe that this type of family exists today? Draw up a plan of your family. Is it conventional? If not, how does it differ from the ideas above? If possible share your ideas with a colleague.

FAMILY STRUCTURES

You may have identified many ways in which your family differs from the idea of the 'norm' or 'conventional'. In this section we will examine the various ways in which the structure of the family has changed over recent years in relation to the characteristics of the conventional family.

The conventional family is headed by married, heterosexual couples

Interestingly, statistics show that, in 1991, 71% of children lived in married couple families with both natural parents (Table 1.1). However, this is a decline from the figure of 83% in 1979 (Condy, 1994). So although it may be argued that the family is in decline, the majority of children experience this type of family at some stage of their lives.

Marriage rates (Table 1.2) have declined overall with a drop of 24% between 1979 and 1991 to 340 000 with a slight rise in 1992 to 347 000: 38% of these were second marriages compared with 14% of all marriages in 1981. This points to the idea that marriage is still seen as important, with most men and women eventually marrying (CSO, 1995).

Table 1.1

Percentages of families with dependent children by family type (1991). (Adapted from OPCS, 1995)

	Couple families			Lone-parent families	All families
	Married	**Cohabiting**	**All**		
Children living with their natural mother and natural father with					
No step-brothers/sisters	72.8	2.7	75.5	–	75.5
Step-brothers/sisters	1.8	0.3	2.1	–	2.1
Children living with one natural parent					
Mother	2.9	1.5	4.4	14.8	19.2
Father	1.0	0.4	1.4	1.8	3.2

Country	1981	1992
UK	7.10	5.40
Belgium	6.50	5.80
Denmark	5.00	6.20
France	5.80	4.70
Greece	7.30	4.70
Irish Republic	6.00	4.50
Italy	5.60	5.30
Luxembourg	5.50	6.40
Netherlands	6.00	6.20
Portugal	7.70	7.10
Spain	5.40	5.50

Table 1.2

Marriage rates: 1981 and 1992 EC comparison (rates per 1000 population). (Adapted from OPCS, 1992)

Activity

Using the material in Table 1.2, compare marriage rates in the various EU countries. What factors might be responsible for the differences?

More people are choosing to cohabit although many do eventually marry at some stage. The increase can be deduced by the number of births registered outside marriage, which has risen steeply from 12% in 1980 to 31% in 1992. Of these, one in five births outside marriage in 1990 was registered by both parents living at the same address compared with one in 25 in 1971. This might indicate that more cohabiting couples are providing a stable environment for children. In 1991, 7% of children aged 0–4 were living with their natural cohabiting parents. Cohabitation is increasingly favoured by couples where one or both partners is separated or divorced with children (Utting, 1995). The 1991 Census shows that family heads describing themselves as Black Caribbean or Black Other are more likely to be cohabiting than the general population. The reverse is so for Indian, Pakistani and Bangladeshi households. Although cohabitation is more popular for a variety of possible reasons, it has been suggested that cohabiting relationships are less stable than marriages. Buck *et al.* (1994) suggest that cohabiting couples are four times as likely to separate as married couples.

Alongside the fall in marriage rates has been a rise in the number of divorces. The UK had one of the highest divorce rates in the EC in 1992 with 173 000 decrees registered (Table 1.3). This is the highest rate recorded so far and more than double that in 1971. If the trend is maintained, more than four out of 10 new marriages will end in separation (Walker *et al.*, 1991). Figure 1.1 shows the rise in divorce rates between 1950 and 1992.

Factors leading to rise in cohabitation
- Changes in social attitudes
- Less importance placed on the institution of marriage
- Economic factors – cost of weddings
- Declining influence of religion
- Rising divorce rates

Table 1.3	Country	
	Australia	2.50
	Austria	2.00
	Belgium	2.00
	Canada	2.40
	Denmark	2.80
	Finland	2.00
	France	2.00
	West Germany	2.10
	Greece	0.90
	Iceland	2.20
	Ireland	–
	Italy	0.50
	Japan	1.30
	Luxembourg	2.00
	Netherlands	1.90
	New Zealand	2.50
	Norway	1.90
	Portugal	0.90
	Spain	0.50
	Sweden	2.30
	Switzerland	1.80
	Turkey	0.40
	UK	2.90
	USA	4.80

Divorce – world wide comparison (per 1000). (Source: Jorgensen, 1995)

Several factors have contributed to the rise in the number of divorces including (Jorgensen, 1995):

- changed attitudes – there is less stigma attached to divorce;
- changes in legislation – changes in the law have made it easier for couples to divorce;
- changing roles of women – more than 75% of petitions for divorce are made by women;
- changing expectations of marriage – today the emphasis appears to be on equality and partnership between husbands and wives, perhaps putting more stress on relationships;
- family experience of divorce – it is suggested that you are more likely to divorce if you have experienced the divorce of your parents.

Activity

Consider each of these possible factors. Using your life experiences and reference to literature, how does each reflect the reality of life?

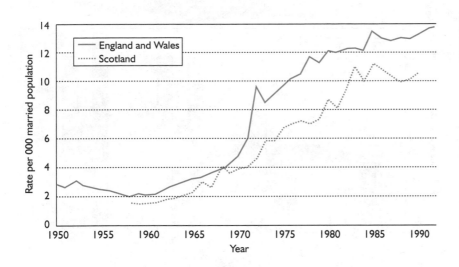

Figure 1.1

Divorce rates 1950–1992.
(Source: Utting, 1995)

An increasing number of children experience living in lone-parent families. The number of dependent children living in one-parent families has risen from 1 million in 1971 to 2.3 million in 1991. Lone-parent families can occur as a result of divorce, separation (from marriage or cohabitation), death, through choice (the woman who deliberately chooses to have a child outside of a stable relationship) or through unplanned pregnancy (Figure 1.2). Most lone-parent families are headed by mothers (18% of all households) with only 2% of households headed by a lone father. Lone-parent families are more frequently found among Black families than other ethnic groups and are least likely to be found among the Indian community. The circumstances in which lone-parent families live can vary tremendously and it is impossible to generalise. However, statistics show that the majority of lone-parent families experience significantly more hardship than couple families. In 1990, 53% of lone-parent families had a weekly income of £100 or less compared with 4% of married or cohabiting families (OPCS, 1993).

Factors leading to rise in lone-parent families

- Rapid rise in divorce
- Demands placed on partners in marriage make single parenthood preferred option
- Women less dependent on men
- Rise in unmarried mothers with increasing sexual activity among the young
- Greater unpredictability during the lives of many people
- Effects of media increasing the acceptability of lone parenthood

Activity

Consider the implications of lone-parent families for practice.

Not all families are headed by a heterosexual couple. Although figures are not available, a small minority may be headed by gay or lesbian couples. A developing freedom allowing gay couples to live openly together has resulted in the controversial issue of children in gay families. Gay families usually come about through one partner having

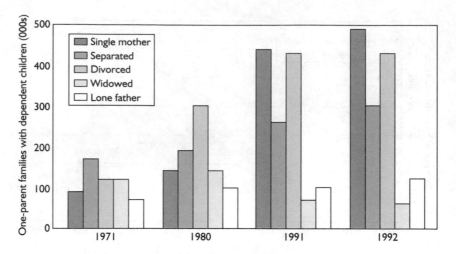

Figure 1.2

Lone-parent families in Great Britain 1991. (Source: Utting, 1995)

been divorced and being given custody of the children from a hetero-sexual relationship. However, there have been incidences of lesbian couples having their own children with the use of artificial insemination. Alternatively both gay and lesbian couples are attempting to adopt children. This change in behaviour requires us to reconsider our views on relationships and the raising of children. Many assumptions about children in gay relationships are based on the maxim that gay parents equal gay children. However, children do not simply follow in their parents footsteps – many other factors influence the way in which they grow and develop. Research has compared children of homosexual and heterosexual couples, and has found no significant difference in their well-being or sexual orientation (Allen and Burrell, 1994, cited by Davidson and Moore, 1996). Many gay couples are as committed to a permanent relationship as married couples.

Activity

Consider your own views on the gay family issue and discuss with colleagues the implications for practice.

The conventional family consists of two or three children genetically and biologically linked with their parents

Whilst this may be true for the majority of children, an increasing number are being raised in families where the genetic links between child and parents have been partially or completely broken.

In 1991, it was suggested that nearly 500 000 *step-families (reconstituted families)* existed in Great Britain, including about 800 000 step-children (most from women's previous relationships) (Haskey, 1994). These data suggest that 30% of children will experience living in step-families during their childhood. Step-families come in many different forms with children from one (or both) partner's previous relationships. At the same time new partners may have children of their own which adds to the difficulties many of these families experience.

A relatively small proportion of families come through *adoption*. This is a common form of family building for those who are unable to conceive and have children naturally. However, the numbers of children adopted are small. In 1988 approximately 1000 babies and 4000 children were adopted out of the 780 000 children born (Humphrey and Humphrey, 1988). In these cases there is normally no genetic link between the child and adopted parents.

An even smaller number of children are born with the aid of *reproductive technology*. Approximately one in seven couples have difficulty conceiving naturally and help is now at hand for some with new fertility treatments. One such treatment is Artificial Insemination by Donor (AID). This method helps to overcome infertility in men by inseminating their partners with either fresh or frozen donated sperm. In this case all children born will have a genetic link with their mothers but not with their fathers. In 1988 approximately 2400 children were born by this method (Humphrey and Humphrey, 1988). Another method leading to disrupted genetic links is surrogacy. This increasingly controversial method exists in different forms but usually involves a surrogate mother being artificially inseminated with the father's sperm. In this case the child will have a genetic link with the father but not with the mother.

There are moral and ethical issues involved with alternative forms of family building. The methods tend to be tightly controlled and limited to those couples considered suitable, as being:

- not too old;
- heterosexual;
- married;
- in long-term stable relationships.

Recent controversy has surrounded applications from gay couples and there is a tendency for single-parent adoption to be shunned. Issues concerned with reproductive technology tend to be centred around the idea that it is wrong to interfere with nature. There are a number of psychological issues that are common to both adoption and reproductive technology which are worth considering:

- With genetic links partially or completely broken, it is suggested that this can interfere with the sense of continuity and commitment to the future that conventional parents may have.
- In the case of adoption, the mother misses out on the experience of birth, which some say is important in the development of relationships between mother and child (White and Woollett, 1992).

Step-family

'A step-family is created when two adults form a new household in which one, or both, brings a child/children from a previous relationship'.
(De'Ath, 1996)

The later the adoption occurs, the more the early experience is missed. The same is true for many step-parents who have to accept that the children have had experiences of which they were not a part. It can be quite difficult to adjust to caring for a child who may have been brought up with a different set of ideals.

- With AID, step-parenting and some forms of surrogacy, the child is clearly genetically linked to only one parent. This may lead to possible conflict within the relationship, especially during stressful times. The child may become 'mine' or 'yours', leading to accusations of blame.

- Parents who have children by alternative methods may choose to keep quiet about their children's origins. For some, the differences are obvious, e.g. parents who adopt older children or suddenly bring home a baby with no previous signs of pregnancy. For others, it may be possible to pass the birth off as entirely natural. Whilst there is no right or wrong, keeping secrets has its disadvantages. Issues related to the rights of children to know their origins are central to the debate. Parents have no legal duty to tell children of their origins. Adopted children have the right to obtain information about their birth parents but only if they have been told of the adoption. However, this may not be a reality for those born by AID due to lack of information.

- A decline in the birth rate has been accompanied by a reduction in the average number of children born to each family. In 1860 there were an average seven children born to each marriage; since 1981 the figure has stabilised to 1.8 (Wise, 1994).

Activity

Consider the implications of alternative methods of family building for your practice.

The conventional family consists of children born to mothers between the ages of 20 and 35

'One of the main features of recent British fertility behaviour is the postponement of parenthood'. (Utting, 1995)

Statistics show that women are choosing to give birth to their first child later in life. In 1971, the mean age at first birth was 24; by 1992 it was approaching 28 (OPCS, 1994). More women are delaying childbirth until their 30s and this applies more to women who have qualifications than those who do not (OPCS, 1993). At the same time there are a growing number of women who are choosing to remain childless. Estimates predict that one in five women born between 1947 and 1957 will be childless at the age of 40 (Church, 1995).

The conventional family lives together in a nuclear household unit

Statistics seem to support the idea that the nuclear family is dominant. However, it does depend on how the statistics are interpreted. Table 1.4 shows us that a quarter of all households consists of people living alone; one-third are households of adults only (about 40% of whom have grown up children); 30% of households contain dependent children but of these one-fifth are lone-parent families. If one considers the data as presented, then it would appear that married couples with children are relatively rare occurrences. However, if one takes into account those families who have yet to have children and those with non-dependent children, nearly two-thirds of households conform to the stereotype nuclear family. Most of us are likely to experience life in a nuclear family at some stage (Muncie *et al.*, 1995).

Nuclear family
- *Conventional* – husband, wife and their children living in same residence
- *Non-conventional* – two adults and children living in the same residence

Households	Percentage
Single person	
pensionable age	15
other	11
Two or more married adults	3
Married couple	
no children	28
dependent children	24
non-dependent children	8
Lone parent	
dependent children	6
non-dependent children	4
Two or more families	1

Table 1.4

Households by type in 1990–1991, Great Britain. (Adapted from OPCS, 1992)

The concept of the extended family offers an alternative family structure which is perhaps more commonly found in its true form among ethnic minorities. In fact it is probably within the ethnic groups that most diversity is found. Evidence suggests that while immigrants adapt to their new environment, the fundamental basis of their beliefs about family life remain intact. For example, Asian households are more likely than White British ones to contain extended family members. Although British housing makes the formation of three-generation households difficult, the extended family remains an important source of mutual support in Asian life. On the other hand, British Afro-Caribbean households rarely contain an extended family (Ballard and Kalra, 1994). However, there is evidence that the extended family continues to be important in Britain. Willmott (1988) identified the 'dispersed extended family' as being members of a family giving support to each other even though they lived some distance apart. Members of the extended family also play a vital role in child care thus allowing mothers to work. A survey by the OPCS showed that half the day care for children under 5 is provided by relatives (OPCS, 1994a).

Extended family
- *Conventional* – more than two generations living in the same household
- *Modified* – extended family members living in close proximity or maintaining contact though living far apart

The conventional family has fathers who are breadwinners and mothers who are full-time housewives

This is no longer necessarily the case. The working pattern of families can be very complex. One or either partner may work part time or full time, from home or outside the home. More mothers are working than ever before and many men are no longer the main or only breadwinner. Increasingly both parents are earning. In 1973 both parents worked in 43% of families. By 1992 this figure had risen to 60% (OPCS, 1994b). The data show that almost three in 10 children under the age of 2 and most secondary school children live in dual-earning families. However, set against the growing number of families where both parents work is the fact that there are a growing number of families in which neither parent works (Gregg and Wadsworth, 1994).

The female work force has been on the increase for some years and rose by 3 million between 1971 and 1990. More than seven out of 10 wives are now considered economically active. More mothers are returning to work; in 1992, 59% of mothers with dependent children were in work. This compares with 49% in 1973 (OPCS, 1994b). Many of these women are in part-time work. It is interesting to note that, although more women are working, there does not seem to be any change in the allocation of household chores. Even where the family has two working parents, most of the chores are left to the woman (Hewison and Dowswell, 1994).

Some fathers remain at home either from choice or through unemployment. In some cases fathers take on role reversal, i.e. they stay at home to care for the children while the partner goes out to work. This usually occurs where the woman's earning potential is more than the man's. Whatever the reason, the father is no longer the 'breadwinner'. This may have psychological effects as many men still see it as their role to provide for their families.

So the debate is: Is the conventional family still the norm? Much of the data examined would seem to support the idea that the conventional family does indeed still exist. Most people in the UK marry and have children, most children are brought up by both birth parents and the nuclear family predominates. What is noticeable is that some modifications have occurred in recent years leading to what some would describe as the 'neoconventional' family. The diverse nature of the family must be taken into account, especially when care for sick children and their families is being planned. Each family will have different needs and will need different kinds of support. At the same time, it is important to recognise that families are not static units, they change and evolve. The conventional family goes through stages (Figure 1.3) beginning with possible cohabitation, then marriage without children, followed by the birth of the first and subsequent children. When the children leave home, the family changes yet again, only to be transformed with the birth of grandchildren. The final stage is one of bereavement, as one or other partner dies. At the same time that one family is changing, others are evolving as children marry.

Figure 1.3

The conventional family life cycle. (Source: Moore, 1996)

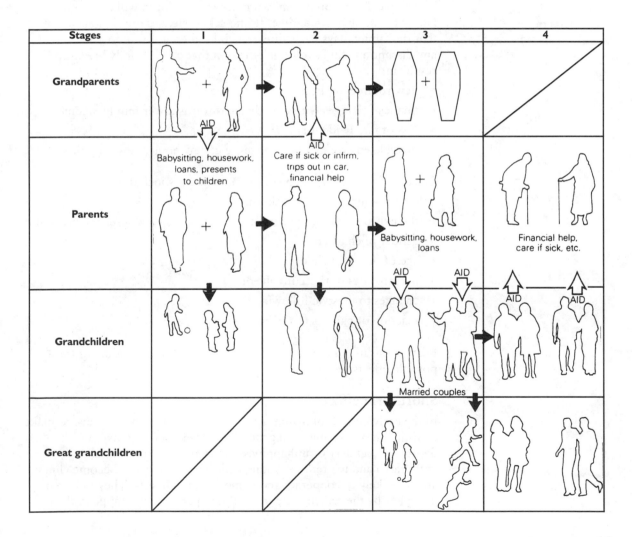

When one considers the non-conventional family, these stages may well overlap. Some families may reshape themselves several times over within the life time of its members.

Activity

John and Jenny Smythe have recently married. John has two children from his former partner who died. Jenny has one child as a result of an unplanned pregnancy and one child from her previous marriage. John and Jenny have one child of their own. Taking each member of the family, map the various forms of family they may have experienced.

Cross reference

Separation – page 203

FAMILY BREAK-UP AND ITS EFFECTS ON CHILDREN

The above discussion has shown that many children will experience family break-up at some time. If one acknowledges the significant role that the family plays in the life of a child, then it is safe to assume that any disruption will have some effect on that child. Family break-up results in:

- new routines and patterns;
- financial changes with a tendency towards lower family income;
- loss of family identity;
- possible environmental changes, e.g. new home, new school.

The consequences will depend on many factors including:

- circumstances of the break-up;
- the existence of family conflict before, during and after the break-up;
- gender of children;
- age of the child/children;
- personalities of those involved;
- changes to lifestyle following disruption;
- reaction of parents to the break-up.

Bearing this in mind it is useful to develop an understanding of the possible effects on children.

Short-term effects

In the early period following family break-up, all members have to make adjustments and changes. In general children react negatively with depression, anxiety or unhappiness. They may become socially withdrawn and inattentive. Young children may regress, become clingy and less likely to cooperate and comply with requests. They may fear being left by the remaining parent. If one parent can disappear, then so could the other one, and they may feel a degree of self-blame (Kurdek, 1988). The reactions can be likened to those following a bereavement, with an initial expression of denial and guilt. Reactions of children to the break-up will be influenced by the way in which the custodial parent deals with the situation. More than 80% of custodial parents are mothers and for most of them the first year of bringing up children alone will be demanding both on emotion and energy. They are more likely to leave children to their own devices, avoid confrontation with them and fail to maintain consistent routines (Hetherington and Arasteh, 1988). This behaviour is likely to make children feel insecure and can change the relationship they have with their mothers. In the short term, girls seem to cope better than boys.

Activity

A 4-year-old boy is admitted to the ward for planned surgery. He has on older brother and a younger sister. On assessing the family you find out that the children's father left home 6 months ago. How might this information influence the care you plan to give this family?

Long-term effects

After the initial period of readjustment, the well-being of all members of the family improves. Routines become re-established as individuals adapt to new circumstances. However, there is evidence that points to long-term influences on children's behaviour. Hetherington (1988) found that children who have experienced family break-up are more likely to be aggressive, non-compliant and underachievers. Wadsworth (1985) studied the impact of divorce on a group of women from broken homes. He compared them with women from intact homes and found that the women from broken homes were more likely to describe their childhood as unhappy or lacking warmth. They demonstrated lower educational achievement and were less demonstrative with their own children. The effects of divorce on girls become more apparent in the long term. They may become rebellious with high rates of depression and have more difficulty with heterosexual relationships than girls from intact homes (Hetherington, 1988).

There can be positive results of family break-up. These include:

- reduction in/removal of conflict;
- children developing a more mature and sensitive approach and benefiting from additional responsibility;
- relationship between custodial parent and children becoming very close;
- siblings becoming closer.

Further reading
COCKETT, M. and TRIP, J. (1994) *The Exeter Family Study: Family Breakdown and its Impact on Children.* Exeter: University of Exeter Press

This study explores the views of children on family break-up

Further reading

JORGENSEN, J. (1995) *Investigating Families and Households*. London: Collins Educational

From a series on Sociology in Action. This book gives a good discussion of the issues raised here. It also gives you an opportunity to interact by completing activities

MUNCIE, J., WETHERELL, M., DALLOS, R. and COCHRANE, A. (1995) *Understanding the Family*. London: Sage

An interesting book that looks at family diversity, policy and the law, and interactions and identity. Also contains activities

Activity

Carry out some further reading on the effects of family break-up on children. You might look especially at the effects of step-parenting. How do children adjust to this new situation? Perhaps you have experienced family break-up yourself? Reflect on how it affected you and other members of your family.

Summary

This part of the module has examined the nature of the family in Britain today. The concept of the 'conventional family' has been explored, examining the changes which have occurred in recent years. Material has been offered to encourage you to reach your own conclusions about the state of the family today and has asked you to consider the implications in family changes for your practice. Try to take the time to explore some of the further reading and to analyse the current trends which affect families today.

Key points ➤

1. Defining the 'family' is difficult to do because of its complex and changing nature.
2. It is important for health professionals to recognise the value of all forms of family unit and to acknowledge individuality.
3. The majority of children live in married family couples with both natural parents *but* an increasing number of children will experience other family forms at some stage during their lives.
4. Most men and women eventually marry *but* the divorce rate has risen markedly in recent years.
5. Alternative forms of family building bring with them considerable ethical and moral issues.
6. Most of us are likely to experience life in a nuclear family at some stage.

ROLES AND RELATIONSHIPS 2

INTRODUCTION

Within each family there is a complex system of relationships and interactions. If we acknowledge the diversity of family form, then these relationships can in themselves be diverse. At the same time as belonging to various subsystems, each member of the family fulfils several roles. Understanding how these roles and relationships work may help you to meet the needs of different family members more appropriately.

It is possible to identify subsystems within all families. These will depend on the type of family but, in a conventional nuclear type, they will consist of (Figure 2.1):

- mother–child/children;
- father–child/children;
- child–child;
- father–mother.

Further reading

RIBBENS, J. (1990) *Accounting for our children: different perspectives on 'family life' in middle income households*. PhD Thesis, CNAA, South Bank Polytechnic, London

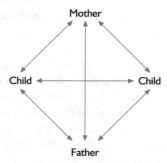

Figure 2.1

Subsystems within the conventional nuclear family.

If one takes into account the extended family then the relationships may become even more complex and, in fact, too complex to draw. Try it for yourself. It is no wonder that families sometimes argue and find it difficult to reach common ground.

Activity

Draw a diagram to reflect the possible subsystems within:
- a step-family
- a lone-parent family
- a step-family with a close extended family

How might an understanding of these subsystems assist your practice?

Many factors will affect relationships and interactions between the different subsystems including:
- number and age of children;
- age gap between children;

- age of parents;
- the family form;
- the presence of twins/triplets;
- the roles each individual fulfils.

It is important to remember that there is no typical family with typical relationships. We must not generalise about families; rather we should look at the issues surrounding relationships and roles so that we are in a better position to understand.

MOTHER–CHILD RELATIONSHIP

Cross reference

Parent–child relationship – page 202

The relationship between a mother and her child has been described as being more highly charged emotionally than others. Personal experience will probably vouch for this. One minute children balk at their mother's constraints, shouting and screaming because they cannot do/have what they want. Perhaps the mother, tired and weary after a hard day's work, begins to shout back, frustrated because the child is misbehaving. A vicious circle builds up. Shortly afterwards, both demonstrate almost overwhelming love and affection, cuddling, and apologise. Not any everyday occurrence perhaps, but one which will ring a bell with many mothers. It is worth exploring for a while this emotional relationship as those of us who care for sick children need to understand it.

Mothers generally give most care, especially to young children, and consequently develop close and strong emotional bonds with them. The bond often seems to have a special quality which no one can describe accurately. Perhaps it begins with the moment of birth? Perhaps it has something to do with a natural tendency for women to feel a close bond with babies and children? Perhaps it is a social expectation? What would be the argument regarding women who adopt, or women who choose not to have children and have a genuine dislike of them. One could argue for and against each of the suggestions. Whatever the special bond is, it is never more so obvious than when a child is ill. Experience has shown that mothers feel intensely about their child's illness, even when the problem may be minor. This can be illustrated by a particular incidence. A very experienced Ward Sister became frustrated with a mother who was very upset about her son's forthcoming circumcision. The Sister declared that she was making a fuss and said 'it's only a circumcision'. Some years later, the same Sister was admitted to the ward with her son for the same operation. She was distraught and crying and obviously distressed about the forthcoming operation. Something had changed her – becoming a mother.

The emotional relationships that mothers have with their children is said to be generally warm, responsive and child-centred. At the same time, their behaviour towards the child has been categorised into one of three types (Baumrind, 1971, cited in Santrock, 1995):

- *Authoritarian* – this type of behaviour is strict and controlling. The mother demands good performance and expects behaviour to be mature. There is no discussion and no reasons given for requests demonstrating unclear communications. When the child misbehaves, the mother punishes and shows little affection. Firm limits and controls are set.

- *Authoritative* – this mother behaves on the assumption that she has more knowledge and skills than the child. A high degree of compliance is expected and, whilst she is not intrusive, she is prepared to impose restrictions. Children's demands and reasons are respected.

- *Permissive* – Macoby and Martin (1983) identified two types of permissive mother. On the one hand, the permissive-indifferent mother is very uninvolved in the children's life. On the other hand, the permissive-indulgent mother is highly involved but places few demands on the children. Children are expected to regulate their own behaviour and generally do as they want.

Baumrind's work has been criticised by Ribbens (1994) who suggests that the study on which the types were based did not take any account of variable social contexts nor was it expressed in terms that women or parents might use themselves.

Research has shown that most mothers recognise the need to remain in control whilst allowing the child autonomy (especially after the age of 4). This can be difficult to achieve especially when the child is ill as there is a tendency to over-indulge the child. The way that a mother behaves with her children will be influenced by a number of factors. Behaviour may change from hour to hour and from day to day, depending on the circumstances. It is possible that many mothers' behaviour is a combination of the above.

Activity

Reflect on some of the mothers you have met. Which type did they seem to fit into? Did their behaviour vary and, if so, what influenced this?

Factors affecting type of parenting
- Depth of understanding of child's ability to understand and reason at different ages
- Pressures on the mother – work, housework, number of children
- Mother's expectations of child
- Social circumstances – lone parent, relationship with father, unemployment

It is interesting to examine the way in which mothers interact with babies and infants. Relationships and interactions are more intense during this stage. The mother uses the same signals as she does in other relationships but in this case they are more exaggerated, e.g. facial expressions are exaggerated. Smiles are broader, eyes open wider, the pitch and pace of the voice is extreme. There is a high level of vocalising with prolonged mutual gazing (Stern, 1977). The language that mothers use has been described as 'motherese'. This language is short, simple, highly intelligible, of high frequency and pitch, and contains more nouns and fewer verbs. It tends to be bossy in nature containing many questions and instructions. It is important to note that the child's behaviour has an effect on the mother. Positive responses make the mother feel she is being a good mother: the baby cries, is cuddled and fed, and then settles back down. The mother feels complete. The baby who cries, is fed and cuddled, but who does not settle and continues to cry, can make the mother feel inadequate and question her own ability and confidence. Interactions between the mother and child are therefore reciprocal.

Activity

Take an opportunity to listen to a mother talking to her baby. Make a note of what she says and then analyse it.

The way that a mother interacts and relates to her child will depend on many factors including:

- mother's personality and sexual orientation;
- confidence;
- mother's state of health;
- support networks available;
- whether the mother works or not;
- cultural diversities;
- the child's gender, age, health, temperament;
- experience of motherhood.

If we really want to give family-centred care, we ought to make time to attempt to assess the mother's relationships with her child.

Activity

Next time you carry out an assessment reflect on how well you were able to assess the mother's relationships with her child.

FATHER–CHILD RELATIONSHIPS

Historically, a father's interactions with his children have been limited. Fathers were very much on the periphery, generally responsible for discipline and punishment. Truby King (1938) suggested that the father's role was very much a supervisory one, ensuring that the mother was able to get out for occasional 'wholesome amusement and fresh air'. Memories of childhood remind me of 'wait until your father gets home'. Fathers were unlikely to become involved in child care. While some things may not have changed very much, fathers are now more likely to have more intimate relationships with their children.

Further reading

MOSS, P. (ed.) (1995) *Father Figures: Fathers in the Families of the 1990s.* London: HMSO

BJRNBERG, U. and KOLLIND, A.-K. (1996) *Men's Family Relationships.* Stockholm: Almqvist and Wiskell

Fathers' relationships with children are influenced by a number of factors as are mothers'. One particular factor is the gender of the child. This does not appear to be as influential for mothers. McQuire (1991) suggests that fathers (and mothers) may not acknowledge gender differences in treatment but that outside observers might pick up on them. Fathers spend much more time with their sons, generally being more involved, particularly as they get older. According to White and Woollett (1992), British fathers express a moderately strong preference for sons. In comparison fathers tend to spend less time with their adolescent daughters and they are more emotionally distant (Steinberg *et al.*, 1989). Fathers interact more through play than do mothers. Play tends to be boisterous, more so with boys. Throwing up in the air or rough and tumble are classic games that fathers play. On the other hand, interactions with girls tend to be quieter, involving more cuddling. Why fathers should show this preference is not easy to answer. Perhaps they feel more comfortable with boys as they know more about the male than about the female. They have more insight into the needs of boys than girls – girls are largely unknown to them.

Activity

Consider the fathers you know. How do they relate to their children? Do they demonstrate a preference for their sons? What implications might this have for your practice?

Russell (1983) identified four types of father:

* traditional – father spends time with the children at home but does not engage in any care giving activities;
* uninterested and unavailable – father is rarely at home;
* the 'good' father – seen as good by their partners because they were willing to help;
* non-traditional highly participative – the father who shares care with his partner.

Although this research was carried out in the USA, Lewis (1986) found similar results in a study carried out in the UK.

Another factor which has been shown to influence the relationship between fathers and their children is the state of marital harmony. When marital harmony is high, fathers are shown to be warmer, more positive and happier with their children than when marital harmony is low. Marital stress leads to less interaction and a feeling of anger and contempt towards the children (White and Woollett, 1992). The quality of relationships before and around the birth is also likely to influence the way fathers behave and interact with the child.

O'Brien and Jones (1996) carried out a survey to study children's perceptions of the role of the father and their relationships with them.

The results showed that girls were more dissatisfied with the amount of time given to them by their fathers than boys. Fewer girls (23%) than boys (44%) felt that their fathers understood them very well.

Fathers' relationships with their children are varied and will depend on many factors. While it is generally the mother who stays with a child in hospital, there are many times when the father will be present and will even stay in place of the mother. It is therefore important to consider and assess the father's relationships with the child as well as the mother's.

Activity

Identify two fathers that you have known while caring for children. Compare and contrast their relationships with their children.

SIBLING RELATIONSHIPS

Relationships between siblings vary tremendously, from family to family, from day to day and from minute to minute. You may be familiar with the following scenario: Tom (aged 7) and Kate (aged 4) adore each other: they tell each other 'I love you' frequently. They play together, watch television together and cuddle. However, by the same token they 'hate' each other frequently, especially when one does something to annoy or tease, or takes a special toy. Generally speaking, however, they are buddies, companions, playmates. They depend on each other when the going gets tough (when one is punished for wrongdoing). A typical sibling relationship perhaps?

Fluctuating emotions

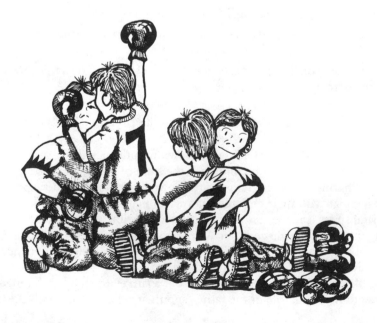

Activity

If you have brothers and sisters, what were your relationships like when you were young and what are they like now?

Relationships between siblings tend to be more reciprocal than those with adults. Children share more jokes, games, role play and pretend play than children and adults together. Tom and Kate love to dress up and play weddings, something they would never get their mother to do. Siblings tend to spend more time with each other than with their parents. They understand each other and have a degree of empathy:

- Kate comes running in from the garden – 'Tom's hurt himself, he needs you'.

- Kate has been told off and begins to cry. Tom puts his arm around her – 'Don't worry darling, Tom's here'.

- Kate has been told off (again) – 'I want Tom!'.

Sibling relationships offer children one of the first contexts in which they can show their feelings for others.

Younger children tend to copy older siblings. At this stage there is an obvious imbalance of skills, physical as well as psychological. The older sibling gives physical and verbal aggression, takes control and leads the play. As the children get older the imbalance of skills becomes less. The younger child takes a more active role and will begin to challenge the older child: this results in fights and arguments.

Dunn (1984) suggests that although sibling relationships are on the whole positive, negative emotions are frequently displayed. They tease and mock each other, quarrel and bicker, hit and pinch one another, take each other's toys, and generally annoy each other. This conflict, companionship, love and affection tend to continue throughout childhood, forming an ideal ground for searching out social rules and forming ideas about social issues.

Some siblings get on better together than others. Perhaps you know some who have no time for each other, even hate each other. There are several factors which will affect sibling relationships:

- *Gender*. Same sex siblings show a tendency to get on better. Perhaps this is because they have similar interests or because parents tend to treat boys differently from girls. I remember when I asked if I could stay out late because my brother did. 'He's a boy' was the reply. I hated my brother for that.

- *Age gap*. A small age gap could mean that there is a greater similarity of interests and perhaps more warmth and closeness. This can be seen in twins. However, at the same time, there is the possibility of greater discord and jealousy. With a large age gap there are few shared interests but there may be fewer arguments as a result.

Activity

Talk to friends, examine your own brother–sister relationships. What is the age gap? How has this affected relationships. Compare and contrast your findings.

- *Mother's facilitation of relationship.* The way in which a mother treats her children can affect their relationships. If there is disparity in treatment and if the mother tends to interfere frequently in sibling conflicts, sibling relationships tend to be more negative. It tends to be the older child who takes the brunt of this interference. Personal experience supports this. Where a mother involves a young child in preparations for the birth of a new baby, sibling relationships are more likely to be positive (White and Woollett, 1992).
- *Middle childhood.* Sibling relationships during this period are often put on hold. The children make more friends outside the home, friends who have the same interests and are dealing with the same experiences.

FATHER–MOTHER RELATIONSHIPS

No two mother–father relationships are the same. None progress the same or end the same. Relationships are directly related to the roles each fulfils and so are complex. It is possible that each partner fulfils several roles depending on the structure and form of the family (Figure 2.2).

Figure 2.2

The complexity of mother and father roles.

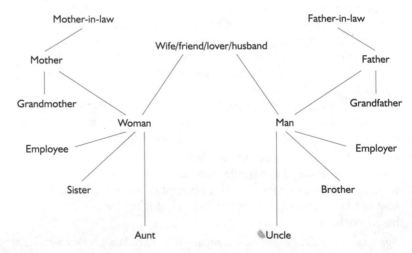

Further reading

DAVIDSON, J.K. and MOORE, N.B. (1996) *Marriage and Family: Change and Continuity.* Boston: Allyn and Bacon

Family Policy Bulletin. Available from: Family Policy Studies Centre, 231 Baker Street, London NW1 6XE. Tel: 0171 486 8211/7680

Each partner will have different relationships within the context of each role and each relationship will be affected by another. One can therefore never really understand how an individual's relationships are formed and develop. What we can do is look at how mother/father roles and relationships have changed.

Moore (1996) shows how sociologists have divided the changing roles and relationships between mothers and fathers into three phases:

- In *preindustrial families*, husband and wife tended to work together on the land. They relied heavily on each other and both worked. However, relationships between them were not particularly close.
- In *industrial families*, men were the breadwinners, women took on the role of housewife and withdrew from the workplace. The father was the head of the household and took charge. The men tended to dominate the relationship.
- In *contemporary families* there has been a move to more equality. Women have moved back into the workplace and have found a degree of financial independence. This, in turn, has made them look for more involvement from the fathers in relation to household chores and child care. This new equality led to the term 'symmetrical family' (Young and Willmott, 1975). This equality has been disputed by many sociologists who argue that male dominance still exists and that there is not equality especially in the area of power and delegation of household chores.

The symmetrical family

'Identified by Young and Willmott as a type of family evolving in the late 20th century in which husbands and wives have a more egalitarian relationship in the home; household and childrearing activities are increasingly shared'.

(Jorgensen, 1995)

Activity

Take a look back at your family. Talk to parents, grandparents, great-grandparents. How would they describe the roles and relationships between them. How have they changed over the generations?

Relationships between mothers and fathers fluctuate and are affected by many things. They fluctuate from day to day and from one stage of the family life cycle to another.

Activity

List the factors which affect your relationships with your partner, or the relationships between your parents.

You may have come up with some of the following:

- *Age gap*. A wide age gap may result in different expectations, interests, even a different approach to life in general.
- *Own parental relationships*. Experience of conflict and fights or conversely warmth and affection.
- *Financial circumstances*. Worries over money can cause conflict and disagreement.
- *Employment or unemployment*. Women going out to work, fathers becoming unemployed.
- *Loss and bereavement*. Loss of a parent, loss of a child.
- *Parenting style*. May differ causing conflict.

- *Sexual relationship.* Different expectations, needs.
- *Birth of a baby.* A transitional stage. Can lead to conflict, stress, less time together, jealousy. More likely to adjust if relationship is stable before birth.
- *Social life.* Friends, hobbies, spending time together.

There may be numerous other factors not mentioned here but this serves to highlight how complex adult relationships can be.

SUMMARY

This section has examined some of the issues surrounding roles and relationships within the family. It is clear that these issues are complex and cannot fully be given justice here. It is also clear that in attempting to implement family-centred care, we must try to understand where the family is coming from. While we are not able to assess all facets of family life we need to acknowledge and be mindful of the various factors which can affect relationships within families.

Activity

Consider a family you have cared for. Analyse the roles and relationships between various family members. How did this affect the care you were able to give? Reflect on how more knowledge of roles and relationships may have helped you.

Key points ➤

1. Within each family, there is a complex system of relationships and interactions.
2. The mother–child relationship has been described as being more highly charged than any other.
3. Fathers are now more likely to have more intimate relationships with their children.
4. Relationships between siblings tend to be more reciprocal than those between adult and child.
5. Relationships between mothers and fathers are directly related to the roles that each fulfils, and so are complex and changing.

FUNCTIONS OF THE FAMILY 3

INTRODUCTION

A variety of views about the role of the family in society exist, ranging from those that are positive and see the family as beneficial, to those that are negative and see the family as a damaging social institution.

The *positive view* is generally that expressed by the functionalist theorists. They believe that the family acts as the link between society and the individual and as such benefits both. The functions of the family are seen as being (Parsons, 1959; Fletcher, 1966):

- *The socialisation of children.* This aspect benefits the individual by preparing the child for his or her role in society. It benefits society by producing individuals who will conform to the rules and regulations of that society. The family teaches its members the roles they will play in society and helps them to accept the rights, duties and obligations accompanying those roles.
- *The stabilisation of the adult personality.* The family serves as a comfortable and secure place within which individuals can deal with the pressures and demands of life outside.
- *The regulation of sexual behaviour and the procreation of children* in a responsible environment.
- *The care of dependent members*, whether young or old.

The *negative view* is held by sociologists who are critical of the functionalist ideas and thus highlight the harmful aspects of family life:

- *Marxist theories* see the family as an instrument of exploitation and oppression particularly of women.
- *Feminist theories* see the family as a patriarchal structure which is the cause of the oppression of women. Radical feminists believe that true liberation for women will only result with the abolition of the family and associated patriarchy.
- *Radical psychiatrists* offer a view which sees the family as the main source of human unhappiness and the root of some psychiatric disorders including schizophrenia. The darker side of family life is emphasised including abuse and violence.

Whichever view one takes of the family it is clear that one major role must be concerned with the development of children. It is the context in which children grow and become adults. Schaffer (1988) suggests that it is not the structure of the family that influences development but the relationships within it. The experiences and relationships within the family in the first years of life are vital if children are to realise their full potential to relate to others – to become social beings.

Marxist theorists
- Karl Marx
- Friedrich Engels
- Loius Althusser
- Eli Zaretsky
- Michele Barrett and Mary McIntosh

Patriarchy

'A system or an instance of social organisation marked by the supremacy of the father in the clan or family, the legal dependence of wives and children, and the reckoning of descent and inheritance in the male line'.

(*Longman New Universal Dictionary*, 1982)

ROLE OF THE FAMILY IN CHILD DEVELOPMENT

The socialisation of children

Socialisation has been described by Booth (1975) as

> *'the process by which an individual born with behaviour potentialities of an enormously wide range is led to develop actual behaviour confined within the narrow range of what is customary for him (her) according to the standards of his (her) group'.*

A simpler definition is given by Sroufe *et al.* (1996) as:

> *'the acquisition by the child of the rules, standards and values of society'.*

Activity

Take 2 minutes to reflect on these definitions. Compare and contrast them.

The first definition acknowledges that human behaviour is the result of an interaction between nature (inborn characteristics) and nurture (experiences). Perhaps the latter does not explicitly impart this aspect, rather seeing behaviour as a result of experience alone. Whichever definition we choose to work with, socialisation of children usually begins within the context of the family. All types of expression are found within family relationships – hate, anger, companionship, despair, aggression. It is within this context that children gain an idea of the causes of various emotions and of the rules which operate inside and outside the family. The family helps children to prepare for life in the wider world and it serves to promote the continuation of cultural beliefs from generation to generation. During the process of socialisation children internalise societal norms, values and roles.

First relationships are held to be important and a prototype for all others. This is generally the mother–child relationship. During the first 8–12 months of life, infants develop attachments to one or more significant others, normally including the mother. Those children who become securely attached are likely to have greater confidence to explore new relationships (Bretherton and Waters, 1985). As relationships between the child and the family develop, interactions help the child to develop social skills.

Cross reference

Attachment – pages 86 and 87

Activity

Reflect on your own childhood. What do you consider you learned from your parents about life outside the family?

You may have come up with some or all of the following. Interactions with parents help children to learn about:

- taking turns, sharing, cooperating with others;
- rules – how to recognise them, why they exist;
- how to interact with others and respond to others' needs;
- moral values – the difference between right and wrong;
- how to act and behave appropriately within social contexts;
- the roles they will play in later life, e.g. as parent, friend, worker;
- cultural beliefs and expectations – the continuity of beliefs.

Parents facilitate the socialisation process by providing a nurturing environment and social contact. The more enjoyable the interactions with parents are, the more likely children are to develop good relationships with others (Pettit *et al.*, 1988).

The earlier a child meets others, the more effective interaction is learnt and the more he or she will be accepted as a companion. To some extent, parents are able to manage children's social lives (especially those of young children) and thus have an impact on peer relationships. They are able to stress the importance of friendship, sharing and playing together. As children develop, so other influences contribute to the socialisation process:

- playgroups and schools;
- mass media;
- play;
- friends/peers;
- religion and culture (sometimes other than those of the parents);
- legal structures.

Socialisation is a life-long process and children need to learn new norms at each stage of the lifespan. They have to cope with learning new rules at school, when they join new groups, on leaving school, going to university, or finding employment. Children also act as socialising agents for their parents, therefore making the process reciprocal.

General aspects of development

The family is the context in which other facets of development take place. There is a tendency for development to be considered without reference to the family, assuming that children's development follows certain patterns and stages regardless of their environment. However, it is important that we acknowledge the social network of the family and recognise that the family is also embedded in a social system.

Parents influence their child's *development of sexual identity* from birth intentionally and non-intentionally (Lott, 1994), directly and indirectly. The direct influence comes from the way the parents behave and the attitudes they hold, and is affected by their own gender role attitudes. These attitudes determine their own behaviour and the way in which they treat sons and daughters (Basow, 1992). Indirect influence comes from the way in which parents control other aspects of life such as the clothes that their children wear, the toys that they play with and even the television programmes that they watch. In their choice of toys for children, parents tend to discourage play with other-sex toys, more so with boys than with girls. A study by Caldera *et al.* (1989) found that, although parents did not actively discourage play with other-sex toys, they showed more enthusiasm when their children were playing with same-sex toys, especially when they were playing with a child of their own sex. It is important to acknowledge the role of other influences in the development of gender identity, for these will have an impact on the way parents treat their sons and daughters. Toys advertised on the television tend to be sex stereotyped, thus encouraging same-sex toys. Parents tend to be much more protective of daughters, whilst allowing boys more freedom and encouraging independence (White and Woollett, 1992). 'Sissy' behaviour in boys is often actively discouraged – 'big boys don't cry' – but, on the other hand, girls are not necessarily discouraged from being tomboys.

Definition – Sex stereotyping

Conforming to general patterns of gender

Activity

Critically reflect on your own childhood. In what ways do you feel that your parents influenced the development of your gender identity? Take opportunities to observe children and their parents, television programmes and advertisements. Is sex stereotyping going on?

As regards *intellectual development*, several studies have shown an association between a child's level of cognitive ability and features of parental child-directed behaviour (Hinde and Stevenson-Hinde, 1988; Teti *et al.*, 1989). The features found to encourage intelligence and cognitive development include the use of varied, developmentally appropriate stimulation, and responsiveness to cues. Guided play with objects helps to develop exploratory skills and imagination (White and Woollett, 1992). According to Bee (1995), several studies have suggested that certain features of family interaction seem to make a difference to a child's IQ level:

- the provision of an interesting and complex physical environment;
- parents who are emotionally responsive towards and involved with their child;
- parents who talk to their child using accurate, rich language;
- parents who avoid excessive restrictiveness and who give the child room to explore;
- parents who expect their child to do well.

The children of parents who are aware of what their child is doing during leisure time and at school are more likely to do well at school and are less likely to have behavioural problems (Crouter *et al.*, 1990). Whilst it is important to consider the role of heredity in the development of intelligence, the influence that the family can have on a child should not be dismissed.

As regards *language development*, parents do not formally teach their children about language; they do it informally and indirectly. They use language to communicate and by doing so they expose children to language. Parents encourage language development by the use of:

- early interactions with the infant encouraging the development of vocalisation and communication;
- word games, telling stories;
- repeating and expanding upon what their child has said (this often includes using more adult forms of speech, thus helping the child to learn);
- explaining and asking questions.

The mother plays an important role in her child's language development. It has been shown that mothers and their babies engage in 'protoconversation' as early as 6 weeks when mutual smiling games have been observed. The mother and baby are seen to take turns, as in a conversation (Tamir, 1984). This is the basis on which further language and communication skills are based. As children begin to talk, so mothers structure their language in order to provide clear, simple and easy-to-understand communications. This type of language has been called 'motherese' and is something that appears to be done unconsciously.

Cross reference
Language development – page 77

SUMMARY

In exploring the functions of the family this section has focused on the role of the family in the development of children. It has skimmed the surface and encourages you to explore more fully some of the ideas raised. When you are working with children, it is important to remember that they are part of a family and that their development goes on within that context. You need to bring together ideas about different family structures and investigate the influences that family life can have upon children. Whether nursing a sick child or promoting health you should assess the child against the family background and take into consideration the different forces acting upon the child. Although the discussion has focused mainly on the role of the parents in child development, other members of the family will play a role in a child's development. These include siblings, grandparents, aunts and uncles, and members of reconstituted families. The family plays a role in all aspects of a child's development, and therefore should be considered in all aspects of a child's care.

'Children are invariably born into a social network, typically a family. The family, too, is embedded in a social system. The family, the primary institution responsible for transforming societal maintenance and perpetuation goals into directives for the new individual, is thus at the core of socialization. Hence the family is society's adaptational unit'.

(Lerner and Spanier, 1978)

Key points ➤

Areas for further study

- The effect of birth order on a child's development
- The effect of reconstituted family life on children
- The role of heredity in intellectual development

1. There are two major views regarding the functions of the family – the positive and the negative.

2. Whichever view one takes, it is clear that the family plays a major role in the rearing of children.

3. The family is regarded by many as being the primary socialising agent for children.

4. The part that nature plays in child development is acknowledged but the role that the family plays should not be dismissed.

5. The importance of assessing the child within the family is stressed.

CHILD-REARING PRACTICES 4

INTRODUCTION

One of the functions of the family is seen by many to be that of rearing children. The *Longman New Universal Dictionary* gives a definition of rearing – 'to raise upright, to build or to construct'. It is within the context of family life – whatever its structure – that parents undertake the responsibility of 'building the individual', helping to 'construct' a person who will reach his/her optimal potential.

Each individual family will have its own beliefs about how children should be raised. These beliefs will be based on many factors including past experiences (especially related to their own upbringing), culture, religion and media influence (programmes and books on 'how to raise children' are plentiful). It is very difficult to make rules about how to bring up children. Each child is an individual and what we do for one child may not work for another.

Patterns of child rearing have changed considerably over the centuries. In the 18th and 19th centuries people had plenty to say about the moral upbringing of children. It was considered important to save them spiritually, given the high death rate among the young. As the infant mortality rate fell, more and more children survived into childhood, and the emphasis was placed on physical upbringing following fairly rigid rules. This rigid approach survived into the 20th century and in the 1930s authors of child-rearing books gave quite authoritative views on the subject. One writer told mothers 'Never kiss and hug them. If you must, kiss them once on the forehead'. Truby King (1938) suggested 'the establishment of perfect regularity of habits initiated by feeding and sleeping by the clock' as being the ultimate foundation of all-round obedience.

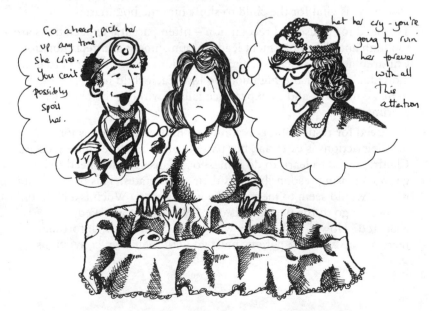

Two views on parenting.

Books for parents on child rearing

GREEN, C. (1990) *Toddler Taming: A Parents' Guide to the First Four Years*. London: Century

JOLLY, H. (1975) *Book of Child Care*. London: Allen & Unwin

LEACH, P. (1989) *Baby and Child*. London: Penguin

SPOCK, B. (1946) *Common Sense Book of Baby and Child Care*. New York: Duell, Cloane & Pearce

Current trends are not so dictatorial and, in fact, often go to the other extreme with the concept of non-advice – do what you find suits the child best. Leach (1989, cited in Swanwick, 1993) suggests that it is impossible to give a child too much attention or love. She believes that rearing a child by any book or set of rules can only work if the rules happen to fit the baby – a minor misfit can cause misery. What parents actually do is to take advice (from books, professionals, from family), and then try to find what suits them and their children best. There is a wealth of knowledge about child rearing upon which today's parents can base their decisions about parenting.

Activity

Reflect on your own upbringing. Talk to your parents about how they found their way through the maze of advice on child care. Who influenced them most?

PRINCIPLES OF CHILD REARING

The principles of child rearing are based on meeting the child's physical (i.e. nourishment, safety, sleep and comfort) and psychosocial needs. Pringle (1980) identifies four main psychosocial needs:

- The need for love and security – the child needs to be valued and cherished for his own sake without any expectation of gratitude. The security of predictability and continuity helps the child to come to terms with his developing self.

- The need for new experience – the child must experience new things and situations if he is to grow and mature. He needs the support and safety of a family in which to explore the world around him. At the same time he needs clear boundaries in which to experiment. Discipline is vital for the child to show him the boundaries.

- The need for praise and recognition – often parental expectations are too high and disappointment leads to punishment and recrimination. Children need an incentive, and expectations must be geared to each individual, neither too high nor too low. Each child needs the right to make mistakes and to experience failure without the fear of reprimand.

- The need for responsibility – allowing children to take responsibility for their actions is essential, but parents often fear the consequences. Children need to learn to do things for themselves and need to be given increasing responsibility as their age dictates. This part of child rearing would seem to me to be the hardest part. When is a child old enough to go to the park on his own? Will he get attacked, abducted? How does he know whom to ask for help? Unfortunately, there are no answers; parents must go with their own convictions.

Green (1991) takes a sensible, no nonsense look at child rearing with particular reference to toddlers. He suggests that 'the important things in child care will always remain the same: love, consistency, example, tension-free homes, sensible expectations and confident parents at the helm'. He believes that child care is natural and that parents have been doing it well for years.

Campion (1995) suggests that there are universal objectives for parents in the rearing of their children which constitute the job of parenting. She sees these as the same for all cultures, although she acknowledges that the specific nature of each will vary depending on cultural norms.

PARENTING STYLES

The way in which the principles of child rearing are put into practice will depend very much on the style of parenting adopted. Macoby and Martin (1983, cited in Bee, 1995) identified two dimensions important in child rearing:

- the level of demand and control;
- the level of acceptance or responsiveness.

By putting these two dimensions together they came up with four types of parenting style (Figure 4.1), each with its own influence on child development:

Level of demand and control

	High	Low
High	Authoritative	Permissive
Low	Authoritarian	Neglecting

Level of acceptance or responsiveness

- *Authoritarian*. Parents tend to exert a high degree of control, are demanding but at the same time display little warmth or responsiveness. They exert power over the child. Children with this type of parent tend to have low self-esteem and may be subdued or out of control.

General objectives for parenting

- Protection from environmental and social dangers
- Development of social skills
- Development of identity
- Development of self-esteem
- Spiritual development
- Cognitive development
- Affection and trust
- Moral guidance
- Economic support
- Self-regulation
- Stability of close relationships
- Adequate nutrition
- Education
- Physical care
- Preparation to be an adult who can contribute to society
- Modelling of socially desirable behaviour
- Development of independent living skills

(Campion, 1995)

Figure 4.1

Parenting styles.

Cross reference

Parental behaviour – page 204

- *Authoritative.* This type of parent, whilst exerting high levels of control and demand, also shows a high level of warmth and is responsive to their child's needs. These children show a higher self-esteem, are more compliant, self-confident and more independent.

- *Permissive.* This type of parent is sometimes referred to as indulgent. Although they show warmth and respond to the child's need, they exert little control. They make few rules and demands for good behaviour; they do not restrict noise, climbing about on furniture; they allow freedom to play without supervision (Mussen *et al.*, 1994). Children tend to show negative outcomes – aggression, immaturity in relationships with peers. They are less independent.

- *Neglecting.* Sometimes this type of parent is referred to as uninvolved. They show little warmth and responsiveness and at the same time little control. Children may show insecurity, difficulty in forming relationships. They are more likely to be impulsive and behave in an antisocial manner (Pulkkinen, 1982).

Activity

Reflect on your own parents, parents of friends. What type are they? If you are a parent yourself, reflect on and try to analyse your own style.

ASPECTS OF PARENTING

There are many aspects of parenting, all of which will be influenced by the factors discussed above. For the purposes of this module, two aspects will be examined in more detail, i.e. discipline and sleep.

Discipline

This is probably one of the most contentious issues in the area of child care. Disciplining children is very difficult; it can be emotionally draining. The problem is that there are no hard and fast rules. Different parents have different views on how to discipline their children. Limit-setting is important for children; unrestricted freedom is often a threat to security and safety.

Activity

Begin by examining your own views about discipline. Do you withdraw privileges, withhold affection, scold, impose unpleasant tasks/penalties?

Discipline is just part of the process of guiding children with the aim of their becoming happy, healthy, fully functioning adults. To try to get it right, Davidson and Moore (1996) suggest that parents need to know why a child misbehaves. Once this is understood he proposes that it is easier to select appropriate methods of discipline.

Other aspects of child rearing worth exploring

- Toilet training
- Weaning/breastfeeding
- Caring practices – hygiene, dental care

Cultural perspective

In the Asian culture there is virtually no discipline for the first 3 years. When it does start, total obedience is expected. Discipline tends to be physical and outside interference is not tolerated

(Mayor, 1984)

Reasons for a child's misbehaviour include:

- *Age of the child.* Knowing what type of behaviour is expected of a child is important when deciding on discipline. For example, we all know about 'the terrible twos'. It is not worth punishing a 2 year old having a temper tantrum. The best way of dealing with this type of behaviour is to tolerate it if you can.

Discipline

'The use of instruction, control, rewards or punishment as a means of training or correcting, in order to instill self-discipline'.

(Davidson and Moore, 1996)

Activity

Consider what actions you might take in the following situation: a 2-year-old child in your care has a tantrum at the top of a flight of stairs in a busy department store. What actions might you take. Discuss this situation with colleagues and explore different ways of dealing with it.

Activity

What other behaviours are age related and should be taken into account when disciplining children?

- *Unsatisfied demands.* Very often, bad behaviour occurs when a child cannot have what he/she wants (or thinks he/she needs). First it is important to decide if the desired demand is legitimate. If it is, then it may be appropriate to acknowledge this but remind the child of how to ask. If the desire is not legitimate, he wants a new toy, then it is important to be consistent – no means no. It is no good changing one's mind just to avoid confrontation. It is better to try some other tactic. Diversion is a useful one. Children, especially young ones, can usually be diverted quite easily.

- *Lack of social knowledge about appropriate behaviour.* It is unwise to punish children for not knowing how to behave. It is far better simply to show them or tell them what to do. It is preferable to indicate what to do rather that what *not* to do, as the latter is very negative.

- *Inappropriate environment.* It is difficult for children to behave when their environment is not suited to their developmental needs. Children are curious, they love to experiment and try out new things. They need to run about and expend energy. If they are restricted they may resort to bad behaviour. Experience has shown that it is better to let children play outside when they want to, even if it is cold, rather than make them come into the house. The latter choice always ends up in a shouting match when the noise and mess become too much.

Activity

For each of the behaviours listed in Table 4.1, indicate whether you find it acceptable or unacceptable. If you find the behaviour unacceptable indicate your reason from the list in the box. Discuss your answers with (a) your mother, (b) a friend and (c) a colleague.

Table 4.1

Acceptable or unacceptable behaviour in children

Behaviour	Yes/No	Reason
A toddler pokes a pencil into an electric socket		
A 4-year-old will not put his toys away		
A 2-year-old swears at his teddy		
A 4-year-old smacks his sister after he has been scolded		
A 3-year-old boy plays with his penis		
A 4-year-old refuses to eat his dinner and hurls it on the floor		
A 5-year-old says he did not do something when he did		
A 5-year-old keeps making rude noises with his mouth		
A 3-year-old will not let a friend have a turn on his bike		
A toddler bashes another toddler with a toy		
A 4-year-old kicks and bites other preschool children		

Reasons for unacceptable behaviour

You think it is:
- dangerous
- unhygienic
- the cause of distress, a nuisance or inconvenience
- the cause of damage, expense or extra work
- against rules or conventions
- babyish
- bad manners or impolite
- disobedient
- irritating or embarrassing
- bad tempered or emotional
- a lie or dishonest

Whatever discipline techniques are used, certain principles apply:
- Discipline is best carried within a warm, responsive caring family.
- To be effective, punishment should either interrupt the undesirable behaviour or take place immediately after it. 'Wait till your father gets home' is of little use as the child will likely have forgotten all about the incident by then.
- The punishment chosen should be worthy of the crime. It should also be feasible. 'We will go out without you if you're not ready in time' is a wasted threat for a 4 year old.
- Discipline must be consistent, between parents and from day to day. Once a rule is set, it must be observed.
- Discipline must not be over-used as it loses its potency and becomes an entertaining game.

Various techniques are suggested from which parents can choose those most congruent with their beliefs and their behaviour:
- *Behaviour modification therapy.* This technique is based on the premise that behaviour reinforced by rewards will be repeated, and behaviour that is not reinforced will probably disappear. Rewards can be in the form of praise, attention and cuddles, or more tangible items such as stickers, stars or small toys.
- *Diversion.* As previously mentioned, this can be quite a useful technique with younger children. Divert the child's attention before the bad behaviour has a chance to take hold.

- *Selective deafness/blindness.* Sometimes it is best just to pretend you did not hear or see what happened. If the behaviour really does not warrant punishment but is something you do not like, ignore it or change the subject.

- *Time out.* This technique can bring rapid response. The aim is to remove the child from a situation and place him in another room for a short time. He then has time to cool off. It also allows time for the parent to calm down so that the situation does not deteriorate further.

- *Removal of privileges.* This technique works for children over the age of about 6. It is of little use for younger children as they do not think much about the future. Privileges such as playing out, watching television, riding a bike, extra pocket money for good behaviour can be withheld. The child needs to know the standard of behaviour expected and the results of misbehaviour.

Activity

It is important to continue with discipline even when a child is ill. Consider how you might deal with discipline for a child in hospital.

Smacking. Article 19 of the UN Convention on the Rights of the Child (1989) states that appropriate measures should be taken to 'protect the child from all forms of physical or mental violence ... while in the care of parent(s), legal guardian(s), or any other person who has the care of the child'. According to Newson and Newson (1989), physical punishment is very common in the UK, with almost two-thirds of a large sample of mothers admitting to smacking their babies before the age of 1. The research found that almost all 4 year olds were being smacked and that 22% of 7 year olds had been hit with an implement. In some countries, smacking is prohibited (Sweden, Finland, Denmark, Norway and Austria). Whilst some measures have been taken to curb physical punishment in the UK, parents have a common law right to use 'moderate and reasonable' means to punish their children. Some carers also appear to retain these rights, e.g. nannies and childminders. This means that whilst it is a criminal offence to use violence against adults, it is acceptable when applied to children.

Activity

Arrange a debate with colleagues – 'Smacking children as a form of punishment should be outlawed in the UK'.

Sleep and sleep problems

Sleep is a complex phenomenon and one that is taken for granted until it is disturbed. It is expected that children should develop 'acceptable'

UN Convention of Rights

The UN Convention on the Rights of the Child was adopted by the UN General Assembly on 20th November 1989. It provides detailed minimum standards against which to test the treatment of the world's children and young people. It was ratified by the UK Government in 1991 'with some reservations'.

Other relevant articles of UN Convention of Rights

- Article 28 states that 'Parties shall take all appropriate measures to ensure that school discipline is administered in a manner consistent with the child's human dignity'.
- Article 37 states that 'No child shall be subjected to torture or other cruel, inhumane or degrading treatment or punishment'.

UK measures against physical punishment

- Physical punishment outlawed in all state-supported schools
- Children in various categories of children's homes protected under the Children Act 1989
- Local authority foster carers prevented from using physical punishment under the Children Act 1989

The case against physical punishment – smacking

- Serves as a model of violence
- Erodes the positive influence of the parent
- Creates a family climate of rejection instead of warmth
- Lowers a child's self-esteem
- Damages parents' self-concept because they lose control of their emotions
- Promotes dependency on external rather than internal control
- For further information contact: FPOCH, 77 Holloway Road, London N7 8JZ

Sleep

'The natural periodic suspension of consciousness that is essential for the physical and mental well-being of higher animals' (*Longman Universal Dictionary*, 1982). The English word *sleep* is of Germanic origin and derives from the Gothic word *sleps*

sleeping patterns, that is they should go to bed when the parent decides, sleep through the night and wake at a reasonable time in the morning. In reality, this expectation is not always fulfilled causing anxiety and stress among families.

When looking at the development of sleep patterns in children (Table 4.2), we see that the sleep pattern of newborns is 'polyphasic' with short cycles of sleep and wakefulness occurring throughout the day and night. Total sleep time (about 15–18 hours) is distributed over the 24-hour period. As the central nervous system matures, the pattern changes and the infant spends more time awake in the day and more time asleep at night. Longer periods of behavioural inhibition become possible and a bulk sleep of 8 hours is usually established by about 4 months of age. As the infant grows and develops so total sleep time decreases and occurs mainly at night. By the age of about 2 years, most children have developed a biphasic sleep pattern with a nap at some stage of the day. A monophasic pattern (the bulk of sleep at nighttime) is generally established by about the age of 4 years. The development of the monophasic sleep pattern of adulthood is affected not only by maturation of the brain but also by environmental and cultural factors. In Mediterranean countries it is common for adults to maintain the biphasic pattern of childhood by taking afternoon siestas to avoid the greatest heat of the day. Thus it is acceptable practice for children to do the same and so have a later bedtime than would generally be accepted in this country.

Table 4.2

Stages in the sleep cycle with age

Age	Sleep pattern	Length of each sleep cycle (min)	%REM	Total sleep time (h)
Newborn – polyphasic	Wake, REM, non-REM	< 45	50	16–18
3 months–1 year – polyphasic	Wake, non-REM, REM	45–50	35	
2–3 years – biphasic	Wake, non-REM, REM	50–60	20–25	12–15
4–10 years – monophasic	As above	60–70	20–25	12 reducing to 7–8
Adult – monophasic	As above	90	20	6–8
Elderly – multiphasic	As above	90	20	Often less than 6

Activity

Consider your own views on what is an acceptable sleep pattern for children. If you have children of your own, how do you manage this aspect of child rearing? If not, explore your parents/friends views.

REM

Rapid eyeball movement associated with paradoxical sleep, increased electrical activity of the brain and dreaming

Sleeping arrangements differ from culture to culture. One of the most interesting features which has been studied is that of *bed-sharing*. It is common practice for Western babies to be placed in their own cot/bed, usually in their own room. It is not generally acceptable to admit to sleeping with babies/children in the marital bed. However, for many cultures there are no special sleeping arrangements for babies. In part of India and Kenya, babies and small children sleep with their parents for several years. In the Philippines, infants sleep with their mothers except during weaning when they are moved to another room with aunts or a grandmother (Conder, 1988). Mayan mothers in Guatemala share their bed with infants during the first year of life and toddlers sleep in the same room (Morelli *et al.*, 1992). The reasons given for not bed-sharing include the possibility of smothering, disturbing parental sleep and preventing sexual intercourse. There may also be a concern that sleeping with children may in itself have sexual connotations. Health visitors and other professionals advise us against bed-sharing and give parents ideas on how to encourage babies to sleep on their own. In societies where bed-sharing is the norm, notably fewer sleep problems are found and the use of transitional objects (e.g. pieces of blanket, soft toys) is unknown (Conder, 1988). There is conflicting evidence as to whether there is a relationship between bed-sharing and sudden infant death syndrome (Carter, 1995) but the Foundation for the Study of Infant Deaths advises against it until the baby is 6 months old (FSID, 1992).

Activity

Talk to children and parents with different cultural backgrounds from your own. Find out their views about sleeping arrangements for infants and young children. Make notes in the margin for future reference.

Concerns regarding an infant's sleeping patterns are often expressed. A number of factors both within the child and the family have been suggested as contributing to the development of sleep disturbances. At the same time it must be recognised that what constitutes a problem for one family may be considered normal for another. This is especially important when considering cultural differences. Physiological factors such as hunger, colic and thermal comfort have been identified as contributing to night waking. Babies who are breast-fed do wake more often at night during the first year of life (Eaton-Evans and Dugdale, 1988). A study of 98 full-term babies by Wailoo *et al.* (1990) found a significant association between thermal environment and waking patterns. The babies who disturbed their parents more frequently were significantly more heavily wrapped and had a significantly higher rectal temperature than those who were still asleep. Affective factors such as fear of the dark and other anxiety-provoking events (e.g. moving house, birth of a sibling) may cause reactions which can be reflected in a child's sleeping pattern. Whatever the cause of the problems, the effects on the family can be devastating.

Ideas for dealing with minor sleep problems

- Give child plenty of exercise during the day – both mental and physical
- Go through the same routine every night
- Try to make the period just before bed a quiet time to allow child to wind down
- Leave a small night light on – some children like the comfort of a light being left on overnight
- Allow the child to listen to music or a story tape, or allow them to play for a short while – offer quiet toy or a book
- If the child cries or makes a fuss, wait 10 minutes and go back in, resettle and leave. Repeat as necessary *but* be firm

Further reading

Dealing with sleep problems

DOUGLAS, J. and RICHMAN, N. (1984) *My Child Won't Sleep*. London: Penguin

HASLAM, D. (1984) *Sleepless Children*. London: Piatkus

Interesting article

SWANWICK, M. (1993) Bringing up baby. *Paediatric Nursing*, **5** (4), 20–23

Cross reference

Children's nursing in a multicultural society – pages 627–634

Sleep problems fall into two main categories:

- frequent waking at night;
- failure to settle at bedtime.

It may be possible to solve sleep problems with some common-sense advice with cultural differences taken into account. However, for more major problems, further professional advice and treatment may be needed.

Behaviour modification has been increasingly advocated as an effective tool for managing sleep problems. The approach requires careful analysis of the individual problem, establishment of goals of treatment and the setting of gradual steps to their attainment. Several studies have attempted to examine the effectiveness of this technique (Richman *et al.*, 1985; Bidder *et al.*, 1986; Farnes and Wallace, 1987). All the studies suggest that the techniques can be an effective therapy for sleep problems provided that the treatment is carried out by professionals with experience and knowledge of the technique. It must also be acknowledged that it may not be suitable for all children and that parental involvement in goal setting and evaluation is essential, with the programme being individually tailored to suit each child.

CULTURAL PERSPECTIVES ON CHILD REARING

Child-rearing practices differ between cultures and ethnic groups, and this is important to remember when assessing and working with children and families. It is wrong to make assumptions based on your own values and beliefs. Studies have shown that styles of parenting among Indian families (Holme, 1984) and Punjabi families (Ghuman, 1975) were significantly different compared with those of indigenous white mothers. Parenting was more relaxed with demand feeding, no fixed bed-times, no plans for potty training. Young babies and infants slept with their mothers. Similarly, Hackett and Hackett (1994) reported a wide range of differences between Gujarati families and indigenous whites. Dosnajh and Ghuman (1997) carried out a study to explore the child-rearing practices of two generations of Punjabi parents. The purpose of the research was to show the effect of acculturation on the child-rearing practices of an ethnic minority community resident in the English Midlands. They found that many of the elaborate customs and rituals had disappeared but there was little difference in feeding and sleeping habits. They concluded that, although there are many factors affecting changing practices, there is a tendency for second generation Punjabi mothers to adopt and adapt some of the customs and practices of white indigenous mothers.

SUMMARY

Rearing children has been described as being fulfilling, frustrating, difficult, rewarding and much more, all at the same time. There are no simple prescriptions about how to rear children. The task for parents is to choose the system which works for them from a range of alternatives. Campion (1995) suggests that there are three criteria which interact and contribute to whether good parenting can take place:

- *The child* – age, personality (some children are more demanding and difficult), sex, health.
- *The parents* – background and upbringing, relationships with each other, employment, income, health, expectations of the child/children.
- *Physical and social environment* – housing, supportive networks, transport, schools, assistance with childcare, cultural perspectives.

Activity

Take each of the criteria above. For each one reflect on issues which facilitate and inhibit good parenting. How might this have implications for your practice?

> **Key points**

1. Each family will have its own beliefs concerning child rearing, influenced by many factors including past experience, culture, religion, society and the mass media.
2. The general objectives of child rearing are universal to all parts of the world but the specific nature of practices will depend on culture and the needs of the society in which the child lives.
3. The principles of child rearing are based on meeting the physical and psychosocial needs of the child.
4. The style of parenting adopted will influence the way in which the principles and objectives of child rearing are achieved.
5. Limit-setting is important for children as unrestricted freedoms offer a threat to security and safety.
6. There is no correct way to rear children but there are many suggestions as to how it might be done.
7. Child-rearing practices differ between cultures and ethnic groups.

References

BALLARD, R. and KALRA, V. S. (1994) *The Ethnic Dimensions of the 1991 Census: A Preliminary Report*. Manchester: University of Manchester.
BASOW, S. A. (1992) *Gender Stereotypes and Roles*, 3rd edn. Pacific Grove, CA: Brooks/Cole.
BEE, H. (1995) *The Developing Child*, 7th edn. New York: Harper Collins.
BOOTH, T. (1975) Growing up in society. In HERRIOT, P. (ed.), *Essential Psychology*. London: Methuen.

BRETHERTON, I. and WATERS, E. (eds) (1985) Growing points in attachment theory and research. *Monographs of the Society for Research in Child Development*, **50**, 209.

BUCK, N., GERSHUNY, J., ROSE, D. and SCOTT, J. (1994) *Changing Households: The British Household Panel Survey 1990–1992*. Essex: ESRC Research Centre on Micro-social Change, University of Essex.

CALDERA, Y. M., HUSTON, A. C. and O'BRIEN, M. (1989) Social interactions and play patterns of parents and toddlers with feminine, masculine and neutral toys. *Child Development*, **60**, 70–76.

CAMPION, M. J. (1995) *Who's fit to be a Parent?* London: Routledge.

COCKETT, M. and TRIP, J. (1994) *The Exeter Family Study: Family Breakdown and its Impact on Children*. Exeter: University of Exeter Press.

CONDY, Y. A. (1994) Family Index. *Family Policy Bulletin*, May 1994.

CROUTER, A. C., MacDERMID, S. M., McHALE, S. M. and PERRY-JENKINS, M. (1990) Parental monitoring and perceptions of children's school performance and conduct in dual and single-earner families. *Developmental Psychology*, **26**, 649–657.

CSO (1995) *Social Trends*, 1995 edn. London: HMSO.

DAVIDSON, J. K. and MOORE, N. B. (1996) *Marriage and Family: Change and Continuity*. Boston: Allyn & Bacon.

De'ATH, E. (1996) Family change: step-families in context. *Children and Nursing*, **10**, 80–82.

DOSNAJH, J. S. and GHUMAN, P. A. S. (1997) Child rearing practices of two generations of Punjabi parents. *Children and Society*, **11**, 29–43.

DUNN, J. (1984) *Sisters and Brothers*. London: Fontana.

FLETCHER, R. (1966) *The Family and Marriage in Britain*. Harmondsworth: Penguin.

GHUMAN, P. A. S. (1975) *The Cultural Context of Thinking: A Comparative Study of Punjabi and English Boys*. London: NFER.

GREEN, C. (1991) *Toddler Taming: A Parents' Guide to the First Four Years*. London: Century.

GREGG, P. and WADSWORTH, J. (1994) *More Work in Fewer Households?* London: National Institute of Economic and Social Research.

HACKETT, L. and HACKETT, R. (1994) Child rearing practices and psychiatric disorders in Gujrati and British children. *British Journal of Child Psychology and Psychiatry*, **32** (5), 851–856.

HASKEY, J. (1994) *Stepfamilies and Stepchildren in Great Britain. Population Trends* 76. London: HMSO.

HETHERINGTON, E. M. (1988) Parents, children and siblings: six years after divorce. In HINDE, R. A. and STEVENSON-HINDE, J. (eds), *Relationships with Families*. Oxford: Clarendon Press.

HETHERINGTON, E. M. and ARASTEH, J. (1988) *The Impact of Divorce, Single Parenting and Step-Parenting on Children*. New Jersey: Lawrence Erlbaum Associates.

HEWISON, J. and DOWSWELL, T. (1994) *Child Health Care and the Working Mother*. London: Chapman & Hall.

HINDE, R. A. and STEVENSON-HINDE, J. (1988) *Relationships within Families: Mutual Influences*. Oxford: Clarendon Press.

HOLME J. (1984) Growing up in Hinduism. *British Journal of Religious Education*. **6** (3), 116–120.

HUMPHREY, M. and HUMPHREY, H. (1988) *Families with a Difference: Varieties of Surrogate Parenthood*. London: Routledge.

JORGENSEN, J. (1995) *Investigating Families and Households*. London: Collins Educational.

KING, T. (1938) *Mothercraft*. Meredith Press: New York.

KURDEK, L. A. (1988) A 1-year follow up study of children's divorce adjustment, custodial mothers' divorce adjustment, and postdivorce parenting. *Journal of Applied Developmental Psychology*, 9, 315–328.

LEACH, P. (1989) *Baby and Child*. London: Penguin.

LERNER, R.M. and SPANIER, G.B. (1978) *Child Influences on Marital and Family Interaction: a Lifespan Perspective*. New York: Academic Press.

LEWIS, C. (1986) *Becoming a Father*. Milton Keynes: Open University Press.

LOTT, B. (1994) *Women's Lives: Themes and Variations in Gender Learning*, 2nd edn. Pacific Grove, CA: Brooks/Cole.

MACOBY, E. E. and MARTIN, J. A. (1983) Socialisation in the context of the family: parent–child interaction. In MUSSEN, P. H. (ed.), *Handbook of Child Psychology*, 4th edn, vol. 4. New York: Wiley.

MAYOR, V. (1984) Pregnancy, childbirth and child care. *Nursing Times*, 13 June, pp. 57–58.

McQUIRE, J. (1991) Sons and daughters. In PHEONIX, A., WOOLLETT, A. and LLOYD, E. (eds), *Motherhood: Meanings, Practices and Ideologies*. London: Sage.

MOORE, S. (1996) *Sociology Alive!*, 2nd edn. Cheltenham: Stanley Thornes.

MUNCIE, J., WETHERELL, M., DALLOS, R. and COCHRANE, A. (1995) *Understanding the Family*. London: Sage.

MUSSEN, P. *et al.* (1994) Dimensions of parent behaviour. In GOTT, M. and MALONEY, B. (eds), *Child Health: A Reader*. Oxford: Radcliffe Medical Press.

O'BRIEN, M. and JONES, D. (1996) Fathers through the eyes of their children. *Family Policy Bulletin*, November, 4–5.

OPCS (1992) *Social Trends 22*. London: HMSO.

OPCS (1993) *General Household Survey 1991*. London: HMSO.

OPCS (1994a) *Day Care Services for Children*. London: HMSO.

OPCS (1994b) *General Household Survey 1992*. London: HMSO.

OPCS (1995) *Social Trends 25*. London: HMSO.

PARSONS, T. (1959) The social structure of the family. In ASHEN, R. N. (ed.), *The Family, Its Functions and Destiny*. New York: Harper & Row.

PETTIT, G. S., DODGE, K. A. and BROWN, M. M. (1988) Early family experience, social problem solving patterns, and children's social competence. *Child Development*, 59, 107–120.

PRINGLE, M. (1980) *The Needs of Children: A Personal Perspective*. London: Hutchinson.

PULKKINEN, L. (1982) Self-control and continuity from childhood to adolescence. In BALTES, P. B. and BRIM, O. G. (eds), *Life-span Development and Behaviour*, vol. 4. Orlando: Academic Press.

RIBBENS, J. (1994) *Mothers and their Children: A Feminist Sociology of Childrearing*. London: Sage.

RUSSELL, G. (1983) *The Changing Role of Fathers*. Milton Keynes: Open University Press.

SANTROCK, J. W. (1995) *Lifespan Development*, 5th edn. Wisconsin: Brown and Benchmark.

SCHAFFER, H. R. (1988) Family structure or interpersonal relationships: the context for child development. *Children and Society*, 2, 91–101.

SROUFE, L. A., COOPER, R. G. and DEWART, G. B. (1996) *Child Development:*

Its Nature and Course, 3rd edn. New York: McGraw-Hill.

STEINBERG, L., ELMEN, J. D. and MOUNTS, N. S. (1989) Authoritative parenting, psychological maturity and academic success among adolescents. *Child Development*, **60**, 1424–1436.

STERN, D. (1977) *The First Relationship: Infant and Mother*. London: Fontana.

SWANWICK, M. (1993) Bringing up baby. *Paediatric Nursing*, **15** (4), 20–23.

TAMIR, L. (1984) Language development: new directions. In LOCK, A. and FISHER, E. (eds), *Language Development*. London: Routledge.

TETI, D. M., BOND, L. A. and GIBBS, E. D. (1988) Mothers, fathers and siblings: a comparison of play styles and their influence upon infant cognitive level. *International Journal of Behavioural Development*, **11**, 451–432.

UNITED NATIONS (1989) UN Convention on the Rights of the Child. New York: United Nations.

UTTING, D. (1995) *Family and Parenthood: Supporting Families, Preventing Breakdown*. York: Joseph Rowntree Foundation.

WADSWORTH, M E. (1985) Parenting skills and their transmission through generations. *Adoption and Fostering*, **9**, 28–32.

WAILOO, M. P., PETERSENS, A. and WHITAKER, H. (1990) Disturbed nights and 3–4 month old infants. The effects of feeding and thermal environment. *Archives of Disease in Childhood*, **65**, 499–501.

WALKER, J., SIMPSON, B. and McCARTHY, P. (1991) *The Housing Consequences of Divorce. The Family and Community*. Newcastle upon Tyne: Dispute Research Centre, University of Newcastle upon Tyne.

WHITE, D. and WOOLLETT, A. (1992) *Families: A Context for Development*. London: Falmer Press.

WILLMOTT, P. (1988) Urban kinship past and present. *Social Studies Review*, November 1988.

WISE, G. (1994) The changing family. In LINDSAY, B. (ed.), *The Child and Family: Contemporary Nursing Issues in Child Health and Care*. London: Bailliere Tindall.

YOUNG, M. and WILLMOTT, P. (1975) *The Symmetrical Family*. London: Penguin.

Further Reading

BJRNBERG, U. and KOLLIND, A.-K. (1996) *Men's Family Relationships*. Stockholm: Almqvist and Wiksell.

DAVIDSON, J. K. and MOORE, N. B. (1996) *Marriage and Family: Change and Continuity*. Boston: Allyn and Bacon. Although this book is American it explores many issues which are relevant to relationships between adults in our society.

DOUGLAS, J. and RICHMAN, N. (1984) *My Child Won't Sleep*. London: Penguin.

HASLAM, D. (1984) *Sleepless Children*. London: Piatkus.

JOLLY, H. (1975) *Book of Child Care*. London: Allen & Unwin.

MOSS, P. (ed.) (1995) *Father Figures: Fathers in the Families of the 1990s*. London: HMSO.

Family Policy Bulletin. Available from the: Family Policy Studies Centre, 231 Baker Street, London NW1 6XE. Tel: 0171 486 8211/7680.

RIBBENS, J. (1990) *Accounting for our children: differing perspectives on 'family life' in middle income households*. PhD Thesis, CNAA, South Bank Polytechnic, London.

SPOCK, B. (1946) *Common Sense Book of Baby and Child Care*. New York: Duell, Cloane & Pearce.

SWANWICK, M. (1993) Bringing up baby. *Paediatric Nursing*, **5** (4), 20–23.

THE GROWING CHILD

Tina Moules

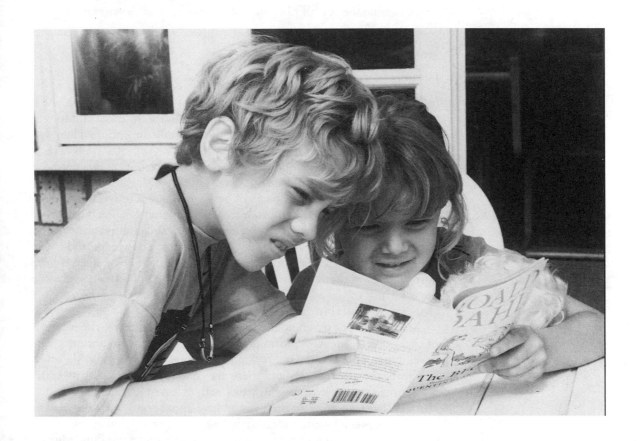

Learning and growing together

OBJECTIVES

The material contained within this module and the further reading/references should enable you to:

- Explore the nature of childhood and how it has changed over recent years.
- Investigate the factors which can influence the growth and development of children.
- Develop an understanding of life before birth and implications for the care of sick children.
- Develop a knowledge of the way in which children grow and in which the body systems mature with time.
- Analyse critically the various theoretical views on cognitive and social development.
- Examine the role of play and education in child development.

INTRODUCTION

In China an individual's age is determined not by his date of birth but by his date of conception. This is an apt concept in the study of children as growth and development begin at the moment of conception. Then follows a process which is both fascinating and mysterious to observe.

The growth and development which takes place during this period is common to nearly all children but occurs at different rates and with different outcomes. Some aspects of development are universal, others are affected by the child's environment and experiences. Each baby develops an individual personality, intellect and social disposition, within the context of a 'family', developing skills, knowledge and attitudes to equip the baby for the society into which he or she has been born. The baby changes from the infant 'mewling and puking in the nurse's arms' to the adolescent ready for independence and the challenge of adult life.

Many different psychologists have attempted to unravel the mysteries of child development, exploring the influence of environment on developmental processes and trying to make sense of the child's world. Whatever the answers are (and there are certainly no correct answers), it is essential that those of us who work with children understand the changes that take place so that we can give appropriate age-related care. A child is a precious gift and as such deserves to be treated as an individual, nurtured and cared for by responsive understanding adults. To do this we need to be aware of the way in which a child thinks about the world and the people around him.

This module can only hope to give you an overview of the various aspects of child development, but it aims to encourage you to explore further by providing you with ideas for additional reading and by inspiring within you a thirst for more knowledge. The module begins by exploring the nature of childhood and the factors that influence growth and development, moving on to consider life before birth. Some discussion follows on growth and maturation, examining the way in which various systems of the body mature. The module moves on to analyse some of the various theoretical views on development, considering first cognitive development (including language development) and then the social world of the child. To conclude the module, we look at the role of play and education in the development of the child with special reference to children with special needs.

Growth, development, ageing and maturation

- *Growth* – an increase in size and number of cells resulting in an increase in size and weight of the whole or any of its parts
- *Maturation* – an increase in competence and adaptability; a change in the complexity of a structure that makes it possible for that structure to work
- *Development* – an increase in complexity; the emerging of an individual's capacities through learning, growth and maturation

1 THE NATURE OF CHILDHOOD

INTRODUCTION

Important dates in the development of childhood

- Elementary Education Act 1870
- Sandon Act 1876 (made parents responsible for ensuring their children went to school)
- Mundella Act 1880 (established School Attendance Committees)
- United Nations Convention on the Rights of the Child 1987
- The Children Act 1989

It would seem from the extensive literature on childhood, that the nature of this concept is complex and continuously evolving. There is very little consensus among writers, some suggesting that childhood was evident as early as the fourth century BC (Watt and Mitchell, 1995) and others that it did not really emerge until the 17th century. Aries (1962) suggested that childhood was invented in the 13th century.

The nature of childhood is dependent on and relative to the views that adults have about children at any one time. Childhood for the children of poor in previous centuries was always brief. Children born into poverty were a burden to their parents and were put to work as soon as was possible. Children as young as 4 years old worked in the textile mills, picking up waste cotton from underneath unguarded machinery. Young children worked up to 12 hours a day in coal mines. Infant and child mortality was high but not dwelt on too much as other children were soon born to take their place. Children of the more affluent were a different kind of investment, cementing social status through marital alliances (Lester, 1993). There was little, if any, state intervention in the lives of children – they were their parents' possessions.

According to Heward (1993), profound changes in the nature of childhood began to take place in the 19th century. This century saw developments which contributed to a change in the way adults viewed their children. One of the most important of these was the introduction and enforcement of compulsory education, and with it a move towards acceptance of state intervention. The enforcement of school attendance made childhood more standardised with all children beginning to have a settled period at school. Education finally served to separate children from adults, giving them their own place in society. Secondly, there was a steady decline in child labour brought about by rising standards of living, and technological advances in agriculture and industry (Nardinelli, 1990). Thirdly, as the status of children and the concept of childhood changed, studies of child development began. One of the earliest studies was made by Charles Darwin of his own son. Darwin believed that by observing children one could reveal the descent of man. Finally, the health of children began to improve. Services specifically designed for children began to emerge in Europe and in Britain. Children's dispensaries were opened in London (1816), Manchester (1829) and Liverpool (1851), and these were followed by the founding of the Hospital for Sick Children, Great Ormond Street, in 1852 (Kosky and Lunnon, 1991).

The 20th century has seen further changes as smaller families allow deeper relationships between children and their parents. The birth rate has fallen and children have become more 'precious'. There is a general acceptance that children need to be protected and guided. The views of children are being taken more seriously as we deal with issues of children's rights and their role in society. Although gender differences remain, they are becoming less important. Opportunities and education are seen as being just as important for girls as they are for boys. Numerous theorists have pondered the nature of children giving us views on how children become adults. We are more interested in ensuring that all children grow up healthy and that they are given every opportunity to develop to their full potential.

Activity

Talk to your parents and grandparents. What was childhood like for them? Compare their stories with that of your own childhood.

FACTORS INFLUENCING GROWTH AND DEVELOPMENT

Many of the debates about child development have centred around the nature versus nurture controversy. Those who favour the former believe that human behaviour is guided by inborn biological factors. They would argue that individual differences are a result of heredity. Those who favour the concept of nurturing stress the importance of acknowledging the influence of a child's physical and social environment. According to them, individual differences are a result of the various experiences that children have. In truth the reality is probably somewhere in-between, with both inherited and environmental factors playing an important role. Development is a complex process and occurs as a result of the interaction of many variables, the effect of which will be different for each child. No two children are the same, even when they have the same parents and a similar home environment.

Many factors have been identified as being influential in the development of children (Figure 1.1) but generally they fall into two categories – inherited and environmental.

HEREDITY

This refers to the transmission of characteristics from one generation to the next. Many of our characteristics or traits are influenced by our genotype – a unique genetic blueprint which each of us has, based on the mix of genes from our parents. Identification of many specific genes and their loci on specific chromosomes has progressed rapidly over recent years. As well as knowing the locus of some genes that control characteristics such as hair and eye colour, blood group, etc., researchers now know the loci for those that lead to genetic disorders such as cystic fibrosis. This brings diagnosis and treatment of these conditions ever

Cross reference

Genetic factors – page 131

Figure 1.1

Factors influencing growth and development.

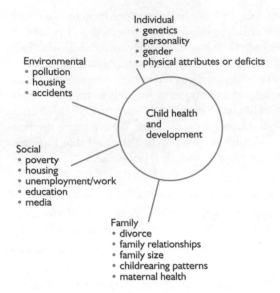

Individual
• genetics
• personality
• gender
• physical attributes or deficits

Environmental
• pollution
• housing
• accidents

Child health and development

Social
• poverty
• housing
• unemployment/work
• education
• media

Family
• divorce
• family relationships
• family size
• childrearing patterns
• maternal health

nearer. Genes are classed as either *dominant* or *recessive* and as such result in various patterns of inheritance.

Dominant inheritance

A dominant gene exerts its influence over the other gene with which it is paired. For example, parents who have different coloured eyes each pass on different genes to their offspring. In this case whichever gene is dominant will exert its influence and will therefore determine eye colour.

This principle can also be applied to those diseases passed on through dominant inheritance, for example (Figure 1.2).

Figure 1.2

Dominant inheritance. Each pregnancy has a 1 : 2 risk of an affected child of either sex. X_0 = affected gene.

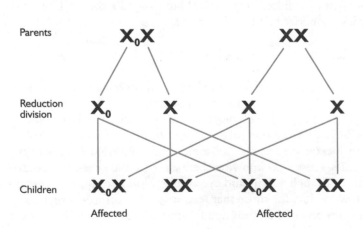

Parents X_0X XX

Reduction division X_0 X X X

Children X_0X XX X_0X XX

Affected   Affected

Recessive inheritance

A recessive gene needs to be paired up with another carrying exactly the same information for it to influence a characteristics outcome. For example, the gene for blue eyes is recessive; therefore, each parent must themselves carry the gene (although they may not have blue eyes) and there must be a successful pairing of these genes in the offspring (Figure 1.3).

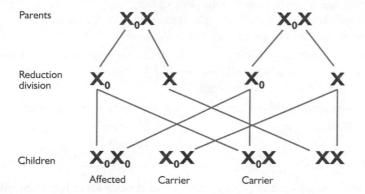

Figure 1.3

Recessive inheritance. There is a 1 : 4 chance of each child inheriting recessive genes from each parent, and a 1 : 2 chance of each being a carrier. X_0 = affected gene.

The inheritance of some disorders follows the same principles, e.g. Tay–Sachs disease, cystic fibrosis and sickle cell anaemia. It is possible in this instance for a characteristic (or disease) to appear 'out of the blue' with no recent family history or to miss generations.

Sex-linked inheritance

Some characteristics (and diseases) are carried on the female chromosome. Genes on the X chromosome have no counterpart on the Y chromosome, so a characteristic determined by a gene on the X chromosome is *always* expressed in the male and so always acts as a dominant gene. A woman who is a carrier of a recessive gene (e.g. haemophilia) has a 1:2 chance of all her male sons having the disease and a 1:2 chance of all her daughters being carriers. An affected male will always pass on the affected gene to his daughters meaning that any daughters he has will be carriers (Figure 1.4).

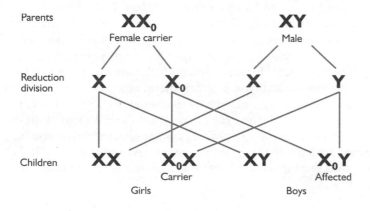

Figure 1.4

Sex-linked inheritance. With each pregnancy there is a 1 : 2 chance of each girl being a carrier or unaffected, and a 1 : 2 chance of each boy having the disease or being unaffected.

Chromosomal abnormalities

Sometimes there is a disruption on one or more of the chromosomes when they unite following fertilisation in the ovum. The precise cause of chromosomal abnormalities is not known but much of the information suggests a link with maternal age (Campbell and Glasper, 1995). The incidence of Down's syndrome, for example, increases markedly with maternal age regardless of the number of pregnancies. There is also some evidence to suggest that some teratogens may cause defects. Chromosome defects are mainly caused by:

- *Non-disjunction* – this is the failure of chromosomes to separate during meiosis. There follows unequal distribution of chromosomes between the two resulting cells.
- *Translocation* – this occurs when two chromosomes exchange material.

ENVIRONMENT

The extent to which any child's growth and development is influenced by his environment will depend on many complex interactions. Some factors will influence the child both before and after birth. Others will only come into play as the child grows (Figure 1.1). It is impossible to give due consideration to all factors so only the major ones will be examined.

Nutrition

This is considered by many to be the most influential factor at any stage of development from the moment of implantation. The fetus receives nutrition from the maternal system and therefore any deficiencies will manifest in fetal development. Severe malnutrition in pregnancy has been cited as being responsible for a permanent reduction in the total number of fetal brain cells thereby influencing the child's later intellectual functioning (Campbell and Glasper, 1995). However, Bee (1995) suggests that there is evidence to contradict this idea. She proposes that malnutrition during pregnancy results in an infant who is more vulnerable to a lack of stimulation and life experiences. Those who are reared in a stimulating environment have been shown to overcome fetal malnutrition (Zeskind and Ramey, 1981). Other effects of malnutrition in pregnancy include a greater risk of stillbirths, low birth weight babies and infant death during the first year of life.

A link between adult health problems (e.g. ischemic heart disease, stroke, hypertension and type 2 diabetes) and nutrition in early life has been suggested by various researchers (Barker *et al.*, 1990; Hales *et al.*, 1991; Fall *et al.*, 1992). The explanation for these links may lie in the role of nutrition in the programming of organs during development. Nutritional inadequacy may prevent organs developing to their full potential thus predisposing the infant to chronic disease in later life (DoH, 1994).

Nutritional elements	Non-pregnant (19–50 years)	Pregnant
Energy (kcal)	1940	+ 200
Protein (g)	45	+ 6
Thiamin (mg)	0.80	+ 0.1ᵃ
Riboflavin (mg)	11.1	+ 0.3
Folate (μg)	200	+100
Vitamin C (mg)	440	+ 10
Vitamin A (μg)	600	+100
Vitamin D (μg)	–	10
Vitamin B12 (μg)	1.5	–
Niiacin (mg)	13	–
Calcium (mg)	700	–
Phosphorus (mg)	550	–
Magnesium (mg)	270	–
Zinc (mg)	7	–
Copper (mg)	1.20	–
Selenium (mg)	60	–

Table 1.1

Nutritional requirements in pregnancy. (Adapted from DoH, 1991)

ᵃ Last trimester only.

Teratogens – diseases and drugs

Prenatally, the effect of any teratogen will depend on the time at which it occurs. Each organ is most vulnerable to disruption when it is developing most rapidly. These periods are known as 'critical' or 'sensitive' periods (Moore, 1988) (Table 1.2).

There are many diseases which, if they occur during pregnancy, can cause disruption to one or more of the developing organs:

* *Rubella.* The effects of this infectious disease during pregnancy are becoming rarer due to the national immunisation programme. Rubella is a relatively mild infectious disease but one which can have devastating effects on the fetus if contracted within the first 3 months of pregnancy. Damage includes congenital cataracts, blindness, underdeveloped eyes and sometimes congenital deafness.

Cross references

Immunisation schedule – page 498

Incubation/infectious period – page 489

Week of gestation	Common sites of damage from disease, drugs, or other outside disturbances
3	Central nervous system and heart
4 + 5	Eyes, heart, limbs
6	Ears, teeth
7	Palate
8	Palate, ears, external genitalia
12	Central nervous system, external genitalia
16	Central nervous system
20–36	Brain
Note: the embryonic period is generally the time of greatest vulnerability	

Table 1.2

Critical periods of organ development before birth. (Adapted from Moore, 1988)

- *Toxoplasmosis*. This infection is caused by a parasite found in the faeces of infected cats and in infected meat. The mother is not affected and may not know she has been in contact with it. However, it can cross the placental barrier and can lead to stillbirth, damage to the developing eyes or brain. Infection in later pregnancy can lead to an enlarged liver or spleen, jaundice or convulsions. Problems can even arise some years after birth.
- *Listeriosis*. This mild feverish condition in adulthood is caused through a food-borne infection commonly associated with soft cheeses and undercooked chicken. If contracted during pregnancy it can lead to premature birth, meningoencephalitis, hydrocephalus or even intrauterine death.
- *Cytomegalovirus* (CMV) is a virus in the herpes group. Very few babies whose mothers have the CMV virus become infected prenatally but those who do have a variety of severe problems including deafness and damage to the central nervous system leading to retardation.
- *AIDS*. A proportion of babies born to HIV-positive mothers are themselves seropositive (European Collaborative Study, 1991).

There are a number of drugs which if taken during pregnancy can cause abnormal development of the fetus.

Activity

List the drugs that you know can cause problems and why, if taken during pregnancy. Make your notes in the margin. Check your list against that given on page 59.

Sociological factors

There are a variety of sociological factors which impact upon a child's development before and after birth:

- The family including family structure, the loss or absence of parents, the size of the family.
- Housing, poverty, unemployment.
- Access to preschool education.
- Culture and ethnicity.
- Social inequalities.
- Relationships.

Cross references

Family – pages 5–18

Relationships – page 20

Activity

Explore each of the above and critically analyse the effect each may have on child development.

The media

The degree to which children are influenced has been a topic of debate for some time. There are many who believe that the mass media have negative influences on children and a there is a growing concern of the effects of violence seen on television and in the cinema. There is no doubt that all forms of media exert a strong influence on children. Media in all their forms are part and parcel of children's everyday lives. The development of the computer and the Internet have opened up even more avenues for children to explore a huge range of material through the media. Lindsay (1994) summarises the suggested undesirable influences of the mass media but counters each with positive arguments:

- Mass media take children away from other more fulfilling and interactive occupations. To counter this Fishbein (1987) found that the activities which suffered as a result of watching television were other media activities such as reading. Hobbies, such as sport, and time spent with friends did not suffer.

- The mass media promote unrealistic stereotyping which can lead to undesirable attitudes. However, while this may be true in some instances, it is suggested that television can and is presenting more positive representations of some groups (e.g. women or ethnic minority groups) leading to positive ways in which children view both sexes and other minority groups (Gunter, 1986).

- The mass media use marketing strategies specifically aimed at children thereby encouraging consumerism. Children are subjected to marketing in many forms, through programmes featuring media characters such as 'Thunderbirds' and 'Barbie', and through advertisements for anything from sweets to clothes, and even undesirable commodities such as cigarettes and alcohol. Whilst this is generally a concern for all involved with children there may be some positive effects of marketing. If children's consumption of sweets and use of toys is influenced by the media, might it not be possible to positively influence their lifestyles? Nutbeam (1989) suggest that this might be so and that the media play an important role in raising awareness about many health issues.

- The mass media encourage young people to develop antisocial behaviour. Evidence to support this is slim but a link has been noted between mass media use and risk-taking behaviours in adolescence (Klein *et al.*, cited by Campbell and Glasper, 1995). Once again it may be possible therefore to use the mass media to exert a positive influence and to encourage prosocial behaviour.

Drugs that can cause problems in pregnancy
- Aspirin
- Anticonvulsants
- Pesticides
- Radiation at high doses
- Lead
- Cocaine
- Alcohol
- Nicotine

Cross reference
Parental behaviour – pages 204–205

Activity

You might try to investigate any of the above by carrying out small-scale research – talk to children that you know. Make some analysis in relation to the comments made here.

SUMMARY

There are certainly many more factors which impact upon child growth and development. What is certain is that development occurs within a complex context where factors interact with each other to exert a variety of influences. It is probably impossible to identify all the influencing factors in a child's life. What we can do is to try to assess each child as an individual, and take into account aspects of his/her life and experiences which may impact upon development. The preceding discussions aim to encourage you to be aware of influencing factors when caring for children, and to explore issues raised in more detail.

Activity

Identify two children whom you have cared for. Reflect on each child's growth and development, and identify factors which may have been influential. Compare and contrast your ideas.

Key points ➤

1. The nature of childhood is a complex and evolving concept – our understanding is based on the views that adults have (had) of children at various times throughout history.

2. The growth and development of children is influenced by both genetic and environmental factors.

3. Heredity accounts for some of our physical characteristics but other inherited features can be influenced by environmental factors and life experience after birth.

4. There are environmental factors that can influence growth and development today, including aspects of the family and relationships, lifestyle, disease and sociological issues.

5. Whilst the mass media have been accused of exerting a negative influence on development, there are some who would argue that there could also be positive outcomes.

GROWTH AND MATURATION 2

INTRODUCTION

According to the Chinese, life begins at conception and this is the point from which age is calculated. This belief acknowledges the importance of life before birth and the fact that intrauterine life and neonatal life constitute a continuum. It therefore seems appropriate when exploring child growth and development to start at the moment of conception. Life before the moment of birth is usually divided into the following phases.

Germinal stage – days 1–14. On day 1 fertilisation occurs and the zygote divides into two cells. By day 3 there are several dozen cells, now called a blastocyst, and by day 5 the blastocyst divides. A cavity forms within the ball of cells and the cells divide into an outer layer of cells which will become the support for the developing embryo, and the inner mass which will become the embryo (Figure 2.1, page 62).

Implantation of the blastocyst in the wall of the uterus begins at about 7 days and is complete within the first 2 weeks.

Embryonic stage – 2–8 weeks. This is an extremely crucial time as the basis of all the major organs develop during this stage. The supportive structures develop. These consist of the amnion (the sac in which the fetus floats), the placenta (fully developed by about 4 weeks after conception) and the umbilical cord (connecting the embryo's circulatory system to the placenta). The placenta acts as the embryo's lifeline, providing nutrients and oxygen, and disposing of waste products. It also acts as a barrier that filters out many harmful substances, e.g. viruses. However, there are some that can cross the placental barrier, such as drugs, anaesthetics and some diseases.

By day 16 the blastocyst differentiates into three layers of cells called the embryonic plate (Figure 2.2, page 63).

Cells of the ectoderm will become the brain, nervous tissue and epidermis; cells of the mesoderm will give rise to connecting tissue, kidneys and genitals; cells of the endoderm will become other internal organs including the digestive tract. By 4–5 weeks, folding of the embryonic plate transforms the plate into a tiny embryo which has a primitive heart, the beginnings of a nervous system, embryonic eyes and ears, and the first suggestion of developing limbs (Figure 2.3, page 64).

Activity

Consider the implications of adverse effects on the embryo during the folding of the neural plate.

By 8 weeks the embryo is about 1.5 inches long and all the basic structures of the organs are formed. No further fundamental changes

Figure 2.1

Days 1–5 of gestation.

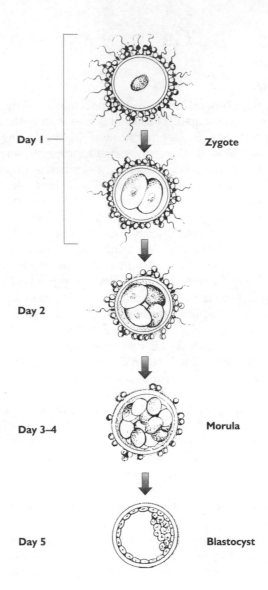

Day 1 — Zygote

Day 2

Day 3–4 — Morula

Day 5 — Blastocyst

will take place. The embryo begins to look human and is floating in a fluid-filled cavity.

Activity

Considering that all the basic structures are present and formed by 8 weeks, what are the implications for the care of pregnant women?

Fetal stage – 9 weeks to birth. Maturation of the systems continues during this stage. Between 9 and 12 weeks the kidneys begin to produce

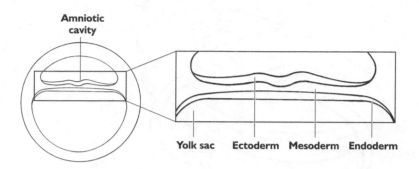

Figure 2.2

The embryonic plate.

urine, the bones grow and ossification begins, and the genitalia develop. The fetus becomes active as the nervous system begins to mature. Neurones begin to appear at about 12 weeks and are virtually all present by 28 weeks. However, the axons are only very short and there are no dendrites. By month 5 the fetal ovaries have produced *all* the 5 million ovarian follicles and a soft downy hair – lanugo – covers the skin. During the last 3 months the fetus grows rapidly and gains most of its birthweight. If the baby continued to grow at such a rapid rate after birth he would weigh 73 kg (160 lb) on his first birthday. Hair begins to grow on the baby's head and the lanugo is shed. By the 7th month, the testes in the male fetus have reached the scrotum. During the 8th month the fetus develops an insulating layer of fat which helps to keep him warm after birth. It is during this time that antibodies and gamma globulin are passed from the mother across the placenta to the fetus. This gives the baby protection from infections for the first 6 months of life. In the last 2 months the nervous system matures considerably as the axons lengthen and the dendrites grow giving rise to a vast number of synapses.

The moment of birth. The fetus usually stops growing by day 260 probably because the ageing placenta loses much of its efficiency. Although many suggest that it is the ageing of the placenta which brings about the change in maternal hormone balance which sets off labour, Nathaniels (1996) argues that there is evidence to support the idea that the fetus decides when it is time to be born. It is thought that the fetus does this by releasing hormones which convert progesterone to oestrogen; this in turn stimulates the mother to produce oxytocin. Oxytocin stimulates the production of prostaglandin which enhances the ability of the uterus to contract.

BIOLOGICAL MATURATION, GROWTH AND DEVELOPMENT AFTER BIRTH

Universal, predictable patterns of growth are basic to all human beings. However, children differ in the rate at which they grow and in their ultimate size, which makes each child unique. It is important for

Figure 2.3

(a) Folding of the embryonic plate. (b) Embryo at 4–5 weeks' gestation.

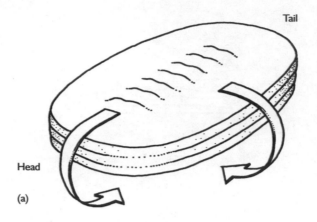

Tail

Head

(a)

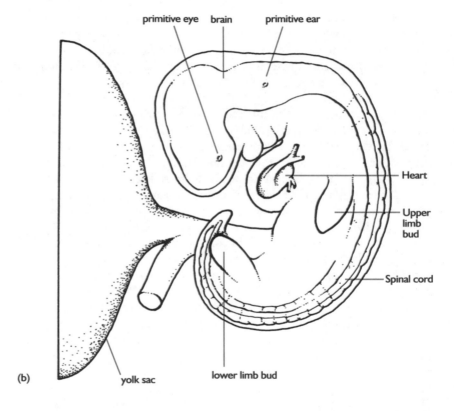

primitive eye   brain   primitive ear

Heart

Upper limb bud

Spinal cord

(b)   yolk sac   lower limb bud

children's nurses to have an understanding of how children grow and the development of physical abilities in order that they can recognise the abnormal. At the same time a knowledge of the maturation process of systems of the body assists the nurses in planning appropriate care.

MATURATION

Whilst all the organs' basic structures are laid down by 8 weeks of intrauterine life with more maturation occurring prior to birth, there are still aspects which require further maturation:

Bones. Development of the bones begins early in embryonic life and is usually complete by the late teens or early 20s. During the growth of long bones, a thin strip of cartilage persists between each epiphysis and diaphysis called the epiphyseal plate. The bones will continue to grow as long as new cartilage develops to maintain this plate. Cessation of bone growth occurs when it becomes ossified and fusion occurs. The growth and development of bone consists of two processes which occur at the same time, i.e. the creation of new cells and tissues (growth) and the consolidation of these tissues into a permanent form (maturation). An increase in the number of bones occurs in the hands and feet, e.g. a 1 year old has three bones in the wrist, an adult has nine. The skull plates are not fused at birth – the posterior plate closes at about 2 months and the anterior at about 16–18 months.

Muscles. All muscles are virtually present at birth. After birth they become thicker, longer and less watery until adolescence, when there is a growth spurt in muscles. A noticeable increase in strength accompanies this growth and is greater in boys than girls.

Neurological system. Most systems grow rapidly after birth but not so the nervous system. The two most rapid periods in the development of the nervous system occur during fetal life. At birth the brain is approximately 25% of adult volume and by 2 years, approximately 75% (Dobbing and Sands, 1973). The cranium continues to expand until about 7 years. Post-natal growth and maturation is mainly related to an increase in communication ability by the advancement of peripheral axons (thereby increasing control over reflexes), and to an increase in the amount of cytoplasm round the nuclei. Most of the dendritic growth occurs in the cortex during the early years aiding the development of imagination and language (Nowakowski, 1987). Myelination is crucial to the development of the nervous system. Myelin sheaths protect the axons and improve conductivity. Myelination is normally complete by about 2 years of age, developing in the cephalocaudal direction.

Renal system. Most kidney growth occurs during the last 20 weeks of fetal life with all the nephrons formed by 28 weeks. After birth kidney size increases in size in proportion to body length, the weight doubling in the first 10 months of life as a result of tubular growth. The glomerular filtration rate (GFR) increases after birth to reach adult values by the age of 3 years. In the first few hours after birth there is a high urine volume with low concentration as a result of immaturity of the sodium and water regulatory systems. Following a diuresis of water the volume gradually falls and the concentration rises. The newborn infant is able to excrete amino acids and conserve sodium and glucose as well as the adult but the ability to excrete free water and to concentrate water is immature. Therefore the infant is less able to excrete large

Question

What are the implications for practice of closure of the fontanelles?

Question

The cranium expands until the age of 7 years – what are the implications for practice?

Cephalocaudal

Head to toe direction

water loads and less able to concentrate the urine in response to dehydration. The regulation of acid base balance is relatively efficient in infancy, but the ability to secrete hydrogen ions is relatively immature and this leads to a limited renal concentration for metabolic acidosis. Dehydration, hypotension and hypoxaemia all produce a marked fall in glomerular filtration rate (GFR), so renal function becomes compromised quickly in a crisis.

Respiratory system. Every component of the respiratory system is immature at birth. The lungs mature after birth with an increase in the size of airway dimensions and the number of alveoli. The airways of the infant are small and easily blocked. By the age of about 10 the increase in alveoli ceases and is followed by an increase in size. By this time there are about nine times as many alveoli as there were at birth. It is also important to recognise that from 0–4 weeks the infant breathes through its nose. In the young infant the chest wall is very compliant, gradually becoming more rigid. It is therefore easily distorted and this increases the work of respiration (Muller and Bryan, 1979).

Gastro-intestinal system. Most biochemical and physiological functions are established at birth. Secretary cells are functional but depend on a specific relationship which is gradually acquired with age; therefore, efficiency may be reduced. Only small amounts of saliva are produced by the glands in neonates, reaching full size and function by the age of 2 years. Acidity of the gastric juice is low in infancy rising to adult levels by about 10 years. The mechanical functions are relatively immature. The oesophageal sphincter is functionally immature during the first 4–6 months of life. Swallowing is an automatic reflex for the first 3 months until the striated muscles in the throat establish cerebral connections. By 6 months the infant is capable of swallowing, holding food in the mouth or spitting it out. The stomach lies horizontally and is round in shape until about 2 years. It then gradually elongates until it assumes the adult position by about 7 years. The capacity of the stomach changes with age (Table 2.1). The immaturity of the digestive system in the infant is shown by the rapidity with which food is propelled through the gastro-intestinal tract. Emptying time in the newborn is 2.5–3 hours;

Glomerular filtration rate

The rate at which fluid is filtered by the glomerulus. It is measured by determining the excretion volume and plasma concentration of a substance that is readily filtered through the glomeruli but not secreted or reabsorbed by the renal tubules

(Watson, 1979)

Question

Infants of 0–4 weeks are nose breathers – what are the implications for practice?

Cross reference

Maintaining fluid balance – pages 339–347

Table 2.1

Stomach capacity

Age	Capacity (ml)
Newborn	10–20
1 week	30–90
2–3 weeks	75–100
1 month	90–150
3 months	150–200
1 year	210–360
2 years	500
10 years	750–900
16 years	1500
Adult	2000–3000

in older infants and children it is 3–6 hours. Peristalsis is more rapid in infancy than at any other time and can reverse resulting in posseting.

Body water. Water is the largest constituent of body tissues – about 70% in the infant and about 60% in the young adult. Water is found in the cells (intracellular) and outside the cells (extracellular). In the adult most water is found inside the cell (67%) but in the infant the larger proportion of water is found outside the cell and there is a higher turnover of water (due to heat production and an inability of the kidneys to conserve water).

Other important points to note related to maturation of the systems include:

- Infants and young children have large surface area/volume ratios.
- Infants under 6 months cannot shiver to generate heat – they produce heat through 'non-shivering thermogenesis'.
- Children have a higher metabolic rate.
- The liver is immature during infancy – it is less able to metabolise toxic substances.
- Infants frequently develop hypoglycaemia during periods of stress because they have high glucose demands and low glycogen stores.
- Heart rate is more rapid, stroke volume smaller than in the adult.
- Child's circulating blood volume is larger per kilogram than that of an adult but volume is small. Therefore a small blood loss may affect blood volume significantly.

Activity

A knowledge of the maturation of the body systems can be invaluable when sick children are being cared for. Using the information given here, and following further reading, explain, giving rationale, why an infant is more prone to dehydration than an adult.

Growth

The rate at which children grow varies from child to child with periods of rapid growth alternating with ones of slow growth. The rapid growth before and after birth slows down gradually, levelling off during early childhood, remaining relatively slow during middle childhood and then increasing at adolescence. Research has shown that normal growth (particularly height) may occur in short (even 24 hour) periods that come in-between long periods with no growth (Lampl, 1992).

Variations in the rate of growth of different tissues and organs produce significant changes in body proportions. A cephalocaudal trend is evident. During fetal life the head is the fastest growing part of the body. In infancy growth of the trunk predominates. In childhood it is the leg growth that predominates, and in adolescence it is again the

---

Non-shivering thermogenesis

The breakdown of brown fat to create heat. The process requires energy so that the infant's oxygen requirement will increase. The regeneration of brown fat requires good nutrition. A poor calorie intake will mean that brown fat is not replaced and the infant will be less able to maintain body heat in a cool environment

---

Further reading

GODFREY, S. and BAUM, J. (1979) *Clinical Paediatric Physiology.* Oxford: Blackwell Science.

HAZINSKI, M. F. (1992) *Nursing Care of the Critically Ill Child*, 2nd edn. St Louis: Mosby.

WATSON, J. E. (1979) *Medical–Surgical Nursing and Related Physiology.* Philadelphia: Saunders.

Increase in height and weight with years

- *Height* – at 3 years there is a steady rate of growth of 5–6 cm/year. At about 12 years of age there is a growth spurt lasting about 2 years. During this time girls can grow as much as 16 cm, boys 20 cm
- *Weight* – birth–6 months: 140–200 g/week; 6–12 months: 85–140 g/week; 1 year–adolescence: 2–3 kg/year

trunk and also the hands and feet. In infancy and early childhood the face is small in relation to the skull. After the first year the bones grow more rapidly than the braincase. Main growth is in the muscles and in the jaws as they enlarge to accommodate the teeth.

Activity

Take time to observe children around you. Note their age and their body proportions. Analyse your results.

Growth charts

New growth charts are available from:

Child Growth Foundation
2 Mayfield Avenue
London W4 1PW

Growth is usually measured in terms of height and weight. It is interesting to note that at birth a baby is one-third of its adult height and by 2 years he is one-half of his eventual adult height. In 1995, new child growth standards were issued based on seven sets of growth data collected between 1978 and 1990 from over 25 000 children. These confirm that mean height has been increasing steadily over the last generation. It is important to note that children from ethnic minorities were excluded from the studies (Hulse, 1995).

Activity

Check that the paediatric areas in your Trust are using the new growth charts. Try to compare them with the old ones. What might be the implications for children who have been measured using the old charts?

Physical development

As children grow and mature so their bodies develop, and they are able to perform more skilful and complex movements. This is often referred to as motor development, and is usually divided into gross motor and fine motor development. The stages at which children reach different milestones will vary and it is always important to look at the whole child and not just one aspect of their development. Knowledge of the milestones helps us to measure the progress that children are making and to identify any deviations from the norm as quickly as possible.

Further reading

More detailed information about motor development can be found in:

BEAVER, M. et al. (1994) Babies and Young Children. Book 1. Development 0–7. Cheltenham: Stanley Thornes.

SHERIDAN, M. (1975) From Birth to Five Years: Children's Developmental Progress. Oxford: NFER-Nelson

Gross motor skills involve whole body movements: crawling, sitting, walking and running. Fine motor skills involve the manipulative skills associated with hand and eye coordination; finger play, grasping objects and pincer grasp. Nearly all the basic skills of both types are achieved by the age of about 6–7 years. Figure 2.4 gives an overview of the milestones in motor development.

SUMMARY

The development of the individual from conception to maturity is a marvellous, complex process. It is important to acknowledge that life begins at conception and that there are many influences acting upon the

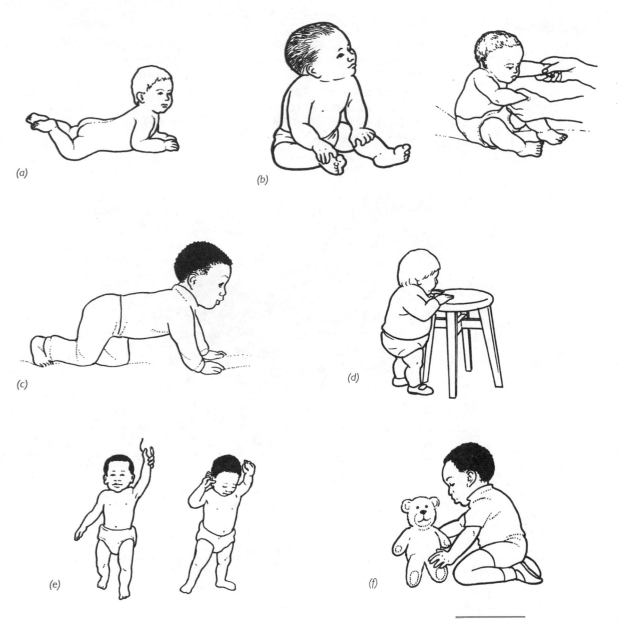

(a)

(b)

(c)

(d)

(e)

(f)

Figure 2.4

*Milestones in motor development. (a)
at 3 months the baby can raise its
head and look around; (b) at 6
months the baby can sit unsupported
for a short while; (c) at 9 months the
baby can crawl quite well; (d) at 10
months the baby can pull itself up by
the furniture; (e) at 12 months the
baby is beginning to walk; (f) at 18
months the baby can walk well, bend
down, push and pull their toys.*

developing fetus. The exciting moment of birth is but one stage and
signifies the beginning of independence. Infants continue to grow and
mature throughout childhood but achieve much of their abilities within
the first few years of life. Consider the first year. The child is born with
little capacity for body control and by 1 year is nearly ready to walk. It
is worth observing children in different settings in an attempt to learn
more about the way in which they grow and develop motor skills.

Activity

Find a family with a baby under 6 months (use your own family where possible). You need to be able to have access to the baby at about monthly intervals for about 4–6 months. On each occasion make observations of the infant, noting aspects of growth and physical development. Use charts to plot the infant's progress. On completing the observations, compare your findings with those given in Figure 2.4. Where time permits repeat with another child and compare the two.

Key points ➤

1. Intrauterine life and neonatal life constitute a continuum – life begins at conception.
2. Life before birth is divided into three stages: germinal (0–2 weeks), embryonic (3–8 weeks) and fetal (9 weeks–birth).
3. Universal predictable patterns of growth and maturation are basic to all human beings.
4. All the organs' basic structures are laid down by week 8 of gestation. The systems continue to mature up until and after birth.
5. A knowledge of the maturation process is vital as it forms a basis on which to rationalise care.
6. The rate at which children grow varies from child to child, but follows a predictable pattern.
7. Children have achieved nearly all the basic motor skills by the age of 6–7 years.

THEORETICAL PERSPECTIVES – 3
COGNITIVE DEVELOPMENT

INTRODUCTION

The development of thought and understanding in children is a fascinating and mysterious process. How often have you wondered what children are thinking or asked yourself how they see the world around them. Whilst all of us have been there, it is unlikely that we can consciously remember how we developed an understanding of our world. In studying cognitive development we can only make assumptions based on what children say, so we are in fact relying on adult explanations of children's thinking. Perhaps that is why some of the theories seem difficult to assimilate as they are adult's perceptions of children.

Cognition is the term generally used in developmental theory to refer to thought and understanding. However, there is more to cognition than just these two aspects as we can see in Figure 3.1. All these aspects interact together to enable children to make sense of their world.

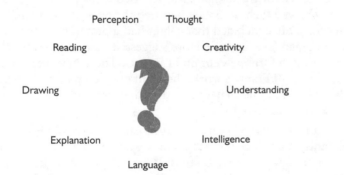

Figure 3.1

What is cognitive development?

For the purposes of this module the discussion will concentrate on three aspects of cognitive development – the development of:

- Visual perception
- Thinking
- Language

VISUAL PERCEPTION

Perception refers to the way in which the brain interprets sensory information. According to Gibson and Spelke (1983): 'perception is the beginning of knowing and so is an essential part of cognition'. There are two main views on the development of perception in children. The nativists believe that a baby senses the world like an adult from birth and therefore sees things as we do. The empiricists, however, believe that the baby has to learn how to perceive things.

Visual perception includes a number of abilities such as pattern and depth perception, size and colour constancy. Research has shown that whilst babies do not have the same visual acuity as adults, they do have some innate visual capabilities:

- Bower *et al.* (1970) investigated infants' abilities to judge distance and direction. They found that babies could tell the direction of an approaching object and that they became distressed if an object appeared to be heading straight for their face. They concluded that the defensive reaction was innate. Ball and Tronick (1971) reported a similar result and came to the conclusion that this aspect of depth perception was innate.

- Bower (1965) also conducted research to test size constancy. His sample consisted of babies who were only a few weeks old. He found that babies were able to recognise the same object at different distances and concluded that size constancy was innate. Slater *et al.* (1990) came to a similar conclusion.

- In the early 1960s, Frantz carried out a number of experiments to test infants' ability to discriminate between patterns and their preference for the human face. He used three pictures (Figure 3.2) and showed them to babies between the ages of 4 days and 6 months. He concluded that babies had a preference for the picture of the human face, and therefore suggested that there is an unlearned meaning in form perception of infants. There have been many criticisms of Frantz's work, the main one being that just because a baby looks at one shape more than another does not mean that that picture is preferred.

- Walton *et al.* (1992) carried out research which allowed newborn infants to produce the images they wanted on a TV screen by sucking on a pressure sensitive dummy. When the infant sucked hard an image appeared on the screen. Which image appeared (mother or

Figure 3.2

Frantz faces.

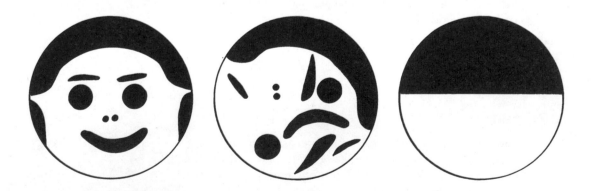

stranger) depended on the rate of sucking. They concluded that not only did newborns behave in a very competent way but that they were able to distinguish a familiar face from a strange one.

Activity

Find out more about these experiments and critically review the methodology of each. Make your own criticisms of the research.

Evidence to support the empiricists' views is also available but appears to be less well defined and often based on animal experiments. Research has been conducted which suggests that early visual experience is important in the development of binocular vision and in the ability to perceive horizontal and vertical lines. Gregory (1966, cited by Mitchell, 1992) found that an individual's susceptibility to the Muller–Lyer illusion (Figure 3.3) was dependent to some extent on the environment. He reported studies which showed that people who live in environments containing few straight lines or corners (rural areas of underdeveloped countries) are less susceptible to the illusion.

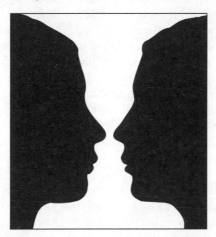

Figure 3.3

Muller–Lyer illusion.

The third possible view, and the one which seems to be supported by many psychologists today, is that the development of perceptual skills is a result of both innate and learned experiences. We now know that babies can see quite well at birth but that their visual abilities do develop over time as a result of visual experiences.

THINKING

According to Campbell and Olsen (1990), thinking is 'an effortful activity, involving mental "work", in which the organism forsakes its normal outward orientation on the presented world and struggles instead with a world indexed only imperfectly by a shadowy inner structure of mental symbols'. Thinking is also about making meaning

Question

Ponder this: 'I think it is going to rain'. What might be the basis for your thoughts?

out of what goes on around us and understanding concepts. Thinking is something you and I do quite often during our everyday lives. We know what we are thinking about and are able to use symbols and imagery to carry out quite complex work in our minds.

Activity

Think of a number, double it, add 3 and then take away 4. What is your answer? It is quite likely that you carried out this activity without having to use any form of visual aid. Try the same exercise with children of different ages. How do they work it out?

The development of thinking is a mysterious process and one which we can only judge on the basis of adult speculations for we will never truly know what a young child is thinking. Three views on cognitive development are offered for you to consider.

Jean Piaget (1896–1980)

Jean Piaget is perhaps the most well-known psychologist in this field and one who has influenced the care of children through his work. Piaget was a biologist who became interested in children's thinking whilst carrying out tests on intelligence. In his work he attempted to find explanations for the way in which children come to understand their world and make judgements about it. His studies were based on the qualitative development of children's ability to solve problems. This involved clinical interviews which used an open-ended, conversation-like technique for eliciting children's responses. From these studies Piaget concluded that children's thinking develops in stages and that each stage is a prerequisite for the next one. He gave approximate age ranges for each stage. With each stage, thinking becomes more complex until the child reaches maturity. His theory is based on the premise that children learn largely unassisted through interaction with the world around them, using experiences to build on their understanding.

Sensori-motor stage: birth–2 years. At this stage babies learn through the senses and through movement. Piaget believed that, at the beginning of this stage, a baby has no concept of the difference between self and non-self and has no understanding of the permanent existence of anything other than himself. It is during this stage that the child develops object permanence. Piaget claimed that babies under 8 months of age do not have the concept of permanence, i.e. once an object is out of sight, they do not understand that it still exists. His explanation for this was that they do not have the necessary ability to conjure up an image of the object in its absence. Between 8 months and 2 years, this concept develops, so that by the age of 2 the child understands that things go on happening and objects have their own independent existence. Piaget concluded that, by the end of this stage, children are

Key terms used by Piaget

- *Schema* – all the ideas and information that a child might have about an object, formed through the child's interaction with the outside world
- *Assimilation* – the way in which a child takes in important elements of any experience
- *Accommodation* – the process of fitting what has been learned into existing schema
- *Adaptation* – the result of interaction between assimilation and accommodation; the child has learned more about the world and can act upon it

Criticisms of Piaget's view of object permanence

Bower (1981) carried out experiments in which he concluded that infants younger than 8 months know that objects exist even when they are occluded. He found that the infants in his study demonstrated this knowledge with their eyes but not with hand or arm movements. This work only suggests that Piaget underestimated the abilities of young infants and does not necessarily negate Piaget's theory able to make mental predictions about their actions through the use of symbolism.

Pre-operational stage: 2–7 years. The ability to form and use symbols is the main feature of this stage. The symbols Piaget described include language, drawing, music and dance. Through the use of these symbols, the child continues to learn about the world and develops the ability to solve problems. However, the child's thinking is intuitive and subjective rather than logical and objective. Piaget suggested that children are egocentric at this age and are incapable of seeing things from somebody else's point of view. Linked to this is an inability to understand and apply principles. Piaget reached his conclusions about this stage by setting children tasks and seeing whether they gave correct or incorrect answers. Children under 7 years nearly always gave incorrect answers. One example of the tests used is that related to the concept of conservation. The child watches as two short wide jars are filled with water to the same level. The contents of one of the jars is then poured into a tall narrow jar and placed next to the remaining short wide jar. The level of water in the tall, narrow jar is much higher. Piaget found that nearly all the children under 7 said that there was more water in the tall jar than in the short one. Instead of attending to a principle, i.e. no water was added or taken away therefore, the children gave intuitive answers based on what they could see, i.e. an increased water level.

Activity

Try out some of these tests on children in your family or on children in your care (remember to get permission before you start). Analyse your results. How do they compare with those of Piaget?

Piaget subdivided the pre-operational stage into two:

- *Preconceptual stage: 2–4 years*. Concepts are not fully formed. Children are not able to distinguish the different properties of objects within a different class. Hence all men are 'daddy', including the milkman! This might explain why young children seem capable of believing in Father Christmas. Even when they see a number of Father Christmases in different places and they all look subtly different, they believe that they are one and the same person.

- *Intuitive stage: 4–7 years*. Ability to classify and organise develops but they are still unaware of the principles that underlie the concepts.

Stage of concrete operations: 7–12 years. According to Piaget children in this stage use logical thinking based on principles to solve problems. Children over 7 give the correct answers to the tests of conservation and realise that their view of something is only one of many possible views. However, they cannot deal with abstract or

---

Conservation

' ... understanding that transformation of appearance need not result in alteration of the underlying reality. The underlying reality remains constant and is therefore conserved'.

(Mitchell, 1992)

Other conservation tasks were related to

- Mass
- Length
- Number

Criticisms of Piaget's tests

Donaldson (1978) felt that the reason so-called pre-operational children gave the wrong answers was because they misunderstood the questions and not because they did not have any logical abilities. She argues that Piaget's questions did not make sense to the children and that they answered according to how they thought he wanted them to

---

Further reading

MITCHELL, P. (1992) *The Psychology of Childhood*. London: Falmer Press.

hypothetical dilemmas – they are firmly rooted in the real world and cannot handle a problem which asks them 'just suppose … '.

Stage of formal operations: 12 years onwards. Characteristics of this stage include the ability to think logically and to deal with abstract ideas. Problems can be solved on a purely mental level with no visual aids. Problems are approached in a logical, systematic and patterned manner with reasoning based on a clear understanding of the underlying principles. Piaget suggested that not everybody reaches this level of thinking.

Many psychologists have attempted to assess the accuracy and appropriateness of Piaget's work. There are many who would argue that his theory should be rejected, others who accept it but feel that it needs modification. There seems to be a consensus that Piaget probably underestimated the abilities of young children.

Lev Vygotsky (1896–1934)

Vygotsky provides an alternative view and challenges those of Piaget. Whilst Piaget saw children as being largely unassisted in the development of their thinking, Vygotsky emphasised the role of the social context and, in particular, the role of direct intervention by others who are more knowledgeable. He believed that it was wrong to judge children merely on what they could do alone, but that what they were capable of doing with help should be also taken into account. The central concept of Vygotsky's theory is that of the *zone of proximal development* (ZPD) (Figure 3.4).

The ZPD is the distance between the child's actual cognitive level and his potential level under the guidance of more knowledgeable adults or collaboration with more competent peers. Any intervention that aims to increase a child's existing repertoire of cognitive skills is most effective when it is within the ZPD, i.e. it should be at a level beyond the child's existing abilities but not so far above that level that it is

Figure 3.4

Vygotsky's zone of proximal development.

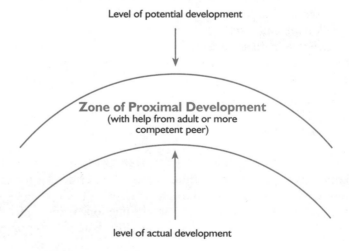

Level of potential development

Zone of Proximal Development
(with help from adult or more competent peer)

level of actual development

incomprehensible. It would appear from the work of Vygotsky that, if we were to judge a child's cognitive level on what he could do with help, then Piaget's description of the ages at which children could do things could be seriously underestimated. The suggestion is that young children have representational powers but can only exercise them with prompting or adult help.

A second important concept in Vygotsky's work was the emphasis he placed on the role of language in the development of thinking and thought. Whilst Piaget argued that thinking develops out of action, not language, Vygotsky thought the opposite. He suggested that by 7 years speech becomes internalised, allowing dialogue with oneself which in turn helps to guide actions.

Jerome Bruner

Bruner (1966) developed Vygotsky's ideas and identified three stages of cognitive development:

- *Enactive: 0–2 years.* The child represents the world around him by actions.
- *Iconic: 2–6 years.* The child begins to use images.
- *Symbolic: 7 years upwards.* The child is freed from the present and real world and is able to use symbols. This ability, largely dependent on language, is at the centre of the child's ability to deal with the abstract.

Activity

Carry out further reading on the ideas of Vygotsky and Bruner. Analyse your findings and compare and contrast their ideas with those of Piaget.

LANGUAGE

The use of language is the main way in which humans communicate. Language is a complex organised system of symbols which can be spoken, written or signed (used by people who are deaf and who have no speech). There are four main areas of language competence which children must acquire:

- *Phonology* – the rules of sounds (phonemes). These are the basic sounds which make up a language. Each language has its own phoneme system.
- *Syntax* (grammar). This refers to the way in which words are put together to make grammatically correct sentences.
- *Semantics.* This refers to the meaning of words and sounds.
- *Pragmatics.* Refers to knowledge about how language is used in different contexts. Children will need to be able to adjust and adapt their language according to the situation in which they finds themselves.

By the time a child reaches the age of 5–6 years he has grasped the essentials of his language and is in fact highly competent in its use. The acquisition of language appears to proceed with no real effort on behalf of the child and no formal education. Sequential stages in the development of language are identifiable (Table 3.1). It is interesting to note that children learning any language seem to progress through the same stages, in the same order and at approximately the same ages (Slobin, 1973).

Table 3.1

Age-related development of language

Approximate age	Characteristics of language development
Birth–1 month	Crying: three distinct types identified: basic – usually from hunger, at first quiet and intermittent but becoming louder; angry – same sequence as basic cry but characterised by differences in length of sound and pauses between sounds; pain – sudden and loud from the onset – long cry followed by long silence and series of short gasping sounds (Smith and Cowie, 1991).
1–6 months	Infant's repertoire increases and includes laughing and 'cooing'; uses mainly vowel sounds with a developing variety of pitch; turn-taking evident between infant and carer (Tamir, 1984).
6–9 months	Begins to babble, a combination of vowels and consonants with no meaning, e.g. dadadadada, mamama, bababa; may be identifiable sounds; important for practising sound-producing mechanisms; can understand simple words, e.g. 'No!'.
9–12 months	Babbling continues, beginning to reflect intonation of speech; by 12 months first words appear, usually names of people or objects with which they are familiar; responds to simple commands; 0–12 months considered as the prelinguistic stage in language development.
12–24 months	By 18 months, vocabulary increased to about 10 words, by 20 months to about 50 words and by 24 months to about 300 words – mainly nouns (Mitchell, 1992). Uses holophrases – one word utterances used to convey many different meanings, e.g. 'Cat' could mean 'There is a cat' or 'Where is my cat?'
2–3 years	Sentences become longer but tend to be telegraphic – uses mainly content words and misses out function words such as 'to', 'at', 'of'. Order of words sometimes incorrect; tends to over-generalise and see all men as 'daddy', all animals as 'dog'.
3–4 years	Speech becomes less telegraphic, beginning to acquire the finer points of language. Uses the past tense and 3–4 word sentences. Has a vocabulary of about 1000 words (Smith and Cowie, 1991); enjoys the use of rhyming poems.
4–5 years	Uses longer sentences with complex constructions; tendency to over-regulate, e.g. assumes that ' … ed' is added to all words to make the past tense, e.g. 'I goed to the park'.
5–6 years and upwards	Good grasp of language although still makes some mistakes with grammar, e.g. 'It was the bestest'; average 6-year-old has a vocabulary of about 14 000 words; continues to develop and refine language; develops the ability to use embedded sentences and negative forms.

Activity

Tape conversations with children of various ages. Analyse what they say; compare and contrast your findings with the information given above.

Theories of language development

Several psychologists have attempted to explain how children learn a language. Once again, as with many areas of development, there are two main views: nature versus nurture. The debate is inconclusive and it seems most likely that in reality there are elements of both.

Nurture. Skinner (1957) believed that language development occurs as does other learning, i.e. through reinforcement of appropriate behaviour. When an infant makes sounds and words they are greeted with a positive response which acts as a reinforcement. Language is then progressively shaped by adults who reward and reinforce correct usage. More recent research appears to give us evidence that the acquisition is far more complex than this. In reality it has been found that mothers rarely correct the grammatical structure of their children's speech, being more interested in the content (Brown *et al.*, cited by Smith and Cowie, 1991). However, the role of adults in a child's acquisition of language is clearly important as has been shown by research into the use of Baby Talk Register by mothers and fathers.

Nature. Naom Chomsky (1986) argued against Skinner's views and suggested that babies are born with an innate ability to acquire language. He claimed that the process of acquiring language was so easy for children because the rudiments of language already exist in their brains in the form of a 'language acquisition device' (LAD). He believes that children learn language on their own and that the environment plays little part.

Cross reference

Role of family in development – page 33

Further reading

GRIEVE, R. and HUGHES, M. (1990) *Understanding Children.* Oxford: Blackwell.

LOCK, A. and FISHER, E. (1984) *Language Development.* London: Routledge.

Activity

Consider how a knowledge of language development would help you in your practice.

SUMMARY

This exploration has tried to give an overview of three important areas in cognitive development. It is important to acknowledge that no one aspect of development occurs in isolation and all are interlinked in some way. Children are an exciting mixture of innocence and maturity. Even 4 year olds have a large degree of understanding of the world around them. They develop an acute awareness of subtle innuendoes and can articulate their feelings very clearly. Their thirst for knowledge is sometimes overwhelming. It is fascinating to observe at close quarters the development of a child's thinking, but at the same time, one can

Other areas related to cognitive development worth exploring

- Children's drawings
- Children's story telling
- Children's explanations
- Intelligence
- Development of writing and reading

easily overlook the important developments. If you have children, reflect back on the way they developed – it is likely that you have forgotten much of what happened. Consider your practice and try to focus on what children are thinking and how their cognitive processes are developing. It is important to attempt to see into the child's world in order to plan and implement care appropriately.

Key points ➤

1. In the study of cognitive development, we can only make assumptions based on what children say. Therefore, wc rely on an adult's explanation of children's developing minds.
2. The term 'cognition' encompasses language, perception, thinking, creativity, memory, concentration and intelligence.
3. Research has shown that, while babies do not have the same visual acuity as adults, they do have some innate capabilities.
4. We can only speculate as to what children are thinking – but it is better to attempt to understand how they view the world in which they live so that we can give appropriate care.
5. The process of the development of language is unclear; however, stages in language acquisition have been identified and can be related to nearly all children.
6. Each aspect of cognitive development is interlinked – development in one area does not occur in isolation.

THERETICAL PERSPECTIVES – THE SOCIAL WORLD OF THE CHILD 4

INTRODUCTION

Becoming a social being is an important process for all children whatever culture they are born into. There is a wealth of evidence to suggest that the quality of a child's early relationships will affect the development of social competence (Howe, 1995). Thus it is important to acknowledge the role of the family and others in a child's social development. For the purposes of this module the discussions will concentrate on three aspects of social development:

- the development of the concept of self and a child's personality;
- the development of social relationships with parents and others;
- the development of social cognition (moral development).

Cross reference

Roles and relationships – pages 19–28

THE CONCEPT OF SELF

Activity

Before reading further, spend 2 minutes to consider your answer to the question 'Who am I?'. Attempt to give 20 answers.

It is likely that you will have identified a variety of characteristics about yourself which you see as being 'you'. These could range from physical characteristics to other qualities such as stubbornness, aptitudes or even ideas about your sex role. These are aspects of your self-concept which shape and influence how we respond to others and how we deal with social relationships. Our ideas about our sex role form a powerful part of our self-concept.

Ideas about how this concept develops have been influenced by Piaget and Freud. Both believed that a baby begins life with no sense of separateness. Their work was developed by Lewis (1991) who identified two steps in the development of the self-concept:

- *The subjective self.* Babies must first work out that they are separate from others and that this endures over time. The key would seem to be the idea that 'I exist'. Lewis believes that this occurs within the first 2–3 months and is achieved through learning from experimentation that 'I can make things happen'. For example, smiling at mother will evoke a response, touching a mobile will make it move. Lewis sees the development of object permanence as being a crucial step and that only when this has occurred at about 8–9 months will the real subjective self have emerged. This coincides with Piaget's ideas on object permanence and, whilst these ideas are somewhat controversial, they could go some way to explaining the sudden onset of a wariness of strangers which occurs at this age.

- *The objective self.* The infant needs to move on to develop self-awareness and to understand that the self has properties and qualities. One way in which the development of the objective self has been studied is through the use of the mirrors and the 'rouge' test (Smith and Cowie, 1991). (You could try this test out for yourself.) Children of various age groups (9–24 months) were placed in front of a mirror. They were then removed from the front of the mirror and their noses discreetly rubbed with rouge. Then they were placed in front of the mirror again. The results, which have been replicated several times, show that, although all the children smiled at the image, only those aged between 21 and 24 months reached for their own noses (Figure 4.1). This would suggest that, by about this age, an infant has a fairly good idea that the reflection in the mirror is a representation of himself. During the second year children become much more aware of themselves and it is now that we begin to see embarrassment, pride, shame, plus the inevitable insistence on doing things for themselves. The child is learning about himself.

Figure 4.1

Mirror recognition and self-naming. Percentage of children who reached for their noses after the rouge had been applied. (Adapted from Lewis and Brooks, 1978, cited by Bee, 1995)

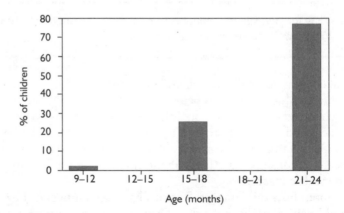

Initially the self-concept is very concrete and linked to visible characteristics such as 'Where I live', 'What I look like' or 'What I am good at doing'. Over the school years this gradually changes as children become more abstract in their thinking and they become focused more on internal qualities.

Activity

Try the last activity with children in a range of age groups. Record what they say and then compare and contrast with the ideas mentioned here.

There is some suggestion that there is a crisis of identity at adolescence. The psychologists most noted for his ideas in this area is Erikson. He thought that it was during this period that the most turmoil could be expected and that many adolescents went through a period of redefining themselves, of trying out new aspects of identity. He called this *crisis identity versus role confusion* and considered it to be normal. Various criticisms have been made of these ideas, largely because Erikson's ideas were based on observations and on clinical practice. Since then attempts have been made to test his ideas using research. The findings seem to suggest that the sense of self changes gradually and not necessarily as a result of adolescence.

Tied in with the development of self-awareness is the concept of self-esteem – the global value of one's worth. We tend to compare ourselves with others and make evaluations about our own worth from that. Harter (1987) suggests that self-esteem is a product of what children think they ought to be and what they think they are. When the difference between the two is low, self-esteem is high and vice versa. Children's self-esteem can be influenced by their beliefs about themselves and the support of others around them.

Activity

Reflect on your own self-esteem. What factors have influenced the value which you place upon yourself?

DEVELOPMENT OF PERSONALITY

Four approaches related to the development of personality are offered for you to consider.

The biological approach

Theorists who support this view have tended to look more closely at temperament, that part of the personality pertaining to mood, activity and general level of energy. They propose that:

- Each individual is born with characteristic patterns of responding to the environment and to people.

- These behavioural dispositions are based in variations in fundamental physiological processes and are therefore influenced by the way the brain, nervous system and hormones work. In other words we inherit tendencies to react in particular ways.

- Temperamental dispositions persist through childhood into adulthood and, although subject to change through experience, a bias for certain patterns remains.

- Temperamental characteristics influence the way a child responds to people and vice versa.

Personality

It is difficult to find a consensus definition of this term. However, the idea that seems to underlie different theoretical perspectives is that 'each individual has a relatively unique and enduring set of psychological tendencies and reveals them in the course of his or her transactions with various social environments ... '.

(Berryman et al., 1991)

Further reading

DAVENPORT, G. C. (1994) *An Introduction to Child Development*, 2nd edn. London: Collins Educational.

OATES, J. (ed.) (1994) *The Foundations of Child Development*. Open University: Milton Keynes

Bates (1989) suggested that temperament 'consists of biologically rooted individual differences in behaviour tendencies that are present early in life and are relatively stable across various kinds of situation and over the course of time'. Evidence to back up this view comes from studies on identical twins who are more alike in temperament than non-identical twins, even when reared apart. Kagan (1988) proposes that there are specific sites in the brain which regulate emotional behaviour and are responsible for differences in temperament. However, this approach does not take account of the developmental nature of children over time.

The learning approach

Learning theorists, although they do not reject the biological basis for behaviour, stress the importance of reinforcement patterns in the environment. Children also learn from modelling themselves on others and therefore develop personality characteristics as a result of this learning. Basic points emphasised by these theorists are:

- Behaviour is strengthened by reinforcement. A child who is reinforced for aggressive behaviour is more likely to express this type of behaviour than one who is not reinforced.
- Inconsistent reinforcement is likely to lead to highly persistent behaviour.
- Children learn new behaviour through modelling (Bandura, 1973).
- As well as learning overt behaviour by modelling, children also learn ideas, expectations, standards and self-concepts this way.

The learning theory helps us to explain why children are so inconsistent in their behaviour, something that would be hard to explain using biological approaches. A child may be calm, well behaved, introvert and do as he is told at school, but be aggressive, wilful and disobedient when he gets home. Learning theorists would explain this as being the result of a variety of reinforcement patterns. There is also room for change within this theory. Many programmes based on reinforcement exist for a variety of behaviour problems, e.g. sleep, bowel training and aggressiveness.

The psychoanalytical approach

The basic premise of this approach is that a child's personality is influenced by an interaction between inborn patterns and environmental influences. These theorists also suggest a clear developmental pattern as children grow older (Tables 4.1 and 4.2). They propose that:

- Behaviour is governed by unconscious as well and conscious motives. Freud identified three sets of motive – sexual (libido), life-preserving and aggressive, whilst Erikson identified only one – identity.
- Personality develops over time as a result of interaction between inborn drives and the responses by key people in the child's life.

Age (years)	Normative crisis	Tasks and activitites
0–1	Trust versus mistrust	To develop trust in central caregiver(s); an early secure attachment
1–2	Autonomy versus shame and doubt	Physical development leads to more free choice, e.g. walking, grasping; toilet training; more control
3–5	Initiative versus guilt	Become more assertive; Oedipus-like feelings may lead to guilt
6–puberty	Industry versus inferiority	Main social interaction outside home; absorb all basic cultural norms
Adolescence	Identity versus role confusion	Main social interaction with peers; identity crisis; search for new values

NB Erikson proposed three additional stages during adulthood.

Table 4.1

Erikson's psychosocial stages in the development of personality

Stage and approx. age (years)	Erogenous zone	Main characteristics	Tasks to achieve (potential source of conflict)
Oral (0–1)	Mouth	Main source of pleasure is mouth; main concern is with immediate gratification of urges	Satisfactory feeding/weaning
Anal (1–2)	Anus	Controlling bowels and bladder	Toilet training
Phallic (2–6)	Genitals	Playing with genitals; Oedipus and Electra complex	Successful solution to Oedipal and Electra conflicts
Latency (6–11)	None – sexual energy quiescent	Same-sex parent identification	None
Genital (11 on)	Genitals	Increasing concern with adult ways of experiencing sexual pleasure	Mature sexual intimacy

Table 4.2

Freud's psychosexual stages of personality development

- The development of personality occurs in stages, each stage centred on a particular task.
- The specific personality a child develops will depend on the success in dealing with the stages.

The interactive approach

Bee (1995) gives us a model which attempts to integrate the three previous approaches (Figure 4.2). She suggests that the basis for the development of a child's personality is the inborn temperament. Thereafter there is a complex interaction of a variety of factors that influences personality.

Activity

Take each of the approaches offered above and critically analyse each one. Attempt to make your own model from the ideas given.

Figure 4.2

A model of personality development. (Adapted from Bee, 1995.)

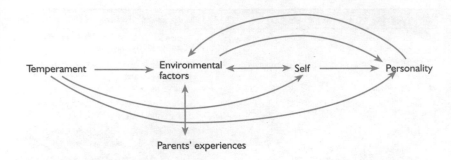

THE DEVELOPMENT OF SOCIAL RELATIONSHIPS WITH PARENTS AND OTHERS

Hartup (1989) describes two types of relationships which he considers vital to the child:

- *Vertical.* Relationships with others who have greater knowledge and power. These could include parents, teachers, older siblings. These relationships give protection and security and enable the development of basic social skills.

- *Horizontal.* Relationships which are egalitarian and reciprocal, e.g. with same-age peers. These relationships give children the opportunity to practise social skills that can only be learnt by interaction with equals, e.g. cooperation, competition and intimacy.

Vertical relationships

The formation of attachments with caregivers is perhaps one of the most important early social relationships. Others, considered as being 'beyond attachment', become important as the child grows older. The discussion which follows will concentrate on early attachment relationships.

Much of the work on attachment theory has been based on ideas developed by John Bowlby during the 1950s and 1960s. In 1969, Bowlby described four phases in the development of a child's attachment (ages are approximate):

- *Birth to 2–3 months.* Little evidence of attachment. The infant signals without discriminating between different people. Behaviours include crying, smiling, responding to caregivers, but they are not directed towards anybody in particular.

- *2–3 months to 6 months.* The infant begins to aim attachment behaviours more narrowly, directing them towards one or more individuals. The infant displays no special anxiety at being separated from parents or being with strangers.

- *7–8 months.* Secure base behaviours. The infant uses the secure base (generally mother but could be another caregiver) as a base from which to explore. Watch the behaviour of children over the age of 8

Cross reference

Separation anxiety – page 210

months, especially those who can crawl. You might see evidence of attachment behaviours – the child crawls away for some distance but occasionally checks out the secure base to look for reassurance and protection. He may cry or protest if his mother leaves. It is at this time that the infant becomes wary of strangers.

- *2–3 years*. The child begins to accommodate the mother's needs. He will be more willing to wait alone if requested until mother returns. However, he still shows attachment behaviours such as cuddling. By the age of about 4 years the child understands that the relationship exists even when his mother is not there. Attachment behaviours become less noticeable but may occur at times of stress.

Activity

The next opportunity you get, try an experiment with a baby aged between 3 and 7 months. Separate him from his mother and/or pass him round a few strangers. Observe his reactions. Then try to repeat the test with an older infant (9–10 months). Compare and contrast the results.

Ainsworth *et al.* (1978) went on to develop a method for testing the strength of attachments – the strange situation. From this research three main types of attachment were identified:

- *Secure attachment*. This type of attachment is evident in about 50–67% of relationships in industrialised countries (Mitchell, 1992). The infant greets mother warmly on her return from any absences. He does not display aggressive behaviour towards her.

- *Unsocial attachment*. The infant is more likely to cry when his mother leaves him but less likely to greet her warmly on her return. Appears to be susceptible to temper tantrums. After a period of separation the infant may avoid contact with his mother.

- *Anxious attachment*. The infant appears to want comfort and attention from his mother but then reacts in a hostile fashion. The infant reacts coolly to mother's attention.

Cultural perspective

According to Oates (1994) the establishment of either one or a small number of ongoing relationships between baby and carer(s) is a virtually universal feature

Activity

Consider the implications of attachment theory for your practice.

Further reading

HOWE, D. (1995) *Attachment Theory for Social Work Practice*. Basingstoke: Macmillan.

MITCHELL, P. (1992) *The Psychology of Childhood*. London: Falmer Press.

SMITH, P. K. and COWIE, H. (1991) *Understanding Children's Development*. Oxford: Blackwell.

From the observation of children, it is clear that they show differing behaviours, demonstrating that the quality of attachment differs. This is perhaps because they have different internal working models of their relationships with their parents. The internal working model comprises the way in which they see the attachment, including the confidence that they have in the attachment, expectations of rebuff or affection and the quality of the secure base. Some theorists have pondered the question,

'Does the quality of attachment remain stable over time?'. The answer appears to be 'yes' and 'no'. If the child's environment is stable, then it would seem that the quality remains stable. However, if circumstances change (change of caregiver, divorce, abuse, bereavement), then the secure attachment and its quality may change also.

Questions for further consideration:
- What happens when attachment fails?
- What are the effects of long-term deprivation and can they be reversed?
- What can the effects of bereavement be on a child's attachments?
- What are the implications for care outside the home?

Activity

Critically reflect on some of the children you have cared for. Attempt to identify those who appear to have maintained the quality of their attachments and those who have not. What were the reasons?

Horizontal relationships

Peer relationships are vitally important in the development of social behaviour, values and personality. In fact much of what a child learns about social behaviour comes from their association with peer groups. The peer group enables a child to learn things that cannot be learned in the same way from parents by sharing problems and feelings. It is usually within this level of relationship that friendships occur. Table 4.3 gives an overview of the development of friendships throughout childhood.

Activity

Take opportunities to observe children in their relationships with their friends. Compare and contrast what you see with Table 4.3

Table 4.3

Age changes in the development of friendships

Age range	Friendship behaviour	References
< 2 years	Clearly interested in other infants of same age. Looks at them, smiles, makes noises, shows toys. Many short overtures to different children. Low level of peer interaction. Playing together is usually around common toys	Brownnell and Brown (1992); Howes (1987)
3–4 years	Prefers to play with peers rather than alone, play is more cooperative. Friendships become clearer and more stable *but* based on proximity and shared interests	Hartup (1992); Hinde *et al.* (1985)
School age	Peers even more important and more perferable than being with older people. Sex segregation appears as a clear pattern in many cultures. Boys play with boys and girls with girls, each sex with own games. Friendships also sex segregated. Boys' relationship tend to be extensive; girls more intensive	Harkness and Super (1985); Gottman (1986)
Adolescence	Mixed-sex friendships appear, more sharing of feelings. Peer group becomes the vehicle for the transition to adulthood. Conformity to group is essential *but* some research suggests that, in reality, peers have much less influence than we believe them to have	Bernt (1992)

The development of moral reasoning and social cognition

Learning the difference between what is right and what is wrong, the rules of good and bad, are an important part of becoming a social being. According to Berryman *et al.* (1991) moral awareness consists of at least four interrelated facets:

- *Resistance to temptation.* This enables an individual to resist bad behaviour even when not being watched.
- *Guilt.* This refers to the emotional discomfort which is felt following wrongdoing.
- *Altruism.* Prosocial acts, such as kindness, helpfulness, service to others.
- *Moral belief and insight.* Covers all aspects of what people say and do with relation to morality.

Several psychologists have investigated this area of development. Kohlberg built on Piaget's ideas, agreeing with him that moral development is one aspect of general cognitive development and as such occurs in stages. Kohlberg's work (1964–1981) concentrates on justice and fairness. He pioneered the practice of assessing moral development by giving children a series of hypothetical dilemmas in story form, each one with a specific moral theme. One of the most famous of these is the story of Heinz.

From his work he identified three levels of moral reasoning:

- *Preconventional morality.* Children are at this level until about 9–10 years of age. The child is concerned with the consequences of an act and judges what is wrong on the basis of what is punished. Reasoning is in relation to himself and not based on societal rules.
- *Conventional morality.* This is the level of moral reasoning which most adults reach. It is concerned with upholding rules, expectations and conventions. Being good is seen as important for its own sake. Judgements about moral issues are based on what most people would think.
- *Postconventional morality.* According to Kohlberg this level is reached by a minority of adults who are able to judge issues by an individual set of beliefs based on principles rather than rules. It is concerned with achieving the greatest good for the greatest number.

Critics of Kohlberg's work say that he looks at how children make moral decisions and justify them, but that he does not look at how they behave in the real world when faced with their own dilemmas. They argue that behaviour may vary depending on the circumstances. Other criticisms are based on the fact that he used only males in his study and that the clinical method of interviewing that he used was very subjective. Others would argue that he underestimated the ways in which young children see moral issues, owing to methods which relied on understanding of

The story of Heinz

A woman was near to death from a special kind of cancer. There was one drug that the doctors thought might save her. It was a form of radium that a chemist in the same town had recently discovered. The drug was expensive to make but the chemist was charging ten times what the drug cost him to make. The sick woman's husband, Heinz, went to everybody he knew to borrow the money but he could only get together about £1000, which was half of what it cost. He told the chemist that his wife was dying and asked him to sell it cheaper or let him pay later. But the chemist said 'No; I discovered the drug and I'm going to make money from it'. So Heinz became desperate and considered breaking in to steal it. Should Heinz steal the drug? What are the reasons for your answer?

Cultural perspective

Snarey (1985) reviewed a number of studies related to those of Kohlberg. The studies had been carried out in a variety of different countries including Canada, Turkey, India, Israel, Indonesia and New Guinea. The results all broadly confirmed that the stages of moral development described by Kohlberg occur in other societies language and the ability to communicate. Lastly, social learning theorists would ague that the development of moral reasoning in a stage-like way is impossible, because children learn from other people and thus could vary in their reasoning depending on the circumstances.

Eisenberg (1986) tried to ascertain the type of reasoning used by children in making decisions about right or wrong. The dilemmas she presented to children included the difficult decision of choosing between self-interest and helping others. For example, would a child choose to stop and help someone who had fallen over if it meant missing ice-cream and jelly at a birthday party. She identified two types of reasoning:

- *Hedonistic reasoning (preschool)*. At this stage the child is more concerned with the self-oriented consequences of actions.

- *Needs-oriented reasoning*. Children at this stage express concern for other people's needs. They do not use principles to make decisions but respond to needs. This develops further during adolescence into doing things because it is expected, and then on to internalising the values that guide them.

The work of Eisenberg bears a similarity to that of Selman (1980) who investigated children's ability to adopt a social perspective or viewpoint, that is, their development of social cognition. Social cognition is an area related closely to moral reasoning and is concerned with the child's ability to understand social relationships, i.e. empathy, self-control and social problem solving. Selman proposed five levels of social understanding:

- *3–6 years*. Children take an egocentric view. They cannot understand that people think or feel differently from themselves.

- *5–9 years*. Capable of appreciating other people's perspectives but do not appreciate that others also perceive the same things about them.

- *7–12 years*. Capable of taking self-reflective and reciprocal perspective.

- *10–15 years*. Capable of adopting a third-person perspective. Able to stand back and view a relationship as if they are outsiders.

- *12–adult*. Capable of adopting an in-depth perspective, understanding that other people's actions are influenced by a variety of factors (e.g. social forces, personality) and are able to take these into account.

Activity

Try Selman's dilemma out on children of various age groups.

It would appear from these last two studies that there is a change in children's social awareness at round about 5–6 years of age when they begin to entertain ideas about the well-being of others. Work by Piaget

A moral dilemma – Selman's story

Holly is 8 and likes to climb trees. She is the best tree climber in the neighbourhood. One day while climbing down from a tall tree she fell off the bottom branch but did not hurt herself. Her father saw her fall. He was upset and asked her to promise not to climb trees anymore. Holly promises. Later that day holly meets her friend Shawn. Shawn's kitten is caught up a tree and can't get down. Something has to be done or the kitten will fall. Holly is the only one who climbs well enough to reach the kitten but she remembers her promise to her father.

- Does Holly know how Shawn feels about the kitten? Why?
- How will Holly's father feel if he finds out she climbed the tree?
- What do you think Holly should do?

also found that pre-operational children could not take account of someone's intentions because they were egocentric. They were more likely to make judgements based on appearances, e.g. how big a lie has been told or how many things have been broken.

Activity

Here are two stories that Piaget used to test children's moral development. Try them out on pre-operational and post-operational children, recording the children's responses if you can. Analyse the results in light of the theories discussed above.

Story 1: John is in his bedroom when called for dinner. He enters the dining room, but does not know that there is a tray with 15 cups on it just behind the door. The door knocks the tray over and all the cups are broken.

Story 2: Henry decides to have some jam one day when his mother is out. He climbs onto a chair to try to reach the jam jar that is in a high cupboard. While stretching up he knocks over a cup which falls to the floor and breaks.

Questions:
1. Which would you say was the naughtier child?
2. Why?

Both Piaget and Kohlberg agree that there is an association between moral reasoning and moral action and that, as children's moral awareness grows, they are able to make judgements about right and wrong and to behave accordingly. However, Kohlberg (1978) makes the point that 'one can reason in terms of one's principles and not live up to them'. In reality, moral behaviour is probably the result of many interacting influences and is, therefore, dependent on the circumstances in which people find themselves (Figure 4.3).

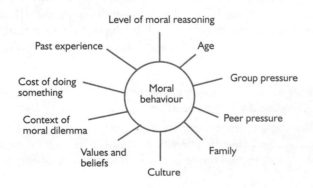

Figure 4.3

Interacting influences on moral behaviour.

Stage and approximate age (year)	Type of empathy	Characteristics
Stage 1 (0–1)	Global	Infant may match the emotions of others, e.g. when another baby cries
Stage 2 (1–2)	Egocentric	Child reponds to other's distress with some distress of own. May try to help by offering what they know works for self
Stage 3 (2–13)	Empathy for another's feelings	Child notes other's feelings and responds in non-egocentric ways. Over the years, child displays wider and wider range of emotions
Stage 4 (adolescence)	Empathy for another's life conditions	Responds not only to other's feelings, but also to their general situation or plight

Activity

Reflect on your own childhood; can you recall any times when your moral behaviour was influenced by any of the discussions above?

Factors which can facilitate the development of moral and social awareness

- Strong ties of affection between parents and children
- Firm moral demands made by parents on their children
- The consistent use of sanctions
- Psychological techniques of punishment
- The use of reasoning and explanations
- Giving responsibilities to young children
- Encouraging the child to see other people's points of view
- Increasing child's level of moral reasoning by discussion

(Berryman et al., 1991)

SUMMARY

This part of the module has tried to give an insight into a child's social development. Children need to know the expectations of the society into which they were born, if they are going to function to their full potential. It is possible that they are born with some inherited, inborn ability to be social. However, it is clear that so much of social behaviour will depend on the child's environment and cultural background. Every child is unique and develops their own self-concept and personality. As parents we all hope that they will develop an acceptable moral code of conduct based on the rules and expectations of society. For some children, fitting into society can be difficult, perhaps because they are influenced by adverse circumstances. What happens in the lives of children who lie, cheat, bully and murder? Is this behaviour inborn or is it a result of social forces and influences on young lives? What we do know is that a child's relationships, especially in the early years, are an important basis on which all future relationships and social behaviour are built. However, it is important to acknowledge that other areas of development will influence social development, that is, cognition and language development. It is important to look at the whole child and not just the social being.

Key points ➤

1. Evidence suggests that the quality of a child's early relationships will affect the development of social competence.
2. Initially self-concept is very concrete and linked to visible characteristics – this gradually changes as children become more abstract in their thinking and more focused on internal qualities.

3. Although the basis for the development of personality may be the inborn temperament, a variety of factors interact thereafter in a complex way to influence it.

4. The formation of both vertical and horizontal attachments is important for a child's social development.

5. As children's moral awareness grows, they can make judgements about what is right and wrong, and are able to behave accordingly.

5 PLAY AND EDUCATION

PLAY

The extent to which play influences development continues to be debated. It is clear that children seem to spend a great deal of time 'playing' but the purpose and nature of this activity is unclear. Views on play have changed during the last century. In the early 1900s play was seen as dangerous in that it presented sensual impulses which ought to be guarded against. Although in the 1930s play became less taboo it was suggested that it be confined to certain times of the day. Now play is part of all the activities of life and, having ceased to be wicked, has become harmless and good and almost a requirement (Wolfenstein, 1955). In order to explore the role of play in a child's development we should try to explore the nature of play.

Activity

What do you understand by the term 'play'? List as many characteristics of play as you can and then try to write your own definition.

As children play outside, they ride their bikes, talk together, run and jump. Sometimes they do not have any specific toys with them but clearly have a good time and do not appear to be trying to achieve anything in particular. How much of what they do is play is the vital question. Most theorists do not attempt to define play using one sentence. Instead they look at the characteristics of play and try to distinguish between what is play and what is not. Garvey (1977) suggests that the characteristics of play are that it:

- is pleasurable and enjoyable and valued positively by the child;
- has no extrinsic value. It is motivated intrinsically and is not directed at achieving any particular end;
- is spontaneous and voluntary, freely chosen by the child;
- involves action;
- has systematic relations to what is non-play. Garvey sees play as a 'non-literal' activity and one which can be contrasted with the 'real' thing. Children recognise when something is the non-real situation but this can often be misinterpreted by adults. For example, they often tease each other and then one begins to 'cry'. The crying appears real and, if an adult intervenes, is told 'We're only playing!'.

Tamburrini (1981) agrees that three of these appear to be generally accepted as being characteristic of play, i.e. it is a spontaneous, voluntary and pleasurable activity. However, she goes on to suggest that this can be true of other activities, e.g. work. Dearden (1968) claims that play is different from other activities in that it is 'non-serious'. By this he means that play is an activity carried out for its own sake and, as Garvey suggests, has no extrinsic goals. A child does not set out in play to find out the answer to a problem or to learn about anything in particular. Piaget (1951) agrees with this characteristic of play in that he sees it as mainly an assimilatory activity. A child's purpose in play is to gain pleasure from mastery of a skill (in sensory play) or to make aspects of the real world subserve his purposes. Hutt (1971) distinguished play from exploration. She suggested that, although play could lead on from exploration, the two were distinctly different in that exploration was serious and focused on 'What can this object do?' whilst play was relaxed and diverse and essentially asked 'What can I do with this object?'.

Although the nature of play is complex and difficult to define, it is clear from observations that children use different types of play at different ages:

- *0–2 years.* Play is mainly used to explore the environment and to master skills. Actions are repetitive and are usually those which give the infant pleasure: shaking, rattling, building and knocking down, filling and emptying containers. As language develops play with sounds becomes evident. Motor development results in the practice of motor skills: running and jumping. Piaget suggests that play during this time enables the child to achieve a sense of mastery and coincides with his sensory motor stage of cognitive development.

- *1–6/7 years.* Towards the end of the first year the development of pretend play begins to emerge. To engage in pretend play children need to be able to distinguish play from reality. Fenson and Schnell

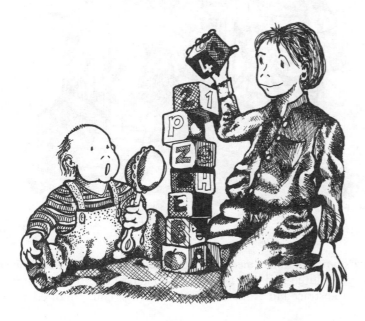

Children playing aged 0–2 years

(1986) identified three parallel aspects of this development The first is *decentration*. Initially, the child's actions are directed towards the self – pretend drinking from an empty cup. Then the same actions begin to be directed towards others – perhaps giving a doll a pretend drink. Finally by about the age of 2 the child is able to get the doll to pretend to drink from the cup. The second aspect is *decontextuali-sation*. To begin with the child relies on real objects – the cup. He then moves on to be able to represent the cup with something else – perhaps an empty yoghurt pot or a shell. Finally by about the age of 3 he is able to use imaginary objects. It is around this time that imaginary friends appear on the scene. Imaginary play is a means of subjecting things to the child's activities without roles or limitations. Vygotsky (1976) terms this as 'an emancipation from situational constraints'. The third aspect in the development of pretend play is *integration*. Initially the child uses one action – feeding the doll. By the age of 2 the child is able to use multischeme combinations and become engrossed in mini-stories. This enables him to progress to more complex sociodramatic play, such as mummies and daddies, cowboys and Indians.

Children playing aged 2–7 years

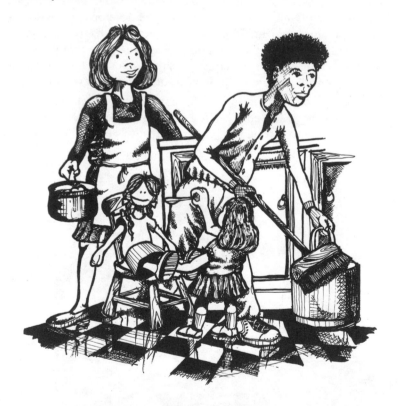

- *7 years onwards.* The emergence of games with formal rules. Prior to this age children find it difficult to understand the properties of rules or their abstract and artificial nature. Although children often have rules in their games, the boundaries frequently change according to the moment, and the rules are particular to that game. Now they are able to take part in games with more formal, public rules with little scope for change, e.g. football and boardgames.

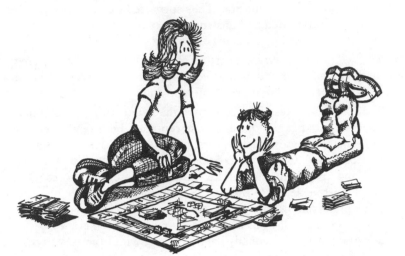

Children playing aged 7 years onwards

Although these distinct periods of development exist, the change is gradual and some forms of play will persist into adulthood. There is a degree of overlap between the stages and some play activities can be seen to fit into each of the stages, e.g. physical play. Pretend play does not necessarily stop at 7 years of age, rather it becomes more complex.

Play with others – stages

Solitary play → Parallel play → Collaborative play

Activity

Carry out an observational exercise – this could be with a group of children whom you know or in a structured setting such as a playgroup. There needs to be a range of age groups. Observe the children's play activities for a designated period of time. Make notes as to the activities of each child. Analyse your findings with reference to the suggested stages in the development of play.

The way a child plays will be influenced by a number of factors:

- *The role of adults*. It is often suggested that adult intervention in a child's play will inhibit it (Tamburrini, 1981). This is based on an assumption that play is universal and spontaneous. Feitelson (1977) claims that pretend play does not develop spontaneously, as it does not exist in some communities where it is actively discouraged. She therefore suggests that it arises as a result of interaction with adults who suggest it. Research into the effect of adult tutoring in play has been carried out and seems to indicate that adult participation in play can facilitate and enhance play (Christie, 1986). Tizard (1977) found

Alternative views on play

- *Froebel (1906)* – 'Play, truly recognised and rightly fostered, unites the germinating life of the child attentively with the ripe life of experiences of the adult and thus fosters the one through the other'.
- *Karl Groos (1900)* – Practice theory of play: 'Play provides exercise and elaboration of the skills needed for survival'.
- *Maria Montessori (1920s and 30s)* – She did not value pretend or sociodramatic play, and thought that this was escape from reality. More emphasis was put on real-life play and the use of constructive play materials
- *Susan Isaacs (1929)* – She saw play as essential for emotional and cognitive growth of young children

Further reading

CHAMBERS, M. (1993) Play as therapy for the hospitalised child. *Journal of Clinical Nursing*, **2**, 349–354.

McMAHON, L. (1992) *Handbook of Play Therapy*. London: Routledge.

VESSEY, J. A. and MAHON, M. M. (1990) Therapeutic play and the hospitalised child. *Journal of Paediatric Nursing*, **5**, 228–333.

Cross reference

Use of play in hospital – page 268

that, in nurseries where adults adopted a passive role, play was frequently of short duration with limited use of available materials. Sylva *et al.* (1980), in a study conducted in Oxfordshire playgroups, made suggestions as to how playgroup leaders could enhance the meaning of play for children. They suggested that there should be a balance of structured and unstructured play, with adults being actively engrossed in some play activities.

- *The child's personality.* Singer (1973) identified children as being of 'high fantasy' and 'low fantasy' dispositions. He suggested that those with the former were more creative in some respects than the latter.
- *The child's sex.* Research has shown that even quite young children select toys and games that fit sex stereotypes. Boys tend to choose more masculine toys such as cars, guns, 'Action Man', building blocks, 'Lego'. Girls tend to engage in more feminine play such as dressing up, soft toys and dolls, imitating household chores (O'Brien and Houston, 1985; O'Brien, 1992). Rough and tumble play seems to be preferred by boys (Smith and Cowie, 1991). Experience suggests that, whilst this is the case, young children are less constrained and are equally happy playing with other-sex toys.
- *The environment.* The degree to which a child plays will depend on numerous environmental factors including cultural contexts. Cross-cultural studies show that children in some cultures may be required to take care of younger siblings, tend crops or help with household chores (Hobsbaum, 1995).

THE PURPOSE OF PLAY

Sylva and Lunt (1982) suggest that play is 'one of the activities most significant' in the overall development of the preschool child. Many different views on the purpose of play have been suggested by various theorists.

Freud believed that play compensated for the frustrations and anxieties encountered in everyday life. Within play, the child's desire for mastery could be acted out in a safe, secure environment. This idea is the basis of play therapy in which children use play for the release of tension. Piaget believed that play was important in, and linked to, the development of cognitive and intellectual skills. In play, reality is moulded to fit in with the child's own experiences and understanding. Social learning theorists see play as important for learning those social skills needed as adults.

Sylva *et al.* (1980) identified two types of play – ordinary, which merely helps to keep children occupied and expend surplus energy, and challenging, which contributes to development (Table 5.1).

Some researchers have attempted to find out what children learn through play by comparing the performances of children who have been given play experiences and those who have not. Dansky and Silverman

Challenging play	Ordinary play
A child playing with 'Lego' spreads the bricks out onto the floor. He carefully chooses the bricks he wants and proceeds to build a model. The child is playing in a systematic and purposeful way.	A child playing 'Lego' builds a tower of bricks – he does not choose any specific bricks but just uses bricks as they come to hand. He takes the bricks apart and then builds another tower in the same way. Routine, repetitive play with no new elements or ideas.
A child sets up an obstacle course around which he rides his bike. This behaviour is challenging as the child is required to use his skills to steer the bike and not bump into the obstacles.	A child rides his bike up and down the track. He does not try to steer the bike round obstacles but looks as if he is letting off steam.

Table 5.1

Challenging versus ordinary play. (Adapted from Sylva et al., 1980)

(1973) showed that free play promotes creative thinking, whilst Sylva *et al.* (1976) found that it improved the problem-solving skills of 3–5 year olds. They and others have concluded that children learn through play. Simon and Smith (1985) urge caution when interpreting the results of research in this field. They concluded that, whilst certain play activities undoubtedly result in certain types of learning, play is only one way in which children learn and it is important not to overgeneralise.

'Play is indeed the child's work and the means whereby he grows and develops'.
(Issacs, 1929)

Activity

Consider ways in which you could research the role of play in development. Analyse the problems inherent in this type of research.

EDUCATION

For most children, school is an important part of the socialisation process providing social contacts outside the home. At the same time as 'teaching' children different subjects, the school acts as a form of social control, transmitting values through formal and informal (hidden curriculum) control (Moore, 1996) (Figure 5.1).

The history of education

Prior to 1870 there was no organised education system. The rich employed private tutors or sent their children to private schools. Most children had no formal education. The Elementary Education Acts of 1870 and 1880 saw the development of a basic network of state-supported elementary schools with compulsory attendance up to the age of 10 years. Following this the school leaving age rose to 14 and then to 15 years in 1944. Prior to 1944 attendance at school was based on ability to pay. The 1944 Butler Act attempted to ensure equality of opportunity and introduced grammar schools and secondary modern schools. Children were sent to one or other of these depending on their academic ability judged by the 11+ exam. The option of staying on until

Figure 5.1

How school teaches social control. (Adapted from Moore, 1996)

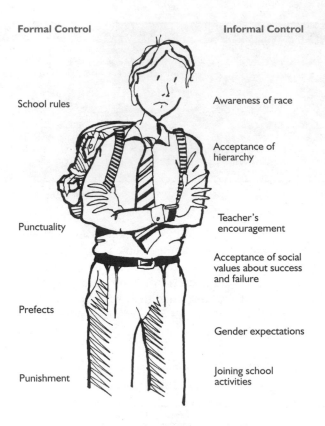

Formal Control

School rules

Punctuality

Prefects

Punishment

Informal Control

Awareness of race

Acceptance of hierarchy

Teacher's encouragement

Acceptance of social values about success and failure

Gender expectations

Joining school activities

the age of 17 was offered. A change of government in 1964 brought about the shift towards comprehensive education which was intended to remove the division between grammar and secondary modern, thus enabling all children to have access to equal opportunities. Whilst this principle still exists, many areas have retained grammar schools and some have developed their own approaches. The 1988 Education Act introduced some significant reforms including the establishment of a National Curriculum, and the opportunity for schools to opt out from the control of local education authorities to become 'independent state schools'. Schools now:

- are run by the governing body, head teacher and staff working as a team;
- are responsible for managing their own budgets;
- must follow the National Curriculum, including new rules on sex education;
- can be compared with other schools by means of national assessments;
- must publish a school prospectus and annual report;
- are subject to inspections.

Public schools (private fee paying institutions) were left untouched by the 1944 Act. They are exempt from the National Curriculum and are only nominally subject to state supervision.

Activity

At the time of writing this text, a new Labour government had been voted into power. What changes, if any, have been made to the education system since then? Analyse the results of any changes.

Compulsory education in Britain begins the year in which a child is aged 5. Some children start school the term in which they are 5, others start at the beginning of the school year. This means that some children, whose birthdays fall in the summer months, will only just have turned 4 when they begin school, quite a young age to start school. Starting school brings a dramatic change in certain aspects of a child's life. Resocialisation to a new culture is one of the most vital aspects of this transition. Children have to learn new rules and routines; they meet many new people, adults and children, and have to find their way round a new environment. Even negotiating the toilets and the dining room can cause alarm and fear in the young child.

Activity

Reflect, if you can, on your own first day at school. If this proves too distant a memory, reflect on your own children or those of family and friends. What was it like for them, how did they cope?

The transition to school will be affected by various factors:
- age of the child;
- siblings already at school;
- the child's personality;
- preparation for school, including attendance at nursery or playgroup, parental views on school;
- the philosophy of the school;
- expectations of the child, teachers and parents.

Once a child has made the transition to school life, many factors will impact upon his education including (Figure 5.2):
- *Parental attitudes*. The degree to which parents show parental attitudes. The degree of encouragement and interest in their children's schooling plays an important part in academic success. It may even help to overcome deprivation and poverty (Moore, 1996). Douglas (1969) found that educational success was closely related to

The National Curriculum

This is a framework that states legally what subjects should be taught in schools and to what standards. Pupils' education is arranged in four phases – the Key Stages:
- *Key Stage 1 (ages 5–7) and Key Stage 2 (ages 7–11)* – consist of three core subjects (English, Maths and Science) and seven foundation subjects (History, Geography, Design and Technology, Information Technology, Art, Music, and Physical Education)
- *Key Stage 3 (ages 11–14) and Key Stage 4 (ages 14–16)* – the same subjects with the addition of languages

Figure 5.2

Factors impacting upon a child's education.

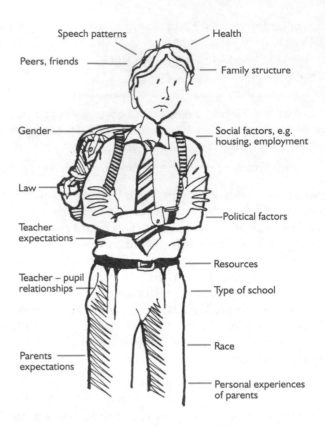

parental encouragement in all classes. He also found that middle class parents were more likely to give encouragement and help.

- *Culture, race, ethnicity.* Black pupils on average tend to do less well in the British educational system than White children. The Swann Report of 1985 (cited by Giddens, 1993) indicated that whilst 13% of the White population obtained one or more passes at A level in 1981/2, only 5% of West Indian school-leavers achieved similar results.

- *Gender.* Many studies have been conducted which indicate gender differences in educational attainment. Girls tend to do better than boys during primary school years and in the early secondary years. However, after this the girls tend to fall behind. A suggestion for this is that the majority of primary school teachers are women whereas women are heavily under-represented in secondary schools, colleges and universities (Giddens, 1993). They are also disproportionally represented in some subject areas such as science, engineering and medicine.

- *Speech patterns.* Bernstein (1975) argues that children from varying backgrounds develop different speech codes. He identifies two – the restricted code of the working class and the elaborated code of the middle class. He suggests that children with the latter are more able to deal with the demands of formal academic education than the former. Tough (1976) and Tizard and Hughes (1984) back up this idea that lower class children tend to have less experience of having their questions answered or being given reasons.

- *Relationships between teachers and pupils.* Rutter (cited by Giddens, 1993) studied the educational achievement of a group of boys over several years. He concluded that schools have a direct influence on the academic achievement of children. Among the factors which impact upon children are the quality of teacher–pupil interaction, an atmosphere of cooperation and caring between teachers and children, and well organised preparation. Lacey (1970) found that the attitudes of teachers affected a child's level of achievement. Most of the teachers in his study disliked teaching the lower streams and this showed in their attitudes towards the children.

Activity

Critically reflect on how a knowledge of the education system in Britain could contribute towards care of the sick child.

Educational provision for children with special needs

The 1981 Education Act states that local education authorities have a duty to:

- ensure that special education provision is made for children who have special educational needs;
- identify and assess children in order to determine their needs;
- respond to reasonable parental requests for assessment;
- involve parents in the assessment process.

The act also emphasises the need for early education for those children with special needs (as early as 2 years). As a result of the 1993 Education Act, a *Code of Practice on the Identification and Assessment of Special Educational Needs* was approved by Parliament in 1994. The purpose of the Code is to give 'practical guidance to Local Education Authorities, and the governing bodies of all maintained schools … on the discharge of their functions under Part III of the Education Act 1993' (DfEE, 1994). The principles of the code are:

- The needs of all children who have special educational needs must be addressed: the Code recognises a continuum of needs and provision.
- Children with special educational needs require access to a broad and balanced education (including the National Curriculum).
- The needs of most children (with or without statements of special need) will be met alongside their peers in mainstream schools.

Cross reference

Educational needs and disability – page 235

Cross reference

Living with a disability – page 232–238

- A child may have special educational needs which require the intervention of the LEA before he reaches compulsory school age.
- A partnership between the parents, their children and schools, LEAs and other agencies is vital to ensure effective assessment and provision.

The provision of education for children with special needs will depend upon the degree to which they are able to be integrated into mainstream schools. For some children the advantage of a specialist school may be the provision of specialised equipment, professional support and peer support from others who share similar difficulties. Whatever the outcome, the Code of Practice ensures that the child and carers will be fully involved in all decisions affecting the child's future.

SUMMARY

Play and education are a major part of a child's life. They both impact upon a child's development and serve to enable a child to grow up to reach his full potential. There are many aspects of play which are still puzzling to many theorists. However, it would appear that most reach a consensus that play is important in a child's development and in his learning of life and the world around him. An understanding of how children play can serve a useful basis for playing with sick or chronically ill children, or with children who have special needs. As a children's nurse you should be able to appreciate the many facets of play so that you can enhance play for children in hospital, and also use play as therapy to help overcome some of the psychological trauma associated with hospitalisation. Each child's education will be unique to him, as the impact of education on him will be influenced by many factors. The education of our children provides them with a basis for ongoing education in adulthood and helps to prepare them for a future role in society. The importance of education is recognised in the provision of schooling for sick children.

Cross reference

Play in hospital – pages 259 and 268

Activity

Contact your hospital school teacher and discuss hospital in school. Find out about legislation and the organisation of schooling for children who are in hospital. Analyse some of the issues related to school in hospital.

Key points ➤

1. The extent to which play influences development continues to be debated, especially as the nature of play is so complex and unclear.
2. Different types of play are evident at different ages.

3. The way a child plays will be influenced by the role of adults, the child's personality, age and gender, and the environment.

4. The purpose of play has been suggested by various theorists as being important in all aspects of development. However, it is important to note that it is only one way in which children learn.

5. For most children, education is an important part of the socialisation process and is influenced by a variety of factors that are unique to each child.

6. Education for children with special needs is based on assessment of need in partnership with parents and is provided where possible alongside peers in mainstream schools.

References

AINSWORTH, M. D. S., BLEHAR, M. C., WATERS, E. and WALL, S. (1978) *Patterns of Attachment: A Psychological Study of the Strange Situation.* Englewood Cliffs, NJ: Erlbaum.

ARIES, P. (1962) *Centuries of Childhood.* London: Penguin.

BALL, W. and TRONICK, E. (1971) Infant responses to impending collision: optical and real. *Science*, **171**, 818–820.

BANDURA, A. (1973) *Aggression: A Social Learning Theory.* Englewood Cliffs, NJ: Prentice-Hall.

BARKER, D. J. P., BULL, A. R., OSMOND, C. and SIMMONDS, S. J. (1990) Foetal and placenta size and risk of hypertension in adult life. *British Medical Journal*, **301**, 259–262.

BATES, J. E. (1989) Concepts and measures of temperament. In KOHNSTAMM, G. A., BATES, J. E. and ROTHBART, M. K. (eds), *Temperament in Childhood.* Chichester: Wiley.

BEE, H. (1995) *The Developing Child*, 7th edn. New York: Harper Collins.

BERNSTEIN, B. (1975) *Class and Pedigree: Visible and Invisible.* London: QECD.

BERNT, T. J. (1982) The features and effects of friendship in adolescence. *Child Development*, **53**, 1447–1460.

BERRYMAN, J. C., HARGREAVES, D., HERBERT, M. and TAYLOR, A. (1991) *Developmental Psychology and You.* London: British Psychological Society.

BOWER, T. G. R. (1965) Stimulus variables determining space perception in infants. *Science*, **149**, 88–89.

BOWER, T. G. R. (1981) Cognitive development. In ROBERTS, M. and TAMBURRINI, J. (eds), *Child Development 0–5.* Edinburgh: Holmes McDougall.

BOWER, T. G. R., BROUGHTON, J. M. and MOORE, M. K. (1970) Infant responses to moving objects: an indicator of response to distal variables. *Perception and Psychophysics*, **8**, 51–53.

BOWLBY, J. (1969) *Attachment and Loss,* vol. 1. London: Hogarth Press.

BROWNELL, C. A. and BROWN, E. (1992) Peers and play in infants and toddlers. In HASSELT, V. and HERSEN, M. (eds), *Handbook of Social Development: A Lifespan Perspective.* New York: Plenum Press.

BRUNER, J. (1966) On cognitive growth. In BRUNER, J. S., OLIVER, R. R. and GREENFIELD, P. M. (eds), *Studies in Cognitive Growth.* New York: Wiley.

CAMPBELL, R. and OLSEN, D. (1990) Children's thinking. In GRIEVE, R. and HUGHES, M. (eds), *Understanding Children*. Oxford: Blackwell.

CAMPBELL, S. and GLASPER, A. (1995) *Whaley and Wong's Children's Nursing*. St Louis: Mosby.

CHOMSKY, N. (1986) *Knowledge of Language: Its Nature, Origin and Use*. New York: Praeger.

CHRISTIE, J. F. (1986) Training of symbolic play. In SMITH, P. K. (ed.), *Children's Play: Research Development and Practical Applications*. London: Gordon & Breach.

DANSKY, J. L. and SILVERMAN, I. W. (1973) Effects of play on associative fluency in pre-school children. *Developmental Psychology*, 9, 38–43.

DEARDEN, R. (1968) *The Philosophy of Education*. London: Routledge & Kegan Paul.

DfEE (1994) *Code of Practice on the Identification and Assessment of Special Educational Needs*. London: Central Office of Information.

DOBBING, J. and SANDS, J. (1973) Quantitative growth and development of human brain. *Archive of Diseases in Childhood*, 48, 757.

DoH (1991) *Dietary Reference Values for Food Energy and Nutrients for the United Kingdom. Reports on Health and Social Subjects 41*. London: HMSO.

DoH (1994) *Weaning and the Weaning Diet*. London: HMSO.

DONALDSON, M. (1978) *Children's Minds*. London: Fontana.

DOUGLAS, J. W. (1969) *The Home and the School*. London: Panther.

EISENBERG, N. (1986) *Altruism Emotion, Cognition and Behaviour*. Englewood Cliffs, NJ: Erlbaum.

EUROPEAN COLLABORATIVE STUDY (1991) Children born to women with HIV-1 infection: natural history and risk of transmission. *Lancet*, 337, 253–260.

FALL, C. H. D., BARKER, D. J. P., OSMOND, C., WINTER, P. D., CLARKE, P. M. S. and HALES, C. N. (1992) Relation of infant feeding to adult serum cholesterol concentration and death from ischemic heart disease. *British Medical Journal*, 304, 801–805.

FEITELSON, D. (1977) Cross cultural studies of representational play. In TIZZARD, B. and HARVEY, D. (eds), *The Biology of Play*. London: Heinemann.

FISHBEIN, H. (1987) Socialisation and television. In BOYD-BARRETT, O. and BRAHAM, P. (eds), *Media, Knowledge and Power*. London: Croom Helm.

GARVEY, C. (1977) *Play*. London: Fontana/Open Books.

GIBSON, E. J. and SPELKE, E. (1983) The development of perception. In MUSSEN, P. (ed.), *Handbook of Child Psychology, III*. New York: Wiley.

GIDDENS, A. (1993) *Sociology*, 2nd edn. Oxford: Blackwell.

GOTTMAN, J. M. (1986) The world of co-ordinated play: same and cross-sex friendship in young children. In GOTTMAN, J. M. and PARKER, J. G. (eds), *Conversations of Friends: Speculations On Affective Development*. Cambridge: Cambridge University Press.

GUNTER, B. (1986) *Television and Sex-Role Stereotyping*. London: John Libbey.

HALES, C. N., BARKER, D. J. P., CLARK, P. M. S., COX, L. J., FALL, C. and OSMOND, C. (1991) Fetal and infant growth and impaired glucose tolerance at age 64. *British Medical Journal*, 303, 1019–1022.

HARKNESS, S. and SUPER, C. M. (1985) The cultural context of gender segregation in children's peer groups. *Child Development*, 56, 219–224.

HARTER, S. (1987) The determinations and mediational role of global self-worth in children. In EISENBERG, N. (ed.), *Contemporary Topics in Developmental Psychology*. New York: Wiley-Interscience.

HARTUP, W. W. (1989) Social relationships and their developmental significance. *American Psychologist*, **44**, 120–126.

HARTUP, W. W. (1992) Peer relations in early and middle childhood. In HASSELT, V. and HERSEN, M. (eds), *Handbook of Social Development: A Lifespan Perspective*. New York: Plenum Press.

HEWARD, C. (1993) Reconstructing popular childhoods. *Children and Society*, **7**, 237–254.

HINDE, R. A., TITMUS, G., EASTON, D. and TAMPLIN, A. (1985) Incidence of friendship and behaviour toward strong associates versus nonassociates in preschoolers. *Child Development*, **56**, 234–245.

HOBSBAUM, A. (1995) Children's development. In CARTER, B. and DEARMAN, A. K. (eds), *Child Health Care Nursing*. Oxford: Blackwell Scientific Publications.

HOFFMAN, M. L. (1988) Moral development. In BORNSTEIN, M. H. and LAMB, M. E. (eds), *Developmental Psychology: An Advanced Textbook*, 2nd edn. Englewood Cliffs, NJ: Erlbaum.

HOWE, D. (1995) *Attachment Theory for Social Work Practice*. Basingstoke: Macmillan.

HOWES, C. (1987) Social competence with peers in young children: developmental sequences. *Developmental Review*, **7**, 252–272.

HULSE, T. (1995) Growth monitoring and the new growth charts. *Health Visitor*, **68**, 424.

HUTT, C. (1971) Exploration and play in children. In HERRON, R. E. and SUTTON-SMITH, B. (eds), *Child's Play*. London: Wiley.

ISSACS, S. (1929) *The Nursery Years*. London: Routledge & Kegan Paul.

KAGAN, J. (1988) Temperamental contributions to social behaviour. *American Psychologist*, **44**, 668–674.

KOHLBERG, L. (1978) Revisions in the theory and practice of moral development. *New Directions for Child Development*, **2**, 83–88.

KOSKY, J. and LUNNON, R. J. (1991) *Great Ormond Street and the Story of Medicine*. London: The Hospitals for Sick Children.

LACEY, C. (1970) *Hightown Grammar*. Manchester: Manchester University Press.

LAMPL, M. (1992) Saltation and stasis: a model of human growth. *Science*, **258**, 801.

LESTER, J. (1993) Changing attitudes to children. *Health Visitor*, **66**, 162–163.

LEWIS, M. (1991) Ways of knowing: objective self awareness of consciousness. *Developmental Review*, **11**, 231–243.

LINDSAY, B. (1994) Influencing development: the media. In LINDSAY, B. (ed.), *The Child and Family: Contemporary Nursing Issues in Child Health and Care*. London: Bailliere Tindall.

MITCHELL, P. (1992) *The Psychology of Childhood*. London: Falmer Press.

MOORE, K. L. (1988) *Essentials of Human Embryology*. Ontario: Decker.

MOORE, S. (1996) *Sociology Alive!*, 2nd edn. Cheltenham: Stanley Thornes.

MULLER, N. I. and BRYAN, A. C. (1979) Chest wall mechanics and respiratory muscles. *Pediatric Clinic of North America*, **26**, 503.

NARDINELLI, C. (1990) *Child Labor and the Industrial Revolution*. Bloomington: Indiana University Press.

NATHANIELS, Z. P. (1996) *Life Before Birth: The Challenges of Fetal Development*. New York: Freeman.

NOWAKOWSKI, R. S. (1987) Basic concepts of CNS development. *Child Development*, **58**, 568–595.

NUTBEAM, D. (1989) *Health for All Young People in Wales*. Health Promotion Authority for Wales: Cardiff.

O'BRIEN, M. (1992) Gender identity and sex roles. In HASSELT, V. B. V. and HERSEN, M. (eds), *Handbook of Social Development: A Lifespan Perspective*. New York: Plenum Press.

O'BRIEN, M. and HOUSTON, A. C. (1985) Development of sex-typed play behaviour in toddlers. *Developmental Psychology*, **21**, 866–871

OATES, J. (ed.) (1994) *The Foundations of Child Development*. Milton Keynes: Open University Press.

PIAGET, J. (1951) *Play, Dreams and Imitation in Childhood*. London: Routledge & Kegan Paul.

SELMAN, R. L. (1980) *The Growth of Interpersonal Understanding*. New York: Academic Press.

SIMON, T. and SMITH, P. K. (1985) Play and problem solving: a paradigm questioned. *Merrill-Palmer Quarterly*, **31**, 265–277.

SINGER, J. L. (1973) *The Child's World of Make-Believe*. New York: Academic Press.

SKINNER, B. F. (1957) *Verbal Behaviour*. New York: Appleton Century Crofts.

SLATER, A., MATTOCK, A. and BROWN, E. (1990) Size constancy at birth: newborn infants' responses to retinal and real size. *Journal of Experimental Child Psychology*, **51**, 395–406.

SLOBIN, D. (1973) Cognitive prerequisites for the development of grammar. In FERGUSON, C. A. and SLOBIN, D. (eds), *Studies in Child Development*. New York: Holt Reinhart and Winston.

SMITH, P. K. and COWIE, H. (1991) *Understanding Children's Development*, 2nd edn. Oxford: Blackwell.

SNAREY, J. R. (1985) Cross-cultural universality of social-moral development: a critical review of Kholbergian research. *Psychological Bulletin*, **97**, 202–232.

SYLVA, K. and LUNT, I. (1982) *Child Development: A First Course*. London: Grant McIntyre.

SYLVA, K., BRUNER, J. S. and GENOVA, P. (1976) The role of play in the problem-solving of children 3–5 years old. In BRUNER, J. S., JOLLY, A. and SYLVA, K. (eds), *Play: Its Role in Development and Evolution*. Harmondsworth: Penguin.

SYLVA, K., ROY, C. and PAINTER, M. (1980) *Childwatching at Playgroup and Nursery Schools*. London: Grant McIntyre.

TAMBURRINI, J. (1981) What is play? In ROBERTS, M. and TAMBURRINI, J. (eds), *Child development 0–5*. Edinburgh: Holmes McDougall.

TAMIR, L. (1984) Language development: new directions. In LOCK, A. and FISHER, E. (eds), *Language Development*. London: Routledge.

TIZARD, B. (1977) Play – the child's way of learning. In TIZARD, B. and HARVEY, D. (eds), *The Biology of Play*. London: Heinemann.

TIZARD, B. and HUGHES, M. (1984) *Young Children Learning, Talking and Thinking at Home and at School*. London: Fontana.

TOUGH, J. (1976) *Listening to Children Talking*. London: Ward Lock Educational.

VYGOTSKY, I. S. (1976) Play and its role in the mental development of the child. In BRUNER, J. S., JOLLY, A. and SYLVA, K. (eds), *Play: Its Role in Development and Evolution*. Harmondsworth: Penguin.

WALTON, G. E., BOWER, N. J. A. and BOWER, T. G. R. (1992) Recognition of familiar faces by newborns. *Infant Behaviour and Development*, **15**, 265–269.

WATSON, J. (1979) *Medical, Surgical Nursing and Related Physiology*. Eastbourne: Saunders.

WATT, S. and MITCHELL, R. (1995) Historical perspectives. In CARTER, B. and DEARMUN, A. K. (eds), *Child Health Care Nursing*. Oxford: Blackwell Scientific Publications.

WOLFENSTEIN, M. (1955) Fun morality: analysis of recent American child-training literature. In MEAD, M. and WOLFENSTEIN, M. (eds), *Childhood in Contemporary Cultures*. Chicago: University of Chicago Press.

ZESKIND, P. S. and RAMEY, C. T. (1981) Preventing intellectual and interactional sequelae of fetal malnutrition: a longitudinal, transactional, and synergistic approach to development. *Child Development*, **52**, 213–218.

Growth and maturation

Further reading

BEAVER, M., BREWSTER, J., JONES, P., KEENE, A., NEAUM, S. and TALLACK, J. (1994) *Babies and Young Children. Book 1. Development 0–7*. Cheltenham: Stanley Thornes. Contains some good line drawings of motor development.

GODFREY, S. and BAUM, J. (1979) *Clinical Paediatric Physiology*. Oxford: Blackwell Science.

HAZINSKI, M. F. (1992) *Nursing Care of the Critically Ill Child*, 2nd edn. St Louis: Mosby. Especially Chapter 1: Children are different. The beginning of other chapters contains sections on essential anatomy and physiology.

SHERIDAN, M. (1975) *From Birth to Five Years: Children's Developmental Progress*. Oxford: NFER-Nelson

WATSON, J. E. (1979) *Medical–Surgical Nursing and Related Physiology*. Philadelphia: Saunders. Chapter 11: Age implications for nursing.

Thinking development

MITCHELL, P. (1992) *The Psychology of Childhood*. London: Falmer Press. Chapter 2: An assessment of Piaget's Theory – this gives an interesting and research-based assessment of the work of Piaget.

Language development

GRIEVE, R. and HUGHES, M. (1990) *Understanding Children*. Oxford: Blackwell. Chapter 2: Children's Language – takes a different approach and considers more theoretical aspects of development taking a deeper look at how children learn language.

LOCK, A. and FISHER, E. (1984) *Language Development*. London: Routledge. This book contains papers by various authors and covers many interesting aspects of research into language development.

Temperament

DAVENPORT, G. C. (1994) *An Introduction to Child Development*, 2nd edn. London: Collins Educational.

Attachment

HOWE, D. (1995) *Attachment Theory for Social Work Practice*. Basingstoke: Macmillan. Many of the chapters in this book are relevant to the theory of attachment. It is interesting to read and opens up new perspectives for us to think about.

MITCHELL, P. (1992) *The Psychology of Childhood*. London: Falmer Press. Chapter 9.

SMITH, P. K. and COWIE, H. (1991) *Understanding Children's Development*. Oxford: Blackwell. Chapters 3 and 4 give a good overall view of the development of relationships inside and outside the family.

Play therapy

CHAMBERS, M. (1993) Play as therapy for the hospitalised child. *Journal of Clinical Nursing*, **2**, 349–354.

McMAHON, L. (1992) *Handbook of Play Therapy*. London: Routledge.

VESSEY, J. A. and MAHON, M. M. (1990) Therapeutic play and the hospitalised child. *Journal of Paediatric Nursing*, **5**, 228–333.

PROMOTING CHILD HEALTH

Tina Moules

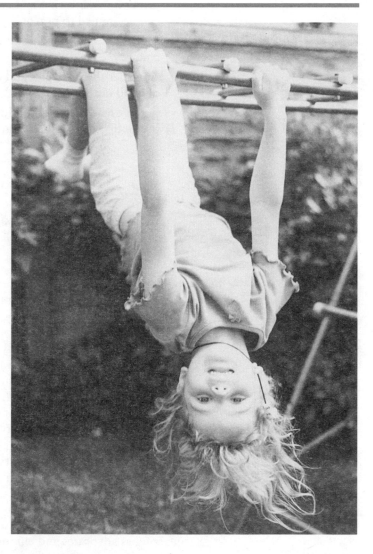

Active and healthy

OBJECTIVES

The material contained within this module and the further reading/references should enable you to:

- Explore the state of health of children in the UK today and investigate changing patterns of illness and disease.

- Examine the factors and trends which impact upon children's health.

- Explore children's beliefs about and concepts of health.

- Analyse and critically review various models of health promotion/education and consider how theoretical underpinnings can be applied to practice.

- Investigate the changing role of the nurse in promoting health in children.

- Consider the strategies and interventions implemented for a range of child health issues.

- Act as an advocate for children's health and contribute to promoting healthy behaviours among children.

INTRODUCTION

> *The health of children is of major importance not only in its own right but also as a determinant of adult health and of the health of the next generation*
>
> (DoH, 1990)

There has been an upsurge in interest regarding the health of our children in Britain today. It is now well recognised that children's health is important because they are tomorrow's adults. What they take with them from childhood in the way of health or ill health may influence their health for the rest of their lives. Children are the future and as such need to be able to reach their full potential to meet the demands that adulthood brings with it. In 1991 the Government made a major step in recognising the importance of child health when it ratified the UN Convention on the Rights of the Child (1989). Article 24 states that each child has the 'right to the highest level of health possible and to access to health and medical services, with special emphasis on primary and preventive health care, public health education and the diminution of infant mortality'. However, action is more important than words and children need advocates to ensure that their rights are upheld. Children's nurses, in whatever setting they work, can play a major role in acting as advocates and empowering children and their carers.

The emerging health demands on the health service in the 1990s are dominated by the demand for care rather than cure. One of the most

Cross reference

Nurse's role as an advocate – page 590

influential developments in the past two decades has been the World Health Organisation's *Health for All* by the year 2000 resolution. The central theme in this is that people must be enabled to be in control of the factors which influence their life. The role of the nurse is therefore changing to incorporate an increased concern with health promotion. In order to fulfil this role, nurses must have an understanding of theories and models of health promotion so that they can become effective health educators. This change in role is clearly defined in Rule 18 of the *Nurses, Midwives and Health Visitors Rules* (Statutory Instrument No. 1456, 1989, p. 5) which states that the Registered Nurse must be competent to 'advise on the promotion of health and the prevention of illness and to recognise situations that may be detrimental to the health and well-being of the individual'. Amendment rules to the above allow for the implementation of Diploma programmes (Project 2000) and give a more specific outcome for the student nurse to achieve. They state that the nurse should be able to identify the health-related learning needs of patients, clients, families and friends, and to participate in health promotion.

This module concentrates on issues related to health and its promotion. It begins by examining the health of children in the UK and discussing the changing patterns of childhood illness. Some of the factors which impact upon child health are reviewed with special reference to poverty and its effects on health. Children's beliefs about health and its meaning are explored, encouraging you to ascertain their views regarding their own health behaviours. Different age groups have different views of health and this needs to be recognised when health is promoted. An outline of some of the views regarding health promotion and education are given. Several models are put forward for you to consider, helping you to analyse critically health promotion in practice. Several issues of child health which were particularly relevant at the time of writing are explored and will give you an insight into how health promotion is put into practice. The role of the nurse in health promotion is discussed, the roles of children's nurses examined and also of other nurses who have contact with children. Finally several aspects of health are considered with the purpose of enabling you to contribute effectively to encouraging children (and carers) to make healthy choices.

1 TRENDS IN CHILD HEALTH

INTRODUCTION

- *Mortality rate* – the number of deaths as a proportion of the population of a given age
- *Morbidity* – all forms of ill health including acute and chronic conditions

Over the last four decades the health of children in the UK has improved markedly. In the middle of the last century many children suffered severe ill health and lived in appalling conditions. One-third of children died before the end of childhood. Childhood was a fragile time and engendered a kind of indifference.

Now childhood death and serious infections are increasingly rare and living conditions have improved in general. Advances in medical technology have improved the life chances of premature infants and children with serious illness. However, detailed analysis of data reveals that, whilst infant mortality rates have decreased, morbidity has increased. Child poverty continues to affect health. In 1987, over 3 million children (26% of all children in the UK) were living in poverty. This was an increase from 12% in 1979 (Woodroffe *et al.*, 1993). Wilkinson (1994) suggests that widening income differentials, which lead to differences in relative poverty, are the single most important determinant of health. Numerous studies continue to reveal social class differences in mortality and morbidity (Whitehead, 1988; Wilkinson, 1989; Power *et al.*, 1991). Reading (1997) ascertains that virtually all aspects of health are worse 'among children living in poverty than among children from affluent families'.

This section looks critically at the trends in child health and considers the epidemiology of childhood illness and disease in the 1990s.

MORTALITY RATES

Trends in mortality rates (particularly infant mortality rates) have long been considered one of the best indicators of children's health. It is suggested that mortality reflects the cumulative interaction of biological and social factors over time. As mortality data have been well documented for many years, trends can be traced and analysed. However, one must recognise that these data are only the tip of the iceberg and other factors contribute to the judgements made about child health, including data on morbidity.

Infant mortality rates (deaths under 1 year per 1000 live births)

In England and Wales there has been a steady decline in infant mortality rate (IMR) since the 1940s. In the period 1941–1945, the rate was 50 per 1000 live births. Between 1971 and 1991 the rate fell by 52% to 7.9 but, as shown in Figure 1.1, the rate was higher for males (8.8) than females (6.8).

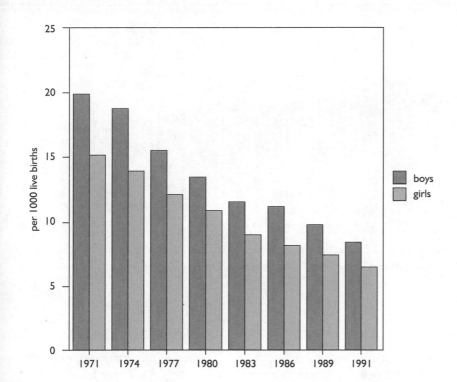

Figure 1.1

Decline in infant mortality rates, 1971–1991. (Adapted from OPCS DH 1/19, 1971–1991, Birth Statistics, Mortality Rates.)

Between 1991 and 1992 the IMR for both sexes fell by 11%. The mortality rate in boys fell from 8.3 per 1000 live births to 7.4, and in girls from 6.4 to 5.8. By 1994 the IMR had fallen to 6.2 (ONS, 1996). Although a general decline in the IMR is evident there are still variations among social groups and regions of the country. Regional variations reflect partly the ethnic and social class make-up of populations. Health districts with higher than average IMRs tend to have above average proportions of mothers born in Pakistan and the New Commonwealth and an above average population of fathers in social classes IV and V (Britton, 1989). The IMR is lowest (6.8) in the South West and highest (9.9) in the West Midlands (Figure 1.2). Social class variations in the IMR have existed for many years and data show that inequalities persist.

Activity

Take some time to look critically at the possible factors which lead to regional differences in the infant mortality rate. Try to trace back the data to see how the differences compare with previous years.

A baby born to a father in social class V is twice as likely to die than a baby born to a father in class I (Whitehead, 1992). It is likely that the social class differential is significantly greater than that revealed by

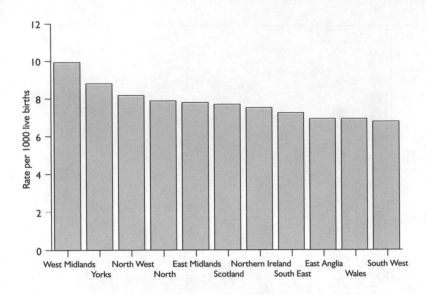

Figure 1.2

Infant mortality rate per region, 1990. (Adapted from OPCS Monitor DH3 91/2, 1992, Regional Trends.)

'The other group'

This group contains several disparate groups such as 'inadequately described' and others who are unoccupied

Stillbirths

Fetal deaths after 24 weeks' gestation

official statistics because only infants registered within marriage, or by both parents living together, are included in the data. Those born outside marriage, whose birth is registered by the mother alone, and those in the 'other' group are not included. This constitutes about 8% of babies.

Infant mortality is subdivided into:

- *perinatal deaths*: still births and deaths in the first week of life;
- *neonatal deaths*: deaths within the first 27 days of life;
- *postneonatal deaths*: deaths at 28 days and over (but under 1 year).

Activity

Before reading on, take a few minutes to consider what might be the major causes of death in the neonatal period and why there has been a large decline in mortality rate.

Infancy remains the most vulnerable period of a child's life. Of all deaths under the age of 20, half occur under 1 year. Of these deaths a third occur during the neonatal period. It is encouraging to see that it is in this group that the largest decline in mortality rate is evident. Between 1971 and 1989 the neonatal death rate fell by 60% (OPCS DH6/3, 1989). By 1994 the neonatal death rate was 4.1 per 1000 live births (ONS, 1996). The major causes of neonatal death are prematurity, congenital abnormalities and respiratory conditions (Figure 1.3).

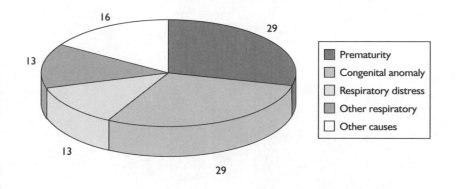

16

29

13

13

29

Prematurity
Congenital anomaly
Respiratory distress
Other respiratory
Other causes

Figure 1.3

Causes of neonatal death (%), 1990. (Adapted from OPCS DH 6/3, 1989, RG Scotland, 1990; RG N. Ireland, 1991.)

Several factors have contributed to the fall in neonatal deaths. Recent advances in the care and management of low birth weight babies has led to an increased survival rate. The numbers of babies born with a congenital defect has fallen and can be attributed in part to antenatal screening and the provision of terminations. An example of this is a reduction in the number of babies born with spina bifida. In 1979 the number of births registered as having spina bifida was 13 per 1000. This rate had fallen to 7 per 1000 by 1990 (OPCS MB3/5, 1990).

The trend in postneonatal mortality rate has shown a much flatter rate of decline. Between 1971 and 1990 the rate fell by 37% (OPCS DH6/3, 1989). One reason suggested for the slow improvement in this death rate is that mortality after birth is perhaps much more influenced by social and environmental factors and therefore much more reliant on social policy. The main underlying cause of death in this period is sudden infant death syndrome (SIDS). In 1989 46% of deaths in this age group were classified as SIDS (OPCS DH6/3, 1989). A higher incidence is reported among boys in many studies in various regions and countries. Once again considerable social class differences are evident. Although SIDS affects all social classes, infants in families in social class V are three times more likely to succumb to SIDS than those in social class I families. A considerable decrease in the number of deaths from SIDS has been evident since a peak in 1988 when the rate was 2.3 per 1000 live births. By 1991 the rate had fallen to 1.3 per 1000 (Figure 1.4), and by 1994 the rate had fallen to under 1.0 per 1000 (OPCS, 1995). The decline has been rapid and has been attributed in part to campaigns to make parents aware of the dangers of the prone position for sleeping babies.

The remaining causes of death in the postneonatal period are congenital anomalies (16%), respiratory disease (10%), diseases of the nervous system and sense organs (5%), infectious diseases (4%), and neoplasms (1%) (Figure 1.5).

Both the neonatal and postneonatal mortality rates are higher in social class V than in I (Figure 1.6).

Factors contributing to the decline of spina bifida

- Reduction in the natural incidence for reasons which are so far unexplained
- Administration of folic acid supplements prior to conception and in the first 12 weeks of pregnancy – based on studies by the Medical Research Council
- Advent of techniques for detecting neural tube defects during pregnancy (screening) and the option of termination

Cross reference

SIDS – page 43

Figure 1.4

Decline in sudden infant death syndrome, 1987–1992. (Adapted from Gilbert, 1994.)

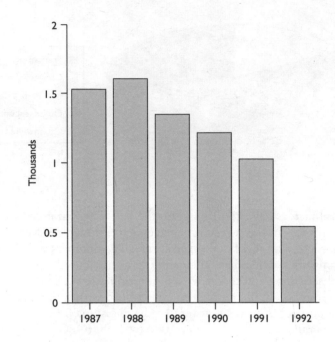

Figure 1.5

Causes of post-natal death (%, UK), 1990.

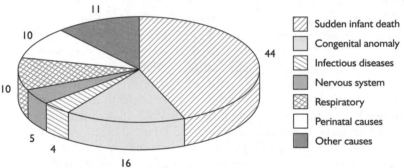

Childhood mortality (based on the estimated population in the relevant age group)

Childhood mortality figures are generally given within the following age ranges:

* 1–4 years
* 5–9 years
* 10–14 years
* 15–19 years.

The death rates for children aged 1–14 are based on small numbers so should be examined with care

The risk of death in childhood is significantly less than the risk in infancy. In general, the rate of decline in childhood mortality has been slow particularly since the early 1980s. Figure 1.7 shows the deaths for each age range in 1990.

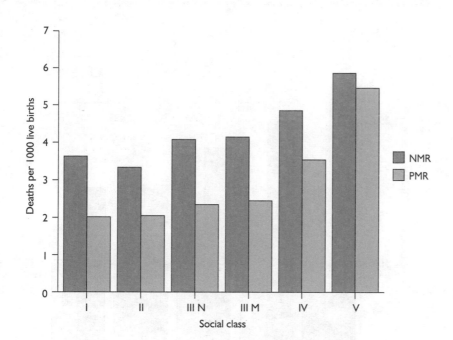

Figure 1.6

Social class variations in neonatal (NMR) and post neonatal (PMR) mortality rates, 1990. (Adapted from Kumar, 1993.)

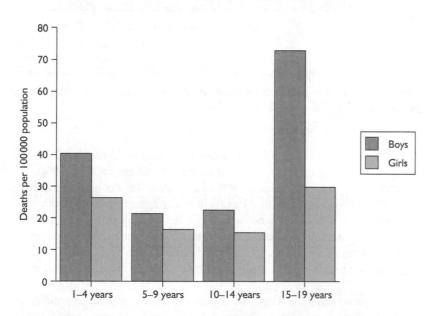

Figure 1.7

Deaths in childhood per age group, 1991. (Adapted from Botting, 1995.)

The trend in mortality by age group from 1963 to 1991 is shown in Figure 1.7. It can be seen that the steepest decline has been in the 1–4 age group, which at the beginning of the period exceeded that of the 15–19 age group. The graph also shows that mortality is twice as high among preschool children and teenagers than school-age children. Among older children a gender differential is seen, with the death rate in boys (2:10 000) being double that in girls (1:10 000) (Platt and Pharoah, 1996).

Figure 1.8

Trends in mortality in the 1–19 age group, 1971–1991. (Adapted from Botting, 1995.)

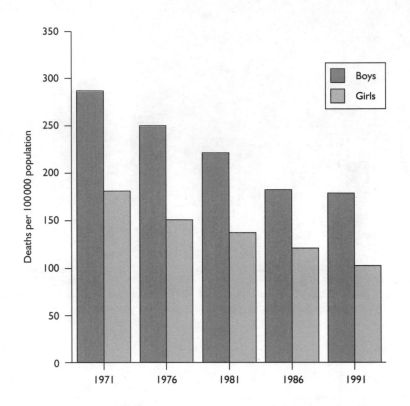

Activity

Take some time to consider the factors which may have contributed to changes in childhood mortality since 1963.

Cross reference

Factors influencing accidents in childhood – page 152

Accidents are the major cause of death in childhood causing 24% of deaths in the age group 1–4; 37% of deaths in age group 5–9; 39% of deaths in age group 10–14 and 60% of deaths in age group 15–19 in the UK in 1990 (Woodroffe *et al.*, 1993). In every age group, the death rate from accidents is higher for boys than it is for girls. Although there has been a steady decline in the number of deaths, the rate of decline has slowed considerably since 1980. Many accidents are preventable meaning that much work is still to be done to make childhood a safer time.

Other main causes of death in childhood are congenital anomalies (over two-thirds of which are heart and circulatory system malformations) and neoplasms which accounted for 16% of all childhood deaths in 1989.

Social class differences are evident in child mortality but are not quite so marked. Recent data are as yet unavailable but data from 1982 to 1983 show an advantage for children in the higher social groups especially in the 1–4 age group (Figure 1.9).

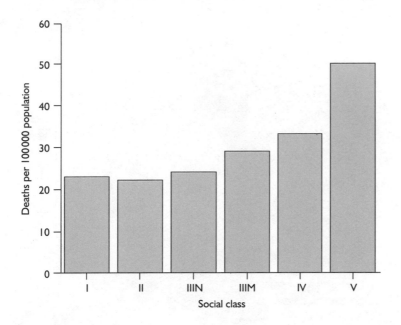

Figure 1.9

Social class differences in child mortality.

Class differences are particularly evident in relation to accidents. According to Jarvis *et al.* (1995), accidental injury is the cause of death with the steepest social gradient. Reasons for this are multifactorial but are likely to include lack of safe areas to play and lack of resources to make homes safe. In 1892–1893 children in social class V were six times more likely to die in fires than those in social class I. A study by Constantinides (1987) found that children in the most deprived ward of one area were four times more likely to be involved in accidents than those in the most affluent ward. Data from 1982–1983 show that children aged 1–14 in social class V were four times more likely to die from injuries than those in class I (Figure 1.10).

MORBIDITY

Morbidity is the second major indicator used for measuring health. It looks at the prevalence or incidence of disease. Information regarding child morbidity is gained from population surveys [particularly the General Household Survey (GHS)], notifications of infectious diseases, registers of children with specific conditions (e.g. cancer) and hospital admission data.

Morbidity

The relative incidence of disease and illness

Activity

Each of the methods of gaining data on morbidity has strengths and weaknesses. Critically review each of the methods and analyse the role of each in its contribution to knowledge regarding the incidence and prevalence of disease in childhood.

Figure 1.10

Social class variations in deaths from injury (%) in the 1–14 age group, 1978–1980 and 1982–1985.

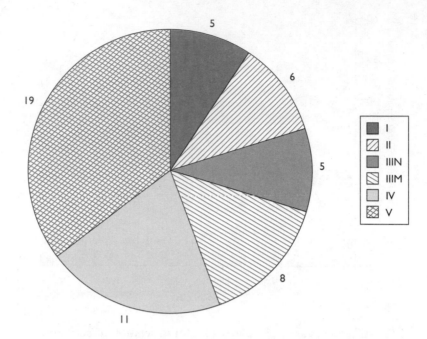

Many of the data presented here are from the GHS conducted by OPCS. This survey was introduced in the 1970s. It surveys 10 000 private households sampled from the electoral register. Participants in the survey are asked to report any long-standing illness, disability and visits to the GP.

According to the GHS (OPCS, 1991), there was a two-fold increase in chronic illness in children between 1972 and 1991. Alongside this there has been a rising trend in disability reported in all age groups.

Factors which have influenced childhood morbidity include:

- *Improved management and treatment of children with childhood cancers.* The survival rates for lymphoblastic leukaemia have improved dramatically since the 1970s. However, at the same time concerns have been raised about possible long-term side effects of treatment.

- *Improved management and treatment of low birth weight infants.* Unfortunately this improvement has brought with it increased risks of blindness, deafness and cerebral palsy. For children born in 1984–1988, the rate of deafness in survivors to 28 days was 15 times higher in babies who weighed less than 1500 g at birth than it was for all babies (Oxford Register, 1991, cited by Woodroffe *et al.*, 1993). The incidence of cerebral palsy in very low birth weight babies (under 1500 g) has increased markedly (Woodroffe *et al.*, 1993).

- *Improved survival rates for children with cystic fibrosis.* This has contributed to an increase in chronic illness. The median life

Cross references

Treatment of leukaemias – page 556

Cerebral palsy – page 500

Cystic fibrosis – page 515

expectancy for a child born with cystic fibrosis in 1990 is estimated at 40 years (Elborn *et al.*, 1992, cited by Woodroffe *et al.*, 1993).

- *Possible increased incidence of respiratory diseases.* Respiratory diseases are a major cause of long-term illness and disability in childhood. Chest infections and asthma predominate. Asthma is the most common chronic disease of childhood affecting about 10% of schoolchildren (Valman, 1993). In 1991 there were an estimated 2 million asthma sufferers of whom more than 700 000 were children under 16 (HMSO, 1991). It has been suggested that deaths from asthma are on the increase. However, data do not support this except in the 15–19 year age group. Hospital admissions on the other hand have doubled since the mid-1970s (Strachan and Anderson, 1992). This may reflect an increased prevalence of the disease perhaps related to environmental pollution or parental smoking. Alternatively, it could be due to changes in the use of diagnostic labelling or to changes in care. It may be that an increased awareness of the disease prompts more cases to be diagnosed. Burney *et al.* (1990) studied a representative sample of primary schoolchildren. The results showed a definite increase in the prevalence of diagnosed asthma and of 'wheeze on most days and nights' from 1973 to 1986.

Cross reference

Respiratory problems – page 513

As with mortality, social class differences still exist although they are not as significant (OPCS, 1989). One of the difficulties in interpreting the data is that parental self-reporting (the major method of data collection in the GHS) can lead to under-reporting of children's illness by mothers in the lower social classes (Blaxter, 1990). A study by Butler and Golding (1986) found that more than twice as many children in social class V had suffered pneumonia by the age of 5 than those in classes I, II and IIIN.

OTHER INDICATORS OF CHILD HEALTH

Dental health

There has been considerable improvement in the dental health of children during the last 20 years largely due to the fluoridation of toothpaste and drinking water. However, dental caries remains a major health problem. It is preventable and there is no reason why it should not be eradicated in childhood. In the 10 years from 1973 to 1983 improvements were seen in all ages from 5 to 15 and in all regions of England and Wales. The proportion of 5 year olds with dental caries fell from 73 to 48%. The most recent survey published by OPCS (Todd and Dodd, 1994) shows a continued improvement with dramatic falls in the prevalence of dental caries. The survey was carried out in 1993 and shows that by the age of 15 years, 40% of children were free from tooth decay compared with only 8% in 1983. Just 16% of children aged 10 years had one or more permanent teeth filled compared with 45% in

Cross reference

Dental hygiene – page 184

1983. However, the survey showed that half of the children in England still experienced some dental decay in their teeth by the time they were 15. Hinds and Gregory (1995) investigated the dental health of children aged 1.5–4.5. They found that 16% had active decay on examination and a further 2% had teeth filled; 2% had teeth missing from decay. Social class variations are again evident in that the percentage of children with caries is greater in classes IV and V than it is in classes I and II. Silver (1987) found a higher rate of tooth decay in 3 year olds in classes IV and V than in class I. Regional variations in dental health also exist throughout the country. Hinds and Gregory (1995) and Pitts and Evans (1996) found that children in Scotland and the north of England experienced almost double the decay seen in children living in central and southern England.

Growth

Height is taken as a sign of the state of health of a population. Over recent centuries the average height of people in the UK has increased and the trend continues. In general children's heights are increasing but a class differential has been identified. A study in Newcastle in 1974 found that 15 year olds in classes I and II were on average 4.5 cm taller than their counterparts in classes IV and V. Reading *et al.* (1993) surveyed the heights of 5–8 year old schoolchildren in Northumberland and found a significant difference between those in the most affluent ward and those in the most deprived area. The mean height differential varied between +0.1 SD in the former and –0.2 SD in the latter.

Nutrition and diet

The nutritional status of children is a key indicator of health status. Whilst the nutritional intake of children has improved there is mounting evidence to justify a growing concern about children's diets in the 1990s.

Breastfeeding gives an infant a healthy start in life protecting against infection and allergy. It also provides the correct amount and balance of nutrients for healthy growth and development. In the early 1970s the incidence of breastfeeding was at its lowest level but this had increased by 1980 when the proportion of mothers breastfeeding was 67%. However, since then the rise has not continued and in fact a decline in numbers is noted. In 1995 only 39% of babies were wholly or partly breastfed at birth. Social class differences are evident in that four times as many infants are breastfed at 6 weeks in class I than in class V.

Cross reference

Weighing children and babies – page 282

Standard deviation

A measure of the extent to which values of a variable are scattered about a mean value in a frequency distribution

Breastfeeding and cognitive development

Studies have investigated the role of breast milk in neurological development and suggest that there may be a small advantageous effect of breastfeeding (see Further Reading at the end of this module)

Further reading

LANTING, C. I., *et al.* (1994) Neurological differences between 9-year-old children fed breastmilk and formula as babies. *Lancet*, **344**, 1319–1322.

LUCAS, A., *et al.* (1992) Breastmilk and subsequent intelligence quotient in children born preterm. *Lancet*, **339**, 261–264.

Cross references

Nutrition – pages 177–184
Breastfeeding – page 178

Activity

What factors may contribute to the social class differences with regard to breastfeeding? How might some of these be overcome?

Obesity in childhood is likely to lead to obesity in adulthood. Many diseases are linked to obesity, e.g. heart disease and stroke. Obesity is increasing in adults and there is some evidence to suggest that the trend in the proportion of young people who are too heavy for their height is increasing. In 1986 to 1987, 18% of young men and women were overweight. This is an increase from 1980 (Figure 1.11). The number of obese young men has not changed but the number of obese young women has doubled (Woodroffe *et al.*, 1993).

Definition – Body Mass Index (BMI)

This summarises the relationship between height and weight:

- Obesity = BMI of over 30
- Overweight = BMI of 25–30

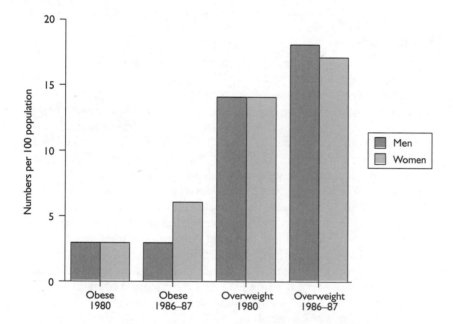

Figure 1.11

Increases in overweight and obese young men and women (16–24 years old in Great Britain, 1980 and 1986–1987).

The first major study to highlight the nature of children's diets was commissioned by the DoH in 1983. Interestingly the full report was not published until 1989. This study found that the main source of dietary energy for British schoolchildren was bread, chips, biscuits, milk, meat, cakes and puddings. Three quarters of the children in the study had fat intakes above the recommended level. However, the Department deduced that the diets of children were satisfactory.

A more recent study by Doyle *et al.* (1994) looked at a group of schoolchildren aged 12–13 living in an inner city socially deprived area of London. They found that there was little variety in the foods children ate. Very few ate fresh fruit and/or vegetables: 40% of girls and 34% of boys ate no fresh fruit during the week of the study. Only a few children (17% of girls, 20% of boys) ate a portion of fresh or frozen vegetables (other than potatoes) on a daily basis. One-third of the children ate no breakfast before going to school. There was a high consumption of crisps, chips, sweetened fizzy drinks and sweets. The study concluded that most of the children were eating unhealthy diets when compared with recent recommendations. The latest study (Hinds and Gregory,

Food Poverty Network
National Food Alliance
5–11 Worship Street
London, EC2A 2BH
Tel: 0171 628 2442
Fax: 0171 628 9329

Cross reference

Immunisation schedule – page 498

Cross reference

Immunisation – page 186

1995) examined the food intake of nearly 2000 children aged 1.5–4.5. The study showed that children are eating too much salt, not enough fruit and vegetables and insufficient iron.

Activity

Arrange to talk to a group of children about their eating habits. Compare different age groups. What are your findings and how do they compare with the above research?

Immunisations

Immunisation is one of the best documented ways of protecting children's health. Deaths from infectious diseases have reduced markedly since the early part of the century due in part to public health reforms in the 19th and early 20th centuries. However, the role of immunisations in the eradication of many diseases and the reduction in incidence of others must not be negated. Measles notifications reached an all time low of less than 10 000 in 1991 in England and Wales, and in 1990, for the first time, there were no deaths from the disease. Deaths from pertussis (whooping cough) were seven in 1990 with none in 1991, 1992 and 1993. Mumps is now considered a rare disease in this country and there has been an overall reduction in the number of cases of rubella both in children and pregnant women. The number of tuberculosis (TB) cases notified in 1990 showed little decline in comparison with earlier years and the number of deaths was 390. Fears that the incidence of TB is rising led to an examination of the data in 1992–1993. This showed a slight increase in the numbers of TB cases (up from 6000 in 1987 to 6500 in 1993 (OPCS, 1994). By 1994, however, this had fallen back down to just over 6000.

Target 5 of the WHO European Region's *Health for All 2000* strategy states that 'by the year 2000 there should be no indigenous polio, neonatal tetanus, diphtheria, measles and congenital rubella syndrome'. The Government set its own targets in 1985 to achieve the 90% WHO coverage target. This target was revised in 1991 to achieve 95% immunisation coverage nationally by the year 1995. In 1993 the immunisation uptake was at an all time high (Figure 1.12).

The average uptake among 1 year olds of diphtheria, tetanus and polio vaccination was 94% and of pertussis 91%. Among 2 year olds, 93% had received measles, mumps and rubella (MMR) vaccine (Bedford, 1993). A huge campaign in November 1994 was implemented to immunise 7 million children between the ages of 5 and 16 against a threatened epidemic in 1996.

Although national immunisation coverage is high there is evidence to suggest that uptake is not equal across social groups. Reading *et al.* (1994) investigated four birth cohorts of children in Northumberland. Activities for improving the uptake of immunisations were implemented

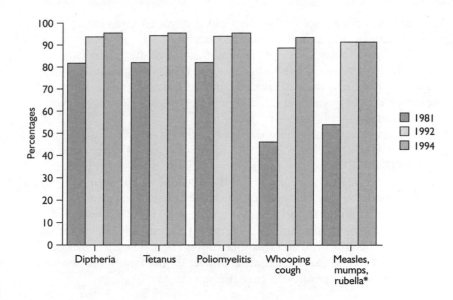

Figure 1.12

Immunisation uptake 1981–1994. *Includes data for both measles-only and combined vaccines. (Source: CSO, 1996.)

and the differences between social classes examined. The activities were successful in raising the uptake levels but there remained differences between the most deprived areas and the most affluent. Uptake was poorest in the former. These lower uptake rates tend to pull down the national average figures.

A high uptake rate is essential for all children if infectious diseases are to remain a thing of the past. However, with the near elimination of these diseases can come complacency. Parents who have never experienced measles, diphtheria and pertussis may question the need for immunisation. There then comes the danger that uptake rates will fall and epidemics will flare up once more. Health professionals may have to work harder to convince some parents that immunisations are necessary. Sustained efforts to achieve the national targets and to reduce inequalities in uptake are required.

Activity

Find out what the uptake figures are for the area in which you work. Compare the figures with the national average. What are your conclusions?

Changing patterns of health and disease

An examination of the data has revealed that the epidemiology of childhood diseases, though changing, remains the same in some respects. The incidence of infectious disease remains fairly low whilst deaths from accidents remain extremely high. Chronic illness has and is increasing as medical advances prolong the life of children with congenital disorders and of low birth weight infants. In 1990, 14% of children under 16 had a long-standing illness and 3% had a disability.

Childhood cancer is one of the major causes of death particularly in the older age group. In 1986, the National Cancer Registration system reported 1482 new cases in children under 19. Leukaemia is the most common cancer in younger children whilst Hodgkin's disease is the most common in adolescence.

The most recent infectious disease requiring sensitive handling is HIV and AIDS. Up to October 1996 there were over 450 reported cases in the UK of HIV infection in children aged 14 and under (PHLS, 1996). Francis (1994) predicts that HIV infection in children will escalate in the future. Contraction of the virus has been through transfusion of blood factors (e.g. for haemophilia) (60%), through mixing of the blood during birth – vertical transmission (33%), through blood transfusions (6%) and by other routes (1%). The diagnosis of HIV infection in a child has a devastating impact on the family and resources will be required to ensure effective management.

Cross reference

Caring for children with HIV disease – page 493

FACTORS AFFECTING CHILD HEALTH

Many factors exist which affect children's health and development today. The purpose of this section is to identify and examine some of these factors and encourage you to explore the issues more fully. Before reading on try the next activity.

Activity

List as many factors as you can which you think have an impact on child health and development. Then try to put them into categories. Compare your thoughts with those in Figure 1.13.

Environmental

Concerns have been raised about the impact of many environmental issues in recent years. The threat to children from leaded paint has been known for many years with cases of lead poisoning reported up until 1982. Various regulations now exist in the UK which limit the lead content of paint applied to surfaces that children might chew or suck. However, the main problem now is from old lead paint which may still exist, e.g. in old buildings. Other sources of lead include motor vehicle exhaust fumes. Whilst the levels of lead in the air are decreasing from the introduction of lead-free petrol, it still remains a major source of lead. High levels of lead are particularly found near motorways and in large urban areas (especially during the rush hour). A growing body of evidence suggests that low levels of lead exposure do have an effect on

'Vastly increasing numbers of people, on a vastly increasing scale, now dig the earth to take and make what they want: they cut down forests, breed animals, grow crops and fish the seas; and from everything that is made or eaten pollution is generated'.

(DoH, 1970)

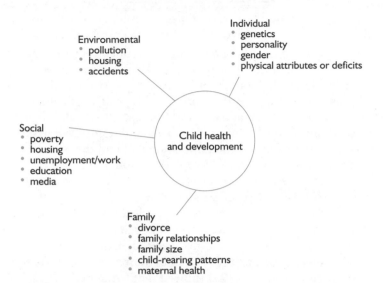

Figure 1.13

Overview of factors affecting health.

children's intelligence with evidence of reduced IQs in children with high levels of lead (Lansdowne and Yule, 1986).

Other sources of air pollution are industry and agriculture. The link between air pollution and lung disease has been acknowledged since the 1930s. This poses a serious health threat. The long-term effects of a high exposure to motor fumes are thought to include asthma, chronic obstructive airways disease, coughing, wheezing and chest pain.

The 1980s saw the emergence of concerns related to excessive exposure to sun in childhood and the links to skin cancer in later life. Children and adolescents who have frequent and long periods of exposure to intense rays causing painful blistering sunburn are at risk from developing malignant melanoma later in life. Malignant melanoma is largely preventable and curable if recognised early. Children and carers should therefore be educated about safety in the sun including the use of hats and sunscreens.

Social issues

- *Poverty*. It is difficult to gauge the extent of the problem in the UK because of the lack of a clear definition of poverty. However, if one uses the measure taken as an unofficial poverty line in national surveys (Oppenheim, 1993) – families with incomes below 50% of the average household income – then the results are very worrying. Figures suggest that in 1979, 1.4 million children (10%) were living in poverty. By 1991 this figure had trebled with some 3.9 million children (31%) growing up in poverty (DSS, 1993). Of these the majority belong to one-parent families and those in which there is unemployment (House of Commons, 1993). The direct effects of poverty on children's health and development have not been studied to any great extent. However, studies have shown that the issues related to poverty can have far-reaching effects on children.

- *Housing deprivation and homelessness.* Families living in poverty are more likely to find themselves in unsuitable accommodation, e.g. high rise flats, with poor amenities (heating, cooking and sleeping facilities), in multiply deprived areas. Such properties are more likely to be cold, damp and mouldy (Kumar, 1993). Although the standard of housing has improved in general terms over recent years, certain sections of the population still find themselves living in poor accommodation. In 1993, 1.3 million homes in England were found to be unfit (i.e. defective in one of nine areas such as drainage, food preparation area, state of repair) (DoE, 1993). Overcrowding and lack of amenities can lead to an increased likelihood of accidents, acute infections such as gastroenteritis and respiratory infections. The link between the latter and poor housing is well known (Graham, 1989, cited by Kumar, 1993). Platt *et al.* (1989, cited by Kumar, 1993) showed that living in damp and mouldy conditions could have severe effects on children's health (independent of the effect of low income and smoking in the house). The effects included symptoms of infection and allergy: fever, sore throat, headaches and respiratory problems. Blackman *et al.* (1989, cited by Kumar, 1993) found that children and adults living in poor housing were likely to experience psychological distress. Martin and Hunt (1989, cited by Kumar, 1993) found a significant relationship between death in 0–4 year olds and low socioeconomic status and poor, high density housing. More recently it has been shown that the average mortality rate is significantly higher in the most deprived 25% of District Health Authorities than it is in the least deprived (Judge and Benzal, 1993, cited by Kumar, 1993). The National Child Development Study (Davie, 1993) demonstrated an association between social disadvantage and poor educational attainment. This in itself can result in a cycle of poverty from generation to generation. Families who live in temporary accommodation (e.g. bed and breakfast) often find if difficult to enrol children in school or register with a GP.

- *Unemployment.* Whether this occurs as a result of poverty or is the cause, unemployment within the family can contribute to physical and psychological problems for children as well as adults. Studies have shown a higher incidence of low birth weight in babies of unemployed fathers (Whitehead, 1987), and children of unemployed fathers to be shorter than those of employed fathers (DoH, 1989, cited by Kumar, 1993). Children may be affected by the stigma of unemployment which in turn can affect their relationships with peers (Madge, 1983, cited by Kumar, 1993). The impact of unemployment can have far-reaching effects on a family and can lead to a greater relative deprivation for the children in such families.

GENETIC FACTORS

Each of us has our own individual genetic make-up, the only exception being identical twins. Recent advances in biochemistry, molecular genetics and cytogenics have raised awareness of the importance of hereditary influences on health. Many disorders and diseases in children have a genetic link. In some there is a definite genetic cause which is known (cystic fibrosis and Down's syndrome are just two examples) and the disorder is apparent at birth. In others the effects of the disorder do not become apparent until some months or even years after birth (e.g. sickle cell anaemia and phenylketonuria).

There are three broad categories of genetic disease:

- *Chromosome abnormalities (cytogenic)*. These disorders occur when there is a deviation in the number or structure of one or more chromosomes.

- *Single-gene (monogenic) disorders*. In these disorders there is a definite single gene mutation. The consequences of such a mutation can be mild with no effect on the child, or can lead to serious disability or be incompatible with life. Genes are classed as either dominant or recessive in their effect. For a dominant gene to be passed on, only one parent need carry the gene. For a recessive gene to be passed on, both parents must carry the gene. This latter scenario is less likely than the first, unless the parents are blood relatives when the likelihood increases.

- *Multifactorial disorders*. These disorders show an increased incidence in some families but do not show a definite inheritance pattern. Individuals appear to have a genetic susceptibility for a certain disorder, e.g. some congenital abnormalities such as spina bifida, diabetes and hypertension.

As research into genetics increases it is becoming more possible to identify those fetuses which have abnormalities. This in turn poses ethical and moral questions, as one has to deal with the consequences of finding out that a child carries a genetic disorder. Some would argue that knowing about problems enables early detection and subsequent treatment (e.g. phenylketonuria) or termination of pregnancies should that be an alternative. Others show concern about genetic screening in that in some instances it is difficult to know the extent to which a child will be disabled and that terminating abnormal fetuses is a contradiction of human rights. Nevertheless, genetic screening is offered to families who have reason to believe that they may be carriers of certain genes. This must only be done against the backdrop of an effective counselling service, the purpose of which must be to help the family of an individual child to:

- understand the facts – the diagnosis, course of the disorder and available management;

Gene

'A large complex molecule of a protein compound (deoxyri-bonucleic acid – DNA) which is capable of self-duplication. Genes contain information necessary for controlling the development and activity of cells'.

(Watson, 1979)

Cross reference

Heredity – page 53

Examples of chromosome disorders

- Down's syndrome (Trisomy 21)
- fragile X syndrome
- Kleinfelter's syndrome
- Turner's syndrome

Examples of single-gene disorders

Autosomal dominant
- Marfan's syndrome
- achondroplasia
- Huntingdon's chorea

Autosomal recessive
- cystic fibrosis
- phenlyketonuria
- galactosaemia

X-linked recessive
- Duchenne muscular dystrophy
- haemophilia

X-linked dominant
- hypophosphataemic vitamin D-resistant rickets

- appreciate how heredity contributes to a disorder and how it may affect specified relatives;
- choose an appropriate course of action in view of the risks and family situation;
- adjust as well as possible to the disorder in an affected family member and/or the risk of recurrence (Fraser, 1974).

Activity

Because the ethical and moral issues related to genetic screening are huge, we suggest that you explore this area more fully. Try discussing issues with your colleagues either in the ward or in college. Remember to make notes of any references. They could be useful to you in the future.

SUMMARY

Whilst the health of the nation's children has improved in many ways, there remain children whose health status is compromised by a poor environment, inadequate diet and inequalities. Health in a child's early years is of paramount importance and these issues must be addressed if all children are to be given the best possible chance of a healthy future. As the pattern of illness and disease changes, so the health needs of children will change. An increasing prevalence of chronic disease will require a reallocation of resources into the community. Debates will continue over the moral and ethical issues related to the treatment of low birth weight infants and of those children requiring multiple organ transplants. Many factors influence the health of our children today both before and after birth. By being aware of these factors it may be possible to address some of them and contribute to the future health of all children.

Key points ➤

1. The infant mortality rate has fallen by 52% since 1971.
2. The number of babies born with congenital defects is decreasing.
3. The survival rates for some cancers are improving.
4. The survival rates for cystic fibrosis are improving.
5. Accidents continue to be the major cause of death in 1 year olds and over.
6. There is a rising trend in the numbers of children with disabilities and long-standing illness.
7. Marked inequalities exist in nearly all areas of child health.
8. A variety of factors influences the health of children today including environmental issues, social issues and individual factors.

HEALTH 2

INTRODUCTION

To consider the theoretical aspects of health promotion and education we should first consider the meaning of health.

Activity

Consider what the term 'being healthy' means to you. List all the factors which contribute to your health.

Many people have attempted to define health over the years and the only concrete notion to emerge is that there is no simple, obvious definition. Health is a complex, multidimensional idea the interpretation of which differs from person to person. The word is derived from the old English term *hoelth* meaning 'a state of soundness' and has been used to refer to soundness of the body. One commonly quoted definition is that from the WHO (1946, p. 2) which states that health is 'characterised not only by the absence of disease but also by a state of complete physical, mental and social well-being'. This definition describes an ideal state.

More recently various definitions have been proposed. A few will be offered here for the reader to consider. The definitions fall into three categories.

- Definitions which emphasise actualisation. These stress the realisation of human potential through purposeful action. Health is seen not merely as a state free from illness but as a much more dynamic, emergent process. Among the nurse theorists who hold this view is Orem (1985). In her self-care theory she describes health as consisting of two characteristics. The first is soundness of human structures and bodily functions. The second is movement towards fulfilment of one's self-ideal and personalisation.

- Definitions which emphasise adaptation. These view health as being concerned with the ability of the individual to adapt to the environment. Neuman (1982) describes health as being a condition in which the physiological, psychological and sociocultural systems are in balance. The central concept of Roy's model of nursing (1984) is one of adaptation and she defines health as a state and process of successful adaptation.

- Definitions which embrace both actualisation and adaptation. The definition which demonstrates this view is that of King (1981, p. 5). King sees health as a dynamic process which involves 'continuous adaptation to the internal and external environment through the optimum use of one's resources to achieve maximum potential'.

Further reading

DINES, A. and CRIBB, A. (1993) *Health Promotion, Concepts and Practice.* Oxford: Blackwell Scientific.

Chapter 1 gives a good analysis and discussion on the meaning of health

One idea that has been proposed by several authors is that health can be viewed in many different ways by the same person. Individuals can change their perception of health depending on the situation in which they find themselves at any given time. Health could therefore be defined as being what the individual says it is. This can present difficulties for health professionals when trying to implement health promotion activities.

Hanna (1989) explored student nurses' views of health. They described health as an awareness of physical abilities, appearance and energy level as well as a mental state of happiness, contentment and clarity of thinking

Activity

Analyse each of the definitions given above. Identify the strengths and weaknesses of each. Talk to friends and patients about what health means to them. Then try to write your own definition of health.

HEALTH PROMOTION AND EDUCATION

Until the 1980s, health education was the main way in which individuals were encouraged to adopt healthy behaviours. Health education arose out of the traditional concern with the treatment of illness rather than with its prevention. Much of the activity in this area took on an individualistic approach. It used as its basis the assumption that individuals have control over their own health. This approach has been criticised for failing to acknowledge the social influences on health and for assuming that individuals have free choice. It has engendered a tendency towards victim blaming. In reality there is much to suggest that there are often factors mitigating against personal change. The health of people in Britain has generally been improving over the last 10–20 years. However, two well publicised reports have demonstrated that inequalities in health still exist making it difficult for many individuals and families to opt for health behaviours (Townsend, 1980; Whitehead, 1992).

Homelessness and unemployment also impact quite strongly on the health of the nation. Researchers over the last decade have shown how low income increases the individuals exposure to health hazards like poor housing, pollution and unsafe environments. Blaxter's study (1990), analysing data from a large survey of health and lifestyles, found that the health of low income groups improves substantially as income increases. According to Acheson (1991) there is a limit to the extent to which an individual can change his behaviour in the absence of wider strategies to reduce deprivation and improve the environment.

Tannahill (1990) suggests that health education has tended to be a combination of a disease-orientated approach and a risk-factor approach. He argues that these focus on disease and the negative aspects of health neglecting the positive dimensions.

Health For All 2000

One of the major contributing factors in the development of the concept of health promotion has been the *Health For All* movement initiated by the World Health Organisation (WHO) in 1977. The key to attaining health was identified as primary health care. The Ottawa Charter for action, drawn up in 1986, strengthened the idea that the promotion of health was much more than an individual responsibility. It led to the development of the New Public Health movement. This is emerging as an approach which embraces environmental change *and* individual responsibility thereby seeking to avoid victim blaming. Underlying many of today's health problems are issues of local and national public policy which the New Public Health seeks to address.

Health promotion

The above factors have all contributed to the development of the concept of 'health promotion' as distinct from 'health education'. Various definitions have been proposed over recent years. All have as their core the view that health promotion is a global term which incorporates the promotion of health through a wide range of initiatives and policies and campaigns. Emphasis is placed on putting energy into dealing with the underlying problems which lead to negative health behaviours. This is achieved by building healthy public policy, and empowering individuals and groups within society. Some of the views of health promotion are considered in more detail.

WHO's principles of health promotion

The WHO (1986) defines health promotion as '... the process of enabling individuals and communities to increase control over the determinants of health and thereby improve their health'. Five principles underpin this definition:

- health promotion focuses on the population as a whole rather than on individuals who are at risk;
- health promotion should be aimed at the factors which influence health;
- health promotion must combine a wide variety of complementary approaches including education, legislation and organisational change;
- health promotion requires full community participation;
- health professionals have a key role to play in nurturing and promoting health through education and advocacy.

The Ottawa Charter elaborates some of these principles and especially emphasises the importance of achieving equality in health. It stresses that health promotion must aim at reducing differences in health. It must ensure that equal resources and opportunities are open to all in order for them to achieve their full potential.

A model for health promotion

One model widely acknowledged is that of Tannahill (1985). Tannahill's model sees health promotion as consisting of three overlapping activities (Figure 2.1):

WHO Resolution 1977

The main social target of governments and the WHO in the coming decades should be the attainment by all citizens of the world, by the year 2000, of a level of health that will permit them to lead a socially and economically productive life

Ottawa Charter for Action (1986)

- healthy public policy
- supportive environments
- strong community action
- develop personal skills
- preorientate health services

New public health

To find out more about this you should look at ASHTON, J. and SEYMOUR, H. (1988) *The New Public Health*. Milton Keynes: Open University Press

Figure 2.1

A model for health promotion. (From Downie et al., 1990. Reproduced by permission of Oxford University Press.)

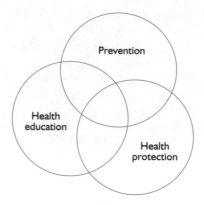

- Preventive care
- Protection
- Education

Preventive care is aimed at reducing the likelihood of the onset of a disease process, illness or disability (or some other unwanted state). Individuals are provided with information and advice to enable them to avoid health damaging behaviours. It is an area with which the nurse should be familiar and is of particular importance to the community team. It is generally taken to consist of intervention at three levels:

- Primary prevention. This includes immunisations and specific actions to prevent accidents, curb smoking and encourage a balanced healthy diet.

- Secondary prevention. This is concerned with the early detection of disease or illness *before* it manifests itself. This then allows early treatment to be initiated. Screening plays an important role in the prevention of disease and illness in children. One example is the routine test for phenylketonuria. This test is carried out on all babies at 10 days of age. It has been instrumental in detecting the condition early so that effective treatment can be started as soon as possible. Developmental surveillance is another example of secondary prevention. Every child is seen at regular intervals. Checks are made on developmental progress and deviations from the norm are identified.

- Tertiary prevention is concerned with curing disease, preventing complications and the prevention of spread of disease. Action at this level includes medical and surgical interventions and rehabilitation. Specialist nurses work at this level to teach individuals how to cope with a disease or illness so as to limit the development of complications.

Protection. According to Downie *et al.* (1990, p. 51), health protection comprises 'legal or fiscal controls, other regulations and policies, and voluntary codes of practice aimed at the enhancement of

Phenylketonuria

Phenylketonuria is a relatively rare autosomal recessive metabolic disorder. The conversion of phenylalanine to tyrosine is blocked. Increased levels of phenylalanine lead to severe mental deficiency and seizures

(See also Figure 4.1 – page 448)

positive health and the prevention of ill-health'. The aim is to make it less likely that individuals will meet hazards in the environment and behave in an unhealthy way. It is about making the healthy choices the easy ones:

* legal control – this is concerned with legislation, e.g. the use of child and infant restraints in cars;
* fiscal control – this is concerned with the imposition of healthy monetary policies by the government, e.g. the imposition of more tax on leaded petrol to make unleaded petrol cheaper and therefore more attractive;
* other policies – these are policies which are implemented by agencies other than the government (one example is the implementation of no-smoking policies in the work place);
* voluntary codes of practice – these are agreed codes as in the advertising of tobacco products. However, with no legal backup these can be broken with no redress.

Health education is the third activity in Tannahill's model. It is a long-established activity which has been defined by many authors over recent years. Within the new concept of health promotion, education is seen as being aimed at influencing behaviour, promoting positive health and preventing ill-health. It is important that education is carried against the individual's background taking into consideration their social and cultural situation. Thus it moves away from the victim blaming approach and acknowledges the underlying influencing factors.

The model suggests that each of the three activities can occur in isolation. Examples of these have been given previously. However, in reality they overlap giving rise to a further four health promotion activities (Figure 2.2):

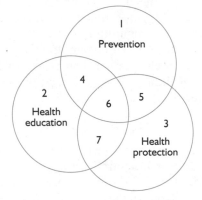

* Preventive health education (4, see Figure 2.2) – education related to available preventive measures. Immunisations are a valuable preventive measure but without education parents may not realise the benefits of taking up the programme. Thus education is aimed at

parents and carers. One recent example of this has been the television advertisement campaign for the haemophilus influenza type B (HIB) vaccine. Education is also carried out with the use of posters and leaflets.

- Preventive health protection (5, see Figure 2.2) – this includes legal, fiscal or other policies which are preventive in nature. One example of this is the fluoridation of water supplies to promote healthy teeth.

- Health education for preventive health protection (6, see Figure 2.2) – although many preventive policies exist, individuals need to be educated about them so as to gain the maximum benefit. Using the above example, parents and carers need to be given the facts about fluoridation and its benefits. In this way more will be enabled to make informed choices about their child's care.

- Health education aimed at health protection (7, see Figure 2.2) – this entails raising the public's and policy makers' awareness of the need for protection measures. One recent example of this has been the lobby for the introduction of traffic calming measures outside schools. As a result of public pressure in many areas, speed restrictions have been imposed outside schools.

Activity

What other views/models/theories of health promotion can you find? Look for names like Keith Tones, Ian Sutherland and Russell Caplan. Analyse and explore each view that you find. How do they compare with Tannahill's views and those of the WHO?

Health education

To Tannahill then, health promotion is a composite concept to which health education is simply one of the contributors. It serves principally as the communicating channel for influential ideas and seeks to empower individuals and communities by providing information, developing skills and a healthy self-esteem. In this way people can come to feel in control of themselves rather than by external forces outside their influence. Several authors have explored the concept and have offered models of health education.

Beattie's model of health education

Beattie (1986) identifies two factors which he sees as fundamental to health education, i.e. the *mode* and the *focus* (Figure 2.3).

The *mode* is where ownership of the appropriate knowledge in health education, and therefore the control, lies. At point A, control lies with the expert. It is the expert who decides what it is that the client needs to know. At point B, control is determined by the client(s). The client identifies what it is he/she needs to learn, taking into account

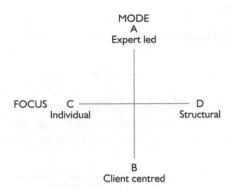

Figure 2.3

Factors fundamental to health education. (Adapted from Beattie, 1986.)

his/her needs, circumstances and beliefs. The importance of this mode is stressed as it contributes to a feeling of empowerment.

The *focus of intervention* is concerned with where/who the education is aimed at. At point C, the education is aimed at the individual – the *individualistic approach*. At point D the focus is the community, an institution or even society – the *structural approach*. Beattie shows these factors as two intersecting lines giving rise to four categories of education (Figure 2.4):

- *Paramedic advice* – this is expert-led and is directed at the individual. An example is giving health education to a child and carer related to diabetes and its complications.
- *Personal growth* – a young mother realises she does not know enough about weaning and feeding her son. She asks the health visitor for advice. This is client-led and client-centred and encourages a feeling of being in control.
- *Public agenda setting* – a group of experts agree on the need for a plan for education related to HIV and AIDS. They attempt to educate the policy formers and decision makers. This is expert-led and structural in its focus.
- *Popular outreach* – a group of parents lobby their MP regarding the need for traffic calming methods outside a local school. This is client-led and structural in its focus and encourages empowerment.

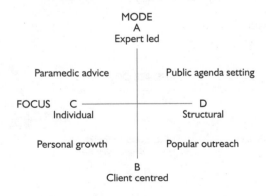

Figure 2.4

Four categories of health education. (Adapted from Beattie, 1986.)

Activity

Take each category shown in Figure 2.4 and identify an example from your own field of work.

Tones' model of health education

Tones and Tilford (1990) describe the contribution that health education makes to health promotion. In doing so they identify three main categories (Figure 2.5):

- The traditional approach – this has always been focused on the individual and its aim has been to encourage a change of behaviour to prevent disease. Tones still sees a place for this approach providing that the individual is not blamed for his/her actions. It should concentrate on influencing attitudes and beliefs and empowering people rather than changing behaviour.

- Raising public awareness – Tones splits this into two. (1) Agenda setting – this relates in some way to Beattie's public agenda setting and is used to describe the process of generating public awareness about a specific health problem before legislation is introduced. An example is the general advertising campaign conducted prior to the implementation of the back seat belt law. (2) Critical conscious raising – the aim of this type of education is to encourage individuals/communities to look critically at themselves and their environment. It is hoped that they are then empowered to take action to pressure for policy making. An example is a campaign to make individuals and groups look at the effects of smoking. As a result non-smokers have pressurised for more non-smoking environments.

Figure 2.5

The contribution of health education to health promotion. (From Tones and Tilford, 1990. Reproduced by permission of Chapman & Hall.)

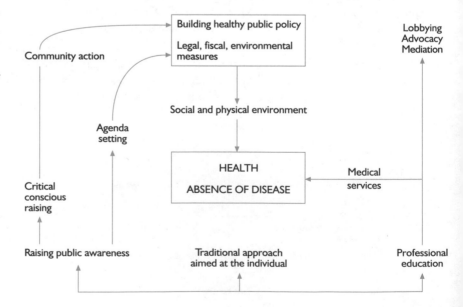

- Professional education attempts to educate health and other professionals so that they in turn can become effective health educators.

The health-oriented approach (Downie *et al.*, 1991)

This model is based on two main principles, i.e. the prevention of ill-health and the enhancement of positive health (Figure 2.6).

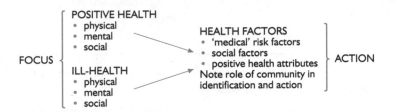

Figure 2.6

Health-oriented approach. (From Downie et al., 1990. Reproduced by permission of Oxford University Press).

It acknowledges the underlying factors which influence health. Action is aimed at the risks and is applicable at both the structural and the individual level. It is not merely led by professionals but involves public (and group) participation, especially in identifying the risks, thus highlighting the importance of empowerment.

The three views on health education described here have certain similarities which can act as principles:

- They all acknowledge that individual approaches have a role to play providing that the individual's circumstances are taken into consideration. It is important to start where the client is, to consider his/her social circumstances, beliefs, values and culture.

- They each see a role for public agenda setting and for involving individuals and communities in securing action.

- Finally, they each have as a central theme the concept of empowerment.

Activity

Set yourself the task of analysing each of the views covered here. Explore any other theories and or models that you find in your reading.

Empowerment

Empowerment is a popular term in use today in many different arenas. This makes it difficult to simply define the term as it can take on different meanings for different people in different contexts. The word is derived from the Latin *potere* meaning 'to be able'. Today the term is particularly relevant to the current health promotion movement and can be defined as the social process by which people are enabled to take control of their own health. It involves helping people to take a critical look at a situation and facilitating a realistic plan of action. In doing this

Cross reference

Empowerment – page 173

health educators need to be aware of the complex array of political, social, economic and demographic factors which influence health and illness. However, it is necessary to attempt to change the conditions which create powerlessness at the same time and to be proactive. An example of this is installing a suggestion box on the ward, and encouraging children and parents to participate in the improvement of the environment. Thus the process of empowerment must include not only individual change but also change in the social setting itself (Wallerstein, 1992).

Activity

How feasible is the definition of empowerment shown in the box to the left? What are the reasons for your conclusion?

Empowerment

'... a social process of recognising, promoting and enhancing people's abilities to meet their own needs, solve their own problems and mobilise the necessary resources in order to feel in control of their own lives'.

(Gibson, 1991)

Within the arena of child care, obstacles to the empowerment of children exist. The first is to do with the developmental stage of children and the second with the social context in which children live.

The amount of responsibility which children can assume for their own health must be considered. Too much too soon can create demands which children are not developmentally ready to meet. However, it is important to acknowledge that children have their own views and ideas about health and to accept these as valid. The children's nurse, therefore, needs an understanding of the changing perceptions that children have of health as they develop. This then enables the nurse to promote empowerment where appropriate (see the chapters on the role of the nurse and the child's perceptions of health).

Within the social context children are assumed to be cognitively and socially immature. While the health needs of children are recognised in policy and planning documents their role is one of passive recipient (Kalnins *et al.*, 1994). Children are not generally given the opportunity to participate in health making decisions. Factors which act against empowerment include:

- Parental attitudes – whilst many parents are willing to involve their children in the decision making process, they can feel threatened by the competence of the children (Lewis and Lewis, 1990).

- Non-participation in clinical interviews – interactions between doctors and carers can often ignore the child. Attitudes of health professionals can influence the child's perceptions of his/her role and can lead to silent cooperation rather than questioning.

- Professional jargon – this can exclude children and carers from participation in decision making. Language must be interactive and encourage open participation both by carers and children.

It is important that children have a voice in their future health. They often have very firm views on health issues and will participate in community projects with great enthusiasm. It is necessary to encourage a shift in thinking as children are encouraged to participate in health promotion. Empowerment is for all, not just for the adults in society.

SUMMARY

It is essential that you have an understanding of the theoretical basis of health promotion if you are to fulfil your role as a health promoter. This section has given you an overview of theories and you should now read further to expand your knowledge and understanding. Material in this section will help you to look critically at some of the health promotion interventions related to child health.

> ➤ *Key points*

1. Defining health is complex. The concept is viewed in different ways by the same person. Each individual will have his own views about what it means to be healthy.

2. The health promotion movement incorporates promotion of health through a wide range of initiatives and activities. Building a healthy public policy is one of the central concepts.

3. Health education is just one part of health promotion. It can be considered as the communication channel for influencing ideas and behaviours.

4. Empowerment of people and of communities is central to all health promotion. People need to feel in control of their own lives and need to be enabled to make healthy choices. This concept is applicable to adults and children alike.

3 CHILDREN'S CONCEPTS OF HEALTH

INTRODUCTION

As we have seen, defining health is difficult to do. Each of us has our own definition based on experience, knowledge and developed concepts, and influenced by culture, society, family and personal beliefs. The concepts that we have as adults are formed from our experiences during the maturation process and then refined and adapted as we grow and mature. Children's ideas about the world in which they live change and develop as these concepts are formed. Hence their ideas about health change. To meet the health care needs of children, nurses must understand how these ideas change with age. It is essential that health promotion activities are pertinent to a child and are related to the way in which he or she interprets health. Only then can the promotion of healthy behaviours begin to be successful. A knowledge of how children view health can also be useful when caring for them during periods of ill health. Their ideas may affect how they interpret information about disease and can lead to alarming misconceptions. Take for instance that a child is told that his tonsils will have to be removed from his throat. He becomes quite frightened as he thinks that his throat will be cut to remove the tonsils. Compliance with treatment may also be affected by a lack of understanding. For example a young child who does not understand the function of the gastro-intestinal tract may be reluctant to take an oral pain killer for a headache.

The fact that children's perceptions change as they grow and develop presents us with a challenge – to understand each child and to value his or her beliefs and ideas, acknowledging that what they believe is important.

DEVELOPING IDEAS ABOUT THE HUMAN BODY

Studies which explore children's beliefs about the human body are limited. Table 3.1 draws on some of the studies and shows how a child's ideas might develop.

McEwing (1996) and Gaudion (1997) concur that young children have most knowledge about the heart, bones and brain, and that as cognitive ability develops children are more able to understand more abstract concepts.

DEVELOPING IDEAS ABOUT HEALTH

It is interesting to note that there is less research available about health beliefs than there is about illness beliefs. Perhaps this is because of the traditional ideas that put more emphasis on cure and treatment than on prevention and health. As the importance of promoting health in

Cross references

Children's concepts of illness – page 214

Children's perceptions of pain – page 351

Age	Knowledge of inside of body	Knowledge of function of organs
3–5 years	Draws pictures that show food, bones and sometimes blood. These are all things that the child can 'see' or 'feel'.	Limited understanding of body functions. Unclear about body boundaries.
5–10 years	Drawings often include the heart and brain. Not until 10 years are children likely to regularly include the stomach and the lungs.	Believe that organs can only have one function, e.g. the heart is for loving, the brain is for thinking. Do not identify the role of the brain in the senses or motor behaviour. Not able to relate the various parts of the body together.
Adolescence	Now aware of liver, kidneys and the internal reproductive organs.	Understand that organs can have more than one function. Relate parts of the body together so would understand the workings of the digestive system.

Table 3.1

Children's developing ideas about the human body

childhood is recognised and as the views of children are acknowledged, we may be more interested in finding out what they have to say about health. Two major approaches to the study of children's health beliefs are evident from the available literature.

Cognitive–developmental approach

This approach is based on the belief that the development of concepts follows a pattern that is the same in all children, albeit at different rates. It assumes that as children mature, they gradually develop expanding and more differentiated concepts. It would seem that the formation of many concepts, e.g. time, space and number, follow the patterns outlined by cognitive psychologists. The approach questions 'how' behaviour comes about, analysing the thinking, cognitive processes of children. It relies on the interviewer probing children's minds to find out reasons for saying what they say about health. The difficulty here is that the results of such an interview are affected by the effectiveness of the interviewer. If he or she does not probe well enough insufficient information may be gained on which to make a judgement. The interviewer may also misinterpret what is said by the child. The technique really calls for an ability to interpret what children say. This can be difficult as no adult can really know exactly what is going on inside a child's head. However, it is an approach that is used frequently, perhaps because of the popularity of cognitive psychologists in child development. The framework that has been used most frequently by researchers in this area is that based on Jean Piaget's work. Studies show that the quality of children's thoughts about health do change developmentally, reflecting the stages of cognitive development as described by the Swiss psychologist Piaget and that their ideas become more complex and abstract as they mature (Table 3.2).

Pre-operational stage (up to age 7). Children at this stage of cognitive

Age	Cognitive development	Concept of health
Up to 7 years	Pre-operational – egocentric, present-oriented, intuitive, magical thinking, unable to reverse processes.	Find health difficult to define – tend to list activities and behaviours centred on self. Health in others judged by external cues (rosy cheeks, clear eyes). Health and illness unrelated. Rely on others to tell them when they are sick. Health vulnerable to external forces, e.g. magic.
7–11 years	Concrete operational – begin to consider causal relationships. Develop reversibility and conservation. Can think through a chain of events. Classify objects and concrete ideas. Able to shift from part to whole and back again. Remain present-oriented until about 9 years.	Health viewed as a broad whole body concept – feeling good, being fit and strong. Possible to be part healthy, part not healthy. Still see health vulnerable to external forces but see that ill-health can be caused by physical contact, e.g. with dirt. Understand that illness can be prevented to some degree.
11–16 years	Formal operations – future-oriented, can formulate hypotheses, consider abstractions. Develop deductive reasoning.	Aware of problems associated with defining health. Use internal cues as well as external ones to judge people's health – consider the abstract points. See health and sickness as related. Consider mental health important.

(Adapted from work by Bibace and Walsh, 1980, and Natapoff, 1982.)

Concept

'something conceived in the mind; a thought, notion; a generic idea abstracted from particular instances'.

(*Longman New Universal Dictionary*, 1982)

development find it difficult to define health. Eiser *et al.* (1983) asked 6 year olds 'what does it mean to be healthy?' – 65% of them were unable to answer the question. Natapoff (1982) found that children in the pre-operational stage gave general, undifferentiated answers to questions about health and had to use visual cues to judge whether somebody was healthy or not. However, when it came to judging their own health they often relied on other people to tell them if they were ill. They based their own health on what they were able to do, play outside, go to school. Health at this age is seen as a series of unrelated activities of which eating the right food is seen as important. So children at this age tend to list things that make them healthy. According to Piaget, children in this stage are unable to reverse processes. This is evident in their inability to see health and ill-health as part of a continuum or existing together. They see health as an absolute and believe that if you are healthy you cannot get sick. The maintenance of health relies on external forces. Explanations for the cause of illness are often magical in nature (Bibace and Walsh, 1980) and so it is not surprising that children have little perception or understanding of illness prevention (Eiser *et al.*, 1983). The future is too abstract for children of this age to think about so any discussion about the consequences of non-healthy behaviours would be meaningless.

Concrete operations stage (7–11). As children develop their cognitive abilities they begin to be able to classify pieces of information into a whole. Therefore they define health as a total body state. Being healthy is feeling good, being in good condition, fit and strong (Natapoff, 1982). Health is seen as a broad concept developed from an integration of learned material and information. As children of this age have learned to conserve, they see the possibility of being part healthy and part not healthy. They can shift from the whole to part of the whole. Therefore somebody with a broken leg can still be healthy. Operational children still see health as being vulnerable to external forces but are beginning to understand that illness can be contracted through physical contact with a source, e.g. dirt (Bibace and Walsh, 1980). They therefore understand that illness can be avoided and can identify rules for maintaining health.

Formal operations stage (11–16 onwards). Young people at this stage of development are aware that defining health is very difficult to do. They can now see that it is possible to be part healthy and part sick at the same time. The children in Natapoff's study (1982) described health as 'lasting a lifetime', and involving both the body and the mind. This was the first time that children had mentioned the importance of mental health. They saw sickness as something temporary and therefore something that it was possible to avoid and or prevent by taking proper care of oneself and by avoiding certain behaviours that were unhealthy (Bibace and Walsh, 1980). Children in the formal stage are becoming capable of abstract thinking and now do not rely on visual cues to judge health in other people. They acknowledge the importance of questioning an individual to find out how they feel about their health. There has been a shift from the use of external cues to the use of internal ones.

The developing complexity of cognitive processes identified above enable the adolescent to engage in self-care and to take more responsibility for his or her own health, taking actions and making decisions about health behaviours (Maddux *et al.*, 1986). This has implications for health promoters as it is vital to find the right time in a child's development to use initiatives that focus on healthy behaviours and the prevention of ill-health.

Health belief model approach

The health belief model (Rosenstock, 1974) was developed to attempt to explain why individuals differ in their health-related behaviours. The model (Figure 3.1) starts from the premise that any actions will be influenced at the outset by age, sex, social and cultural factors. These factors in turn influence an individual's perception of their vulnerability to ill-health. Together with the individual's reception of the benefits of health-related actions will then influence the degree to which they intend to take actions.

The use of this model in the study of children's concepts of health addresses the action component of that concept. It concentrates on the child's beliefs about one or more aspects of health and does not try to look at the underlying causal relationships between action and thought.

Figure 3.1

Health belief model.

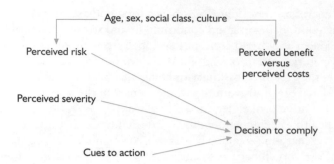

Instead it studies actions that children take. The advantage of this approach is that it is easy to implement. Children of different ages are asked a series of questions to determine their beliefs about particular health issues in relation to:

- perceived vulnerability;
- perceived benefits of healthy behaviours and or illness avoiding behaviours;
- intentions to take actions.

The frequency with which certain beliefs are held are then analysed.

In the 1970s Gochman (cited in Kalnins and Love, 1982) carried out a number of studies using this approach. He developed a series of tools that measured:

- salience – the degree to which children were aware of health issues;
- vulnerability – how vulnerable the children thought they were to 16 health problems including fever, rash, sore throat and dental problems;
- motivation;
- potential behaviour – measured children's awareness behaviours that were beneficial to health.

Locus of control

- Individuals with an internal locus of control tend to believe that they can exert influence over their lives and their health
- Individuals with an external locus of control tend to believe that nothing they can do will alter the outcome for them, in relation to health and even their future. They believe in luck and what will be will be

The results of these studies suggested that children are not generally motivated by health and that their perceived vulnerability is low. Beliefs about vulnerability become stable at around 10–11 years of age. Only a small number of children perceive themselves as vulnerable to various health problems. Perhaps this relates to the fact that young children can only deal with the present and the future is too abstract a concept to deal with. If this is so then promoting illness avoiding behaviours may be ineffective in children unless their perceived vulnerability can be increased. Gochman's studies also showed that children's perceived vulnerability and their potential for health behaviours is influenced by age, sex, class and locus of control. Boys in the study had a lower level of expectancy of health problems than the girls as did the younger children compared with the older children. Children living in inner city areas had a higher level of expectancy of health problems than did children living in rural areas. Dielman *et al.* (1980) found that young children's beliefs about health and illness differed more among them than in older children. This finding relates well to findings from the cognitive development studies and serves to suggest that health teaching should begin early before a differentiated belief system is established at the age of about 12.

Activity

Take an opportunity to talk to well and sick children of different ages about health. Ask them questions such as :

- what does being healthy mean to you?
- what food is healthy?
- what things do you do that are not healthy?
- how do you know when you are ill?

Ask them to draw pictures about health. Analyse what they say and what they draw. How does it compare to the findings from the above studies?

Whichever approach is used to assess children's concepts of health, it is important to remember that all children are individuals and are influenced by their families, peers and significant others. Few studies have explored the influences on children's beliefs about health, but Lewis and Lewis (1974) showed that television advertisements had a considerable impact. Children aged 10–13 years of age thought that 70% of advertisements relating to health were true. Nearly half of the children believed all the messages conveyed in advertisements. Social and cultural factors must also impact on children's beliefs about health. For example, the Romany rituals of body cleanliness and the system of wash bowls are introduced to children from an early age and are strictly adhered to from puberty (Taylor, 1991). Children vary in their cognitive abilities and it would be dangerous to assume that all children of a particular age held the same views and beliefs. It may be useful to try to put the two approaches reviewed here together. It would seem that 'what' children believe about a certain health issue must be influenced by 'how' they think. This in turn depends on the complexity of their cognitive processes. Generally researchers have found that there is a distinct change in the way children perceive health (and illness, their bodies and treatment) at around the age of 8–9 years with an improved ability to think in a reality-oriented causal manner.

It is important that children's nurses, who are in an ideal situation to influence the health beliefs and behaviours of children, understand the development of the concept of health through the ages. In order to empower children and encourage them to take responsibility for their own health, their views and ideas about health must be acknowledged as being valid by other people. Spend time talking to children to find out what they believe and understand about health. Then you can begin to incorporate your findings into the care that you implement.

Key points ➤

1. Children's ideas about the world in which they live change and develop as concepts are formed.

2. This presents children's nurses with a challenge – to understand each child and value his/her beliefs about health, acknowledging them as valid.

3. The cognitive development theorists suggest that beliefs about health develop in an orderly staged manner. The approach questions how behaviour comes about.

4. Studies based on the health belief model are more interested in the action component of the concept of health.

DEVELOPING STRATEGIES FOR HEALTH 4

INTRODUCTION

Putting effective health promotion into practice presents a challenge for all professionals. Strategies need to be appropriate for the audience, stimulating and educative. This section examines some important child health issues and looks at the way in which health promotion has been implemented and evaluated.

Activity

Take a few minutes to list the child health issues that you believe to be particularly important today.

Your list may include some of the following issues:
* smoking;
* physical exercise;
* diet;
* sex education;
* HIV and AIDS;
* dental caries;
* accidents;
* skin care in the sun;
* respiratory diseases, e.g. asthma;
* drug and alcohol abuse.

The following discussion will concentrate on those particular issues highlighted as being pertinent to children in the Government's *Health of the Nation Strategy* (DoH, 1992a). These are:
* accidents;
* smoking;
* sexual health, HIV and AIDS.

In each case the size and nature of the problem will be explored in order to give some idea of the scope for health promotion. Some of the activities that have been or are being implemented for each will be examined and an evaluation made where possible. This will give you an opportunity to explore a variety of activities, critically reviewing their effectiveness and the relationship, if any, to the theories and models discussed earlier in the module.

ACCIDENTS

Accidents are the leading cause of death in children aged 1–15 and as such are a major public health problem. In 1990, in England and Wales, a total of 646 children died as a result of accidents, the majority being involved in motor vehicle accidents (50% – 322 deaths) (Beishon, 1993). The remaining causes of death were fire and flames (14%), drownings (8%), falls, suffocation, inhalation, and poisoning. Deaths from accidents represent only the tip of the iceberg as they also account for a considerable amount of morbidity in children. In 1991, 6079 children were seriously injured on the roads. In 1989, 647 000 children under 5 were estimated to have been injured in the home (DTI, 1992) the most severe injuries being from fires, burns and scalds, and falls. Each year approximately 10 000 children are permanently disabled, and one in six children attends hospital accident and emergency departments as a result of accidents at a cost to the NHS of nearly £150 million a year (Hall *et al.*, 1994). It is feasible to suggest that many more children are injured daily as a result of accidents in and around the home but remain outside the statistics due to home treatments.

The government has recognised the importance of placing accident prevention high on the list of priorities and has set a target of a reduction of the rate of deaths in children under 15 by at least 33% by the year 2005.

Factors influencing accidents in childhood

- *Developmental*. The types of accidents that occur in any age group are generally related to the child's developmental stage. Table 4.1 shows the major developmental factors and associated accidents that occur in the various age groups.
- *Sex*. It is a statistical fact that boys are more likely to be involved in accidents than girls above the age of 9 months. This does not necessarily mean that boys have more accidents because they are male. It does, however, seem to point to the fact that boys are more likely to be involved in accidents. Perhaps boys are more likely to be exposed to situations that predispose towards accidents. For example, they are more exposed to risk-taking activities than girls. To what extent do you think this is influenced by upbringing?
- *Social and environmental factors*. Various socially related factors have been identified as contributing to the huge number of accidents that happen in childhood. Quantitative and epidemiological research into childhood accidents has revealed a definite social class gradient. Townsend (1980) showed that children in social class V are five times more likely to die as a result of accidents than children from social class I. According to Avery and Jackson (1993) boys in social class V are seven times more likely to be killed in pedestrian

Age group	Significant development factors	Related accidents
Infants 0–1 year	• Increasing locomotor skills: rolling, sitting, crawling, cruising unsteady in locomotion • Improving manipulative skills.	Falls, e.g. off beds, down stairs
	• Curiosity about the environment	Burns, e.g. from unguarded fires; drowning in baths, toilets; suffocation, e.g. from plastic bags
	• Mouthing of objects	Aspiration and choking, e.g. from small toys
Toddlers and preschoolers	• Unrestricted freedom through locomotion • Unaware of dangers • Undeveloped visual field – limited peripheral vision	Motor vehicle accidents, e.g. caused by running into the road, misjudging speeds
	• Can open some doors and gates • Explores, curious • Climb up and down stairs, limited depth perception	Falls, e.g. down stairs, from windows, off climbing frames
	• Helpless in water, unaware of depth	Drowning
	• Able to reach heights by climbing, standing on tip-toe and/or on objects • Unaware of potential sources of heat.	Burns, e.g. by pulling at pan handles, flexes
	• Explore objects by putting them in their mouths (becomes less likely through this age group)	Choking, poisoning
	• Generally clumsy	General bodily injury
School age	• Achieving social acceptance, peer pressure • May attempt hazardous feats without planning or realising consequences	Ingestion of poisonous material, e.g. glue sniffing, tablets Falls, e.g. from trees, walls; drowning, e.g. when playing near rivers, canals
	• Becoming more independent in daily activities, e.g. walking/ cycling to school • Limited understanding and application of road safety measures, misinterpretation of traffic signs, speed of traffic • Lack of concentration when playing, limited range of vision	Motor vehicle accidents, e.g. crossing busy roads; cycle accidents
Adolescents	• Clear physical, sensory and psychomotor function • Feelings of strength and confidence • Increased energy that must be released through action often at the expense of common sense	Motor vehicle accidents as a passenger or driver; moped and/or motorbike accidents; sporting injuries
	• Propensity for risk taking, especially among boys • Access to more complex tools, objects, locations	Drowning
	• Stress from peer pressure, exams, social acceptance	Suicide

Table 4.1

Developmental factors and associated accidents

road accidents, 15 times more likely to be killed in accidental death by fire and nine times more likely to drown than boys in social class I. A study by Sparks *et al.* (1994) suggests that there are social class differences in the successful use of safety measures. The study puts forward social deprivation and a lack of material resources as being a potential reason for this difference. Although the sample used in the study was small (32 families) it used a qualitative approach that investigated the social and material environment in which children and families live their lives, focusing on people's accounts of factors involved in keeping children safe. It therefore contributes to an understanding of the reasons for the social patterning of accidents within the context of the family and the community.

Activity

Having identified that there are social class variations in the accident rates for children, spend some time analysing the possible reasons for this. To help you do this carry out a literature search for any research or papers that might relate to the subject. To get you started two references:

AVERY, J., *et al.* (1990) Geographical variations in mortality due to childhood accidents in England and Wales, 1975–1984. *Public Health*, **104**, 171–182.

CHANDLER, S., CHAPMAN, A. and HOLLINGTON, S. (1984) Fire incidence, housing and social conditions: the urban situation in Britain. *Fire Prevention*, **172**, 15–20.

Some of the points you may have analysed might have included:

- Children in the lower social classes are perhaps more likely to live in poor quality housing in which they are more at risk from: fire and burns, unsafe and faulty electrical wiring, injury from non-safety glass in windows, and hazardous forms of heating (e.g. paraffin stoves).
- It is perhaps likely that children in working class families live in a more dangerous physical environment than middle class children leading to the risk of injury from: deserted canals, railway lines, derelict houses, factories, rubbish tips and busy streets.
- Lack of safe areas to play.
- Poverty and an inability to afford to buy expensive safety equipment, e.g. car restraints. It may be also that second hand safety devices are used which may be broken and unsuitable.
- Differences in child-rearing patterns. Children with mothers who work and who cannot afford appropriate child care may leave their older children unattended after school. Possible different parental perceptions about what is safe and how much supervision children need.

Cross reference

Child-rearing practice – pages 35–45

	Education	Engineering	Enforcement	Equity
Primary prevention				
Secondary prevention				
Tertiary prevention				

Figure 4.1

*Accident prevention matrix.
(From Machie, 1993.
Reproduced by permission of
PMH Publications.)*

How many of these factors did you examine? Are there many studies that corroborate them or disprove them?

Accident prevention

To prevent accidents in childhood, interventions need to concentrate on changing children's behaviour and the environment in which they live using a multi-agency approach. Mackie (1993) suggests the creation of an accident prevention matrix (Figure 4.1) in which he identifies four types of intervention, i.e.

- Education – increasing knowledge of problems and their solutions;
- Engineering – changing the design and construction of products;
- Enforcement – using regulations, standards and legislation;
- Equity – ensuring equal access to accident prevention activities;

at three levels: primary, actions to prevent accidents occurring (e.g. the fitting of stair gates); secondary, actions to decrease the severity of an accident (e.g. the wearing of cycle helmets); and tertiary, actions to limit the severity of the final outcome of an accident (e.g. teaching first aid).

These types of interventions clearly relate to some of the ideas and concepts that we have examined already in looking at theories and models. This will become evident as we move on to examine some of the initiatives that have been implemented within these four areas at various levels.

Education

The Eastern Region Children's Traffic Club, aimed at preschool children and their carers, is an example of education at the primary level. The idea originated in Scandinavia and was developed in the UK by the Transport Research Laboratory and sponsored by General Accident. The club aims to teach children and their carers about road safety using activities designed to involve children in learning by 'doing'. The material consists of five booklets each one designed by teachers and psychologists to meet the developmental needs of a specific group:

- To know that traffic might appear from places other than the road, e.g. driveways
- To recognise that the kerb is a boundary at which he or she must stop
- To recognise whether objects are moving or stationary
- To ride wheeled toys in safe places
- To use a restraint in car if fitted
- To sit in the rear of cars
- To name, recognise and match colours
- To recognise the sounds that identify the approach of traffic
- To continue developing their perceptual and motor skills such as visual search, attention, memory and coordination

(Downing et al., 1991)

Significant differences between behaviour of children in experimental group compared with a control group

- More carers of club members reported that their children held hands when out walking
- More club members were reported to always stop when told to
- More carers of club members were likely to plan safe routes to school
- More club members were adept at tracing safe routes from a picture
- More club members identified safe places to play
- More club members described the correct procedure for crossing the road

(Bryan-Brown, 1994)

Book 1	3–3.5 years
Book 2	3.5–4 years
Book 3	4–4.5 years
Book 4	4.5–5 years
Book 5	5–5.5/6 years

Each book is based around a number of objectives related to the particular age group. The objectives for Book 2 are shown in the box.

The activities begin by looking at 'stopping', 'looking' and 'listening', and then move on to putting all three together. Each page concentrates on a particular aspect giving things to do at home and things to do outside. Brightly coloured pictures encourage discussions about the road and the traffic on it. A check list enables carers to evaluate their child's progress. Activity cards in each book give games to play, cut out vehicles to make and pictures to colour.

The club was launched in May 1990 in seven Eastern Counties after a series of pilot studies. All children in the participating counties were sent a copy of Book 1 on their third birthday and invited to join the club by returning a registration card. At this time there was no charge for membership. Surveys were carried out at the end of the first year and towards the end of the first series of books to evaluate the success of the club (West *et al.*, 1993; Bryan-Brown, 1994). Overall the surveys have found that the effect of the club is beneficial. Uptake of the programme was approximately 50%. Some significant differences between club members and non-club members were found. However, the effectiveness of such a club depends on membership. The first series was issued free of charge. In 1995, the charge introduced to carers was £9.95.

Activity

Look back to part 2 of this module (Health), Theories and models of health promotion. How does this programme relate to the various ideas and models of health promotion discussed?

You may have picked up the following points:

- Education is one of the activities that contributes to health promotion (Tannahill, 1985). This particular programme is at the primary level in that it attempts to reduce the number of road accidents by influencing children's behaviour. It therefore falls into the category of preventive education. By giving information to carers it could promote empowerment and help them to feel more in control over their child's safety on the roads.

- According to Beattie's model of health education this programme fits into the category of paramedic advice. The club was designed by professionals (teachers and psychologists) and is aimed at the individual.

- According to Tones and Tilford (1990) the programme would be one of the traditional approach as it is aimed at the individual to encourage a change in behaviour.

- It is possible, since the programme is aimed at the individual, that it could be seen as victim blaming in that it sees carers as being responsible for their child's safety on the roads. It is not easy to judge how the individual's social and cultural situation can be taken into account in such a broadly aimed programme.

- One important aspect of health promotion is that it should be accessible to all. That a charge is now made for this programme could detract from its effectiveness.

Activity

Another example of the educative approach to the reduction of accidents is the *Play It Safe* television campaign that ran in the early 1980s and again in 1991. Find out about this campaign and its effectiveness. Analyse it in relation to theories and models.

Engineering

Educating individuals about safety, be it inside the home or outside, is insufficient by itself. Children are at the mercy of their environment and so the design of product and of the environment must be done with safety in mind. This involves alliances between designers, politicians, architects, health professionals, businessmen and the children and carers themselves. Improvements in product design have been numerous in recent years. It has been shown that changes in design can have positive effects on injury reduction (Towner *et al.*, 1993).

One specific engineering project introduced measures to redistribute traffic in an attempt to reduce road accidents. The Urban Safety Project in the 1980s identified five experimental locality areas and a similar number of matched control areas. Measures introduced included more roundabouts, central refuges on wide roads, banned right-hand turns and closed roads. Although there were wide variations in accident reduction between the schemes, the overall rate was 13% and vulnerable road users such as children and cyclists benefited from the schemes (Mackie *et al.*, 1990; Tillman, 1992).

Enforcement

It is often not enough to advocate changes in design and to try to educate about safety. Laws are needed to try to enforce measures to protect children from the dangers in our everyday lives. Legislation relevant to child safety exists in many areas, e.g.

- Toy safety – the Toy (Safety) Regulations (1989) govern the design of toys made specifically for use by children.

Safety

Domestic engineering to improve home safety

- prohibition of open tread stairs
- installation of regulation safety glass
- compulsory handrails on stairs

Improved product design

- redesign of front loading washing machines
- warnings on plastic bags
- redesign of pen tops to prevent asphyxiation when swallowed
- coiled kettle flexes
- safety devices for use around the home
- child-proof packaging

- Safety at school – several acts cover the safety of children at school, e.g. the Education (School Premises) Regulations Act 1981 and the Education Reform Act 1988.
- Children in cars – since 1983 the use of seat belts in the front of cars has been a legal requirement. In 1989 legislation was passed which made it compulsory for children under 14 to be restrained in the rear seats providing one was available.

Activity

In what other areas does legislation exist which is designed to protect children from accidental injury? How easy is it for this legislation to be upheld? Next time you are out for a drive, see how many children are properly restrained in vehicles. Have a discussion with a colleague as to why children may not be restrained adequately.

Equity

Equity is about ensuring that health promotion reaches everybody. Many of the activities related to accident prevention call for resources, e.g. the fitting of smoke alarms and the purchase of safety items many of which are expensive. This can mean that not all families can have access to these resources particularly those that live in poverty. Several schemes have been set up which make it easier for carers to borrow or buy safety equipment at cost price. One such scheme in Stockport has been described by Crew and Fletcher (1995). The Brinnington Action for Safety Equipment (BASE) scheme was set up in a socially deprived area of Stockport in January 1994. It sells safety equipment at cost price to families who would otherwise not be able to afford it. Crew and Fletcher identify the advantages of the scheme as:

- making equipment available at affordable prices;
- raising awareness of safety issues;
- making equipment accessible;
- empowering people to have more control over the safety in their homes;
- improving community networks by healthy alliances;
- payment can be spread over a number of weeks.

Activity

Using the accident prevention matrix in Figure 4.1 identify alternative health promotion activities for accident prevention in each of the sectors. They can be ones that you know of or ideas for activities that you have developed.

SMOKING

According to the Royal College of Physicians (1992), tobacco smoking does far more harm than any other addictive drug. It is identified as being the single most important cause of preventable ill-health in the UK today contributing to 95 000 deaths every year. Yet the young in our society continue to smoke and most recruits to smoking are under 18. In 1990, statistics show that one-quarter of all 15 year olds smoked with little change over the last decade except that the present figures suggest that more girls than boys now smoke (Lader and Matheson, 1991). See Figure 4.2.

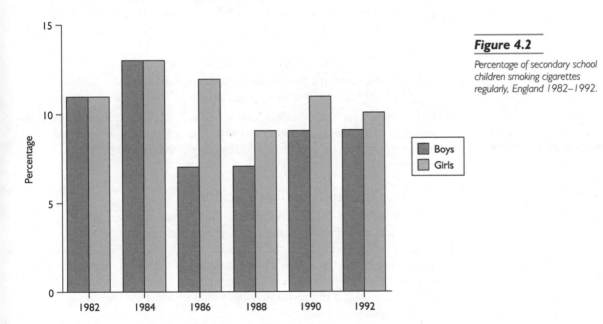

Figure 4.2

Percentage of secondary school children smoking cigarettes regularly, England 1982–1992.

The average consumption for boys is 56 cigarettes per week and for girls 49 per week. Statistics indicate that approximately 450 children start smoking every day with only one-third of 15 year olds never having smoked (Lader and Matheson, 1991). In 1992, Action on Smoking and Health estimated that the illegal sale of cigarettes to children under 16 was worth £100 million a year. The total consumption of cigarettes by children aged 11–15 in England is estimated at 17 million per week (Lader and Matheson, 1991).

The effects of tobacco on health have been well documented and can be divided into the effects of passive and active smoking.

Passive smoking and children's health

Exposure to environmental tobacco smoke (ETS) is a fact for over 3.5 million young children who live with at least one adult who smokes. Until recently it has been difficult to quantify the amount of ETS that passive smokers inhale. Recent studies have used biological markers to quantify exposure (Jarvis *et al.*, 1985). One such measure is cotinine, the main metabolite of nicotine and a sensitive indicator of exposure to tobacco smoke. Whilst it cannot provide verification of past exposure or cumulative exposure, it can provide valuable information concerning exposure and the data collected have made it possible to identify a number of important health effects on young children:

- Studies in England (Golding, 1993) and Sweden have identified a clear association between maternal and other passive smoking and sudden infant death syndrome (SIDS).
- Various studies have shown that the incidence of hospital admission for acute respiratory illness in infancy is increased where one or both parents smoke (Colley *et al.*, 1974; Fergusson *et al.*, 1980; Chen *et al.*, 1986).
- There is considerable evidence that passive smoking aggravates asthma symptoms in children with an established disease (Weitzman *et al.*, 1990; Murray and Morrison, 1986).
- Other effects on health include increased school absenteeism in the children of smokers, heightened risk of injury from house fires and long-term effects on health in adulthood, e.g. heart disease and cancer.

Active smoking and children's health

Although the most common serious complications of smoking (coronary artery disease, chronic bronchitis, emphysema and lung cancer) are rarely seen before middle age there is evidence that problems start soon after smoking is taken up. The earlier smoking is started the greater the risk of serious effects. The effects on young smokers can mainly be divided into those on the respiratory system and those on the cardio-vascular system.

Development of smoking in children and young people

Activity

List the factors that you think may influence children to smoke. Reflect on your own experiences of childhood and the extent to which you were persuaded to smoke or not as the case may be.

You may have listed some or all of the following factors that have been shown to influence smoking in children:

- personality – risk-taking, rebelliousness, poor self-image (Lader and Matheson, 1991);
- perceptions of smoking as 'fun' combined with a disregard for the long-term effects of smoking;

The effects of active smoking

- Increased respiratory disease (Charlton and Blair, 1989)
- Increased rates of cough, sputum, wheeze and shortness of breath
- Increased heart rate, blood pressure and peripheral vasoconstriction
- Decreased physical fitness – reduced oxygen carrying capacity of haemoglobin
- Activation of platelets
- Increase in blood cholesterol and triglycerides

(Royal College of Physicians, 1992)

- parental and sibling smoking – young people are more likely to smoke if other people at home smoke and siblings seem to be more influential than parents (Bellew and Wayne, 1991);
- best friends who smoke (Murray *et al.*, 1983);
- social activities, e.g. dancing, discos, parties, etc.;
- teachers smoking at school;
- smoking in public places where smoking is seen as the norm;
- availability of tobacco – illegal sales to children under 16 persist; a survey by the Office of Population Censuses and Surveys (OPCS, 1994) found that 82% of children who smoked identified newsagents and confectioners as their usual source of cigarettes;
- advertising in magazines, films, soap operas, sports sponsorship publicity, bill boards.

Reducing the prevalence of smoking

Considering the numerous and varied factors that influence smoking in young people, it is necessary to use a number of different approaches to:

- improve knowledge;
- develop personal skills to resist social pressures;
- create supportive environments within the family and within the wider community;
- strengthen community action;
- raise public awareness and promote non-smoking among adults;
- build healthy public policy.

Much of the educative work to reduce smoking in young people goes on in schools. Bellew and Wayne (1991) identify three phases of smoking in young people and suggest the appropriate focus for the curriculum in each phase (Table 4.2). They propose that the content of school education programmes should include:

- information on short- and long-term health effects of smoking;
- exploration of social influences – peers, family, the media;
- development of skills in decision making and saying no;
- development of alternative coping strategies;
- sessions to meet the different needs of boys and girls.

Many projects have been or are being implemented which attempt to address some of the issues and topics mentioned above. Two such initiatives are:

- *The Smoking and Me Project* (Health Education Authority). This programme is aimed at 12–13 year olds and attempts to develop personal skills in resisting social pressures to start smoking. It is a

Table 4.2

Phase, curriculum focus and examples of resource in smoking education

Phase	Curriculum focus	Resource	Age
Before typical age of onset	Health and attitude information	*Hooked*	9+
		C932	9–10
		My Body Project	7–11
At typical age of onset	Lessons on social influences	*Smoking and Pollution, Smoking and Me, Seven Ages of Moron*	11–12
			12–13
After onset of smoking	More sophisticated informaton; lessons about social influences to maintain non-smoking; early cessation support, in and out of school		13–14
		Pack it In	15+

From Bellew and Wayne (1991). © 1991 *Health Education Journal* (reproduced with permission).

person centred education programme in which the pupils work in groups. The group leaders are selected from the class by the pupils and their role is to lead discussions, role play exercises and decision making activities. The project materials consist only of a teacher's guide that gives an outline of the five lessons and information on how to manage the sessions. Newman *et al.* (1991) explored teachers' views of the programme. They concluded that teachers found the programme a useful teaching aid that captured the interests of the pupils. The use of peers as group leaders was positively evaluated.

- *SmokeBusters England* (Health Education Authority). This initiative has been in existence since 1985 and consists of clubs for 10–14 year olds. It uses out of school activities such as youth clubs, religious groups, the Scouts, etc., as its medium helping adults to devise stimulating ways of persuading young people not to smoke. Members receive an introductory pack and a quarterly newsletter. Conferences, fun days and workshops are arranged for both members and organisers. The value of clubs such as these lies in their ability to raise public awareness, attract publicity and most important of all encourage participation among young people. The extent to which they can contribute to a reduction in smoking however is difficult to establish (RCP, 1992).

Activity

Explore in more detail the programmes identified above. Have they been evaluated, what are the findings? In your reading you may come across other interventions – make a note of them. Try to analyse the interventions to identify what area of the curriculum they address and how they aim to contribute to a decline in teenage smoking.

Other programmes that exist are identified in the box on the left.

Additional health promotion activities aimed at reducing smoking among the young

- Family Smoking Education Project (Health Education Council)
- The Brigantia Smoking Prevention Programme (Charlton, 1986)
- Teenage Smoking Mass Media Campaign (Health Education Authority)
- Educational programmes to make shopkeepers, parents and children more aware of the laws governing the sale of cigarettes to young people
- Health warnings on tobacco products
- Restrictions on smoking in public places

SEXUAL HEALTH, HIV AND AIDS

The sexual behaviour of adolescents has long been a concern to adults. Early sexual activity can have effects on the physical, mental and social well-being of young people of both sexes in the shape of:

- unwanted pregnancies (associated with increased risk for the mother and child);
- sexually transmitted diseases (including HIV and AIDS);
- an increased risk of cancer of the reproductive organs in later life.

Cross reference

Caring for children with HIV disease – page 493

It is very difficult to obtain accurate data regarding the sexual behaviour of young people but certain trends are evident:

- the age at which teenagers begin sexual intercourse has gone down;
- there is no evidence to suggest that they are more likely to have casual sex – only a small proportion of teenagers have multiple sex partners (Ford and Morgan, 1989);
- the use of contraceptives has increased but according to Bowie and Ford (1989) contraceptives are used mainly for the prevention of pregnancy rather than disease prevention as only about a third of sexually active teenagers use condoms – in light of the advent of HIV and AIDS this is a worrying fact;
- the number of teenage pregnancies continues to be high. In 1989, 9.5 per 1000 girls aged 13–15 became pregnant (DoH, 1993).

Adolescence is a transition between childhood and adulthood and as such brings with it curiosity not least in the area of sexual activity. Young people need opportunities to gain knowledge and skills within a supportive environment so that they can make informed choices about their sexual relationships and promote their sexual health. Sexual health is about being empowered to make choices, to say no if that is what you want. It is about being free of disease but also being autonomous and respecting ones' rights and those of others (Massey, 1990). One way of promoting sexual health is through sex education.

Sex education

Sex education in school remains a very controversial issue. Early sex education tended to revolve around factual sessions on reproduction, often in relation to animals. Even now sex education is often somewhat haphazard depending very much on who is prepared to tackle it. This leads to ill-informed young people who are not sure who to trust and are left with feelings of guilt and inadequacy (Massey, 1990). One view against sex education is that it encourages promiscuity. However, studies have shown this not to be the case. The World Health Organisation (WHO, 1993) found no evidence that sex education leads to earlier or increased sexual activity. In fact it led to a delay in the start of sexual activity and increased the adoption of safer sex practices. Similar findings have been noted by Marsiglio and Mott (1986) and Miller (1986).

Sex Education Forum

NCB, 8 Wakely Street, London
EC1V 7QE
Tel: 0171 843 6052

The Sex Education Forum is an independent body representing organisations involved in providing support and information to those who provide sex education to young people. The Forum recommends (1992) that sex education should:

- be an integral part of the learning process for all children, young people and adults including those with physical, learning or emotional problems;
- encourage exploration of values and morals, consideration of sexuality and relationships and the development of decision making skills;
- foster self-esteem, self-awareness, a sense of moral responsibility and the skills to resist unwanted sexual experiences.

Several recent legislative changes have an important bearing on the way in which sex education is carried out in schools today:

- The Education (No. 2) Act 1986 – under this act, all school governors are required to decide whether any further sex education, above that provided in the National Curriculum, should be provided in their school and to maintain a written record of that decision. Any sex education that is given must be given in such a manner as to encourage a due regard for moral considerations and the value of family life.
- An amendment to the Act in July 1993 required the governors of maintained secondary schools to provide sex education to all registered pupils. At the same time all reference to HIV and AIDS and other STDs is to be removed from National Curriculum Science. A controversial part of this amendment is the rights of parents to withdraw their children from sex education that falls outside the National Curriculum in both primary and secondary schools.

Activity

Consider the possible consequences of these amendments to the Education Act.

Sexual health through health promotion

Many initiatives, particularly at local level, have been set up to promote sexual health among young people (DoH, 1993):

- Young persons advice centre – North Staffordshire DHA
- Outreach services for young people led by a senior nurse – Harrow DHA

- Sexual health steering group to develop a strategy for sexual health – Dorset DHA
- 'Sexwise' evening clinics for young people – Rotherham Family Planning Services and education authority
- Peer education project – young mothers trained to give presentations in schools about their experiences and encourage discussions on family planning – Norwich DHA

Elsewhere education initiatives are being piloted and implemented for schoolchildren:

- *Someone Like You* (Women in Theatre Group). This project was sponsored by the Nottinghamshire Health Authorities and developed and performed by the Women in Theatre Group. It is aimed at 14 year olds and consists of a 30 minute play followed by a workshop. The play is about the relationship between two young people and their thoughts as they prepare for their first date. After the play the children are invited to discuss 'what happens next' and the possible consequences of the couple's actions. The two characters stay in role to answer questions from the children. It is only during the following workshop that the girl reveals her HIV-positive status. An evaluation of the project (Denman *et al.*, 1995) found that the programme improved knowledge regarding the spread of HIV infection. Most of the children surveyed found the programme to be interesting and a good way to learn about HIV and AIDS. Many of the issues and aspects were found to be memorable and perhaps left them with strong impressions. However, there was little change noted in the degree to which the children saw themselves at personal risk. It is suggested that this could be because very few of them had experienced sexual intercourse and therefore distanced themselves from the threat of infection.
- Peer education programme (A PAUSE project South Western Regional Health Authority). Peer education has been introduced into many health promotion initiatives on the basis that teenagers may be more willing to accept information about risky behaviour from their peers than from adults. The above project aimed to work with schools to improve pupils' knowledge, tolerance and respect and to improve contraceptive use for those who were sexually active. Following training the peer leaders led four sessions with a class of pupils in which they directed discussions, role play and group work related to sexual issues. The results of the project indicated that pupils' knowledge, skills and beliefs were positively affected as a result of the peer led sessions. The peer leaders, whilst having some reservations to begin with, especially over the issues of class control, were able to manage the sessions well, developing in confidence and gaining knowledge and skills (Phelps *et al.*, 1994).

Further reading and resources

PLANT, S. (1997) *From Needs to Practice – Effective Sex Education and Training Support.* London: NCB.

SMITH, R. (1997) Promoting the sexual health of young people: part II. *Paediatric Nursing*, **9**, 24–27.

Brook Advisory Centre
165 Gray's Inn Road, London
WC1X 8UD.
Tel: 0171 713 9000.

Contraceptive Education Service
2–12 Pentonville Road, London,
N1 9FD.
Tel: 0171 837 4044.

Activity

Arrange visits to your local schools. Talk to the headmaster and school nurse about their sex education policy. Perhaps you could arrange to observe a sex education session.

Activity

As you read and explore you might find it useful to build up a resource collection. This will be useful to you in your career as a children's nurse and will help you in directing children and their carers to useful information.

SUMMARY

This part of the module has attempted to give you some insight into the types of health promotion activities that have been introduced for children and young people. You should now read and explore how health promotion can influence children's lives with regard to some of the other health issues that you identified earlier on.

Key points ➤

1. Health promotion aimed at children and young people must be appropriate to their developmental stage and to their particular needs.
2. A number of different approaches to health promotion must be used to positively enhance health for young people.
3. It is vital that the public become aware of the risks to the health of young people of today so they can be influential in bringing about change.
4. Health promotion requires a multi-agency approach – child health is everybody's business.
5. Children and young people must be allowed and encouraged to participate in health promotion programmes.
6. Health promotion activities for children and young people must promote empowerment, thus enabling them to make healthy choices about their future lifestyles.

ROLE OF CHILDREN'S NURSES IN CHILD HEALTH PROMOTION 5

INTRODUCTION

The promotion of child health is everybody's business if children are to reach their full health potential. All professionals who have contact with children have a responsibility to identify opportunities for the implementation of health promotion activities not only with individuals but also in the context of the community and society.

Activity

Take a few minutes to identify the professionals who come into contact with children and who you believe have a role to play in promoting child health.

You may have listed the following:

- Children's nurses – in hospital and community
- Public health nurses (health visitors)
- School nurses
- GPs
- Practice nurses
- Social workers
- Teachers
- Dentists
- Nursery nurses, playgroup leaders

The discussion here will concentrate on the role that nurses can play with particular reference to children's nurses in hospital and in the community. The role of other community nurses will also be explored.

BACKGROUND

The idea that nurses were potential leaders in the new health promotion movement was first proposed by Hafdan Mahler (WHO, 1986) the then WHO Director General. He recognised that nurses were in an ideal position to influence health not only with individual patients but also on a more global level. The nursing profession responded:

- Health protection and promotion is top of the list of competencies in Rule 18(a) of the Nurses, Midwives and Health Visitors Act (1979).
- The ENB wrote health promotion into their training and policy recommendations (English National Board, 1985).

Cross references

The role of children's nurses as health educators – page 641

The teacher – page 592

Rule 18 (a)

'... acquire the competencies to: (a) identify the social and health implications of pregnancy and child bearing, physical and mental handicap, disease, disability or ageing for the individual, his or her friends, family and community; and (b) recognise the common factors which contribute to, and adversely affect physical, mental and social well-being of patients and clients and take appropriate action'.

- The Royal College of Nursing (1991) urged nurses to incorporate activities related to the promotion of health and the prevention of disease into their care.
- Educational curricula recognise the importance of health promotion as a nursing function. Diploma level nurse education is based on health and the assumptions that nurses fulfil a health promoting role alongside other roles such as carer, technical expert, counsellor and teacher.

In contrast national policy has not recognised the role that nurses can play in health promotion. The UK Government in its White Paper 'Promoting Better Health' identified the importance of the Primary Health Care team in health promotion work. However, it recognised doctors as the leaders as they were seen as the natural health promoters. This failed to recognise that nurses are probably in a far better position to take opportunities for health promotion because of their sustained contact with patients. Nurses were seen as providers of information and the role they can play in health at community level was ignored. Perhaps this is because the role of the nurse in health promotion, whilst talked about, is unclear in practice.

CHANGING ROLE OF NURSES

Traditionally the nurse's role has been illness-oriented with goals aimed at treating and caring for sick individuals. Little emphasis was placed on teaching about health and, when it was, the outcome was often prescriptive and expert-led. Professional dominance was evident leaving no room for patients to participate in decision making. This approach often failed to recognise the social and environmental background of the individual and health education was often unsuccessful. The style of ward management, task-oriented and hierarchical, did not allow for trusting, supportive relationships between staff and patients to be built up. Moving from this state to one where health promotion is seen as an integral part of a nurse's role, in whatever setting, requires a shift in thinking.

Some studies have looked at how this changing role is being incorporated into the nurse's function with particular emphasis on the hospital setting. Johnston (1988) explored the health promotion activities of hospital-based staff and found that although nurses felt that promoting health was part of their work, they were unsure how to do it. The patients on the other hand recognised that they needed to change their behaviours in order to improve their health and that they expected staff to be good at promoting health. However, only four out of the sample of 50 had been given any advice about their lifestyles. Opportunities for potentially successful health promotion were therefore missed. In 1990, Gott and O'Brien examined nurses' perceptions of their health education role and practice. They found that hospital-based nurses were still locked into routine practices and systems with no evidence of partnership and participation which is essential to successful health promotion. The extent to which health promotion had become integrated into practice was explored by Wilson Barnett and Latter (1993). They found that although the response was positive the focus was on giving information and patient education, again with little recognition of collaboration, participation and empowerment.

FACTORS WHICH FACILITATE AND INHIBIT HEALTH PROMOTION IN HOSPITAL SETTINGS

Before looking at how nurses can effectively incorporate health promotion into their work it is useful to examine some of the factors which inhibit and facilitate health promotion.

Activity

Read the activity, then close the book before you do it. Think for a few minutes about your own health promotion activities with children or adults. Then jot down all the factors which you think influence this part of your work. Which inhibit and which facilitate you?

Compare your thoughts with those presented in Table 5.1

Inhibiting factors	Facilitating factors
Lack of time (Wilson Barnett, 1988)	Team nursing or primary nursing
Heavy workload (Honan et al., 1988)	Supportive ward environment
Staff shortage	Appropriate skill mix
Traditional hierarchical ward management	Provision of sufficient health promotion resources
Disempowered staff	Empowered, autonomous staff (Wilson Barnett and Latter, 1993)
Lack of knowledge (Faulkner and Ward, 1983)	Enhanced knowledge
Short length of patient stay	Facilitative sisters/charge nurses

Table 5.1

Factors that inhibit and facilitate health promotion

Cross references

Team nursing – page 719
Primary nursing – page 719

Now let us examine in more detail why these factors might inhibit or facilitate health promotion. Lack of time is often a factor used to explain non-events. How many times have you used this excuse for not doing something? Linked to heavy workloads and staff shortages it serves as a plausible excuse. The 'care' of patients is of the utmost importance and therefore only what has to be done is done. However, promoting health should be an integral part of the caring for sick children. All too often it is seen as an extra role and therefore it is argued that there is no time to 'do it'. Next time you are looking after a child see if you can incorporate some health promotion into your work. Even discussing health issues with a child or carer while you perform a dressing or monitor an infusion is health promotion.

The method of management can influence the extent to which health promotion is carried out on a ward. The traditional hierarchical structure often leaves staff feeling disempowered and unable to take decisions for themselves. If the staff are disempowered they are not in a position to empower the child/carer. Once the structure changes to a more democratic one with team nursing or primary nursing, staff become more autonomous, decision making is devolved giving a better basis for the formation of trusting, supportive relationships between the nurse and the child/carers. This in turn can facilitate health promotion. Even the child and his/her carer can then be involved in promoting health by giving suggestions on how to improve the ward environment. Supportive, facilitative ward managers can encourage staff to be pro-active and to identify health promoting opportunities.

Activity

Analyse the style of management in your own area of work. Do you feel empowered and autonomous? Identify where changes could be made if necessary to improve opportunities for health promotion by adapting the style of management.

Lack of knowledge of health promotion can lead to a reluctance on the part of the nurse to engage in activities. Faulkner and Ward (1983) found that nurses had a poor knowledge base regarding smoking and that this inhibited their willingness and ability to act as health educators. Enhanced knowledge therefore can facilitate the nurse's role in promoting health as can the provision of sufficient resources.

Activity

How would you describe your own level of knowledge of health issues? Take, for example, the issues related to nutrition. What resources do you have on your ward for health promotion?

THE ROLE IN PERSPECTIVE

We have identified the need for health promotion to be an integral part of the nurse's work. Achieving this will need some shift in thinking, a change in attitudes and an enhanced knowledge about health-related issues. How can you begin to incorporate health promotion into your roles? Using health promotion models can help to see where you might start.

Tannahill's (1985) model of health promotion identifies three overlapping health promoting activities as we have already seen:

- preventive care;
- protection;
- education.

Beattie's (1986) model of health education identified four categories of health education:

- paramedic advice;
- personal growth;
- public agenda setting;
- popular outreach.

By integrating these two models together it is possible to see the huge potential for health promotion within the nurse's work.

Preventive care/education – paramedic advice

This is led by the expert and aimed at the individual. Here the nurse is the expert and uses his/her knowledge to provide information, give advice, teach about and take action aimed at the individual in relation to the three levels of prevention (Table 5.2).

Cross references

Beattie's model – page 138

Tannahill's model – pages 135–136

Primary	Explain the importance of protective precautions to a child and carer confined to a cubicle because of an infectious disease
	Give out a leaflet on immunisation to a young mother
Secondary	Carry out a routine test for phenylketonuria on a 10-day-old baby in your care
	Relay your concerns over a baby's developmental progress to the health visitor
Tertiary	Teach a newly diagnosed diabetic youngster about the complications of diabetes and how to avoid them

Table 5.2

Levels of preventive care/education – paramedic advice

Activity

Using Table 5.2, identify health promotion opportunities within your own field of work related to each level of prevention.

Preventive care – personal growth

This type of health promotion is still individualistic but the children/carers are the experts. In other words the activities are centred around what they think they need, not what the nurse *believes* they need. This can be a difficult thing for the nurse to do as the tradition has been for the nurse to be the expert and to prescribe care. However, with the advent of family-centred care and partnerships in care, the children's nurse should be ready to take this aspect of health promotion on board. Assessment of need, negotiation, an understanding of the child's/carer's perceptions of health and empowerment are the key to making this aspect of health promotion successful.

Activity _____

Using Table 5.2, explain how each situation would be different were it to be child/carer-centred rather than expert-led.

Preventive care/protection/education – public agenda setting

This is expert-led but this time the activities are not aimed at the individual but at communities and/or society in general. You may think that you have a minimal role to play here but in fact children's nurses could and should work together to influence the policy and decision makers. To do so you need to recognise the consequences on health of political forces and policies. The issues relating to health and its promotion must be explored and understood if you are to use your skills to convince others that health is important and that it can be improved by community and social programmes. You and your colleagues, either individually or as a group, can influence health at varying levels from within your own cohort of students to a national level. Working as a group will probably hold more sway at all levels. Table 5.3 gives you some ideas of how you might achieve action.

Table 5.3

Ways of influencing health at various levels

Within your cohort	A small group of students in your cohort smoke; the rest of you decide to use your knowledge and experience to put together a package aimed at changing your colleagues' habits
Within your hospital	You notice that the food presented to the children at meal times is inappropriate and unhealthy; using your knowledge of children and healthy eating you draw up a letter to the catering manager; you get the support of the Ward Manager and other staff

One way of becoming politically active and of influencing health at a local level is to send your concerns, as a knowledgeable professional, to your local councillor or MP. The following activity makes you think about this.

Activity _____

You decide to write to your local councillor regarding the lack of safe and appropriate play areas in your town. What main points would your letter contain and how would you back up your arguments? Who is your local councillor? You could check your answer by arranging an appointment with him/her to discuss ways of influencing action.

Preventive care/protection/education – popular outreach

This type of activity is led by the client and aimed at groups or society. The people themselves identify health issues which need addressing and they lobby the appropriate individual/group. As a children's nurse you may well find yourself joining other members of your community in lobbying for change. Whilst you are using your professional knowledge you are also acting as a consumer/client. Examples include joining action groups for safer packaging of dangerous products, for a reduction in the sugar content of yoghurts or for a change in the law regarding the wearing of cycle helmets by children.

The potential role of the children's nurse in health promotion has been examined and shown to be quite wide. You may find yourself working with the individual child/carer or becoming involved in a much wider arena. Whichever it is you should be actively concerned with the empowerment of children and their carers.

EMPOWERMENT

Empowerment is a valuable tool in the fight for children's health. If, as nurses, we want to increase children's responsibility for their own health then we must make them feel more in control. How can you help to empower the children and carers you work with?

- You must take into account the developmental age and stage of the child and his/her perceptions of health.
- The clinical environment needs to encourage children's participation.
- Acknowledge the important role of the child's carers and ensure that partnership in care actually happens and is not just an ideal theoretical concept.
- Acknowledge children's concerns about their health as valid.
- See children as partners in health promotion – accept that children are capable of representing themselves, making decisions about health and participating in their health care.
- Exchange medical and nursing jargon for a more mutually interactive style of communication, one that children can actually understand.
- Children ought to be made aware of their role and responsibilities within the health care system.
- Be proactive in encouraging empowerment. You should not wait for reaction from the children but should take actions to stimulate response. For example, you could allow the children to be involved in teaching each other about healthy lifestyles. Ask children what they want, rather than tell them. Involve them in the decision making process.

Cross reference

Empowerment – page 141

Activity

Look around the clinical area in which you are working for aspects which (a) encourage participation from the children/carers and (b) dissuade participation.

Ideas for research

- Children's views about health in the context of everyday life
- Children's level of participation in health care
- Children's perceptions of health promotion activities
- Children's understanding of health issues

Some research does exist which shows that children are capable of taking an active role in health and that they actually respond very well. The 'healthy schools' campaign has led to empowered children making changes in schools including recycling programmes, efforts to reduce alcohol, drug abuse and smoking (Kalnins *et al.*, 1992). The campaign strives to give children the opportunity to make decisions and has demonstrated that the children often address health issues that have been ignored by adults. Empowering children through education has been shown to be successful enabling children to actively take part in self-care and to encourage the adoption of healthy behaviours (Botvin and McAlister, and Lewis and Lewis, cited in Igoe, 1990). Perhaps you are required to undertake a research project in your studies. This may be one of the areas which you could consider.

THE ROLE OF THE HEALTH VISITOR (PUBLIC HEALTH NURSE)

Public health work within primary care consists of:

- health profiling of the community and practice population;
- the identification of groups with health needs;
- action to meet health needs;
- collaborative action with other agencies;
- facilitating community participation and action;
- evaluating health care interventions.

This work is closely linked with and interdependent on, work with individuals. The role of the health visitor has, in the past, been concentrated on work with families and children and the challenge now is to combine this work with the public health work identified above.

The health visitor is in an ideal position to contribute to community health particularly in relation to children and families. The health visitor is the key community worker in the preventive child health services and the main health advisor during childhood, able to implement health promotion activities with children and mothers either through home visits or through child health clinics. Within the role health visitors can take part in health promotion aimed at individuals and at communities, mainly in the area of prevention and protection. Health visitors are in an ideal position to influence policies affecting child health at national and local level by:

- linking into pressure groups;
- lobbying professional bodies;
- contacting local councillors and MPs;
- linking with other concerned professionals, voluntary groups (Luker and Orr, 1992).

Important aspects of the health visitors role include:
- anticipating in child health surveillance (based on recommendations of the Hall Report, Hall, 1991);
- the provision of health education, proactive advice and ongoing support to parents;
- identification of children with special needs, assisting and supporting parents;
- participating in ensuring that immunisations are taken up;
- following up children who have had serious illness, liaising with the GP.

THE ROLE OF THE SCHOOL NURSE

School nurses play a key role in supervising the health care of children at school, liaising with teachers, parents and health care professionals. They play a central role, within the school health team, in promoting children's health and taking forward the Government's *Health of the Nation* agenda. The school nurse can be highly influential in broadening a school's approach to health, developing trusting and confidential relationships with children. The early interventions of school nurses can be vital in the detection of disabling health problems, e.g. asthma and anorexia, and they play a vital role in identifying child abuse.

The importance of the school nurse was recognised by the UKCC (1994) in its strategy for post-registration education and training, meaning that school nurses take their place alongside other specialist community health care nurses. Recent doubts over the future of the school nursing service have also been tempered by the recognition of the need for further research into school nursing practice, identifying what school nurses do and clarifying roles. It has been suggested that the school nurse should be the leader of the school health service, taking the lead in the screening process, a role that has until now been fulfilled by the school doctor. The potential for the work of the school nurse is huge and could be developed to expand the surveillance and health promoting role. The school nurse is in an ideal position to empower children within the healthy schools campaign. In many instances school nurses have been involved with setting up support groups for teachers who want to give up smoking, promoting healthy eating policies and encouraging exercise among children.

The role of the school nurse involves:

- health promotion normally integrated naturally into the curriculum, e.g. sex education, HIV and AIDS, family planning, smoking and health, alcohol and drugs, exercise;
- inspecting the hygienic conditions of the school periodically;
- participating in immunisations – the use of the school nursing system to immunise children against a threatened measles epidemic in 1994 helped to flag up the importance of having a service that reaches all schoolchildren quickly;
- participating in investigating communicable diseases in the school;
- participating in surveillance programmes;
- acting as an advocate for the children and enhancing empowerment;
- fulfilling an occupational health role with education staff.

In the same way as health visitors, school nurses can play a vital role in influencing health policies which affect children in today's society particularly at a local level but also at national level.

Activity

Analyse changes in the school nurse structure and the effects on the service which have occurred in recent months and years.

Key points ➤

1. The nurse is in an ideal position to influence health on an individual and global level.
2. Health promotion needs to be an integral part of a nurse's role.
3. The factors which facilitate health promotion within the nurse's role should be identified and enhanced.
4. Empowerment is a valuable tool in the fight for children's health.
5. Health professionals working with children must be proactive in empowering children and families.

ASPECTS OF HEALTH IN CHILDHOOD 6

INTRODUCTION

In order for the children's nurse to promote health and healthy behaviours in children it is important to understand some of the key issues related to such behaviours. The purpose of this part of the module is to examine some of these issues in relation to:

- Nutrition
- Dental hygiene
- Immunisation

'Children are people. They grow into tomorrow only as they live today'.

John Dewey

NUTRITION

The nutritional status of children has been briefly reviewed previously. Nelson (1993) concluded from a number of studies carried out since 1979 that 'the diets of schoolchildren are too high in fat, especially saturated fat, and in sugar. They are too low in iron, calcium, dietary fibre and probably in anti-oxidant vitamins such as vitamin E'. The *Health of the Nation* (DoH, 1992) identified diet and nutrition as one of the risk-factor targets for strategies in the UK. Dietary habits formed during childhood may be a factor contributing to the onset of diet-related disease in later life (heart disease and stroke). The *Health of the Nation* targets for diet and nutrition are as follows:

Cross reference

Nutrition – page 124

- To reduce the average percentage of food energy derived by the population from saturated fatty acids by at least 35% by 2005.
- To reduce the average percentage of food energy derived by the population from total fat by at least 12% by 2005.
- To reduce the proportion of men and women aged 16–64 who are obese by at least 25 and 33%, respectively, by 2005.

These targets therefore serve as a starting point from which to consider current views on diet and health in children and young people.

INFANT NUTRITION

Breast milk is the best source of nourishment in the early months of life (DoH, 1994) but it must be recognised that there are mothers who for many reasons are unable to breastfeed. Whilst every effort should be made to encourage mothers to breast-feed for at least 4 months, those who choose not to should be supported in carrying out successful bottle feeding and should not be made to feel inadequate or guilty.

Useful contacts

Association of Breastfeeding Mothers
7 Maybourne Close, London
SE 26 6HQ.
Tel: 0181 778 4769.

La Leche League (GB)
BM 3424, London WC1N 3XX.
Tel: 0171 242 1278.

National Childbirth Trust
Alexandra House, Oldham Terrace,
Acton, London W3 6NH.
Tel: 0181 992 8637.

See *Successful Breastfeeding* (Royal
College of Midwives, 1991). This
small book contains a wealth of well
researched information and many
excellent references for further
reading. It would be useful to have
on your ward

Breastfeeding

Ten facts about breastmilk:

1. The fat content of breastmilk increases as the breast empties.
2. The composition of breastmilk is influenced by the stage of lactation.
3. The mean energy value of human milk is 60–70 kcal/100 ml (Lucas *et al.*, 1985).
4. The fat in human milk is well absorbed.
5. Breastmilk has a lower concentration of protein than other milks with low casein.
6. A high proportion of the whey fraction contains immunologically active proteins which enable the absorption of iron and inhibit the growth of micro-organisms.
7. Passive transfer of immunoglobulins G and M occur during feeding, and breastmilk cells produce immunoglobulin A.
8. Breastmilk alone does not provide sufficient iron, copper and zinc from 6 months of age.
9. Breastmilk is easily digested and contains enzymes which reduce the risk of gastro-intestinal and respiratory infections (Howie, 1990).
10. Breastmilk possibly reduces the risk of gastro-intestinal disorders (e.g. Crohn's and coeliac disease).

In encouraging mothers to breastfeed consideration should be given to the following points:

- Babies should be put to the breast immediately after birth.
- Breastfed babies should be left with their mothers and not removed to the nursery at night. However, it is important to be available to give support during the night. Personal experience of being left with a new baby in the middle of the night without any support served to stress the importance of this for the author.
- Breastfed babies should not normally be given complementary bottle feeds. This will only serve to lessen the supply of breastmilk. Remember, the more a baby sucks, the more milk will be produced. So, if the milk supply is inadequate, increase the frequency of feeding and ensure the mother's intake of fluid and nutrients is adequate.
- Additional water is rarely needed by breastfed babies even in hot weather.
- The mother must be shown how to position the baby for feeding ensuring that the whole of the nipple and areola is taken into the baby's mouth. The baby must be facing the mother's breast (chest to chest) not looking upwards (Figure 6.1). If this position is adopted painful nipples can be avoided.
- Allow the baby to feed on demand. This increases the supply of milk.

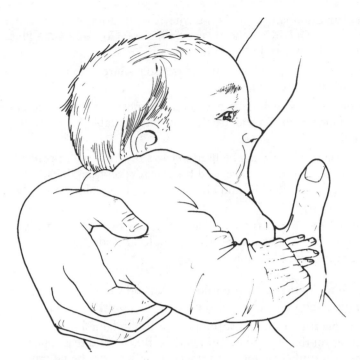

Figure 6.1
Correct position for breastfeeding

- It is a fallacy that breastfed babies do not get wind. Some may do and will need winding in the normal way.
- Support for breastfeeding mothers is always available from the National Childbirth Trust, the La Leche League (GB) and the Association of Breastfeeding Mothers (see list of addresses in the box at the top of the previous page.

Bottle-feeding

Infants who are not breastfed should be given infant formula or follow-on milk although follow-on milk is not recommended for the first 6 months (DoH, 1992b). The range of infant formulas available is wide with the choice of dry powder or ready made bottles/cartons.

Ten facts about infant formulas:

1. Guidelines for the composition of infant formulas were agreed in 1991 in a European Commission Directive.
2. Essential fatty acid alpha linoleic acid is added to infant formula in the UK.
3. Absorption of some minerals from infant formula is less efficient than from human milk therefore levels of iron, zinc and vitamin D are increased to overcome poor bioavailability.
4. The carbohydrate most commonly used is lactose.
5. Whey dominant formula have a whey:casein ratio similar to human milk. Examples include Cow and Gate Premium, Farley's First Milk, Milupa Aptamil and SMA Gold.

6. In casein dominant formula the whey:casein ration is approximately the same as in cow's milk. Examples include Cow and Gate Plus, Milupa Milumil and SMA White.

7. Infant formulas provide a satisfactory sole source of nutrients in the first 4–6 months of life.

8. Follow-on milks generally have higher concentrations of protein than infant formulas and are therefore not suitable for the younger infant.

9. Soya infant formula can be used in cases of cow's milk protein allergy, lactose intolerance, and for vegan/vegetarian diets. Examples include Cow and Gate Infasoy, Mead Johnson Prosbee, and SMA Wysoy.

10. Lactose-free formulas are available and may be used in a variety of conditions, e.g. gastro-enteritis. Examples include Mead Johnson Pregestimil and Nutramigen.

In teaching mothers about bottle-feeding and supporting them consideration should be given to the following points:

- The preparation of infant formula must be explained with special emphasis on the importance of hygiene. Bottles and teats must be washed carefully to remove all traces of milk before being immersed in a sterilising solution. If salt is used to wash the teats care must be taken to ensure that all traces of salt are removed in order to avoid hypernatreamia.

- Enough bottle feeds for 24 hours can be made up in one batch providing they are cooled immediately and placed in the refrigerator.

- Once heated, milk must not be reheated but should be discarded.

- In making up the feeds care must be taken to ensure the correct amount of boiled water is added to the appropriate amount of powder. The general rule is one scoop of formula to 1 fluid ounce of water. If the concentration of formula is too high hypernatreamia can result. A weak solution will lead to failure to thrive.

- Freshly boiled water should be used. Using water that has been repeatedly boiled can result in an overconcentration of minerals.

- Babies must never be left alone with a bottle because of the danger of choking. Encourage mothers to hold babies for bottle-feeding just as they would if they were breastfeeding.

- Bottles of milk should not be warmed in a microwave oven. The distribution of heat is uneven and the baby can be severely burnt by the milk.

- When feeding with a bottle ensure that the teat remains full of milk to avoid the ingestion of too much air.

- Babies will probably need winding during feeds although this will depend very much on the individual baby. Simply sitting the baby up and gently massaging the back is generally all that is needed. Avoid banging his/her back, this is not necessary.

Weaning

Weaning is defined by the DoH (1994) as the 'process of expanding the diet to include food and drinks other than breast milk or infant formula'. It enables infants to meet their changing nutritional requirements at a time of rapid growth. The DoH (1994) recommends that weaning should begin no earlier than 4 months and no later than 6 months of age. By this time the infant's nutritional requirements can no longer be met by milk alone which gives insufficient energy, protein and vitamins A and D. The infant's iron stores also become depleted at this age and additional sources are needed. By the age of 4 months the infant has developed sufficient neuromuscular coordination to allow him to eat solid food and the renal and digestive systems have matured enough to cope with a varied diet.

The 1994 Coma Report (DoH, 1994) makes several recommendations regarding the content of the weaning diet:

- The provision of adequate dietary energy is essential to ensure normal growth and development (Table 6.1).
- An adequate intake of protein with a proper balance of amino acids is essential (Table 6.2).
- As fat provides the major energy source for infants any reduction is likely to give rise to a diet of lower energy density. It is therefore advised that fat reduction should not be considered for children under 2. Semi-skimmed milk can be given after 2 years and skimmed milk after the age of 5. The report recommends a flexible approach to the reduction of fat between the ages of 2 and 5.
- The intake of non-milk extrinsic sugars (added sugars, sugars in fruit juices and honey) should contribute no more than about 10% of total dietary energy. Sugars provide energy but make no other contribution to nutritional needs.
- If energy intake is adequate the amount of starch in the diet should increase as fat decreases.
- Adequate intakes of iron and calcium are essential. The report acknowledges that iron deficiency is the most commonly reported nutritional disorder during early childhood in the UK and other countries. Iron deficiency anaemia is associated with psychomotor delay, apathy and reduced exercise capacity.
- Adequate vitamin intake should be encouraged through a varied diet and moderate exposure to summer sunlight. Vitamin A and D supplements should be given: from 6 months of age where breastmilk is the main drink, to bottle-fed babies if intake is less than 500 ml per day, to bottle-fed babies on cow's milk and to all infants aged 1–5 years unless it is certain vitamin status is adequate.

Weaning

Start weaning no earlier than 3–4 months because before this age:

- babies have poor head control and effective positioning for feeding is difficult
- babies cannot easily form a bolus to move solid food from the front of the mouth to the back
- limited renal function means that water is not conserved efficiently and large solute concentrations cannot be dealt with
- the secretion of intestinal and pancreatic enzymes is not fully developed in the young infant

Weaning

Start weaning no later than 6 months because after this time:

- it may be difficult to teach the baby to chew lumpy foods
- the baby is more likely to refuse foods
- the baby will become underweight and fail to thrive as nutritional needs will not be met

PART ONE Health in Childhood

Table 6.1

Energy requirements for children aged 0–24 months

Age (months)	Energy intake per kg body weight (kJ (kcal) kg/day)
1	480 (115)
3	420 (100)
6	400 (95)
9	400 (95)
12	400 (95)
18	400 (95)
24	400 (95)

Adapted from DoH (1994).

Table 6.2

Recommended protein intake for children aged 0–24 months

Age (months)	Protein intake (g/day)
0–3	12.5
4–6	12.7
7–9	13.7
10–12	14.9
13–24	14.5

Adapted from DoH (1994).

Religious, cultural beliefs and diet

Judaism
- avoidance of pork, shellfish
- foods prepared by special 'kosher' methods
- meat products kept separate from dairy products at all stages of preparation, eating and cleaning up

Islam
- avoidance of pork
- foods either 'haram' (unlawful) or 'hallal' (lawful).
- food prepared by ' hallal' methods
- Ramadan – month long abstinence from food during daylight hours – not practised by children

Hinduism
- may be strict lactovegetarians
- pork (unclean) and meat from cows (sacred) avoided
- milk and ghee (clarified butter) sacred foods
- dairy products usually important part of diet

Rastafarianism
- variable dietary restrictions
- may follow vegan diets
- preserved foods are chemical and avoided

Sikism
- sometimes vegetarians
- pork and beef usually avoided
- meat if eaten must NOT have been bled but killed by stunning 'jhatka'

- Milk or water should constitute the majority of drinks given.

Table 6.3 gives a guide to the foods to use during weaning. It must be remembered that each child is an individual and the diet will need to be flexible in order to meet nutritional requirements as well as any cultural, religious beliefs.

Practical hints for successful weaning are:

- Be flexible, patient and calm. Allow the infant to progress at his own rate in a relaxed and happy environment. Do not force an infant to eat solids but be encouraging and supportive. Do not be afraid to back track. Pick meal times when other members of the family are not demanding attention, e.g. the midday meal. Introduce one new food at a time. Avoid undue praise or punishment during the weaning process. Above all try to make meal times enjoyable.

- Show tolerance. Accept that the infant is an individual and do not impose your tastes on him. Do not force infants (or children) to 'eat up'. Accept food refusal without fuss or try to ignore it. Do not expect a high standard of table manners. Instead prepare the eating area appropriately, e.g. put a plastic cloth under the high chair. Try to tolerate the mess and spills but gently encourage good eating habits as time progresses (Figure 6.2).

- Use appropriate utensils. Ensure that the infant is sitting comfortably in a chair (restrained) or on your knee. Use plastic teaspoons, offer finger foods, use cups with lids. Do not add solid foods to bottles. Never leave an infant alone at meal times.

- Offer a variety from the four main food groups (in a texture appropriate for the infant's age): meat, fish, eggs, beans, pulses; bread, cereals, rice, pasta; fruit and vegetables; and milk and milk

182

Table 6.3 A guide to foods during weaning

Food	4–6 months	6–9 months	9–12 months	After 1 year
Milk	Breast or infant formula	Breastmilk, infant formula or follow-on milk	Breast milk, infant milks	Whole milk as a drink
Dairy products and substitutes	Cow's milk in weaning, e.g. yogurt, custard	Hard cheese cubed or grated as finger food		Soft cheese; low fat milk in cooking
Starchy foods	Low fibre smooth cereals Mash or pureed starchy vegetables	Two to three servings daily introduce wholemeal bread and cereals Foods with a 'lumpier' texture Toast as finger food	Three to four servings daily Encourage wholemeal foods Discourage biscuits and cakes Starchy foods can be normal adult texture	Minimum of four servings daily At least one serving at each mealtime Discourage high fat starchy foods, e.g. crisps and pastry
Vegetables and fruit	Smoothly pureed soft cooked vegetables and fruit	Two servings daily Introduce raw soft fruit, e.g. bananas, melon, tomato Cooked vegetables can be coarser	Three to four servings daily Encourage lightly cooked or raw fruit and vegetables Unsweetened orange juice with meals	Minimum of four servings daily Foods can be adult texture though some fibrous foods may be difficult, e.g. celery
Meat and meat alternatives	Soft cooked meat/pulses Add no salt or sugar to food during cooking or after	One serving daily Soft cooked minced or pureed meat/fish/pulses	Minimum of one serving daily from animal source OR two from vegetable source In vegetarian diet use mixture of vegetables and starchy foods, e.g. macaroni cheese	Minimum of one serving daily or two from vegetable source Encourage low fat meat and oily fish (sardine, herring) Liver pate after 1 year
Occasional foods	Low sugar desserts, e.g. yogurts Avoid high salt foods	Encourage savoury rather than sweet foods Fruit juice not necessary; try to restrict to mealtimes – offer water or milk	Moderate amounts of butter, margarine Small amounts of jam on bread Limit salty foods	Limit crisps and savoury snacks Give bread, fruit between meals Do not add sugar to drinks Limit soft drinks to mealtimes Encourage pattern of three meals a day Discourage frequent snacking on fatty or sugary foods

Adapted from DoH (1994).

Figure 6.2

Tolerate the mess!

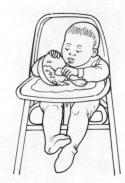

products. Giving a range of foods, either home-prepared or commercially produced, broadens the infant's experience of tastes and will encourage acceptance of a varied diet.

Activity

Making use of the above points, plan a day's menu for:

- a 5-month-old infant;
- an 11-month-old infant whose parents wish to bring up as a vegetarian;
- a 2-year-old toddler.

Healthy eating during childhood

Children's diets are influenced by many factors including their attitude to food, knowledge and understanding of food and nutrition, parental attitudes to eating, and media advertising. If they are to develop healthy eating habits in adulthood they must be given the opportunity to learn and explore the requirements of a healthy diet. The general advice to young people regarding their diet should be (HEA, 1995):

- Enjoy your food.
- Eat a variety of different foods, including starchy foods; meat/alternatives, fish and eggs; fruit and vegetables; dairy products.
- Eat the right amount to be healthy.
- Do not eat too much fat.
- Do not eat sugary foods too often.
- Eat plenty of foods rich in fibre and starch. Meals should be based on fibre-rich starchy foods, bread, pasta, potatoes, rice.
- Look after the minerals and vitamins in your food. Girls particularly need good sources of iron and calcium.

Cross reference

Dental health – page 123

DENTAL HYGIENE

Recent reports show that children's oral health is improving (Todd and Dodd, 1994) with 40% of 15 year olds free from tooth decay (dental caries) in 1993 compared with only 8% in 1983. However, half the children in England still experience caries in their permanent teeth by the age of 15. Children's nurses are in an ideal position to give advice and education regarding dental health in hospital or in the community. Dental caries can be prevented by:

- A diet low in sugar. It has been shown that the frequency of consumption of non-milk extrinsic sugars is the most important factor in the development of dental disease (HEA, 1982). Every time that sugar is consumed acid is generated in dental plaque within seconds. Within 1–2 minutes the pH has fallen allowing enamel dissolution to occur. The return to a neutral pH can take from 20 minutes to 2 hours. Therefore, if consumption of sugars occurs frequently, there is no time for the plaque pH to recover. It is therefore advisable to limit sugary foods and drinks to mealtimes and to avoid sugary snacks between meals. Children should be encouraged to quench their thirst with water.

- Effective teeth cleaning. Teeth are at risk of dental decay as soon as they appear, plaque can form readily covering the teeth with a sticky bacterial coating. The first tooth generally appears between 6 and 9 months and it is vital that effective teeth cleaning begins straight away. The role of toothbrushing is to remove the plaque. In the young infant this can be done with special toothbrushes and a pea sized amount of fluoride toothpaste. This can easily be carried out by holding the infant on the lap with his back resting on the carer's chest. Hold the chin gently with one hand and brush with the other. Every surface of every tooth must be brushed with special attention to the area between the tooth and gums. Children generally need assistance with brushing until about 8 years of age. Brushing should be done twice a day but particularly at night.

- The use of fluoride. Fluoride is a mineral which inhibits the demineralisation of enamel and can strengthen teeth against caries making them more resistance to acid attack. Fluoride is present in drinking water in some areas. Fluoride can also be used topically by using a fluoride toothpaste or can be given as a supplement in the form of drops or tablets. However, these supplements must be taken daily from the age of about 6 months through to adolescence and compliance with this may be difficult. The amount of supplement given will depend on the amount of fluoride in the water supply and advice should always be sought from the dentist. If the local water supply is already well fluoridated overdosage of fluoride can occur giving rise to staining of the teeth.

- Encouraging regular dental attendance. Babies can be registered with a dentist from birth. Mothers should be encouraged to take babies and children with them when they attend for check ups to help build up confidence and trust in the dentist. Regular attendance also makes the detection of problems easier.

Approximate ages at which teeth emerge

Deciduous teeth
- incisors — 6–9 months
- canines — 16–18 months
- 1st molars — 12–14 months
- 2nd molars — 20–30 months

Permanent teeth
- lower incisors — 6–8 years
- upper incisors — 7–9 years
- lower canines — 9–10 years
- upper canines — 11–12 years
- premolars — 9–12 years
- 1st molar — 6–7 years
- 2nd molar — 11–13 years
- 3rd molars — 17–21 years

Dental health resources

British Dental Health Association
Eastlands Court, St. Peter's Road, Rugby, Warwickshire CV21 3QP
Tel: 01788 546365

Brochures
Caring for your teeth and gums
Don't be afraid
Your guide to a better smile

Leaflets
Dental care for mother and baby
Preventive care and oral hygiene
Visiting the dentist

General Dental Council
37 Wimpole Street, London W1M 8DQ
Tel: 0171 486 2171

Leaflets
Diet and your child's teeth
Healthy mouth, happy smile
Danger mouse, tooth sleuth
Wallcharts and posters

Packs
Dental discovery kit teaching pack for 12–15 year olds

British Association for Toothfriendly Sweets
64 Wimpole Street, London W1

Chuck Sweets Off the Checkout Campaign
Iona Smeaton, Chief Community Dietician, c/o The Wislon Hospital, Cranmer Road, Mitcham, Surrey CR4 4TP

Activity

Find out the level of fluoride in your local water supply by contacting the relevant water authority. Do children in your area need fluoride supplements?

IMMUNISATION

Cross reference

Immunisation – page 126

In 1994 immunisation uptake rates were at an all time high and accompanied by an overall reduction in the incidence of infectious diseases. However, as infectious diseases become less prevalent carers may become more concerned with the possible associated risks of immunisation. These may appear to be greater than the risk of contracting a relatively rare disease. If this occurs immunisation uptake rates may well fall with a subsequent increase in the incidence of diseases again. It is essential therefore that children's nurses are able to contribute to the maintenance of the uptake rates by giving accurate and informed information to parents. Immunisations are available against eight infectious diseases:

- diptheria
- measles
- polio
- tetanus
- pertussis
- rubella
- mumps

Cross reference

Immunisation schedule– page 498

- Haemophilus influenza type B infections (HIB)

Immunisation against tuberculosis depends on local policy.

Answering questions commonly asked by parents

- *What is the possibility of my child having a severe reaction to immunisation?* Severe reactions are rare. From 1978 to 1989, 118 anaphylactic reactions were reported out of a total of about 25 million immunisations (DoH, 1992b). Encephalitis following MMR affects less than 1 in a million whereas one in 5000 children suffering a natural measles infection develop complications (HEA, 1993). The incidence of febrile convulsions following DTP is limited to the third dose only and affects one in 12 500 (HEA, 1993). Death or brain damage from the pertussis vaccine occurs very rarely if at all (Griffin *et al.*, 1990; Miller *et al.*, 1993).
- *There are no serious side effects of the HIB vaccine?* One child in 10 has some redness and swelling but this subsides after about 2–3 days (Thompson, 1995).
- *My child is adopted and we do not know his family history. Should we have him vaccinated?* Yes, he should receive all vaccinations appropriate to his age unless there is reason to believe that he may be HIV-positive. In this case contact the adoption agency.

- *I had a bad reaction to my vaccinations. Should my daughter still be vaccinated?* There is no real evidence to suggest that reactions run in families therefore you should go ahead with vaccination.

- *My child has had an infectious disease. Should he still be vaccinated against it?* Only if there is microbiological proof that he has had the disease. There is no harm in him being vaccinated against a disease that he has already had.

- *My baby was born prematurely. Should the timing of his vaccinations be altered to compensate?* No, the timing of vaccinations starts from birth, not the expected date of delivery.

Contra-indications

There are very few contra-indications to vaccination and it is important to dispel any myths that surround this subject. The true contra-indications are:

- Acute illness with fever or systemic upset. Vaccination should be postponed until the child is well. Minor illness without a fever is NOT a reason for withholding vaccination.

- Children who have previously had an anaphylactic shock should only be given vaccinations under hospital supervision if at all. Minor allergic reactions, e.g. to eggs or antibiotics, are NOT relevant.

- If a child is immunocompromised or HIV-positive he should be referred to his consultant for advice.

- Household contacts of children who are immuno-supressed should be given inactivated polio vaccine instead of the oral vaccine because the former is not transmissible.

- Pertussis vaccine should not be given to children who have had a severe systemic or local reaction to a previous dose.

- Children with cerebral damage, idiopathic epilepsy, convulsions have an increased risk of a febrile convulsion after vaccination against pertussis, measles, mumps and rubella. However, they are not at any greater risk for severe reactions and should be vaccinated.

Vaccinations should not be withheld due to asthma, eczema, hayfever, snuffles, failure to thrive, cerebral palsy, Down's syndrome, history of neonatal jaundice (Hall *et al.*, 1994).

➤ **Key points**

1. Children's nurses have a major role to play in promoting healthy behaviours in children and as such need to keep abreast of issues relating to health.
2. Dietary habits formed in childhood may be a factor contributing to the onset of diet-related disease in adulthood.
3. The message to carers and children about healthy eating should be 'eat a variety of foodstuffs from the four main groups, cut down

on sugar and fat, and ensure adequate intakes of fibre, starch and vitamins'.

4. Although the dental health of children is improving, half of all children have experienced dental decay by the time they are 15.

5. Dental caries can be prevented by: low sugar diet, effective teeth cleaning, fluoridation and regular dental checks.

6. Children's nurses play a major role in maintaining high uptake rates of vaccinations by giving accurate and informed advice to parents and carers.

References

ACHESON, D. (1991) The health divide. *The Guardian*, 13 September.

ASHTON, J. and SEYMOUR, H. (1988) *The New Public Health*. Milton Keynes: Open University Press.

AVERY, J. C. and JACKSON, R. H. (1993) *Children and their Accidents*. London: Edward Arnold.

BEATTIE, A. (1986) A mapping of health education. *Radical Health Promotion*, Issue 4.

BEDFORD, H. (1993) Immunisation facts and figures. *Health Visitor*, 66, 314–316.

BEISCHON, M. (1993) Preparing for the unexpected. *Health Lines*, September, 12–14.

BELLEW, B. and WAYNE, D. (1991) Prevention of smoking among schoolchildren: a review of research and recommendations. *Health Education Journal*, 50, 3–8.

BIBACE, R. and WALSH, M. E. (1980) Children's concepts of illness. *Pediatrics*, 66, 912–917.

BLAXTER, M. (1990) *Health and Lifestyles*. London: Routledge.

BOTTING, B. (ed.) (1995) *The Health of our Children. Decennial Supplement*. London: OPCS.

BOTVIN, G. and McALISTER, A. (1990) cited by IGOE, J. Healthier children through empowerment. In WILSON BARNETT, J. and MACLEOD CLARK, J. (eds), *Research in Health Promotion and Nursing*. Basingstoke: Macmillan.

BOWIE, C. and FORD, N. (1989) Sexual behaviour of young people and the risk of HIV infection. *Journal of Epidemiology and Community Health*, 43, 61–65.

BRITTON, M. (1989) Mortality and geography. *Population Trends*, 56, 16–23.

BRYAN-BROWN, K. (1994) *The Effectiveness of the General Accident Eastern Region Children's Traffic Club*. Crowthorne: Transport Research Laboratory.

BURNEY, P. G. J., CHINN, S. and RONA, R. J. (1990) Has the prevalence of asthma increased in children? Evidence from the national study of health and growth 1973–86. *British Medical Journal*, 300, 1306–1309.

BUTLER, N. R. and GOLDING, J. (1986) *From Birth to Five*. Oxford: Pergamon Press.

CHARLTON, A. (1986) Evaluation of a family linked smoking programme in primary schools. *Health Education Journal*, 45, 140–144.

CHARLTON, A. and BLAIR, V. (1989) Absence from school related to children's and adults' smoking habits. *British Medical Journal*, 298, 90–92.

CHEN, Y., LI, W. and YU, S. (1986) Influence of passive smoking on admissions for respiratory illness in early childhood. *British Medical Journal*, **293**, 303–306.

COLLEY, J. R. T., HOLLAND, W. W. and CORKHILL, R. T. (1974) Influence of passive smoking and parental phlegm on pneumonia and bronchitis in early childhood. *Lancet*, **ii**, 1031–1034.

CONSTANTINIDES, P. (1987) *The Management Response to Childhood Accidents*. London: King's Fund.

CREW, K. and FLETCHER, J. (1995) Empowering parents to prevent childhood accidents. *Health Visitor*, **68**, 291.

CSO (1996) *Social Trends 26*. London: HMSO.

DAVIE, R. (1993) The impact of the National Child Development Study. *Children and Society*, 7, 20–36.

DENMAN, S., PEARSON, J., MOODY, D., DAVIS, P. and MADELEY, R. (1995) Theatre in education on HIV and AIDS: a controlled study of schoolchildren's knowledge and attitudes. *Health Education Journal*, 54, 3–17.

DIELMAN, T. E., LEECH, S. L., BECKER, M. H., ROSENSTOCK, I. M and HORVATH, W. J. (1980) Dimensions of children's health beliefs. *Health Education Quarterly*, 7, 219–238.

DoE (1993) *English House Conditions Survey 1991 – Preliminary Report on Unfit Dwellings*. HMSO: London.

DoH (1970) *Government White Paper on Pollution Control*. London: HMSO.

DoH (1989) *The Diet of British School Children*. London: HMSO.

DoH (1992a) *The Health of the Nation: A Strategy for Health in England*. London: HMSO.

DoH (1992b) *Immunisation against Infectious Diseases (The Green Book)*. London: HMSO.

DoH (1993) *Key Area Handbook – HIV/AIDS and Sexual Health*. London: HMSO.

DoH (1994) *Weaning and the Weaning Diet: Report of the Working Group on the Weaning Diet of the Committee on Medical Aspects of Food Policy*. London: HMSO.

DOWNIE, R. S., FYFE, C. and TANNAHILL, A. (1990) *Health Promotion Models and Values*. Oxford: Oxford University Press.

DOWNING, C. S., MURRAY, G. and DUROW, C. (1991) *Trials of a Road Safety Booklet for a Pre-school Traffic Club*. Crowthorne: Transport Research Laboratory.

DOYLE, W., JENKINS, S., CRAWFORD, M. A. and PUVANDERDRAN, K. (1994) Nutritional status of schoolchildren in an inner city area. *Archives of Disease in Childhood*, **70**, 376–381.

DSS (1993) *Social Security Statistics*. London: HMSO.

DTI (1992) *Home and Leisure Accident Research 1989 Data: 13th Annual Report of the Home Accident Surveillance System*. London: DTI.

EISER, C., PATTERSON, P. and EISER, J. R. (1983) Children's knowledge of health and illness: implications for health education. *Child Care, Health and Development*, 9, 285–292.

ENGLISH NATIONAL BOARD (1985) *Consultation Paper: 'Professional Education/Training Courses'*. London: English National Board.

FAULKNER, A. and WARD, L. (1983) Nurses as health educators in relation to smoking. *Nursing Times*, **79** (8), 47–48.

FERGUSSON, D. M., HARWOOD, L. J. and SHANNON, F. T. (1980) Parental smoking and respiratory illness in infancy. *Archive of Diseases in Children*, 55, 358–361.

FORD, N. and MORGAN, K. (1989) Heterosexual lifestyles of young people in an English city. *Journal of Population and Social Studies*, **1**, 167–182.

FRANCIS, B. (1994) The incidence of HIV/AIDS in children and their care needs. *Nursing Times*, **90** (26), 47–49.

FRASER, F. C. (1974) Genetic counselling. *American Journal of Human Genetics*, **26**, 636.

GAUDION, C. (1997) Children's knowledge of their internal anatomy. *Paediatric Nursing*, **9** (5), 14–17.

GIBSON, C. (1991) A concept analysis of empowerment. *Journal of Advanced Nursing*, **16**, 354–361.

GILBERT, R. (1994) The changing epidemiology of SIDS. *Archives of Disease in Childhood*, **70**, 445–449.

GOLDING, J. (1993) Parental smoking and sudden infant death syndrome. In CHIEF MEDICAL OFFICERS EXPERT GROUP (eds), *The Sleeping Position of Infants and Cot Death*. London: HMSO.

GOTT, M. and O'BRIEN, M. (1990) *The Role of the Nurse in Health Promotion: Policies, Perspectives and Practice*. London: DoH.

GRIFFEN, M. R. *et al.* (1990) Risk of seizures and encephalopathy after immunisation with diphtheria–tetanus–pertussis vaccine. *Journal of the American Medical Association*, **263**, 164–165.

HALL, D. M. B. (1991) *Health for All Children*. Oxford: Oxford Medical Publications.

HALL, D., HILL, P. and ELLIMAN, D. (1994) *The Child Surveillance Handbook*, 2nd edn. Oxford: Radcliffe Medical Press.

HANNA, K. M. (1989) The meaning of health for graduate nursing students. *Journal of Nursing Education*, **28**, 372–376.

HEA (1982) *The Scientific Basis of Dental Health Education*, 3rd edn. London: HEA.

HEA (1993) *A Guide to Childhood Immunisations*. London: HEA.

HEA (1995) *Diet and Health in School Age Children*. London: HEA.

HINDS, K. and GREGORY, J. R. (1995) *National Diet and Nutrition Survey: Children Aged 1–4 years. Volume 2: Report of the Dental Survey*. London: HMSO.

HMSO (1991) *The Health of the Nation: A Consultative Document for Health in England*. London: HMSO.

HONAN, S., KRSNAK, G., PETERSON, D. and TORKELSON, R. (1988) The nurse as patient educator: perceived responsibilites and factors enhancing role development. *Journal of Continuing Education in Nursing*, **19**, 33–37.

HOUSE OF COMMONS (1993) *Hansard*, 27 July, col. 1010 and 18 October 1993. London: House of Commons.

HOWIE, P. W., FORSYTH, J. S., OGSTON, S. A., CLARK, A. and FLOFY, C. du V. (1990) Protective effect of breastfeeding against infection. *British Medical Journal*, **300**, 11–16.

IGOE, J. (1990) Healthier children through empowerment. In WILSON BARNETT, J. and MACLEOD CLARK, J. (eds), *Research in Health Promotion and Nursing*. Basingstoke: Macmillan.

JARVIS, M. J., RUSSELL, M. A. H. and FEYERABEND, C. (1985) Passive exposure to tobacco smoke: saliva cotinine concentrations in a representative sample of non-smoking children. *British Medical Journal*, **291**, 927–929.

JARVIS, S., TOWNER, E., and WALSH, S. (1995) Accidents. In BOTTING, B. (ed.), *The Health of our Children: OPCS Decennial Supplement*. London: HMSO.

JOHNSTON, I. (1988) A study of the promotion of healthy lifestyles by hospital based staff. In WILSON BARNETT, J. and MACLEOD CLARK, J. (eds), *Research in Health Promotion and Nursing*. Basingstoke: Macmillan.

KALNINS, I. and LOVE, R. (1982) Children's concepts of health and illness – and implications for health education: an overview. *Health Education Quarterly*, 9, 104–115.

KALNINS, I., McQUEEN, D. D., BACKETT, K. C., CURTICE, L. and CURRIE, C. E. (1992) Children, empowerment and health promotion: some new directions in research and practice. *Health Promotion International*, 7, 53–59.

KALNINS, I., McQUEEN, D. D., BACKETT, K. C., CURTICE, L. and CURRIE, C. E. (1994) Children, empowerment and health promotion: some new directions in research and practice. In GOTT and MALONEY (eds), *Child Health – A Reader*. Oxford: Radcliffe Medical Press. (Abridged version)

KING, I. M. (1981) *A Theory for Nursing: Systems, Concepts, Processes*. New York: Wiley.

KUMAR, V. (1993) *Poverty and Inequality in the UK: The Effects on Children*. London: NCB.

LADER, D. and MATHESON, J. (1991) *Smoking among Secondary School Children in 1990. OPCS*. London: HMSO.

LANSDOWNE, R. and YULE, W. (1986) *The Lead Debate: The Environment, Toxicology and Child Health*. London: Croom Helm.

LEWIS, C. E. and LEWIS, M. A. (1974) The impact of television commercials on health-related beliefs and behaviours of children. *Pediatrics*, 53, 431–435.

LEWIS, M. and LEWIS, C. (1990) Consequences of empowering children to care for themselves. *Pediatrician*, 17, 63–76.

LUCAS, A., EWING, G., ROBERTS, S. B. and COWARD, W. B. (1985) How much energy does the breastfed infant consume and expend? *British Medical Journal*, 295, 75.

LUKER, K. and ORR, J. (1992) *Health Visiting – Towards Community Health Nursing*. London: Blackwell Scientific Publications.

McEWING, G. (1996) Children's understanding of their internal body parts. *British Journal of Nursing*, 5, 423–429.

MACKIE, A., WARD, H. and WALKER, R. (1990) *Urban Safety Project. 3. Overall Evaluation of Area Wide Schemes*. Crowthorne: Transport Research Laboratory.

MACKIE, P. (1993) Health of the Nation Targets: 1. Reducing accidents locally. *Professional Care of Mother and Child*, April, 105–109.

MADDUX, J. E., ROBERTS, M. C., SLEDDEN, E. A. and WRIGHT, L. (1986) Developmental issues in child health psychology. *American Psychologist*, 25–34.

MARSIGLIO, W. and MOTT, F. L. (1986) Impact of sex education on sexual activity and contraception use and premarital pregnancies among American teenagers. *Family Planning Perspectives*, 18, 151–152.

MASSEY, D. (1990) School sex education: knitting without a pattern? *Health Education Journal*, 49, 134–142.

MILLER, D. *et al.* (1993) Pertussis immunisation and serious acute neurological illnesses in children. *British Medical Journal*, 307, 1171–1176.

MILLER, W. B. (1986) Why some women fail to use their contraceptive method – a psychological investigation. *Family Planning Perspectives*, 18, 27–32.

MURRAY, A. B. and MORRISON, B. J. (1986) The effect of cigarette smoke from the mother on bronchial hyperresponsiveness and severity of symptoms in children with asthma. *Journal of Allergy Clinical Immunology*, 77, 575–581.

MURRAY, M., SWAN, A. V., JOHNSON, M. R. D. and BEWLEY, B. R. (1983) Some factors associated with increased risk of smoking by children. *Journal of Child Psychology & Psychiatry*, **24**, 223–232.

NATAPOFF, J. N. (1982) A developmental analysis of children's ideas of health. *Health Education Quarterly*, **9**, 34–45.

NELSON, M. (1993) *Nutritional Content of Children's Diets and the Health Implications in Food for Children: Influencing Choice and Investing in Health*. London: National Forum for Coronary Heart Disease Prevention.

NEUMAN, B. (1982) *Neuman's Systems Model: Application to Nursing Education and Practice*. Connecticut: Appleton Century Crofts.

NEWMAN, R., SMITH, C. and NUTBEAM, D. (1991) Teachers' views of the 'Smoking and Me Project'. *Health Education Journal*, **50**, 107–110.

ONS (OFFICE OF NATIONAL STATISTICS) (1996) *Population Trends – Summer 1996*. London: HMSO.

OPCS DH1/19 (1971–1991) *Birth Statistics, Mortality Rates*. London: HMSO.

OPCS DH6/3 (1989) *Mortality Statistics: Childhood*. London: HMSO.

OPCS MB3/5 (1990) *Congenital Malformation Statistics*. London: HMSO.

OPCS (1989) *General Household Survey*. London: HMSO.

OPCS (1991) *General Household Survey*. London: HMSO.

OPCS Monitor DH3 91/2 (1992) *Regional Trends*. London: HMSO.

OPCS (1994) *Smoking among Secondary School Children in England in 1993*. London: HMSO.

OPCS (1995) *Sudden Infant Death 1990–1994*. DH/3 95/3. London: HMSO.

OPPENHEIM, C. (1993) *Poverty: The Facts*. London: Child Poverty Action Group.

OREM, D. E. (1985) *Nursing; Concepts of Practice*, 3rd edn. New York: McGraw-Hill.

PHELPS, F. A., MELLANBY, A. R., CRICHTON, N. J. and TRIPP, J. H. (1994) Sex education: the effect of a peer programme on pupils (aged 13–14 years) and their peer leaders. *Health Education Journal*, **53**, 127–139.

PITTS, N. B. and EVANS, D. J. (1996) The dental caries experience of 14 year old children in the United Kingdom. Surveys co-ordinated by the British Association for the study of Community Dentistry in 1994/5. *Community Dental Health*, **13**, 51–58.

PLATT, M. J. and PHAROAH, P. O. D. (1996) Child health statistical review, 1996. *Archives of Disease in Childhood*, **75**, 527–533.

POWER, C., MANOR, O. and FOX, J. (1991) *Health and Class: The Early Years*. London: Chapman & Hall.

PUBLIC HEALTH LABORATORY SERVICE (1996) Communicable disease report: HIV and AIDS in the UK. *Monthly Report*, **6**, 42.

READING, R. (1997) Poverty and the health of children and adolescents. *Archives of Disease in Childhood*, **76**, 463–467.

READING, R., JARVIS, S. and OPENSHAW, S. (1993) measurement of social inequalities in health and use of health services among children in Northumberland. *Archives of Disease in Childhood*, **68**, 626–631.

READING, R., COLVER, A., OPENSHAW, S. and JARVIS, S. (1994) Do interventions that improve immunisation uptake also reduce social inequalities in uptake? *British Medical Journal*, **308**, 1142–1144.

ROSENSTOCK, I. M. (1974) Historical origins of the Health Belief Model. *Health Education Monograph*, **2**, 328–335.

ROY, C. (1984) *Introduction to Nursing: An Adaptation Model*, 2nd edn. New York: Prentice-Hall.

ROYAL COLLEGE OF NURSING (1989) *Into the Nineties: Promoting Professional Excellence*. London: RCN.

ROYAL COLLEGE OF NURSING (1991) *Successful Breastfeeding*, 2nd edn. London: Churchill Livingstone.

ROYAL COLLEGE OF PHYSICIANS (1992) *Smoking and the Young*. London: RCPL.

SEX EDUCATION FORUM (1992) *A Framework for School Sex Education*. London: Sex Education Forum.

SILVER, D. A. (1987) A longitudinal study of infant feeding practice, diet and caries related to social class in children aged 3 and 8–10 years. *Nursing Times*, **79** (8), 47–48.

SPARKS, G., CRAVEN, M. A. and WORTH, C. (1994) Understanding differences between high and low accident rate areas: the importance of qualitative data. *Journal of Public Health Medicine*, **16**, 439–446.

STRACHAN, D. and ANDERSON, H. (1992) Trends in hospital admissions for asthma in children. *British Medical Journal*, **304**, 819–820.

SUTHERLAND, I. (ed.) (1979) *Health Education, Perspectives and Choices*. London: George Allen and Unwin.

TANNAHILL, A. (1985) What is health promotion? *Health Education Journal*, **44**, 167–168.

TANNAHILL, A. (1990) Health education and promotion; planning for the 1990s. *Health Education Journal*, **49**, 194–198

TAYLOR, J. (1991) Health behaviour and beliefs. *Health Visitor*, **64**, 223–224.

THOMPSON, J. (1995) Facts, fiction and fears. *Health Visitor*, **68** (7), 92–93.

TILLMAN, M. (1992) *A study of the longer term effects of the urban safety project. The case of Reading, Berkshire*. MSc Transport Operations Group, Newcastle upon Tyne.

TODD, J. and DODD, T. (1994) *Children's Dental Health in the United Kingdom, 1993: A Survey Carried out on Behalf of the United Kingdom Health Departments, in Collaboration with the Dental Schools of the Universities of Birmingham and Newcastle*. London: HMSO.

TONES, K. and TILFORD, S. (1990) *Health Education: Effectiveness Efficiency and Equity*, 2nd edn. London: Chapman & Hall.

TOWNER, E., DOWSWELL, T. and JARVIS, S. (1993) *Reducing Childhood Accidents. The Effectiveness of Health Promotion Interventions: A Literature Review*. London: HEA.

TOWNSEND, P. (1980) *Inequalities in Health: The Black Report*. London: Penguin.

UKCC (1994) *Post-registration Education and Training*. London: UKCC.

VALMAN, H. B. (1993) *ABC of One to Seven*, 3rd edn. London: BMJ.

WALLERSTEIN, N. (1992) Powerlessness, empowerment and health, implication for health promotion programs. *American Journal of Health Education*, **6**, 193–205.

WATSON, J. E. (1979) *Medical–Surgical Nursing and Related Physiology*. London: Saunders.

WEITZMAN, M., GORTMAKER, S. L., WALKER, D. K. and SOBOL, A. (1990) Smoking and childhood asthma. *Pediatrics*, **85**, 505–511.

WEST, R., SAMMONS, P. and WEST, A. (1993) Effects of a traffic club on road safety knowledge and self-reported behaviour of young children and their carers. *Accident Analysis and Prevention*, **25**, 609–618.

WHITEHEAD, M. (1987) *Inequalities in Health in the 1980s*. London: Health Education Council.

WHITEHEAD, M. (1988) The health divide. In TOWNSEND, P., DAVIDSON, N. and WHITEHEAD, M. (eds), *Inequalities in Health*. Harmondsworth: Penguin.

WHITEHEAD, M. (1992) *The Health Divide*, 2nd edn. Harmondsworth: Penguin.

WHO (1946) *Constitution*. New York: WHO.

WHO (1993) *World Health Review*. London: WHO.

WHO (1986) *Ottawa Charter for Health Promotion*. Geneva: WHO.

WILKINSON, R. (1989) Class mortality differentials, income distribution and trends in poverty, 1921–1981. *Journal of Social Policy*, **18**, 307–335.

WILKINSON, R. (1994) Divided we fall. *British Medical Journal*, **308**, 30 April.

WILSON BARNETT, J. (1988) Patient teaching or patient counselling? *Journal of Advanced Nursing*, **13**, 215–322.

WILSON BARNETT, J. and LATTER, S. (1993) Factors influencing nurses' health education and health promotion practice in acute ward areas. In WILSON BARNETT, J. and MACLEOD CLARK, J. (eds), *Research in Health Promotion and Nursing*. Basingstoke: Macmillan.

WOODROFFE, C., GLICKMAN, M., BARKER, M. and POWER, C. (1993) *Children, Teenagers and Health*. Milton Keynes: Open University Press.

Further reading

LANTING, C. I., *et al*. (1994) Neurological differences between 9-year-old children fed breastmilk and formula as babies. *Lancet*, **344**, 1319–1322.

LUCAS, A., *et al*. (1992) Breastmilk and subsequent intelligence quotient in children born preterm. *Lancet*, **339**, 261–264.

MOBLEY, C. E. (1996) Assessment of health knowledge in pre-schools. *Children's Health Care*, **25**, 11–18.

PLANT, S. (1997) *From Needs to Practice – Effective Sex Education and Training Support*. London: NCB.

SMITH, R. (1997) Promoting the sexual health of young people: part II. *Paediatric Nursing*, **9**, 24–27.

Contacts

Association of Breastfeeding Mothers
7 Maybourne Close, London SE 26 6HQ. Tel: 0181 778 4769.

La Leche League (GB)
BM 3424, London WC1N 3XX. Tel: 0171 242 1278.

National Childbirth Trust
Alexandra House, Oldham Terrace, Acton, London W3 6NH. Tel: 0181 992 8637.

British Association for Toothfriendly Sweets
64 Wimpole Street, London W1.

British Dental Health Association
Eastlands Court, St Peter's Road, Rugby, Warwickshire CV21 3QP. Tel: 01788 546365.
   Brochures:
   • *Caring for your teeth and gums*
   • *Don't be afraid*

- *Your guide to a better smile*

Leaflets:
- *Dental care for mother and baby*
- *Preventive care and oral hygiene*
- *Visiting the dentist.*

General Dental Council
37 Wimpole Street, London W1M 3DQ. Tel: 0171 486 2171.
    Leaflets:
- *Diet and your child's teeth*
- *Healthy mouth, happy smile*
- *Danger mouse, tooth sleuth*
- *Wallcharts and posters*
    Packs:
- *Dental discovery kit teaching pack for 12–15 year olds.*

Chuck Sweets Off the Checkout Campaign
Iona Smeaton, Chief Community Dietician, c/o The Wislon Hospital, Cranmer Road, Mitcham, Surrey CR4 4TP.

Brook Advisory Centre
165 Gray's Inn Road, London WC1X 8UD. Tel: 0171 713 9000.

Contraceptive Education Service
2–12 Pentonville Road, London N1 9FD. Tel: 0171 837 4044.

Sex Education Forum
NCB, 8 Wakely Street, London EC1V 7QE. Tel: 0171 843 6052.

PART TWO

HEALTH AND DEVIATIONS IN CHILDHOOD

UNDERSTANDING FAMILIES IN STRESS

Joan Ramsay

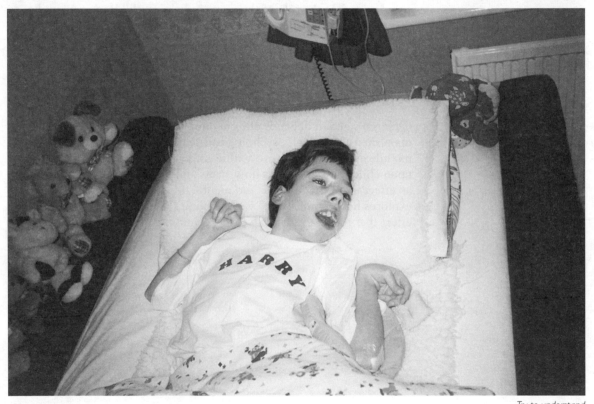

Try to understand

OBJECTIVES

The material contained within this module and the further reading/references should enable you to:

- Appreciate the effect that stress within the family has upon the child.
- Discuss children's perceptions of death.
- Explore how chronic illness and disability impacts upon the child and family.
- Consider how the stress of hospitalisation affects the child.
- Examine the effects of violence upon the child and understand the role of the nurse in recognising and reporting child abuse.
- Appreciate the role of the nurse in helping children and families to cope with stressors.

INTRODUCTION

Children's health depends not only upon their physical health but also upon their individual, psychological, social and spiritual lifestyle. This module explores how stress within these aspects of family living impacts upon children. It discusses how stress and illness within the family has an effect upon the physical and mental health of the child. It also explores how families cope with disability, violence and death, and the effect that these stressors have upon children.

THE INFLUENCE OF FAMILY STRESS UPON THE CHILD 1

INTRODUCTION

Children are born with very few innate behaviours and they rely on their parents to provide the necessary factors for their continued growth and development. Although the structure of the family has changed in recent years, and no longer consists of only a man, his wife and his children who live in a common household, it is generally responsible for the child's physical and psychological health.

In 1946 the World Health Organisation redefined health as the state of complete physical and social well-being, and not merely the absence of disease or infirmity. More recent definitions see health and illness in relative rather than absolute terms. This means that children's state of health will not only depend on their biological fitness but also on personal, psychosocial and spiritual factors.

How much does the family influence these factors? The Chinese calculate the age of their children not by the child's date of birth but by the date of its conception. This seems appropriate when studying the family's influence on the health of the child as some behavioural problems have their origin before birth and even before conception.

MATERNAL HEALTH

Studies have shown that pregnant women under excessive stress have more complications during pregnancy, labour and delivery, and are less likely to have healthy babies than those mothers not under stress. Arehart-Treichel (1980) reported that negative emotions such as grief, fear and anxiety during the last 3 months of pregnancy appear to give rise to irritable, hyperactive children who feed badly. The same author found that a high percentage of mothers of autistic children had been subject to disharmony during pregnancy. Many children who were born to mothers in Central London during the early years of World War II showed a high incidence of delinquency (Stott, 1962). Gunther (1963) found a significant association between psychosomatic symptoms and crises during pregnancy and premature delivery, which is one of the most crucial factors contributing to infant mortality.

Maternal health also influences the unborn child. It is well known that smoking retards fetal growth and increases the stillborn and neonatal death rate (Merritt, 1981). However, it also affects subsequent psychological development. Women who smoke and cough heavily during pregnancy have been found to have more nervous and insecure infants than non-smokers (Butler and Goldstein, 1973). In 1979, Brown and Cooper found that maternal malnutrition could cause cerebellar dystrophy and predispose to clumsiness, hyperactivity and learning

Cross references

Family structures – page 6

Health – page 133

Role of the family in child development – page 30

Factors affecting child health – page 128

disorders. They also discovered that disorders of pregnancy, such as toxaemia, hypertension and hyperemesis or prolonged labour, showed a correlation with a variety of childhood behaviour problems such as hyperactivity, defective concentration, tics and emotional instability. These studies do not clarify whether the effect on the child is due to the physiological effects of stress on uterine function or the attitude of the mother towards the child who has caused the difficult pregnancy or labour.

Activity

Find a child with a behaviour problem such as those described above and discover whether the mother's obstetric history reveals any problems. Talk to the mother about her feelings about the baby during the time of the problems.

PARENT–CHILD RELATIONSHIP

Cross reference

Roles and relationships – page 19

Parental attitude towards a child is an important preconceptual factor as wanted children are more likely to be happy and healthy. A 1975 Czech study (cited by Arehart-Treichel, 1980) found that unwanted children, especially boys, are liable to acute illness, hospitalisation and antisocial behaviour than wanted children. Conversely, Illingworth (1983) describes a very much wanted child born after 17 years of marriage, developing hypochondria as a result of his parents over anxiety and over protection.

Over-protection or smother-love can also occur for other reasons. It may occur as the result of the birth of a healthy child after a series of miscarriages or following the birth of a child of a particular sex after a series of children of the opposite sex. It may occur if the baby is premature or handicapped, especially if initially it was not expected to live. It may also be due to the mother's personality. A mother who had an unhappy childhood or is unhappily married may smother her child to meet her own needs for affection. A child who is over protected is insecure, does not react well to others, lacks confidence, is accident prone and has a tendency towards sleeping and eating problems (Illingworth, 1983).

The parents' desire for a child also affects their ability to relate to their newborn baby. Much has been written about the importance of the reciprocal relationship between parent and child, and the adverse effects of separation of the two because of pre-term delivery or illness. Lynch and Roberts (1977) found that children who had been taken away from their mothers to be nursed in intensive care units showed a higher incidence of child abuse than those cared for immediately by their mothers. Bonding may not occur because of rejection of the child. It may be of the wrong sex or have congenital anomalies, it may be the result of an accidental pregnancy, or it may have caused a difficult pregnancy or labour. Parental attitudes may range from excessive criticism to neglect and cruelty. The rejected child tends to be excessively shy and fearful, more aggressive and quarrelsome and demonstrates severe behavioural problems such as enuresis, head banging, truancy and stealing (Illingworth, 1983). Rejection can also cause physical problems McCarthy (1974) made a special study of children with stunted growth and concluded that children who eventually show physical signs of this syndrome have suffered from rejection from an early age, probably right from birth or even before birth.

SEPARATION

Physical and psychological problems may occur if the bonding relationship is broken by separation of the child from one or both parents later in childhood. Initial studies by Bowlby (1973) indicated that severe long-lasting emotional problems could result from hospitalisation. Separation anxiety is now a well known complication in preschool children who have been separated from their mothers for long periods of hospitalisation. Regression and emotional instability may continue for some time after the child has returned home. The crucial factors appear to be the length of the separation and the continuity of care as there is no indication that daily separation of children from their mothers is harmful, providing the children are cared for in a consistent way by a known carer (Wallston, 1973).

Permanent separation from a parent may be the result of separation, divorce or bereavement. The child's consequent behaviour depends upon the reason for the separation and the quality of the relationship with the remaining parent. Rutter (1971) concluded that although children's behaviour tended to deteriorate immediately after a divorce or separation severe problems such as delinquency were more likely to occur within a discordant family life than a stable one-parent home. Discord also seems to affect the child more than the actual loss of a parent. Analysis of the studies into the characteristics of adolescents who take overdoses show a significant number of these children are from families who have split up (Kingsbury, 1993).

Many studies have been performed on the effect on the child of non-traditional families. Schaffer (1988) describes studies which compare children from single-mother families, social contract families, families living in communes and traditional two-parent nuclear families. Any problems were found to be independent of the type of family group.

The child–parent relationship can also be disturbed by the birth of a sibling. The first child is likely to become more tearful, have difficulty in sleeping and show a regression in toilet habits (Dunn, 1981).

Cross references

Attachment – pages 86 and 87

Family break-up and its effects – page 16

Aetiology of deliberate self-harm in children

- Single-parent family
- Under the care of social services
- Psychiatric disorder and previous overdose among family members
- Not living with either parent
- Significantly high rate of arguments with parents
- Difficulty in communicating with fathers
- Parents seen as controlling

(Russell-Johnson, 1997)

FAMILY DISABILITY AND ILLNESS

Cross reference

Living with a disability – page 232

Chronic physical illness or prolonged severe illness in one parent which affects family life and relationships may also cause behaviour problems in the children, but generally mental illness in the parents has been found to have a more disturbing effect. Parental depression appears to have the more damaging effect. Preschool and schoolchildren of mothers who are depressed show a high incidence of psychiatric problems. Children who have siblings with a chronic illness or handicap generally show more disturbed behaviour than the affected child. The child may feel guilty or fearful and demonstrate behavioural problems in order to regain parental attention (Gath, 1980).

However, there are also positive effects from living with a family member who is disabled. Faux (1991) showed that siblings of a disabled child can demonstrate a greater degree of empathy and kindness than children with healthy siblings.

Activity

Talk to a sibling of a child with a chronic illness or disability and find out the effect this has had upon the sibling's lifestyle. Consider what effect this has had upon the sibling's character.

PARENTAL BEHAVIOUR

Cross reference

Parenting styles page 37

In Western societies the cultural values of independence and relating well to others usually underpin the way in which parents raise their children. Swanwick (1982) suggests that undue pressure on children to develop autonomy and social skills may result in separation fears and nightmares.

In any kind of behavioural problem the attitude of the parent will determine the extent and spread of the behaviours. Patterson (1982) has investigated the acquisition of problem behaviours in children. As a result of his work he developed the coercion theory. Coercion theory suggests that unskilled parents permit young children to use aversive techniques such as crying, demanding and having tantrums to achieve their needs. Without effective and consistent intervention the child continues the aversive behaviour to manipulate the environment. Such children tend to be more aggressive and resort to lying and stealing.

Cross reference

The media – page 59

Parental behaviour will also affect their child's behaviour – children are natural imitators. Social learning theory considers that aggression is learnt through observation and the more such behaviour is reinforced the more likely it is to occur. Bandura (1973) showed that nursery school children readily imitated aggression following either filmed or live models of aggression. Children who watch violence on television are more aggressive and are more likely to think that aggression is a good way to overcome problems.

Activity

Watch a children's TV cartoon and consider what children may learn about verbal and physical violence from seeing this type of programme. Also watch an early evening adult film or comedy and assess what influence this may have upon children.

Activity

Considering your findings from the previous activity; what rules or limits (if any) would you place on children watching TV?

If there is violence in the home the children (especially boys) will be more aggressive. Girls of such homes tend to grow up to be violent and neglectful mothers. Illingworth (1983) describes an Australian study of parental alcoholism where the irrational and violent behaviour of fathers tended to lead to depression, hostility and aggression in the children.

Some studies have also investigated whether parental behaviour can cause children to develop type A behaviour and thus a predisposition to coronary heart disease. Rosenman *et al.* (1975) found that hard working boys had fathers with the same traits. Further studies seem to show that type A behaviour is more likely to develop in children whose mother and father were achievement- and competition-oriented.

PARENTAL ATTITUDE AND PHYSICAL ILLNESS

Other physical illnesses may be exacerbated by parental attitudes. Arehart-Treichel (1980) reports that the underlying cause of ulcerated colitis, asthma and anorexia nervosa may be related to family influences. Her studies have shown that children with ulcerated colitis have domineering mothers and passive remote fathers, neither of whom are able to express their emotions freely. Like ulcerated colitis, anorexia nervosa often has origins in a dominating mother and in a family where emotions are usually repressed. However, mothers of anorexics tend to be pre-occupied with food and may use food as a way of showing affection. Obesity also seems to stem from over-protection and dominating parents. They are often the only or youngest children with a pathological dependence on their parents. A similar situation is seen in origins of asthma which commences during childhood. Retrospective studies suggest that many children with asthma have dominating mothers and ineffective fathers. Childhood asthma is twice as common among boys as girls, and the affected boys, who are usually only children, or the youngest child, tend to have been over-protected and over indulged by their mothers and rejected by their fathers. However, these studies have been largely unsupported as it is always difficult to know whether parental behaviour is the cause or effect of the child's chronic condition.

Cross reference

Parenting styles – page 37

Cross reference

Mental health – page 534

Juvenile rheumatoid arthritis also shows an origin in family influence, but in a different way to those discussed above. Arehart-Treichel (1980) suggests that children with rheumatoid disease tend to be first born children who have one parent who is rejecting, aggressive and punitive. A 1979 American study showed that nearly a third with rheumatoid arthritis had lost a parent through death, divorce or separation, compared with 11% in the control group. Parental loss or separation also appears to be a pre-disposing factor in mental illness. A 1965 study showed that 38% of suicides had experienced the death of one or both parents during childhood and a further 34.5% had parents who had separated or divorced. A 1975 German study found that over 25% of schizophrenics had lost a parent by death or divorce while young. Reactive depression appears to correlate with strict unemotional fathers and mothers who are intrusive and perfectionists (cited by Arehart-Treichel, 1980).

Studies have also been done to discover if events in childhood can predispose to cancer. An American study which has been ongoing since the 1940s (The New York Longitudinal Study) found that 30% of cancer patients report a lack of warm, loving parental relationships (Chess and Thomas, 1984). Most significantly none of these patients were only children. Further studies have suggested that early frustrations in childhood due to the birth of a sibling correlates with the later development of cancer.

Activity

Study the family background of a child with one of the above disorders and see what evidence you find for the link between physical illness and parental attitude.

RELATIONSHIPS BETWEEN STRESS AND DISEASE

Why do childhood experiences cause a person to develop a disease? Although little research has been done in this area, there seem to be three factors involved. Increased levels of adrenal steroid hormones have been found in adults whose mothers had died when they were young. Elevation of adrenal steroid hormones have been found to depress the immune system. Depression and grief also result in a rise of steroid hormones whereas repressed emotions reduce antibody levels (Arehart-Treichel, 1980). Studies of 100 children by Meyre and Haggerty in 1962 seem to give strength to this theory. Throat swabs of each child were taken every 2 weeks and cultured for streptococci. The family kept a diary of events particularly noting upsetting events and illnesses. The researchers found that 25% of the children showed positive throat swabs 2 weeks after stressful events. This does not totally explain why children develop physical or psychological problems related to stressful lifestyle events. Not all only children develop juvenile rheumatoid arthritis and not all unwanted children have behavioural problems. This difference may be due to personality or the individual differences between the children. Psychologists do not agree about the way in which personality develops but, one way, social learning theory, indicates that individual differences result from variations in learning experiences. Some personality characteristics such as moods are inherited biological factors, so it is possible that the family still plays a part in influencing the child.

SOCIAL CLASS AND ENVIRONMENT

It is also known that there are many other pre-disposing factors that influence the development of mental and physical illness. One great influence is social class. In the Newcastle study of 1000 children (Miller *et al.*, 1974) it was shown that effective parental skills increased with social class due to better education and health services. Accidents are more common and more severe in poorer families, especially if there is maternal neglect or an overcrowded home (Miller *et al.*, 1974). Overcrowding tends to give rise to infection more readily and poor children catch these diseases earlier in life when they have less mature body defences.

Environmental factors may also influence behaviour. Rutter *et al.*, (1975) compared children from a stable and cohesive community with a comparable group of children from an inner London borough. He showed how the unsettling influences of city life gave rise to a greater incidence of delinquency.

The availability of social support is also of importance. In a study of battered children and their parents (Smith *et al.*, 1974), social isolation and loneliness were as important as environmental problems such as cramped conditions and lack of amenities.

Thus it appears that although the family does have an important influence on health, there are also other factors to consider. This is perhaps best summarised by The National Child Development Study (Wedge and Prosser, 1973). Ten thousand children were studied from birth until the age of 11. The results showed clearly the interrelationship between physical development, ill-health, accidents, maladaptive behaviour, with social and environmental disadvantages and parental interest.

Activity

Do a literature search to discover more recent research to support or dispute the findings cited in this module. Make a note of your findings.

It seems to follow that there is an increased need for health practitioners to look at the whole family and not just the child. Any action relating to the prevention, maintenance or improvement of children's

---

Factors protecting children from the effects of stress

- A good relationship with at least one parent
- Effective supervision and security
- Clarity and consistency of rules
- Respect as an individual
- Recognition of effort and achievement
- Gradual increase of responsibility and independence
- Good relationships with siblings
- Own adaptable and sociable temperament

Lask and Fossen (1989)
(See also pages 225 and 231)

Cross references

Personality – page 83
Social issues – page 129

---

health should take into account the children's relationship with their carers as well as their home setting and family structure. McMahon (1995) states that it makes sense to use family therapy and work with the family rather than the individual child because the causes of so many childhood problems are found within the families' relationships with each other. Preconceptual advice and education about the factors affecting child health may also help to reduce the psychological and physiological disorders of childhood as well as promote mental and physical health through positive family influences.

Key points ➤

1. Certain characteristics of parental behaviour towards children such as emotions, controlling methods and communication patterns significantly influence psychological development.

2. Families who provide warmth and affection have children who develop better and more secure social relationships than those who are cold and rejecting.

3. The structure of the family affects family functioning. Changes in family structure are associated with significant stress and adversely affect child-rearing patterns.

4. The overall level of poverty or affluence of the family influences family interactions and relationships by affecting health, discipline and levels of stress and support.

5. Authoritative parents who provide warmth, control, communication and security whilst responding to their children as individuals produce children who are more confident, competent, independent and affectionate.

6. Family therapy can be used as a way of gaining insight into the cause and nature of children's psychological problems.

HOSPITALISATION AND ILLNESS 2

INTRODUCTION

Hospitals are strange and frightening environments for everyone. They are associated with real and imagined fears, and actual and potential threats. Since Bowlby and Robertson's studies in the 1950s hospitalisation is known to cause particular anxiety for children, and can lead to short- and long-term emotional and behavioural problems. For children, the unfamiliar environment, numerous strangers, peculiar equipment and the sight and sound of other distressed children is confusing and frightening.

Activity

Take some time to look at your own place of work from a child's viewpoint. Crouch down and consider how it looks for a small child. What changes might make it more welcoming from this view?

It is not only the strange environment of hospital which children find stressful. Bossert (1994) discovered that hospitalised children could identify a range of stressful events. She categorised these stressors into six main areas; intrusive events, physical symptoms, therapeutic intervention, restricted activity, separation and environment. She also found that children with short-term acute illnesses were more likely to name physical symptoms as most stressful. Children with chronic illness had a greater number of stressors and found intrusive events the most stressful.

Children's reactions to hospitalisation are influenced by several factors and are known to be reduced by preparation and explanations. However, familiarity with hospital, for those children with chronic illness, does not reduce fears (Hart and Bossert, 1994). For these children fears may be worse because they know the reality of being in hospital. Although most children experience some stress when in hospital, it can also be a positive experience. It can give children the opportunity for further social interaction and it may help them to cope better with future illness or stressors.

Illness and hospitalisation in childhood affects the whole family and as family stress has its impact on the ill child, the children's nurse should be aware of these effects. Other sections discuss the ways of minimising the traumatic effects of hospitalisation for the child so this section will concentrate mainly on the reactions of the child and family to this trauma.

Cross references

Creating an appropriate hospital environment for children – page 256

Preparation for hospital and procedures – page 264

Cross reference

Vertical relationships – page 86

Separation anxiety – influencing factors

- Sex of the nurse and usual care giver
- Parental response to the separation and the nurse
- Familiarity of the environment
- Friendly attitude of the nurse
- Distance of nurse from the child
- Amount of physical contact by the nurse
- Child used to other carers
- Child's personality – anxious versus confident
- Parenting styles

Children's reactions to hospitalisation

Depend upon:

1 Developmental age
- infancy
- preschool
- school age
- adolescence
2 Previous experience
- illness
- family separation
- hospital
3 Available support
- resident parents
- family and friends
- named nurse
4 Seriousness of the illness

SEPARATION ANXIETY

Infants appear to be fearless for the first 6–8 months of life and the startle reflex of the young baby which occurs in response to a sudden noise or movement is probably the nearest reaction to fear (Marks, 1987). After about 6 months the infant or child becomes wary of strangers and may show anxiety, depending on age and previous experience. At the same time as the development of this stranger anxiety children show evidence of separation anxiety when their usual caregiver is absent. Kagan (1979) explains that this reaction is due to the child losing the usual source of physical and emotional comfort, and not understanding the reason or the temporary nature of the loss. The understanding that people and things still exist even though they cannot still be seen does not develop until 10 months of age. However, separation anxiety occurs after this age and is exacerbated by other unfamiliar events, such as hospitalisation. The amount of distress is determined by parenting styles. Main *et al.* (1985) found that parents who were easily accessible and responsive to their children increased the children's confidence and enabled them to accept brief separations. Children with affectionate parents who are used to being comforted by them tend to be more confident and able to tolerate brief separations (Ainsworth, 1982). The amount of distress is also affected by the parents' response to the separation; if parents are calm and happy with the situation it is likely that the child will be less anxious. This is an important issue for nurses who need to be able to reassure parents at least as much as the child.

Regardless of influencing factors, some separation anxiety will always occur and should be accepted as a normal display of grief at the loss of someone who is important to the child. The child should be comforted and reassured so they still feel secure and loved. If the manifestations of separation anxiety are ignored or punished the child may develop long-term consequences. Ainsworth (1973) suggests that the feelings of insecurity and loss of confidence and trust that the child experiences during separation can result in difficulty in developing and maintaining relationships in adulthood.

Bowlby (1953) observed children in foster care and discovered that, when young children were separated from parents for any length of time, they demonstrated three distinct phases of separation anxiety; protest, despair and detachment. Whilst his observations centred around children between the ages of 8 months and 3 years, older children can also display some signs of anxiety on being separated from their home and parents. Detachment is uncommon because most children stay in hospital for only brief periods and any parental separation is only brief. However, the protest and despair phases can occur after only a brief separation and it is important that nurses recognise and react to these so that long-term effects of separation are avoided (Figure 2.1).

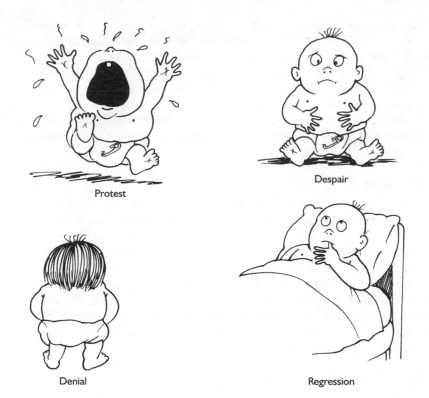

Figure 2.1

Separation anxiety.

Protest

The child first demonstrates separation anxiety by protesting. Protest may be shown in many ways according to the age of the child. Infants and young children will cry loudly for their parents and will be inconsolable, refusing comfort from anyone else. This phase can last for several days and small children may only sleep when they are exhausted by crying.

Older children may express their protest by anger and be aggressive to other children and anyone who tries to console them. Adolescents may show anger and frustration and be generally uncooperative. They do not cry or express their concerns because they do not want to appear weak, childish or dependent, but Hart and Bossert (1994) discovered that the fear of being separated from the family was schoolchildren's greatest cause for concern about hospitalisation.

Despair

At this stage of separation, the young child appears to accept that parents are not returning and shows features of depression. This behaviour can go unnoticed, and the child labelled as quiet and good.

The child is withdrawn, sad and apathetic, showing no interest in toys, food or other children. Usually when parents visit, the child cries bitterly and nurses have used this as evidence that parental visiting is upsetting to children in hospital. However, Robertson (1970) showed that these children were crying to relieve their tension and not because the presence of their parents upset them.

Older children's despair may be demonstrated by stoicism, withdrawal or passive acceptance. They also lose interest in activities and food.

Detachment

At this stage the child appears to have adjusted to the new situation and becomes more active and interested in the surroundings. Detached children will play, eat and sleep as usual and will accept care from anyone. In reality, they have coped with their separation by unattaching themselves from their parents. As a result they lose interest and no longer relate to their parents. Robertson (1970) suggests that at this stage the child represses the fear, sorrow and loneliness and tries to make the best of the alternative situation. Although this stage is rarely seen now children stay in hospital for shorter periods than previously, it is perhaps not recognised because it is less common.

Regression

Children in hospital who feel insecure often display attention-seeking behaviour which may continue on discharge home. This behaviour usually relates to the characteristics of a younger child. If this regression is not recognised and managed appropriately by nurses or parents the child will suffer further stress and insecurity.

There are three important ways of preventing regression: getting to know the child as an individual, being able to anticipate needs and minimising stress. If the nurse knows and maintains normal home routines and does not expect behaviour beyond the child's developmental abilities the child's security is upheld. The nurse who knows the child's preferences and abilities can anticipate needs which provides added security. Further stress can be minimised by consistency of care given by familiar staff. These named nurses can provide cuddles and comfort in the family's absence as well as explanations and preparation for procedures which are adapted to meet the individual child's needs. They can also establish a relationship and work in partnership with the parents to care for the child. The child will also feel more secure if parents appear calm and relaxed.

If a child does show regressive behaviour, the nurse should not insist upon usual behaviour. The situation should be accepted calmly and the reasons for insecurity explored. Parents should be warned that children sometimes show regression once they return home, even if they appeared to adjust well to hospital. They also need to know that if

Regressive behaviour
- Clinging to parents
- Persistent comfort-seeking behaviour
- Temper tantrums
- Unusual aggressiveness
- Refusal to associate with other children or siblings
- Refusal to eat
- Refusal to go to bed
- Waking and crying in the night
- Soiling or wetting although toilet trained

regression is recognised and managed appropriately immediately following their return home, normal behaviour will gradually return.

PARENTAL CONCERNS

It is never easy for parents whose child is in hospital. Even if there are no siblings, parents have other concerns. They tend to feel fearful, anxious and guilty. Fear and anxiety is often related to their lack of knowledge about the illness and its treatment, which may be exacerbated if they had frightening experiences themselves as children in hospital. Remember that resident parents and dedicated children's wards are a relatively new concept which may not have been available when some parents were small. Guilt is a common reaction of most parents to any child's illness; they always wonder if any action or omission could have caused or prevented the illness.

As with any crisis, parents often report feelings of depression after the hospitalisation. They may have been so busy supporting the ill child in hospital as well as managing the home that it is not until they return home that exhaustion occurs. It is then difficult to manage any emotional and behavioural changes that the child or siblings may exhibit. In addition, they now have concerns about the child being at home and whether they have the necessary skills to provide continuing care. Bailey and Caldwell (1997) found that parents always want more discharge information than they receive and suggest that nurses need to look at the effectiveness of their communication and discharge planning.

SIBLINGS OF HOSPITALISED CHILDREN

The effects of childhood chronic illness upon siblings has been widely studied (Morrison, 1997). However, until recently the effect of short-term hospitalisation for acute illness upon siblings has not been considered. Yet, the feelings of loneliness, fear and anxiety still occur. Simon (1993) found that the stress of siblings was equal to the stress experienced by the ill child, with those siblings who visited daily experiencing the most stress. These findings were replicated by Morrison (1997) who found that this stress was demonstrated by feelings of sadness, nervousness and difficulty in sleeping and concentrating at school. The reasons for this stress have not been proven but are thought to relate to parental separation as one parent is likely to remain with the hospitalised child.

Activity

Consider how you could minimise stress for the child whose sibling is in hospital for 48 hours.

Parental reactions to hospitalisation

Depend upon:

1 Parental temperament
- adaptable
- confident

2 Previous experience
- illness
- hospitals

3 Available support
- communication within family
- personal coping mechanisms
- cultural and religious beliefs
- other stresses within the family

4 Seriousness of the illness
- degree of threat to the child
- medical procedures involved

Cross reference

Sibling relationships – page 24

Morrison (1997) suggests that family-centred care should not centre around the parents but should involve siblings. The same methods that have been developed to reduce the stress of the hospitalised child can be used for siblings. Initiatives have taken place to provide siblings of children with cancer the opportunity to learn more about the care of cancer (Woodhouse, 1996) and this idea could be extended. The siblings of those children coming into hospital for a planned admission could also be invited to the pre-admission club and siblings of long-term hospitalised children could be invited to a special open day. Nurses can also explain sibling stress to parents so that they can appreciate the need to keep siblings informed. Evidence shows that parents do not realise that healthy siblings also have concerns about hopitalisation (Craft, 1986) and it seems likely that siblings either do not talk to parents about their concerns or do not have the opportunity to discuss problems with them.

CHILDREN'S CONCEPTS OF ILLNESS

Cross reference

Children's concepts of health – page 144

Carson *et al.* (1992) believe that a child's adaptation to hospitalisation can be determined by their concept of illness. Studies into children's understanding of illness rely heavily about Piaget's theory of cognitive development but recent studies suggest that young children are able to understand more than Piaget's cognitive levels imply (Meadows, 1993). Bird and Podmore (1993) suggest that small children's limited knowledge of illness is more likely to be due to poor or inadequate explanations than their inability to understand the concept. Although nurses are taught to explore children's existing level of knowledge and intellect before any explanation or teaching, it would appear that in practice they accept cognitive development theory and prevent children's understanding of illness through their inadequate information (Alderson, 1993). Rushford (1996) found that most nurses aimed their information giving at mid school-age level regardless of the child's actual age, intellect or previous knowledge and experience.

Concepts of illness begin at the preschool age. These young children tend to accept what they have been told about illness and their lack of experience with language causes them to interpret what is said literally. Because of this, common nursing expressions such as 'taking a temperature' may be viewed with alarm. Equally, their lack of knowledge about body functioning means that explanations need to be carefully phrased and thorough to prevent fear and confusion. They are often told at this age that colds are caught and they may use this rationale for all illnesses unless told otherwise.

School-age children are more concerned about the consequences of the illness than its causation. They usually know that some outside factor causes illness but are not very clear about the exact explanation although school, television, books and life experience have now given them more information about the body and its illnesses. Because of this, they are aware of and worry about disability and death and their greatest fear is being told that they have a chronic illness (Hart and Bossert, 1994). They become frustrated when illness prevents their developing independence and physical activity. At this age they have a thirst for knowledge and take an active interest in finding out about their illness. They cope better with the illness and hospitalisation by finding out as much as possible about it. Given appropriate information most children of this age can give a good account of their illness which would appear to support the idea that children's cognitive abilities are not limited to their age.

Activity

Ask a school-age child to tell you about their chronic illness and consider whether the explanation is related to the child's cognitive age or ability.

Independence, individuality and freedom is important for adolescents. Illness and hospitalisation may take all of these away. They may further isolate themselves from peers and family as they strive to maintain some independence. They are then left with no support mechanisms. Thus illness is seen as a loss of control and power. To help them regain control they also want to know as much as possible about their illness. They now know about the physical and psychological causes of disease and expect to be given information as adults. They will not tolerate or value being treated as a child or having information hidden from them. They are aware of potential problems of illness and treatment and will expect to be told about these. Appearance is important to this age group and they worry about alterations such as scarring and deformity.

MINIMISING SEPARATION ANXIETY

Activity

Read the case studies entitled 'The stressful effects of hospitalisation' and suggest ways in which these problems could be overcome.

Ideally, admission to hospital for children between 6 months and 4 years of age should be avoided. If hospitalisation is essential then day care is less traumatic than an in-patient stay. Allowing a close family member (preferably a parent) to be resident with the child is the best way to overcome separation anxiety but may not always be possible. Parents with other children have the unenviable task of deciding which child benefits from the parental presence and there may not be other family members around to help. Harris (1993) suggests that when this is not possible that a soft article of clothing belonging to the parent

The stressful effects of hospitalisation

1 Bobby, aged 2. Bobby has been admitted to hospital after a car accident in which his father was seriously injured. His mother is trying to divide her time between Bobby, his siblings at home and her husband. She cannot be resident with Bobby and her visits can only be brief. She is distressed by the situation and worried about its effect on Bobby

2 Jane, aged 4. Jane is at home following a brief stay in hospital following a febrile convulsion. Her mother asks you for advice about her behaviour since their return home. Jane, who always went to bed with no fuss, is now refusing to settle and wakes constantly during the night. She is very clingy during the day and making a terrible fuss about leaving her mother to go to nursery

3 Rosie, aged 8. Rosie was admitted earlier today with appendicitis. She is shortly going to theatre. Her mother needs to stay at home with Rosie's twin brothers, aged 6 months, and her father is out of the country. Rosie is in pain and is frightened and very upset at her mother's absence

4 Mark, aged 14. Mark has been in hospital for 3 weeks. He fractured his femur in a road accident on his way to school and is now in traction. He is becoming more and more rude and uncooperative to the nurses. His mother, a single parent, can only visit in the evenings after work. During her visits he is often rude and uncommunicative and she is very upset by his behaviour

provides the young child with a constant and comforting reminder of the parent. Any other comforters (teddy, blanket, dummy) should also be left with the child. To try and prevent the child from feeling unloved and insecure, a consistent figure other than the parent should be available and follow the child's home routine wherever possible. If parents or family cannot stay with the older child links with home may be provided by photographs and a clock to denote times of visits.

Older children's fears of loss of control may be minimised by explanations and involvement with treatment or care and being allowed a choice as much as possible. Burr (1993) believes that in spite of the fact that adolescence is known as a period where independence and self-control develop, little consideration is given to enable these older children to be independent in hospital. Although conflicts with parents tend to occur at this age, parents are still very important, especially at times of stress. Greenberg *et al.* (1983) found that the quality of adolescents' relationships with their parents was central to their sense of well-being and happiness. Therefore, it is important not to presume that hospitalised children in this age group do not need their parents.

The effects of hospitalisation on the older child can be minimised by preparation for the strange environment of hospital and any associated procedures and this helps to overcome some fears of the unknown.

Key points ➤

1. Hospitalisation is traumatic for children of any age, but it particularly affects children between the ages of 6 months and 4 years.

2. When a child is in hospital it affects the whole family and family-centred care should take this into account.

3. Nurses should take care not to mistake the features of separation anxiety for the characteristics of a good child who is settling well into hospital.

4. If separation anxiety is not recognised or managed well the child can have problems maintaining relationships in later life.

5. The behaviour of children who have been discharged from hospital can regress. This can be very distressing for parents if they are not warned of this and given advice on its management.

6. Admission to hospital for very young children should be avoided whenever possible. If hospitalisation is essential, procedures should be in place to minimise the traumatic effects for the whole family.

DEATH AND THE FAMILY 3

INTRODUCTION

Death is an experience within the natural realm of human experience as a necessary part of human life. Hiding death in a shroud of mysticism will not change the inexorable fact that death is the end of the line for every living thing. There is therefore a need to discuss death to rid society and ourselves of the myths and superstitions which surround death. This section aims to help you to begin to examine your own ideas, feelings and beliefs about death so that any fears, anxieties or conflicts which you may have can be diminished. As a result, it should begin to enable you to talk openly about death and accept it as part of life. It is only when you can do this that you can hope to help others cope with death. Parents of children who are dying need help to come to terms with this and also need help to explain what is happening to the child and the siblings. The role of the nurse in this situation will range from giving information and practical advice to providing emotional support for the whole family. Effective psychological care requires the nurse to be aware of personal feelings about death (McKerrow, 1991).

A century ago, people were exposed to death earlier and more often throughout their lifespan. The extended family meant that children were more likely to observe death and that they participated in the emotional and ceremonial aspects. Today, children are often shielded from the trauma of death. Improved living conditions, health care and highly skilled medical and surgical interventions have contributed to longer lifespans, which means that death becomes a distant event which seems too far away to consider. The breakdown of the extended family and the tendency for more people to die in hospital or residential homes means that children are less likely to encounter death. Their grief for a lost pet is often tempered by a replacement. If children are not involved in the reality of death, the development of a realistic concept of death is inhibited and thus, in adulthood, death is surrounded by fear and myths.

Activity

Consider your ideas and beliefs about death by answering the 'Death attitudes' questions listed on the right.

Death attitudes

1 How would your personal lifestyle change drastically if you discovered you had a terminal illness?

2 Are you afraid of death? What do you think has influenced your answer?

3 What are your personal beliefs about death?

4 Do your family and friends discuss death openly? Why do you think this is so?

5 What are your plans for your own death?

6 What things would you like to do before you die?

7 What sentiments would you want to express to your family and friends before you die?

8 What experience of death have you had to date? How much has this influenced your answers to the previous questions?

CHILDREN'S FEELINGS ABOUT DEATH

Children's perceptions of death depend upon their age and, in general, their understanding parallels their cognitive and psychological

Cross reference

Caring for the dying child and family
– page 393

development. They encounter death in various ways and at different ages. This encounter is most likely to be on television, or in games and fantasies which may not give them a realistic idea of death. Some children may have experienced the death of a pet or a grandparent but their understanding of this event may be influenced by their parents' explanations. As Lovell (1987) notes, many adults are too confused about death to be able to give their child a rational explanation.

Activity

Billy, aged 4, tells you about the death of his cat. He asks: 'If Kitty is in heaven and heaven is in the sky, why did daddy bury her in the garden?' How should you reply?

Lovell (1987) suggests that for younger children, such as Billy, death can be explained by relating it through nature and the life cycle of flowers and trees. The concept of heaven is confusing for children who are not able to think in the abstract. It is also difficult for preschool children to appreciate the permanency of death. Michael and Landsdown (1986) found that children wanted to talk about death and those who were not allowed to do so were those who had more difficulty in adjusting to their loss. Extreme fear and phobic behaviour can result from the exclusion of children from family discussions about death (Bentovim, 1986).

Activity

Samantha is 8 years old and her grandmother, of whom she was very fond, has just died. Samantha's parents want your advice about whether she should attend the funeral. What advice should you give?

Children in this age group are often excluded from mourning. Randall (1993) believes that young children grieve differently from adults. In reality, the difference lies not in the grief process but the way in which children express their grief. For young children, whose bereavement occurs at the stage of development when they cannot properly understand the meaning of death or the meaning of their loss, loneliness and fear may be immediate reactions. Their inability to communicate can lead to misunderstandings about the level of grief they feel. This situation and the exclusion from any involvement in the death can cause them more distress. This distress may manifest itself in regressive or aggressive behaviour. Pettle and Landsdown (1986) found that children who were able to participate in the events surrounding the death of a sibling were less disturbed than those who did not. The death of a parent has been found to have long-reaching psychological effects among children (Randall, 1993) and Lovell (1987) suggests that these reactions could be minimised by allowing the child to spend time with the dying parent, help with their care and given the opportunity to discuss what is happening.

TALKING ABOUT DEATH

Talking with parents and children is an emotional, difficult thing to do. Often a nurse is reluctant to approach a dying child and the family because of not knowing what to say. They are worried about answering questions wrongly. There can be no set procedure for this situation and the most appropriate way of learning to cope with this problem is to use role play and discussion.

Activity

You are looking after Bobby, aged 6, who has been admitted for investigations of severe headache, dizziness and vomiting. Investigations indicate an inoperable cerebral tumour but parents have not yet been told. Suddenly, Bobby's mother asks: 'Is Bobby going to die?' Consider your response.

Listening is the most important skills for the nurse. It may be difficult for an experienced nurse to answer direct questions about whether a child is dying, but parents will only choose a nurse whom they can trust to ask such crucial questions. The nurse can accept that trust by enabling them to talk more generally about the issue. Faulkner (1995) suggests such responses as: 'What do you already know about the condition?' or 'Is that what is worrying you?' In this way the nurse can listen to the parents' real concerns and fetch appropriate help if unable to answer all questions personally.

Families' emotions affect the care and support they can give to the dying child. They are in great need of understanding and support from the nurses they meet. Parents need time as individuals and together to work through their reactions to knowing their child is going to die. They will not always feel the same emotions at the same time. Anger, guilt, resentment, blame of the other parent are all common reactions. Hill (1994) recognises that mothers find it easier to express these emotions and that health care professionals expect fathers to cope. Consequently, fathers' needs are often not adequately met.

Children may be well aware of their own death, but choose not to discuss it with their parents because they have learnt that this is not a topic with which the family feels at ease. Children as young as 4 or 5 can usually sense when they are seriously ill and they need simple, honest answers to their questions.

Activity

Peter is a 14 year old who is dying from an inoperable cerebral tumour. His parents have remained adamant throughout his illness that he should not be told of diagnosis and prognosis. During his bath he suddenly asks you: 'Am I dying?' How should you reply?

There is no easy answer to whether parents can override the rights of dying children to be told the truth. Peck (1992) discusses the factors involved in this difficult situation. The need to be honest with the child must be considered alongside the needs of the parents and the legal issues. Ideally, this dilemma should be discussed with parents who wish to withhold information from the child.

Nurses worry about how to answer direct questions about death, but Hill (1994) advises that a response such as 'Is that something which worries you?' enables the child to discuss their feelings, gives the nurse an idea of the child's concerns and provides time to alert others of the child's readiness to explore death.

Parents often ask for guidance about what to tell children and siblings. As with any person, it is useful to listen to what is being said and only to answer the question which is being asked. Long and complicated answers may confuse the child even further. Simple answers may be all the child needs. They may give the impetus for further questions but they allow the child to dictate the pace. It is useful to remember the anecdote about the small boy who asked his mother where he came from. Mother gave a detailed account of the facts of life only for the small boy to explain that his friend came from Scotland and she still had not answered his question!

Children's questions about death

- How do you die?
- Will you and I die one day?
- Will I be able to see Granny again when I am dead?
- Can nurses make dead people come alive again?
- How do dead people on TV come alive again?
- Why do people die?

Activity

Read 'Children's questions about death' and consider how you would answer these.

Children's questions are always asked for a good reason and they should be treated with sincerity (Lindsay, 1994). Discussions about death with young children, when death has affected their family, is possible and may be very helpful to them (Meadows, 1993).

GRIEVING

Grieving means feeling and expressing all the emotions related to the death and the deceased person. It is not about forgetting what has happened but about slowly accepting it and adjusting to it. It is about finding a way to remember the person with love rather than pain. Rather like pain, the intensity of grief is difficult to describe and cannot be compared with the grief of another person. Everyone is different, and one person's grief may be as painful as another's, whatever the circumstances. Feelings of grief may last for a long time and may change from day to day.

There is no right way to grieve and whilst there is a generalised pattern of behaviour which all bereaved people exhibit, the time scale is widely variable and there may not be a steady progression to acceptance. Many bereaved people will move backwards as well as forwards between these generalised patterns (Table 3.1).

Time	State	Behaviour	Helpful responses
1–14 days	Shock Disbelief Relief	Crying/inability to cry Refusal to accept Emotionless	'Permission' to cry Accept feelings Listen
After 14 days	Fear Anger Guilt Denial	Feaful of leaving house Resentment allocating blame Self-reproach Enshrining	Acknowledge fears Reassure 'normal' reaction Listen Be non-judgemental
2–3 months	Yearning Searching	Repetition of death Fear of forgetting, visiting old haunts	Allow to talk Listen Be patient
3–12 months	Depression Loneliness	Withdrawal Clinging to grief	Allow to share despair Be tolerant
1–5 years	Acceptance Adjustment Healing	Recall deceased happily Find 'new' life Renewed self-image	'Allow' grief to stop Encourage Acknowledge

Table 3.1

A generalised pattern of bereavement

Activity

Read the accounts illustrating the stages of grief (see next page). For each one consider why the characters are behaving in this way and how you could help.

Grieving does not always begin at death. For many families this process starts at the moment they know that the person is going to die. In this situation, there are intense feelings of grief at diagnosis which may reach a plateau or even decline if there is any length of time between the bad news and the death. In some cancers these feelings may fluctuate with remissions and relapses. Grief rises again at the actual death but the worst point for many people is during the first 6 months following the death. Grief tends to be at a high level throughout the first year of bereavement. During this time every day is an anniversary of a significant event. The first Christmas, wedding anniversary or birthday can be particularly difficult to cope with.

After the first year, grief usually begins to lessen in intensity but it never goes away; it just becomes more manageable with the passing years. Even then, it may re-surface at specific times of the year which are emotive for the family.

PROVIDING SUPPORT

The exact needs of those who have been bereaved depend upon their individual feelings and personalities, but there are many general needs which nurses can meet. Bereaved parents and children are very sensitive at the time of death and during the early months after the death. Although it is difficult to know what to say, it is important that words are carefully chosen. Brewis (1995) gives examples of statements which were probably meant well but left bereaved parents with negative memories of the carers:

- I know how you feel
- Never mind, it's for the best
- You can always have another child

The bereaved do not want to be told how they feel – only they can know this. But they do sometimes need the opportunity to talk about their needs and feelings. It is important to listen to what they have to say and be sensitive to the thoughts they cannot express. Remember that it is sometimes as difficult for them to express themselves as it for you to know what to say. It may help if you can share your own feelings about the death, always taking care not to overwhelm them with your grief.

Activity

Write a letter of condolence to a friend whose child has just died after a road traffic accident. Afterwards consider the following:

- Did you use platitudes?
- Did you communicate your honest feelings and beliefs?
- Were you tempted to put off writing the letter?

The bereaved often relate how other people avoid talking to them or talk about everything except the death when what they want is to feel comfortable with someone who will talk about their loved one and listen to their feelings of grief. For this reason many parents are comforted by others who have had a similar experience to their own. There are many statutory and voluntary agencies offering emotional support and counselling for bereaved children and parents. Families need to be able to choose how they wish to be supported but information should be readily available for them.

PRACTICAL ARRANGEMENTS

When someone dies the bereaved often do not know what practical arrangements have to be made. Often they are too upset to take control of such matters. It is often the nurse that people turn to for advice about such arrangements. Some parents may want advice about planning the funeral service before the death and may find these decisions easier when the child is still alive (Walter, 1990). It is also useful for the nurse to discuss any religious traditions before death to ensure that no beliefs are ignored and to avoid any confusion.

Activity

Find out the answers to the questions listed overleaf in 'Death – the practical details'.

Faulkner (1995) recommends that, if the death occurs in hospital, a small quiet room be available for the bereaved to receive information about registering the death and finding a funeral director. She stresses the importance of this formality being carried out by a nurse who knows the family well to add the personal element and to provide emotional support. It is useful also to be able to give this information in written form as it likely that the shock and grief felt at this time will prevent retention of facts.

Parents report that being able to see and hold their dead child has helped them to grieve. The nurse should prepare them for this experience and be present to offer support if needed (Thompson, 1992). After their child has died parents sometimes need to feel that they have some lasting memory and may be helped by photographs, hand or foot prints or a lock of hair.

1. Nurses need to come to terms with their own beliefs and emotions about death if they are to able to talk openly about it with parents and children.
2. Children's perceptions of death are more likely to have been gained from the media than any direct experience. As a result, they may have developed unrealistic and confusing ideas.
3. Children need to be involved in the care of the dying sibling or parent and to be allowed to discuss their thoughts and fears. Exclusion only distresses them further and may cause long-term psychological problems.
4. There is no right or wrong way to answer children's and parents'

Supporting the bereaved

Do
- Let your concern and caring show
- Be available to listen, run errands, help with the children
- Say you are sorry about the death and about their distress
- Allow them to share their grief
- Encourage them to be patient with themselves
- Allow them to talk about the dead person
- Talk about the special qualities of the dead person
- Reassure them that they did all they could
- Give extra attention to children who are often forgotten by grieving adults

Don't
- Avoid them because you feel uncomfortable
- Say you know how they feel
- Tell them what they should feel or do
- Avoid mentioning the dead person's name
- Try to find something positive about the death
- Suggest that other members of the family can replace the dead person
- Indicate that the care given before death was inadequate
- Let your own feelings of helplessness stop you from offering support

> ### Key points

Death – the practical details

Do you know:

- When a cremation can take place?
- What practical decisions have to be taken when planning a funeral and who can advise on these?
- How much a funeral costs?
- What sort of financial help is available for low income families?
- How to find out about local support groups for the bereaved?
- The circumstances under which an inquest may be held?
- The names of three national organisations which provide support for the bereaved?
- The circumstances under which the doctor must report a death to the coroner?
- The time period within which a child's death should be registered?
- Which services should be notified of a death?
- Who provides what kind of certificate following an expected death?

questions about death. Listening and providing simple and honest answers are the most helpful ways of dealing with awkward questions.

5. The grief of bereavement is a long and complicated process which is different for each individual and never passes. However, there is a gradual adjustment to a new life which can be helped by a patient and understanding listener.

6. Nurses can help parents after the death by being able to give advice about the practical issues which distressed parents do not have the energy or desire to manage.

CHRONIC ILLNESS – FAMILY STRESS   **4**
AND COPING

INTRODUCTION

When a child has a chronic and debilitating disorder the ongoing feelings of grief, guilt, and sorrow experienced by the parents have been defined as chronic sorrow (Myer, 1988). The intensity of these feelings depends on the family's developmental stage, the age of the child at diagnosis, communication between spouses and the degree of support available from family and physician (Burr, 1985). Mothers often feel guilty at producing a child with a chronic problem and this may cause them to become over-protective whilst resenting the time involved in the child's care and feeling uncertain and anxious about the child's future. In comparison, fathers often feel excluded by the relationship between mother and child. Both parents may feel socially isolated due to their child's condition or time-consuming treatment. Thus parents of a child with a chronic condition often have to cope with their own emotions about the implications of the disorder as well as a complex treatment regime. The affected child and siblings also have to cope with conflicting emotions, often without the support of their parents who are too distressed themselves to provide the usual comfort.

Parental knowledge of a chronic childhood illness is considered important for its effective treatment. Education usually begins as soon as the condition is diagnosed, but this is a stressful time and many parents are too anxious to be able to fully comprehend the significance of information given at this time. Studies suggest that parental knowledge and understanding of their child's illness contributes to the development of independence for the child, treatment compliance, control of the illness and maintenance of appropriate family relationships and lifestyle. However, it has also been suggested that parents of children with life-threatening illnesses resist information about the condition because such knowledge will destroy their denial mechanisms with which they cope with the threat of the potentially fatal outcome. The chronic uncertainty of an unknown outcome is responsible for much of the stress experienced by parents which in turn affects their coping strategies (Cohen and Martison, 1988).

Lazarus and Cohen (1977) define coping in terms of the strategies used in the face of different kinds of threat. Leventhal (1986) identifies three important processes involved in coping; the individual needs to:

- understand the threat;
- compare self with others exposed to the same or similar threat;
- acquire a sense of hope.

Psychosocial stresses of chronic illness affecting the children

Schooling
- disruption due to hospitalisation, out-patient appointments
- learning difficulties, due to excessive disruption or treatment

Relationships
- jealousy with siblings
- disruption of social life

Uncertain future
- employment prospects
- marriage and fertility
- genetic implications of illness

Body image changes
- directly related to the condition
- subsequent to surgery
- retarded growth/puberty
- side effects of treatment (alopecia, weight loss or gain)

Frequent hospitalisation
- pain and discomfort from procedures
- disruption of normal routine
- feelings of dependency

There appear to be two main methods of coping with the threat. Approach coping is concerned with doing something directly about reducing the threat and avoidance coping relates to taking palliative action to avoid confronting the threat.

APPROACH COPING METHODS

Gibson (1988) found that parents of children with a chronic illness used three main approach coping strategies, i.e. social support, problem-solving skills and a belief in the efficacy of medical care. Social support is usually gained from health care professionals or other parents in similar circumstances and enables parents to feel a sense of control. Problem-solving skills and having a system of beliefs are intra-psychic methods of coping which also give parents a personal sense of control which in itself is rewarding.

Social support in the form of support groups can reduce the problems of isolation as well as providing emotional and practical support. However, Llewelyn and Haslett (1986) warn that support groups can have a negative influence by imposing the views of dominant members of the group. Isolation tends to be self-imposed because of society's attitude to disability and these negative attitudes have an impact on the family's coping skills (Geen, 1990). This sense of isolation is heightened by 20th century social factors. Families are now smaller and nuclear and more geographically separated, making family support less available than previously. Affluent families have more resources to overcome these social factors and Macaskill and Monach (1990) note that these families are more likely to adjust to the stress of living with a chronic illness.

The need for social support varies within cultures. In cultures where the family is important their own support networks enable them to cope well and they may resist help from health care professionals or other parents. Conversely, Spinetta (1984) found that Mexican and Vietnamese families cope with difficulty because their culture does not value close communication and sharing of emotions. Similarly, the British culture still tends to consider that males should keep a stiff upper lip, and Faulkner *et al.* (1995) describe how fathers found it particularly difficult to share their emotions and felt they should remain unemotional to support the rest of the family.

Problem-solving skills and a belief in the efficacy of health care depends largely on adequate information being available to all the family. Yet, Whitehead (1995) concludes from studies of parents and children's knowledge of diabetes that there is little relationship between parent and child knowledge of the condition; the length of time since diagnosis does not increase the amount of knowledge and knowledge does not relate to management skills. My own studies of parents of children with cystic fibrosis had similar findings (Ramsay, 1990). My own conclusions were that although families needed more information and advice, they also required a structured teaching programme to help them analyse and evaluate their knowledge to aid their problem-solving skills and management of the condition. Similar programmes have been carried out for families of children with asthma with significant positive effects (Lewis *et al.*, 1984). This teaching needs to take into account the physical and psychological problems of the condition. Studies indicate that health care professionals tend to ignore the psychological concerns and require teaching themselves about identifying and managing these (Faulkner *et al.*, 1995). The inability of health care professionals to give bad news in a sensitive way and to address the psychological concerns of the whole family does not help the family to have trust and confidence in them.

AVOIDANCE COPING METHODS

Denial is a common emotion during the time of diagnosis of a chronic illness and is often seen as a maladaptive reaction to stress. However, parents have to come to terms with the loss of their 'perfect child' and Whyte (1992) argues that the defence mechanism of denial is a necessary response to reduce the impact of the diagnosis and all its consequences, and allow life to continue. Prolonged use of denial can prevent long-term adaptation to the situation and may cause parents to over-protect and over indulge their child and neglect treatment (Tropauer *et al.*, 1970).

Jennings (1992) found that many parents of chronically ill children felt intense anger during the period of adjustment to the condition and demonstrated this by crying, screaming and slamming doors. Whilst these reactions can be helpful in the short-term, they do not help long-term adaptation and may cause further stress for other members of the family. Anger often results from the frustration of trying to cope with all the consequences of the illness and maintaining a normal lifestyle, especially when no one seems to recognise these stresses. Beth, the mother of Tom, who died from a chronic neurological condition, remained angry with the health care professionals 2 years after Tom's death: 'I am still cross that so much of my energy had to be used to get the help and support I needed, when I could have used it to be with Tom'.

Other reactions include shame, guilt, uncertainty and depression. Generally, mothers appear to take on the burden of caring for the affected child as well as for the rest of the family and this responsibility often becomes too overwhelming. I remember one mother who refused to talk to me about her child's illness 'because I cry whenever I talk about it'. This reaction is not unique; Shapiro (1983) found that mothers often experience depression which inhibits their talking to others about their child. This is a very difficult problem as it is likely that these mothers are the very people who need help to talk. Difficulty in open communication often impairs parents' management of the

Pyschosocial stresses of chronic illness for the parents

Finances
- frequent hospital trips
- loss of employment and income

Relationships
- meeting the needs of the affected child and the siblings
- social isolation due to child's treatment needs, finding responsible carer
- decreased time for usual family activities
- role changes

Communication
- ability to share feelings with spouse
- coping with the affected child's questions and fears
- ability to explain to siblings

Maintaining discipline
- treating all the family equally
- avoiding overprotective behaviour

Psychosocial stresses of chronic illness for the siblings

Relationships
- resentment towards ill sibling
- loss of contact with parents
- isolation

Role change
- extra responsibilities
- support for parents

Changes in beliefs
- concerns about infection/inheritance
- feelings of guilt about the cause of the condition
- fear of own death

child's condition (Faulkner *et al.*, 1995) and may cause marital difficulties. Evidence of marital breakdown is conflicting. Some authors believe that existing difficulties will be exacerbated (Jennings, 1992), but others have shown that couples feel closer because of the experience (Macaskill and Monach, 1990).

The sheer physical demands of the child's treatment may cause emotional and physical exhaustion. Families will react to this stress in different ways by an alteration in thoughts, emotions and behaviour. Some of these changes represent attempts to cope but may in themselves become secondary causes of stress and result in physical or mental ill-health (Figure 4.1).

Figure 4.1

Coping with stress

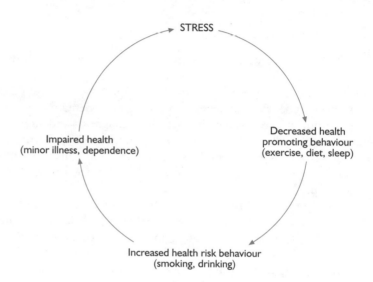

ADAPTATION

McCollum and Gibson (1970) studied families of children with a chronic condition and identified four phases of adaptation:

- pre-diagnostic;
- confrontational;
- long-term adaptive;
- terminal.

In the pre-diagnostic stage parents, especially mothers, felt guilt, despair and even hostility towards the child whom they were unable to rear successfully. There may be conflicts with others over the reality of the child's symptoms. At the confrontational stage, when the diagnosis was confirmed, parents felt initial disbelief followed by intense grief, anxiety and depression. Faulkner *et al.* (1995) found that the way in which health professionals handled this stage clearly affected parents' ability to adapt to the situation. Inept handling can cause such intense fear and anxiety that adaptation to reality is delayed. Diagnosis is often associated with the family's search for a reason why the illness has occurred to them. Faulkner *et al.* (1995) argue that families need to have a belief in a pattern of life events to help them adapt. As parents come to terms with the diagnosis they fluctuate between denial and optimism, grief and chronic anxiety. During this long-term adaptation phase they also reported problems with the management of the treatment regime whilst admitting repression and forgetting of information. The success of the final stage of adaptation seems to depend upon the family's ability to cope positively with the condition. Parents in my own study revealed the problems of the early years after diagnosis and stressed the importance of their own resources and those of other parents in finding solutions (Ramsay, 1990). At this stage, when contact with health care professionals has decreased, help is less available and families feel that they have full responsibility; as one parent described it: 'You either sink or swim'.

COMPLIANCE

Survival into adulthood and beyond for children with chronic illnesses is associated with the avoidance of not only the medical complications of the condition but also the psychological effects of living with a chronic condition. Poor psychological adjustment to the condition often results in depression and poor compliance (Goodchild and Dodge, 1985). There is increasing evidence that compliance with regimes for chronic illnesses is less than optimal. Compliance with treatment regimes for children obviously involves parents until the child is old enough to provide self-care independently. Even then, parental attitude and management of the condition during young childhood are likely to shape the way the older child behaves in relation to the illness. See Figure 4.2(a and b).

Compliance can be defined as a disposition to act in accordance with rules, wishes; to be obedient. Studies on the identification of factors which influence compliance have revealed that compliance behaviour is affected by several issues. Psychological characteristics such as attitudes and perceptions of health and illness affects the individual's concepts of the severity of the disorder and thus the importance and necessity of complying with treatment. Environmental factors such as social support, socioeconomic status and education affect the individual's ability and desire to comprehend the treatment regime. Physician–patient interaction also influences the acceptance and understanding of the illness and its treatment. Ley and Llewelyn (1995) discuss the importance of oral and written communication for understanding and compliance. They stress the need for health professionals to ensure that their communication is effective, memorable and given in a sensitive way. Finally, the therapeutic regime itself will affect compliance. It

---

Positive adaptive responses to chronic illness

- Acceptance of the child's condition
- Realistic expectations for the child
- Day-to-day management of the condition
- Meet the child's normal developmental needs
- Meet the developmental needs of the other family members
- Assist family members to express their feelings
- Educate others about the child's condition
- Establish a support system

(Canam, 1993)

Figure 4.2

Psychological factors and compliance. (a) Poor compliance. (b) Good compliance.

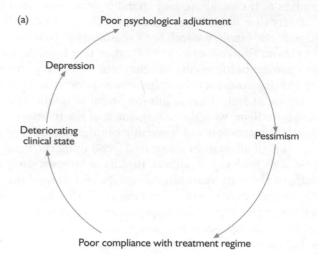

(a)

Poor psychological adjustment

Depression

Pessimism

Deteriorating clinical state

Poor compliance with treatment regime

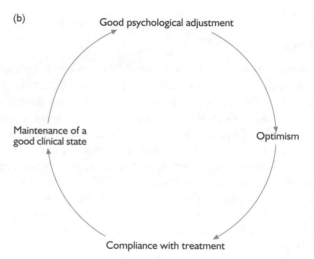

(b)

Good psychological adjustment

Maintenance of a good clinical state

Optimism

Compliance with treatment

Improving compliance by communication

Improving oral communication:

- using shorter words and sentences
- avoiding jargon
- stressing the importance
- breaking down information into categories
- using specific statements
- repeating information
- arranging follow-up visits to test recall

Providing written information

- using symbols, graphics, colour to ensure it is noticed
- ensuring legibility
- using simple terms in short sentences
- explaining technical terms
- stressing relevance
- highlighting areas of specific importance
- addressing counter-arguments

appears that the more complex and lengthy the treatment and the more changes to usual behaviour it involves, the less likely compliance will occur (Ley and Llewelyn, 1995). Again, improved methods of communication can help families to remember and manage complex regimes.

Compliance may be a specific problem in adolescence when chronic illness may be most detrimental to normal growth and development. Illness interferes with the adolescent's need for autonomy and a positive self-image. The adolescent tendency for rebellion and risk-taking may manifest itself in non-compliance with treatment regimes. However, Auslander *et al.* (1991) found that poor compliance in diabetic adolescents was related to stress in the family so it may be that positive adaptation of the family to the condition determines the older child's ability to manage it.

THE ROLE OF THE NURSE

Robinson (1993) has noted that nurses can play a negative role in helping families to adapt to chronic illness. Others believe that the caring, competent and committed attitude of most nurses is enough to support parents to cope positively with the situation (Ray and Ritchie, 1993). Given the importance of social support and the need to believe in the effectiveness of the health care professionals, it seems important that the nurse has the skills to help the family to:

- understand the condition and treatment;
- live as normal a life as possible;
- discuss their feelings with each other;
- include the child and siblings in decision making;
- meet their practical needs;
- establish realistic goals for the future.

How does the nurse learn these skills? Faulkner *et al.* (1995) believe that a thorough understanding can only be gained by working with and listening to families who live with a child with a chronic illness. Certainly, this will add a depth of understanding which teaching alone cannot impart but they propose that nurse education becomes more interactive and experiential so that nurses can role play stressful situations and learn to identify psychological problems. Faulkner *et al.* (1995) also suggest that a named practice nurse, who has been taught these skills of working with families with chronic illness, be assigned to the family at diagnosis. This nurse can identify concerns and help the family to deal with them. This method would provide the family with immediate and long-term credible support.

➤ **Key points**

1. Having a child with a chronic condition changes the lives of the whole family and threatens their plans for the future.
2. Families use a variety of adaptive and maladaptive behaviours during their adjustment to the situation.
3. The family's acceptance of the condition and their adjustment to it is associated with appropriate adaptive behaviours in response to the psychological and physiological management of the condition.
4. Positive adaptation is associated with social support, belief in the efficacy of health care and the ability to problem solve.
5. Positive adaptation is aided by open and honest communication between: all the members of the family, and the family and the health care professionals.
6. Nurses can help families to cope by providing information and recognising psychological and practical problems.

5 LIVING WITH A DISABILITY

INTRODUCTION

Having a child with a disability can often be a positive or negative experience for the rest of the family. Some families gain strengths from the experience but for others it causes disharmony and distress. Nurses can do much to help families cope with the disability and meet the challenge of living with a disabled child.

It is also not easy for the affected child to live with a permanent disability and overcome prejudice, ridicule and discrimination as well as physical problems which influence roles, relationships and life experience. The nurse can help these children to maximise their abilities and to overcome their disability. With the appropriate treatment, education and support disabled children may reach the same goals in adulthood as their 'normal' peers. However, even this does not prevent the disabled child from a constant feeling of being different (Harrison, 1997).

Thus, the role of the nurse is complex. Families need help with the practical issues relating to caring for a child with a disability but they also need counselling and sympathetic and uncritical support. The child also requires emotional and physical help to be able to live as normal a life as possible.

ADJUSTMENT TO DISABILITY

Moos and Tsu (1977) found that there were six factors which were associated with adjustment to disability. Positive adjustment was aided by the ability to:

- change beliefs and goals for the future;
- accept responsibility for the disability;
- seek information about overcoming the disability;
- contain negative feelings.

Poor adjustment was associated with anger and blame directed at others as the cause of the disability and time-consuming fantasies about recovery. Small children growing up with a disability usually take their cues from their parents about their disability. Parents who are able to help their child to live as normal a life as possible will enable their child to adjust and overcome their disability better than the child who is protected from reality (Russell, 1989). Denial of the disability and over-expectations about the future are natural at times but are dangerous if allowed to develop. These fantasies can be accidentally promoted by hospitalisation for surgery or treatment which the child may think will restore normality. If the nurse does not give an honest explanation, the child can feel devastated when the anticipated improvement does not

Sidebar (left column)

- *Impairment* – A stable and persisting defect in the individual … which stems from known or unknown molecular, cellular, physiological or structural disorder
- *Disability* – A stable and persisting physical or psychological dysfunction at the personal level, by necessity again confined to the individual; this dysfunction stems from the limitations imposed by the impairment and by the individual's psychological reaction to it
- *Handicap* – Persisting social dysfunction, a social role assumed by the impaired or disabled individual that is assigned by the expectations of society. Handicap stems not from the individual but from social expectations; it follows from the manner and degree in which expectations alter the performance of social roles by impaired or disabled persons

(WHO, 1980)

Factors which influence adjustment to disability

- Age of acquisition
- Insidious versus traumatic onset
- Stability of condition
- Severity of disability
- Degree of dependency
- Intellectual functioning
- Associated pain or illness

occur. Children with Down's syndrome are now having plastic surgery to correct the characteristic facial features associated with this condition. Whilst some may argue that this provides children with the best chance of normal socialisation, others suggest that such surgery is unnecessary discomfort for the children to appease society's expectations of what is normal (Hinsliff, 1997).

Adjustment is also related to health locus of control. Disabled adults have been found to cope better with their disability if they have an internal locus of control, they have more knowledge of their condition and practise more self-care. Wilkinson (1995) suggests that developing an internal locus of control in disabled children could enhance their satisfaction with life and psychological well-being. It could also help their level of self-care and independence.

Often the care of a disabled child is mainly the mother's responsibility. Complicated, time-consuming and onerous care may use up all her physical and mental resources, leaving little energy for the rest of the family. This can result in social isolation for all the family, loss of maternal care for any siblings and feelings of resentment. This negative scenario does nothing for the disabled child's self-esteem. Maternal reaction to the disability, which appears to be related to adequate support, has been found to significantly influence siblings' acceptance of disability in the family. Inadequate support is associated with neglect of the needs of siblings, and especially girls being given more responsibility for care of the disabled child (Atkinson and Crawford, 1995). The Carers National Association estimates that 40–50 000 children in the UK provide care for a disabled friend or relative. Whilst this can be a positive experience, they are at risk from unrecognised stress and isolation (Syverson, 1997).

ATTITUDES TO DISABILITY

Wright (1983) suggests that the general population assumes that physically disabled people also have a mental disability and tend to treat the disabled with a patronising and pitying manner. Wilkinson (1995) considers that these attitudes arise from idealised images of normality with body image being associated with status, achievement and success. The experience of living with a disability allows some families to reconsider these attitudes to illness and disability. Peace (1996a) cites a mother who said that her definition of disability before she had a child with cerebral palsy was unhappiness. Since her personal experience she now realised that everyone was an individual and no one was perfect.

Although personal attitudes may change, the family still have to cope with others misconceptions. Atkinson and Crawford (1995) found that 70% of siblings had been bullied, teased or avoided because of their brother's or sister's disability. Over half of these children admitted that they were embarrassed, upset or angry by the effect of their sibling's disability on their relationships.

Supporting siblings

Communication
- inform them about the disability and update them as appropriate
- listen to their ideas and concerns
- discuss the future with them

Involvement
- include them in the care of the disabled child
- let them teach their life skills to the disabled sibling
- do not over-burden them with responsibility for care

Appreciation
- treat all children the same in relation to discipline, attention and resources
- provide all children with their own special time alone with parents
- value all children equally
- allow all children to have privacy and solitude
- permit sibling squabbles and disputes

The attitudes of health professionals to disability have also been criticised. Mikulic (1971) found that nurses tended to reinforce dependency rather than independent behaviour. They do not tend to promote normal lifestyles, often seeing such tactics as evidence of the denial of the disability (Robinson, 1993). In this way they may actually prevent families from developing ways of coping (Ray and Ritchie, 1993). Purssell (1994) suggests that such attitudes are due to a lack of education and that nurses need more input about disability and the importance of maximising normalisation.

CARING NEEDS

Wilkinson (1995) argues that hospitals are for sick people and are not best suited to learning to cope with a disability. Rehabilitation and disability management learnt in hospital is not easily transferred into the home. Transitional areas, sometimes found in maternity units, which are more like the home environment, could enable the disabled child and family to develop independence in the skills needed for successful discharge. It would be easier for families to re-discover normality in this kind of environment, giving them a better chance of overcoming the feelings of being different and taking control of their life. To enable this control the family need to have a suitably adapted environment to encourage the child's independence. Many aids and adaptations are available for the disabled and the Disabled Living Foundation can provide useful information about these. Practical advice about clothing for the older child can help the child's independence and still enable them to be fashionable.

Before discharge, parents also need advice about minimising the effect of the disability on family life. Robinson (1993) advocates that the child and family should live a normal family life and that the child should be exposed to the reactions of others so that they can learn to accept these. The family should be encouraged to treat the disabled child as a child and not as a disability. The development of any child is individual and, like any child, the disabled child needs stimulation to aid this development, minimise the disability and maximise abilities. Although parents find it difficult to be strict with their disabled child, it is important to maintain discipline or the child may develop into an immature and spoilt adolescent. Ignoring bad behaviour may also lead to behaviour problems in siblings who will be jealous of what appears to be favouritism. As with any child, the disabled child will need to be able to interact with others as an adult and socialisation should be encouraged. A variety of leisure activities is available for disabled children and participation in these helps socialisation as well as being part of normal childhood.

Activity

Find out what leisure activities are available for disabled children in your locality.

Professional intervention in the care of the disabled child cannot cure the physical problems but it can add to the child's quality of life. Parents of children with a disability often come into contact with a great variety of health care professionals and are frustrated by the lack of continuity and coordination of care (Peace, 1996b). She suggests that a key worker could help to overcome these problems which result in criticisms of inappropriate or duplicate care or none at all. A children's community nurse could be the ideal key worker in these situations and do much to coordinate care whilst enabling the family to take overall control. In addition, a children's nurse would have the skills which families value; an appreciation of the reality of living with a child with a disability and easy accessibility for advice and support (Peace, 1996b). Thorne (1993) also found that families had most confidence and trust in those professionals who could demonstrate competence and effective communication skills.

Farrell (1996) believes that disabled children and their families can benefit from hospice respite care. The huge physical and emotional demands for these families mean that they can become completely physically and emotionally exhausted. This can affect their own physical and mental health as well as the care they provide for their child. Respite care aims to give a supportive environment where the hospice team will share the care usually given solely by the family. It provides an opportunity for the family to rest and to participate in family activities which may have been previously impossible because of the care demands of the disabled child. In addition, respite care may be able to provide the child with new experiences; new treatments or trips out may be possible because the hospice may have access to more resources and skilled help than the home environment.

EDUCATIONAL NEEDS

Learning disability/difficulty are now the terms to describe children with an intellectual impairment who were once known to have a mental handicap. Earys *et al.* (1993) found that this term was prejudicial and did not recognise the specific problems of the child. Whilst some children may only be intellectually disabled, many of them also have associated physical and sensory disabilities. Children with only a physical or sensory disability may have special educational needs in terms of the school environment or the specialist equipment they require.

The Warnock Committee on Special Education Needs did much for the educational rights of disabled children. It made 250 recommendations about the care of children with disabilities, including the abolition of the term handicap and the recognition that parents should be partners in their child's care and education. The 1981 Education Act, which arose from the Warnock report and has since been supported by the Children Act (DoH, 1989), stressed the importance of multi-agency

Practical advice – clothing

- Avoid back fastenings which are awkward to fasten and may cause sores for children in wheelchairs
- Separates can be bought in different sizes and are easier to put on and take off. Velcro strips can be used to hold tops and bottoms together
- Sturdy material which stretches is likely to prolong the life of the clothing
- Bra slips or brassieres which fasten at the front are easier than traditional brassieres
- Capes are more convenient than coats for children in wheelchairs
- Boots and shoes are easier to manipulate if they are elasticated or have laces which open the shoe to the toes
- Most large shoe manufacturers operate an odd-shoe scheme for children with different sized feet. They have to be ordered at an additional charge
- Over-the-knee socks or hold-up stockings are easier to manage than tights, but care should be taken to ensure that these do not compress the top of the leg

Cross reference

Educational provision for children with special needs – page 102

Leisure facilities for the disabled

- *Opportunity playgroups* – for children with any type of disability are available in some parts of the country
- *Toy libraries* – loan toys and play equipment for disabled children
- *Handicapped adventure playgrounds* – throughout greater London and elsewhere
- *Pets* – trained to assist the blind, deaf or disabled
- *Swimming* – advice from the Swimming Teachers Association Guidelines for teaching the Disabled to swim. Many pools have special sessions for the disabled
- *Holidays* – suitable accommodation listed by the Royal Association for Disability and Rehabilitation. Voluntary organisations often have schemes to provide holidays for disabled children. Social Services may help with costs
- *Duke of Edinburgh Award Scheme* – open to disabled and able-bodied children
- *Music* – Disabled Living Foundation has information about courses, teachers and orchestras for the disabled
- *Riding* – The Riding for the Disabled Association has 330 branches throughout the country
- *Sports* – Information from the British Sports Association for the Disabled
- *Scouts and Guides* – County advisor can offer opportunities for disabled children
- *Youth club activities* – organised by the National Physically Handicapped and Ablebodied (PHAB) Association for disabled and able-bodied children over 13

cooperation to identify and meet the needs of disabled children. It promoted the concept of assessment of needs rather than determining requirements by diagnosis, IQ or physical abilities. The Act also enabled children to receive special education in a diversity of settings, including ordinary schools. The importance of integration into ordinary schools is emphasised and defined in many different ways; it can mean a place in an ordinary class, a special unit in an ordinary school or sharing of some facilities between an ordinary and a special school.

Activity

Consider the advantages and disadvantages for a disabled child in an ordinary school.

When I consider this issue I am reminded of the quotation 'Better to reign in hell than serve in heaven' from John Milton's *Paradise Lost*. Is integration really the answer for disabled children? The theory behind integration is that disabled children can gain in self-confidence and independence by the association with able-bodied children in the usual environment of childhood. Evidence of these positive effects have been shown by the National Foundation for Educational Research (Russell, 1989). However, this is not true for all children and there are wide variations between the attitudes of local educational authorities towards resourcing disabled children in ordinary schools. Roger was diagnosed with a degenerative sensory disorder at the age of 8 years. Initially, he was educated at his usual primary school but he became sullen and withdrawn and his previously good schoolwork deteriorated. On investigation, it was found that even with special aids to compensate for his disability, he could not keep pace with his peers. To use his aids he had to sit separately from the rest of the class and he was not allowed to join sports activities, in which he previously excelled, because it was thought to be unsafe. He was eventually transferred to a residential school for the sensory impaired where he has thrived. He integrates with children with a variety of degrees of disability which has helped him appreciate their needs as well as realising that he is not unique. He is able to participate on equal terms with his school friends in a variety of educational and sports activities and, because he is also learning specific life skills for his disability, is able to make realistic future plans.

The Education Act (1981) made provision for the assessment of children's learning needs based on the child's abilities rather than their disabilities. The Act also placed a duty on health authorities to inform the parents and the LEA of any child who has, or is likely to develop, special educational needs. Formal assessment can take place from the age of 2 years, but assessment can take place earlier than this at parents' request. If the LEA considers that a child over 2 requires special educational needs outside that which is usually available through the school services, formal assessment procedures may be initiated. The end product of this assessment is the statement which includes educational, medical and psychological opinion about the child's educational needs and ways of meeting these. Parents have a right to contribute to this written assessment and to use other representatives to provide evidence if they wish. Parents have argued that although they have opportunity to query the draft statement and appeal about the outcome, it is only those who are vocal and able to express themselves well who can make a real impact on the statementing process.

GROWING UP

Adolescence is a difficult time for most children as they struggle to achieve social acceptance as well as independence, self-esteem and autonomy. It is an even more difficult struggle for the disabled adolescent who already has a feeling of being different. Adolescence is often a challenging time for parents who may be reluctant to release responsibility for their child. Parents of disabled children feel this more acutely and are more concerned about the child's ability to be independent.

Local authorities have a statutory obligation to provide special accommodation for the disabled and if the adolescent wishes to live away from home parents need to make sure their name is on the waiting list for this accommodation. A number of surveys now exist to provide information about the available facilities for disabled students within universities. These can be obtained from the National Union of Students. Education authorities are required to award full-time disabled students an additional grant to meet special equipment related to the disability, but the student is expected to apply and explain the need for this extra money.

The Disablement Resettlement Officer (DRO) is employed by the Employment Service specifically to encourage employers to find suitable work for the disabled. Some big companies employ their own DRO. The DRO assesses each disabled person's abilities and compares these with the local job vacancies and the vocational and professional training opportunities. There are also local day facilities for the disabled which may offer some kind of paid employment. These centres tend to be for those who are too disabled to work and can be seen to further segregate the severely disabled.

Activity

Find out what opportunities there are for further education, training or employment for the disabled teenager in your own locality.

Society often considers that sexual relationships for the disabled are inappropriate. Children with a disability may have little understanding

The Warnock Committee of Enquiry (1978)

Recommended that the:

- Single categories labelling a child as handicapped be abolished and replaced by detailed descriptions of the child's special educational needs
- Rigid demarcation between the handicapped and non-handicapped be abolished
- Term sub-normal be replaced by the new descriptive phrase child with special learning difficulties
- Handicapped child should be integrated into normal schools to benefit both the handicapped and the normal child by providing a better opportunity for the development of a constructive attitude to disability

Based on the principles that:

- Handicapped children should be regarded as children first, some having special needs
- A suitable educational programme best suited to the individual child's particular needs should be established
- Children may have several needs which must all be met. One single handicap should not obscure other needs
- Handicap is not static and the child's needs may change over time

Statementing

General advice for parents providing evidence:

- Describe the relevant aspects of the child's functioning at home and at school which contribute to or lessen needs
- Include the child's physical and psychological strengths and weaknesses
- Enclose any relevant aspects of the child's past history (e.g. environments which enabled or prevented the child's development)
- Explain the necessary aims to enable the child to achieve educational development and increased independence
- Describe how the recommended facilities and resources will promote the aims explained above

of sex and sexuality. By the time they reach school leaving age they may have had little opportunity for privacy with other adolescents or to observe the development of usual boy–girl relationships which occur during adolescence. Their ability to get professional advice may be hampered by the constant presence of a carer. Support groups for teenagers with disabilities can help them to overcome this and other problems. Nurses may be able to provide clear explanations in an uninhibited way, and provide information about contraception and other practical issues. However, this is not a subject which all nurses feel at ease with and they tend not to assess or plan care around the issue of sexuality (Van Ooijen and Charnock, 1994). Van Ooijen (1996) suggests that this is because nurses are not at ease with their own sexuality and are uncomfortable listening to others discussing sexual matters.

Activity

Discuss with a colleague your feelings about discussing potential sexual problems with a disabled teenager. Discuss also the reasons for your feelings and the amount of knowledge you have about such problems.

Key points ➤

1. Living with a disabled child can be a positive or negative experience for the family.
2. Children's nurses have an important role in providing families with the necessary skills to accept the disability and adjust to it in an appropriate way.
3. Society holds negative views towards disability and tends to equate a less than perfect body image with failure and loss of status.
4. Children's nurses can act as a resource to provide the practical advice which will help the disabled child to maximise abilities and reach independence.
5. Living with a disabled child can be a huge physical and emotional strain for parents. Respite care can provide them with a rest from their responsibilities whilst helping the child to experience new pursuits.
6. Integration of education can have advantages and disadvantages which depend upon the individual child, the degree of disability and the available facilities. Disabled adolescents need advice and support about all the usual issues related to growing up and the children's nurse may be the most appropriate person to provide this.

VIOLENCE IN THE FAMILY 6

INTRODUCTION

Violence can be defined as behaviour which is intended to hurt another person or to destroy property. Psychologists disagree about the causes of the development of violence. Freud believed that it was a basic instinct and could not be eliminated, only modified by other activities such as sports. Other early psychologists suggested that violence had a biological basis and that frustration induced an aggressive drive which motivated violent behaviour. Social learning theory proposes that violence is no different from any other learned response. It can be learnt by observation or imitation. Bandura (1973) showed that nursery school children learnt violence by imitation and were more likely to repeat the aggressive behaviour if they were reinforced for such actions. This raises the question of the effect of violence watched on television or in films. Most studies agree that viewing violence increases aggression, particularly in young children by:

* teaching aggressive types of behaviour;

* increasing arousal;

* desensitising people to violence;

* reducing restraints on aggressive behaviour;

* distorting views on the resolution of conflict (Bee, 1989).

Violence or abuse in the family falls into five main categories: physical, emotional, neglect, sexual and financial. It can be inflicted against children, young adults and the elderly, and occurs in both the community and in institutional settings. Gelles and Cornell (1985) note that persons who observe violence or who are victims of violence in childhood often become abusers themselves. Additionally, McKibben *et al.* (1989) found that an abused spouse was often an abusing parent.

This section will briefly discuss violence in the family, because of its impact upon any children who are present, but will mainly explore child abuse. It is vital that any professional working with children is able to recognise actual and potential child abuse, and that they know how to react to their findings.

DEFINITIONS

Abuse is difficult to define precisely but may be described as physical and/or psychological harm to another person, either temporarily or over a period of time, and may be inflicted intentionally or unintentionally, or be the result of neglect.

Physical abuse usually means that the attacker causes physical hurt, injury or even kills the subject. It can involve hitting, shaking, squeezing,

---

Definitions of child abuse

Though child abuse defies precise definition, *Working Together*, the guide to inter-agency cooperation in child protection, offers the following definitions:

* *Neglect.* The persistent or severe neglect of a child, or the failure to protect a child from exposure to any kind of danger including cold or starvation, or extreme failure to carry out important aspects of care resulting in the significant impairment of the child's health or development including non-organic failure to thrive

* *Physical injury.* Actual or likely physical injury to a child, or failure to prevent physical injury or suffering to a child including deliberate poisoning, suffocation and Munchausen's syndrome by proxy

* *Emotional abuse.* Actual or likely severe adverse effect on the emotional and behavioural development of a child , caused by persistent or severe emotional ill-treatment or rejection. All abuse involves some emotional abuse

* *Sexual abuse.* Actual or likely sexual exploitation of a child or adolescent. The child may be dependent and/or develop-mentally immature

(DHSS, 1988)

Munchausen's syndrome

Munchausen's syndrome and Munchausen's syndrome by proxy are named after Baron von Munchausen, a legendary 16th century story-teller who told amazing and incredible tales

- *Munchausen's syndrome.* Habitual seeking of hospital treatment for an apparent acute illness, the patient giving a false but plausible dramatic history and presentation of the features of the illness. Some patients may add blood to their urine or ingest poisons to create a more realistic picture. Such patients often undergo many invasive investigations and surgery before a true diagnosis is made
- *Munchausen's syndrome by proxy.* An illness that one person fabricates for another. This is commonly a mother who concocts clinical features of an illness in her child or proxy, to gain the attention of health care professionals or to gain recognition as a dedicated carer who has saved the child's life. Affected children have been known to have been poisoned, to produce chronic diarrhoea and vomiting, or suffocated causing apnoeic attacks, to necessitate medical intervention

Features of neglect

Behavioural observations
- constant hunger
- constant tiredness
- frequent lateness or non-attendance at school
- destructive tendencies
- low self-esteem
- neurotic behaviour
- no social relationships
- running away
- compulsive stealing or scavenging

Physical observations
- poor personal hygiene
- poor state of clothing
- emaciation
- untreated medical problems

burning or biting. It also involves the administration of poisonous substances, inappropriate drugs and alcohol, and attempted suffocation or drowning. It includes use of excessive force when carrying out tasks like feeding or washing a dependent person. Physical abuse includes Munchausen's syndrome by proxy where the abuser induces an illness in another person, usually a child. In children, it is usually the mother who contrives to produce features of illness in the child to gain medical attention (Jones *et al.*, 1987). The fabricated illness can take many forms from suffocation to produce apnoeic attacks to chronic poisoning. Meadow (1989) suggests that this form of abuse continues to affect the child as an adult when they often adopt Munchausen's syndrome.

Sexual abuse involves adults seeking sexual gratification by using others against their will. This may be by having sexual intercourse or anal intercourse (buggery), engaging with the person in fondling, masturbation or oral sex, and includes encouraging them to watch sexually explicate behaviour or pornographic material including videos. Kempe and Kempe (1984) provide the most commonly encountered specific definition of sexual abuse in children: ' ... the involvement of dependent, developmentally immature children and adolescents in sexual activities they do not truly comprehend, to which they are unable to give informed consent, or that violate the taboos of family roles'. This definition includes the following:

- incest;
- sexual intercourse with children in other relationships not covered by current incest legislation, including adopted and step-children;
- other forms of sexual activity.

Neglect is a more difficult area to define but is usually described as a failure to meet the basic essential needs of dependants, like adequate food, clothes warmth and medical care. Leaving young children or dependent adults alone and unsupervised is another example of neglect. Refusing or failing to give adequate love and affection is a case of emotional neglect.

Emotional abuse occurs when a constant lack of love and affection, or threats, verbal attacks, taunting or shouting causes psychological problems. This type of abuse can also take the form of constant ridicule, intimidation or swearing at the victim.

Financial abuse which occurs mostly in the elderly is the withdrawal of finances so that the person becomes totally dependent on the abuser. The victim cannot buy basic necessities, such as food and clothing, and continually worries about money.

EPIDEMIOLOGY

It is difficult to give statistics about violence as much abuse is subtle and many of the abused are too frightened or embarrassed to reveal what is happening. Abuse of adults is usually termed domestic violence and in 95% of cases the abuse takes the form of physical abuse committed by men against women (Smith, 1987). Most abused older people are also women, with the majority of their abusers being men. However, abused men may be less inclined to report violence inflicted upon them by women. In child abuse the abuser is more often female (Stier *et al.*, 1993). Consequently, there is no stereotype abuser or abused person and everyone has the potential for either of these roles (Pritchard, 1996). Nurses also have to accept that some colleagues abuse patients as incidents such as those which occurred at Glasgow's Victoria Infirmary (Clark, 1996), Bassettlaw Hospital (Kenny, 1996), and Grantham and Kesteven District General Hospital (Clothier, 1994) sadly reveal.

No single aetiological factor seems to be responsible for abuse as it is more likely to occur when several variables are involved. The most significant of variables appear to be low wages, poor housing, lack of facilities outside the home, social isolation and overcrowding (Smith, 1987). Recent studies show that domestic violence often begins or increases when the wife is pregnant and that this abuse during pregnancy often continues into child abuse once the baby is born (Bewley and Gibbs, 1994). However, although social factors are linked with abuse, violence is not confined to the lower socio-economic classes. Personality also predisposes people to violence. Those who are aggressive, easily stressed and frustrated, have a need to control, and are accustomed to violence being used freely, are more likely to abuse (Dale *et al.*, 1986).

CHILD ABUSE

The exact incidence of child abuse is not known but in 1996 the National Commission of Inquiry into the Prevention of Child Abuse estimated that in each year at least 1 million children are at risk of significant harm. It is essential that children's nurses be alert to the signs of child abuse (see Figures 6.2 and 6.3 on page 246) and that any concerns are shared with the appropriate people. Wherever you work as a children's nurse, you should have access to your local policies and guidelines and your Area Child Protection Committee (ACPC) procedures.

Activity

Locate, read and identify your own responsibilities in relation to:
- your own agencies' procedures for recording and referring suspected child abuse
- your ACPC manual of policies and procedures.

Most children have falls or knocks which cause minor bruising and grazing and children of school age, who tend to be most active, are

Features of physical abuse

Physical observations
- black eyes without gross bruising of forehead
- bruises on trunk
- bruises on upper arm consistent with gripping
- finger tip bruising – finger marks
- cigarette burns
- human bite marks
- burns caused by lengthy exposure to heat
- scalds with upward splash marks or tide marks
- fractures, particularly spiral fractures
- swelling and lack of normal use of limbs
- any serious injury with no explanation or conflicting explanations, inconsistent accounts

Behavioural observations
- unusually fearful
- unnaturally compliant
- frozen watchfulness
- refusal to discuss injuries – fear of medical help
- withdrawal from physical contact
- aggression towards others
- wearing clothing which covers arms and legs in all weathers

Pre-disposing factors for child abuse

- Parental indifference, intolerance, over-anxiousness towards the child
- History of family violence/socio-economic problems
- Infant premature, low birth weight
- Parent abused or neglected as a child
- Step-parent or cohabitee present
- Single or separated parent
- Mother less than 21 years old at the time of the birth
- History of parental mental illness, drug/alcohol addiction
- Infant separated for more than 24 hours post-delivery
- Infant mentally or physically handicapped
- Less than 18 months between birth of children

(Browne and Saqi, 1988)

The child's fundamental needs

- Basic physical care
- Affection
- Security
- Stimulation of innate potential
- Guidance and control
- Responsibility
- Independence

Vulnerability of the child

- A difficult pregnancy and /or birth may make it hard for mother to relate to the child
- A premature birth or low birth weight may lead to frustrations and anxieties which are displaced on to the child
- One child too many may create maternal overload
- Chronic disappointment about the sex of the child
- A stressful time of day – meal times with children who are slow or fussy eaters, bedtimes, middle of the night, a child who refuses to sleep

Characteristics of parents who abuse

- Hostile background
- Excessive dependency needs
- Role reversal
- Blind to developmental needs
- Rigid, obsessive
- Power, powerlessness
- The saviour
- Stereotyped helplessness
- Violence
- Morbid jealousy
- Drug or alcohol dependency

(Altmeier et al., 1982)

rarely without some mark which has been gained from an accident during play. These accidental injuries are usually easily explained whereas non-accidental injuries are often unexplained and characteristic. There are also characteristic pre-disposing factors of child abuse. Bannister (1992) warns against the uncritical acceptance of these pre-disposing factors. Firstly, because of the danger of only recognising these conditions in families where abuse has occurred, and not responding to other factors, perceived as insignificant, but in reality more crucial. Secondly, some children in high-risk families are well cared for and not abused. However, she still recommends that all professionals who work with children should be aware of the warning signs which can lead to abuse as well as the characteristic features of abuse.

Small children have fundamental needs which may not be perceived by some parents. They are unaware of normal child development and often expect too much from their children. Some children are vulnerable to abuse merely because their mother cannot bond with them after an unwanted or difficult pregnancy and labour or she simply cannot cope with another child (Reder et al., 1993). Other children may be at risk because they have additional needs due to a demanding temperament, chronic illness or disability.

Although child abuse is never restricted to an isolated episode of violence, there is usually a precipitating incident that initiates abuse.

Activity

Think about the day-to-day activities of babies and children. Consider which of these could stress parents, particularly those who are already under some strain.

Many parents can remember how a particular episode of prolonged crying or naughtiness brought them to the brink of violence. The difference between these parents and parents who physically abuse their child is the knowledge of methods other than violence to discipline their child and their ability to recognise and manage their own stress appropriately. It is important that nurses realise the stresses and strains of parenthood and do not make judgements about abusers. Most parents in this situation need to be able to trust the nurse to support them and help them to avoid a reoccurrence. Their feelings of inadequacy and isolation may be exacerbated by a nurse who tries to exclude them from their child's care. Instead the nurse should provide a role model for parents and work with them to support the child.

Activity

Consider how you can encourage an abused child to talk freely to you.

Abused children rarely accuse their abuser. They are often too frightened of the consequences if they reveal what has happened. They may have been threatened or they may fear that they will be taken away from their parents. Even when children have been sexually abused, home may still represent affection and security. The abused child needs to be treated like any other child in hospital. They should not be pressurised into talking about the abuse and any revelations about the abuse should be accepted with equanimity and without criticism of the child or the abuser. Reassure them that the abuse is not their fault and that they are right to tell someone about it. Do not promise not to share the information as it may be required by the courts.

CHILD PROTECTION

Child protection is the specific action taken to protect children from abuse (Home Office *et al.*, 1991). This concept of strategies to protect children was initiated in the UK in 1985 when social services became responsible for investigating allegations of child abuse. Nurses working with children have a responsibility to report to social services all concerns about children whom they suspect are at risk of significant harm (DoH, 1992) (Figure 6.1). The Children Act (DoH, 1989) defines significant harm as that which prevents the child's health or development from meeting the usual standards for a child of similar age and circumstance. If, after an initial investigation, social services decide to pursue the concern the nurse may be expected to:

- provide a written report about the concerns;
- provide copies of relevant nursing records for any court proceedings;
- attend the child protection conference;
- join the inter-agency group to produce a child protection plan;
- attend reviews as necessary.

The DHSS (1988) stress the need for inter-agency liaison in child protection work, and any child protection issue usually involves representatives from social services (as the key agency), education, health, police and, in some areas, the National Society for the Prevention of Cruelty to Children.

In an emergency, concerns may be reported to the police who have powers to ensure the child's safety. The Children Act (DoH, 1989) enabled the police to take children who are at risk into their protection as well as identifying three new child protection orders:

- child assessment order;
- emergency protection order;
- recovery order.

The child assessment order can be obtained by social services when a child is not at immediate risk but significant harm is suspected. It allows

Cross reference

The Children Act (1989) – page 661

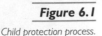

Figure 6.1

Child protection process.

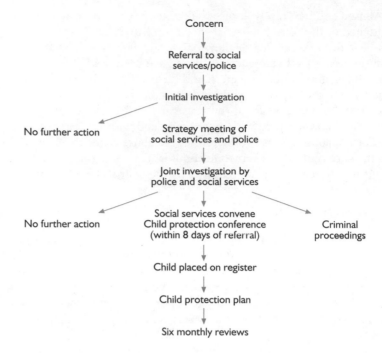

Characteristics of accidental injuries

BRUISES are likely to be:

- few and scattered
- no pattern
- frequent
- same colour and age

BURNS and SCALDS are likely to be:

- treated
- easily explained

INJURIES are likely to be:

- minor and superficial
- quickly treated
- easily explained

FRACTURES are likely to be:

- arms and legs
- seldom to the ribs except for road traffic accidents – rare in very young children
- rarely due to brittle bone syndrome

an assessment of the child's health, development and treatment to determine if any further action is required. The emergency protection order enables a child to be made safe when there is reasonable cause to believe that the child is at risk if not removed from the present environment. The recovery order can be made by the court to discover the whereabouts of a child who has been removed from care.

The Children Act which took effect in 1991 was seen at that time to be an important influence in promoting the rights of the child. However, recent criticism suggests that it prejudices rather than protects children's interests because it does not balance children's wishes with their needs. Dorrell (1997) indicates that although it is important to listen to children's views, it is equally important not to expect them necessarily to be able to make mature judgements about their interests. He believes these judgements should be the responsibility of adults.

Activity

Read the other sections relating to the Children Act (page 661) and the role of the nurse as an advocate of the child (page 59) and discuss Dorrell's point of view with some colleagues.

PREVENTION OF CHILD ABUSE

Activity

Consider what part you can play in the prevention of child abuse.

Children's nurses can play an important role in the prevention of child abuse. In the neonatal unit separation of mother and baby can be kept to a minimum and bonding encouraged. Community nurses can help new parents to appreciate the developmental needs of young children and help them to overcome problems. Studies have found that this type of help is more likely to have an impact on reducing child abuse if aimed at parents of children under 2 years (Olds *et al.*, 1994). Community nurses can refer parents who have no family close by to community services such as mother and toddler groups which will help to provide social support to lonely families. They can also be alert to parents who need help. Jones *et al.* (1987) found that frequent visits to the clinic, GP or hospital with apparently minor problems may indicate parental anxiety and insecurity and represent a cry for help. Some areas have initiated schemes to help parents under stress who can call a help-line for advice if they feel unable to cope.

All nurses can be alert to altered relationships between children and parents and listen carefully to children's concerns. They can also teach parenting skills to meet children's fundamental and developmental needs and give advice about protecting and educating children from sexual abuse. They can be alert to stresses in the home environment which may cause the child to be neglected, for instance when a parent is caring for another dependant or suffering from mental health problems. The parents themselves may be mentally or physically ill and the eldest child may have to be the main carer for the rest of the family. The role of nurse in the prevention of child abuse is strengthened by recent findings about the long-term consequences of child abuse.

ADULT SURVIVORS OF CHILD ABUSE

Cloke and Naish (1997) stress the need for services to support the adult survivors of child abuse so that the experience does not adversely affect the relationship they may have with their own children. The National Commission of Inquiry into the Prevention of Child Abuse (1996) found that only about 30% of child abuse is reported and, whilst all survivors need support in adulthood, serious long-term consequences are more likely in those where the abuse was not recognised or treated. The Commission found that these adults were often dependent on drugs and alcohol, and that pregnancy and childbirth can cause acute distress. In their conclusion, the Commission recommended that existing child health surveillance programmes should include an assessment of the

---

Characteristics of non-accidental injuries

BRUISING is likely to be:

- frequent
- patterned, e.g. finger and thumb marks
- old and new in same place (note colour)
- in unusual positions (see diagram)

BURNS and SCALDS are likely to have:

- a clear outline
- splash marks around burn
- unusual position, e.g. back of hand
- indicative shapes, e.g. cigarette burns, bar of electric fire

SUSPICIOUS INJURIES are likely to be:

- bite marks
- finger nail marks
- large and deep scratches
- incisions, e.g. from razor blades

FRACTURES are likely to be:

- numerous and healed at different times
- always suspicious in babies under 2 years of age

SEXUAL ABUSE may result in:

- unexplained soreness
- bleeding or injury to genital or anal areas
- sexually transmitted diseases

Figure 6.2

Common sites for non-accidental injuries.

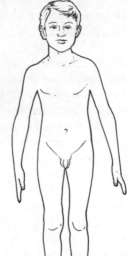

Skull
fractures, bleeding, or bruising
under skull (from shaking)

Ears
bruising, pinch
or slap marks

Eyes
bruising or black (both eyes)

Cheek and face
bruising, finger marks

Neck and shoulders
bruising, grasp marks

Mouth
torn frenulum

Inner and upper arms
bruising, grasp marks

Chest
bruising, grasp marks

Back, buttocks and thighs
linear bruising, outline of
belt and buckle, burns and scalds

Genitals
bruising

Knees
grasp marks

Figure 6.3

Common sites for accidental injuries.

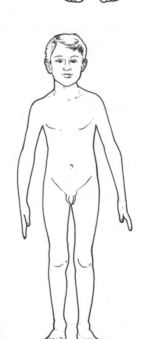

Forehead

Nose

Chin

Bony spine

Elbows

Hips

Forearms

Knees and shins

general welfare of the child and family, thus identifying children at risk and parents in need of advice and support. This could be difficult to implement in view of the lack of recognition given to preventive health in the current NHS (Cloke and Naish, 1997). Consequently, the role of children's nurses is vital in assessing whether children's fundamental physical and psychological needs are met. All nursing assessments should include the observation of children's physical state, emotional behaviour and the parent–child relationship. Any concerns of neglect or abuse should be recorded and reported to social services.

➤ **Key points**

1. There is no accepted single cause for violent behaviour.
2. Violence in the family falls into five main categories of abuse: physical, emotional, neglect, sexual and financial.
3. Violence may be inflicted against and by anyone of any age.
4. It is difficult to give precise statistics about abuse as much of it goes unreported by those who are too embarrassed or frightened to reveal it.
5. Nurses have a responsibility to recognise and report any concerns that a child may be at risk of abuse.
6. There is now a need to have strategic programmes for the prevention of child abuse including the support of adult survivors of abuse.

References

AINSWORTH, M. (1973) The development of infant–mother attachment. In CALDWELL, B. and RICCIUTI, H. (eds), *Review of Child Development and Research, Vol. 3: Child Development and Social Policy*. Chicago: University of Chicago Press.

AINSWORTH, M. (1982) Attachment: retrospect and prospect. In PARKES, C., ATKINSON, N. and CRAWFORD, M. (1995) *All in the Family: Siblings and Disability*. London: Action for Children.

ALDERSON, P. (1993) *Children's Consent to Surgery*. Milton Keynes: Open University Press.

ALTMEIER, W., *et al.* (1982) Antecedents of child abuse. *Journal of Pediatrics*, **100**, 823–827.

AREHART-TREICHEL, J. (1980) *Biotypes*. London: W. H. Allen.

ATKINSON, N. and CRAWFORD, M. (1995) *All in the Family: Siblings and Disability*. London: Action for Children.

AUSLANDER, W., *et al.* (1991) Predictors of diabetes knowledge in newly diagnosed children and parents. *Journal of Paediatric Psychology*, **16** (2), 213–228.

BAILEY, R. and CALDWELL, C. (1997) Preparing parents for going home. *Paediatric Nursing*, **9** (4), 15–17.

BANDURA, A. (1973) *Aggression: A Social Learning Theory*. Englewood Cliffs, NJ: Prentice-Hall.

BANNISTER, A. (1992) *Child Abuse and Neglect: Facing the Challenge*, 2nd edn. Milton Keynes: Open University Press.

BEE, H. (1989) *The Developing Child*, 5th edn. New York: Harper & Row.

BENTOVIM, A. (1986) Bereaved children. *British Medical Journal*, 292, 1482.

BEWLEY, C. and GIBBS, A. (1994) Coping with domestic violence in pregnancy. *Nursing Standard*, 8, 25–28.

BIRD, J. and PODMORE, V. (1993) Children's understanding of health and illness. *Psychology and Health*, 4, 175–185.

BOSSERT, E. (1994) Stress appraisals of hospitalised school-aged children. *Children's Health Care*, 23 (1), 33–49.

BOWLBY, J. (1953) *Child Care and the Growth of Love*. Harmondsworth: Penguin.

BOWLBY, J. (1973) *Attachment and Loss: 2. Separation, Anxiety and Anger*. London: Hogarth Press.

BREWIS, E. (1995) Issues in bereavement: there are no rules. *Paediatric Nursing*, 7 (9), 19–22.

BROWN, K. and COOPER, S. J. (eds) (1979) *Chemical Influences on Behaviour*. London: Academic Press.

BROWNE, K. and SAQI, S. (1988) Approaches to screening for child abuse and neglect. In BROWNE, K., DAVIES, C. and STRATTON, P. (eds), *Early Prediction and Prevention of Child Abuse*. Chichester: Wiley.

BURR, C. (1985) Impact on the family of a chronically ill child. In HOBBS, N. and PERRIN, J. (eds), *Issues in the Care of Children with Chronic Illness*. San Francisco: Jossey-Bass.

BURR, S. (1993) Adolescents and the ward environment. *Paediatric Nursing*, 5 (1), 10–13.

BUTLER, N. R. and GOLDSTEIN, N. R. (1973) Smoking in pregnancy and subsequent child development. *British Medical Journal*, 4, 573–577.

CANAM, C. (1993) Common adaptive tasks facing parents of children with chronic conditions. *Journal of Advanced Nursing*, 18, 46–53.

CARSON, D., GRAVELY, J. and COUNCIL, J. (1992) Children's pre-hospitalisation conceptions of illness, cognitive development and personal adjustment. *Child Health Care*, 21 (2), 103–110.

CHESS, S. and THOMAS, A. (1984) *Origins and Evolution of Behaviour Disorders*. New York: Raven Press.

CLARK, G. (1996) Internal conflicts. *Nursing Times*, 92 (40) 16–17.

CLOKE, C. and NAISH, J. (1997) Save the Children. *Nursing Times*, 93 (14), 34–37.

CLOTHIER, C. (1994) *The Allitt Report*. London: HMSO.

COHEN, M. and MARTISON, I. (1988) Chronic uncertainty: its effect on parental appraisal of a child's health. *Journal of Pediatric Nursing*, 3 (2), 89–96.

CRAFT, M. (1986) Validation of responses reported by school-age siblings of hospitalised children. *Children's Health Care*, 15, 13–16.

DALE, P., DAVIES, M., MORRISON, T. and WATERS, J. (1986) *Dangerous Families*. London: Tavistock.

DES (1978) *Special Educational Needs – Report of the Committee of Inquiry into the Education of Handicapped Children and Young People (Warnock Report)*. London: HMSO.

DHSS (1988) *Working Together: A Guide to Inter-agency Co-operation for the Protection of Children from Abuse*. London: HMSO.

DoH (1989) *An Introduction to the Children Act*. London: HMSO.

DoH (1992) *Child Protection: Guidance for Senior Nurses, Health Visitors and Midwives*, 2nd edn. London: HMSO.

DORRELL, S. (1997) *Social Services: Achievement and Challenge*. Government White Paper.

DUNN, J. (1981) *Sisters and Brothers*. London: Fontana.

EARYS, C., ELLIS, N. and JONES, R. (1993) Which label? An investigation into the effects of terminology on the public perception of and attitudes toward people with learning difficulties. *Disability Handicap Society*, 8 (2), 114.

FARRELL, M. (1996) The role of a children's hospice. *Paediatric Nursing*, 8 (4), 6–8.

FAULKNER, A., PEACE, G. and O'KEEFE, C. (1995) *When a Child has Cancer*. London: Chapman & Hall.

FAULKNER, E. (1995) The importance of communications with the patient, family and professional carers. In ROBBINS, J. and MOSCROFT, J. (eds), *Caring for the Dying Patient and the Family*, 3rd edn. London: Chapman & Hall.

FAUX, S. (1991) Sibling relationships in families with congenitally impaired children. *Journal of Pediatric Nursing*, 6 (3), 175–184.

GATH, A. (1980) How illness in one member of the family affects the children in that family. *Journal of Maternal and Child Health*, 12, 6–8.

GEEN, L. (1990) The family of a child with cancer. In THOMPSON, J. (ed.), *The Child with Cancer – Nursing Care*. London: Scutari Press.

GELLES, R. and CORNELL, C. (1985) *Intimate Violence in Families*. Beverly Hills: Sage.

GIBSON, C. (1988) Perspectives of parental coping with a chronically ill child. *Issues in Comprehensive Pediatric Nursing*, 11, 33–41.

GOODCHILD, M. and DODGE, J. (1985) *Cystic Fibrosis*, 2nd edn. Sussex: Balliere Tindall.

GREENBERG, M., SIEGEL, J. and LEITCH, C. (1983) The nature and importance of attachment relationships to parents and peers during adolescence. *Journal of Youth and Adolescence*, 12, 373–386.

GUNTHER, L. M. (1963) Psychopathy and stress in the life experience of mothers of premature infants. In ILLINGWORTH, L. S. (ed.), *The Normal Child*, 8th edn. Edinburgh: Churchill Livingstone.

HARRIS, A. (1993) *Child Development*, 2nd edn. Minneapolis: West.

HARRISON, C. (1997) Wax, sunlight and X-rays. *Nursing Times*, 93 (22), 52–53.

HART, D. and BOSSERT, E. (1994) Self-reported fears of hospitalised school-aged children. *Journal of Pediatric Nursing*, 9 (2), 83–90.

HILL, L. (1994) *Caring for Dying Children and their Families*. London: Chapman & Hall.

HINSLIFF, G. (1997) The Downs dilemma. *Daily Mail*, no. 31,410,23.

HOME OFFICE, DoH, WELSH OFFICE (1991) *Working Together under The Children Act 1989: A Guide to Arrangements for Inter-agency Co-operation for the Protection of Children from Abuse*. London: HMSO.

ILLINGWORTH, L. S. (1983) *The Normal Child*, 8th edn. Edinburgh: Churchill Livingstone.

JENNINGS, P. (1992) Coping strategies for mothers. *Paediatric Nursing*, 4 (9), 24–26.

JONES, T., PICKETT, S., OATES, T. and BARBOUR, J. (1987) *Understanding Child Abuse*, 2nd edn. London: Macmillan.

KAGAN, J. (1979) Overview: perspectives on human infancy. In OSOFSKY, J. (ed.), *Handbook on Infant Development*. New York: Wiley.

KEMPE, R. and KEMPE, C. (1984) *The Common Secret: Sexual Abuse of Children and Adolescents*. New York: Freeman.

KENNY, C. (1996) Jailed nurse lied to bosses about psychiatric past. *Nursing Times*, **92** (45), 5.

KINGSBURY, S. (1993) Parasuicide in adolescence: a message in a bottle. *ACCP Review and Newsletter*, **15** (6), 253–259.

LASK, B. and FOSSEN, A. (1989) *Childhood Illness – The Psychosomatic Approach*. Chichester: Wiley.

LAZARUS, R. and COHEN, J. (1977) Environmental stress. In ALTMAN, J. and WOHLWILL, J. (eds), *Human Behaviour and Environment*, vol. 2. New York: Plenum.

LEVENTHAL, H. (1986) Health psychology: a social psychological perspective. In BERKOWITZ, L. (ed.), *A Survey of Social Psychology*, 3rd edn. Japan: CBS.

LEWIS, C., *et al.* (1984) A randomised study of ACT (Asthma Care Training for kids). *Pediatrics*, **74** (4), 478–485.

LEY, P. and LLEWELYN, S. (1995) Improving patients' understanding, recall, satisfaction and compliance. In BROOME, A. and LLEWELYN, S. (eds), *Health Psychology*. London: Chapman & Hall.

LINDSAY, B. (1994) Like skeletons or ghosts. Developing a concept of death and dying. *Child Health*, **2** (4), 142–146.

LLEWELYN, S. and HASLETT, A. (1986) Factors perceived as helpful by members of self-help groups: an exploratory study. *British Journal of Guidance and Counselling*, **14**, 252–262.

LOVELL, B. (1987) Sharing the death of a parent. *Nursing Times*, **83** (42), 36–39.

LYNCH, M. A. and ROBERTS, J. (1977) Predicting child abuse; signs of bonding failure in the maternity hospital. *British Medical Journal*, i, 624–627.

McCARTHY, D. (1974) Physical effects and symptoms of the cycle of rejection. *Proceedings of the Royal Society of Medicine*, **67**, 1057–1060.

McCOLLUM, A. and GIBSON, L. (1970) Family adaptation to the child with Cystic Fibrosis. *Journal of Pediatrics*, **77** (4), 571–578.

McKERROW, L. (1991) Dealing with the stress of caring for the dying in the intensive care unit. *Intensive Care Nursing*, **7** (4), 219–222.

McKIBBEN, L., DEVOS, E. and NEWBERGER, E. (1989) Victimisation of mothers of abused children: a controlled study. *Pediatrics*, **83** (2), 531–535.

McMAHON, B. (1995) A family affair – understanding family therapy. *Child Health*, **3** (3), 100–103.

MACASKILL, A. and MONACH, J. (1990) Coping with childhood cancer. The case for long-term counselling help for patients and families. *British Journal of Guidance and Counselling*, **18** (1), 13–26.

MAIN, M., KAPLAN, N. and CASSIDY, J. (1985) Security in infancy, childhood and adulthood. *Monographs of the Society for Research in Child Development*, **50** (1/2), 66–104.

MARKS, I. M. (1987) The development of normal fear. *Journal of Child Psychology, Psychiatry and Allied Disciplines*, **28** (2), 667–697.

MEADOW, R. (1989) Munchausen syndrome by proxy. *British Medical Journal*, **299**, 248–250.

MEADOWS, S. (1993) *The Child as a Thinker: The Development and Acquisition of Cognition in Childhood*. London: Routledge.

MERRITT, T. A. (1981) Smoking mothers affect little lives. In ILLINGWORTH. L.

S. (ed.), *The Normal Child*, 8th edn. Edinburgh: Churchill Livingstone.

MEYRE, S. and HAGGERTY, A. (1962) Stress and physical illness. *Journal of Pediatrics*, 29, 539–561.

MICHAEL, S. and LANDSDOWN, R. (1986) Adjustment to the death of a sibling. *Archives of Disease in Childhood*, 61, 278–283.

MIKULIC, M. (1971) Reinforcement of independent and dependent patient behaviours by nursing personnel: an exploratory study. *Nursing Research*, 20, 148–155.

MILLER, F. J. W., COURT, S. D. M., KNOX, E. G. and BRANDON, S. (1974) *The School Years in Newcastle-Upon-Tyne*. London: Oxford University Press.

MOOS, R. and TSU, V. (1977) The crisis of physical illness; an overview. In MOSS, R. (ed.), *Coping with Physical Illness*. New York: Plenum.

MORRISON, L. (1997) Stress and siblings. *Paediatric Nursing*, 9 (4), 26–27.

MYER, P. (1988) Parental adaptation to cystic fibrosis. *Journal of Pediatric Health Care*, 2, 20–28.

NATIONAL COMMISSION OF INQUIRY INTO THE PREVENTION OF CHILD ABUSE (1996) *Childhood Matters*. London: HMSO.

OLDS, S. D., HENDERSON, C. and KITZMAN, H. (1994) Does pre-natal and infancy nurse home visitation have enduring effects on qualities of parental caregiving and child health at 25–50 months of age? *Pediatrics*, 93 (1), 89–98.

PATTERSON, G. (1982) Coercion theory. In LACHENMEYER, J. and GIBBS, M. (eds), *Psychology in Childhood*. New York: Gardner Press.

PEACE, G. (1996a) Living under the shadow of illness. *Nursing Times*, 92 (28), 46–48.

PEACE, G. (1996b) Chronic complements. *Nursing Times*, 92 (41), 46–47.

PECK, H. (1992) Please don't tell him the truth. *Paediatric Nursing*, 43 (2), 12–14.

PETTLE, M. and LANDSDOWN, R. (1986) Adjustment to the death of a sibling. *Archives of Disease in Childhood*, 61, 278–283.

PRITCHARD, J. (1996) Darkness visible. *Nursing Times*, 92 (42), 26–27.

PURSSELL, E. (1994) The process of normalisation in children with chronic illness. *Paediatric Nursing*, 6 (10,) 26–28.

RAMSAY, J. (1990) *Parental understanding and management of cystic fibrosis*. Unpublished MSc dissertation. City University.

RANDALL, P. (1993) Young children grieve differently from adults. *Professional Care of Mother and Child*, February, 36–37.

RAY, L. and RITCHIE, J. (1993) Caring for chronically ill children at home: factors which influence parents coping. *Journal of Pediatric Nursing*, 8 (4), 217–225.

REDER, P., DUNCAN, S. and GRAY, M. (1993) *Beyond Blame: Child Abuse Tragedies Revisited*. London: Routledge.

ROBERTSON, J. (1970) *Young Children in Hospital*, 2nd edn. London: Tavistock Press.

ROBINSON, C. (1993) Managing life with a chronic disability: the story of normalisation. *Qualitative Health Research*, 3 (1), 6–28.

ROSENMAN, R., *et al.* (1975) Coronary heart disease in the Western Group study. *Journal of the American Medical Association*, 233, 872–877.

RUSHFORD, H. (1996) Nurses' knowledge of how children view health and illness. *Paediatric Nursing*, 8 (9), 23–27.

RUSSELL, P. (1989) *The Wheelchair Child*, 3rd edn. London: Souvenir Press.

RUSSELL-JOHNSON, H. (1997) Deliberate self-harm in adolescents. *Paediatric Nursing*, 9 (1) 29–36.

RUTTER, M. (1971) Parent–child separation: psychological effects on the children. *Journal of Child Psychology and Psychiatry*, **12**, 233.

RUTTER, M., *et al.* (1975) Attainment and adjustment in two geographic areas: III some factors accounting for area differences. *British Journal of Psychiatry*, **126**, 520–533.

SCHAFFER, H. R. (1988) Family structure or interpersonal relationships. *The Context for Child Development*, **2**, 91–94.

SHAPIRO, J. (1983) Family reactions and coping strategies in response to the physically ill or the handicapped child: a review. *Social Science & Medicine*, **17**, (14), 913–931.

SIMON, K. (1993) Perceived stress of non-hospitalised children during the hospitalisation of a sibling. *Journal of Pediatric Nursing*, **8** (5), 298–304.

SMITH, L. (1987) *Domestic Violence: An Overview*. London: HMSO.

SMITH, S. M., HANSON, R. and NOBLE, S. (1974) Social aspects of the battered baby syndrome. *British Journal of Psychiatry*, **125**, 568–570.

SPINETTA, J. (1984) Measurement of family function, communication and cultural effects. *Cancer*, **53**, 2230–2237.

STIER, D., *et al.* (1993) Are children born to young mothers at increased risk of maltreatment? *Pediatrics*, **91** (3), 642–648.

STOTT, D. H. (1962) Evidence for a congenital factor in maladjustment and delinquency. *American Journal of Psychiatry*, **118**, 781–785.

SWANWICK, M. (1996) Child rearing across cultures. *Paediatric Nursing*, **8** (7), 13–17.

SYVERSON, C. (1997) The young ones. *Nursing Times*, **93** (24), 28–29.

THOMPSON, D. (1992) Support for the grieving family. *Neonatal Network*, **11** (6), 73–75.

THORNE, S. (1993) *Negotiating Health Care – The Social Context of Chronic Illness*. London: Sage.

TROPAUER, A., NEAL-FRANZ, M. and DILGARD, V. (1970) Psychological aspects of the care of children with cystic fibrosis. *American Journal of Diseases of Childhood*, **119**, 424–431.

VAN OOIJEN, E. (1996) Learning to approach patients' sexuality as part of holistic care. *Nursing Times*, **92** (36), 44–45.

VAN OOIJEN, E. and CHARNOCK, A. (1994) *Sexuality and Patient Care*. London: Chapman & Hall.

WALLSTON, B. (1973) The effect of maternal employment on children. *Journal of Child Psychology and Psychiatry*, **14**, 81–85.

WALTER, T. (1990) *Funerals and How to Improve Them*. London: Hodder & Stoughton.

WEDGE, P. and PROSSER, H. (1973) *Born to Fail*. London: Arrow Books.

WHITEHEAD, N. (1995) Behavioural paediatrics and childhood cancer. In BROOME, A. and LLEWELYN, S. (eds), *Health Psychology*. London: Chapman & Hall.

WHYTE, D. (1992) A family nursing approach to the care of a child with a chronic illness. *Journal of Advanced Nursing*, **17**, 317–327.

WILKINSON, S. (1995) Psychological aspects of disability. In BROOME, A. and LLEWELYN, S. (eds), *Health Psychology*. London: Chapman & Hall.

WOODHOUSE, S. (1996) Do siblings need a special day? *Paediatric Nursing*, **8** (3), 8–9.

WORLD HEALTH ORGANISATION (1980) *International Classification of Impairments, Disabilities and Handicaps (ICIDH)*. Geneva: WHO.

WRIGHT, B. (1983) *Pyschosocial Aspects of Disability*. London: Harper & Row.

PRINCIPLES OF CARING FOR SICK CHILDREN

Joan Ramsay

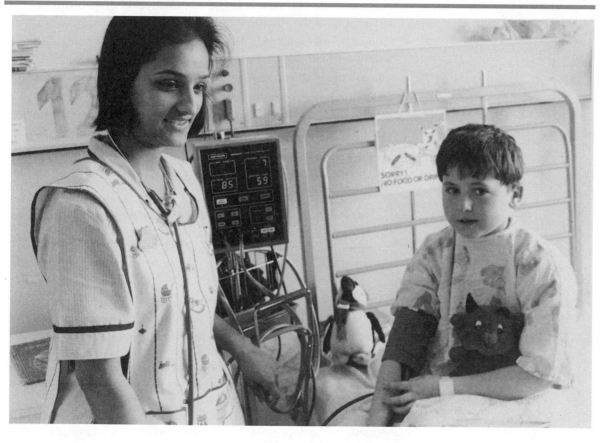

OBJECTIVES

The material contained within this module and the further reading/references should enable you to:

- Evaluate the suitability of hospital environments for children.
- Discuss the value of different types of preparation of children for hospital and procedures.
- Appreciate the importance of the assessment process.
- Explore the process of day surgery for children and families.
- Consider the care of children in the accident and emergency department.
- Appreciate the differences in the administration of medicines to children from the administration to adults.
- Consider how to provide adequate nutrition and maintain fluid balance for children in hospital.
- Discuss the problems associated with caring for children in pain.
- Examine the surrogate role of the nurse.
- Explore the provision of paediatric community nursing in the UK.
- Discuss the specific pre- and post-operative care of children.
- Explore the provision of paediatric intensive care in the UK.
- Consider how to meet the psychological and physical needs of the dying child.

INTRODUCTION

Sick children need the care and skills of a specially trained nurse who has a clear understanding of the special needs of children and their families and can therefore assess, plan, implement and evaluate appropriate family-centred care. This module examines the principles of caring for sick children to provide you with this necessary understanding that children are not just small adults but unique individuals with specific needs of their own. The module begins by exploring the requirements of an appropriate hospital environment for children. It also considers the care of children in particular areas of the hospital – the day care ward, the intensive care unit and the accident and emergency department. It discusses the particular need of children for clear and age-appropriate preparation for hospital and hospital procedures to help to allay their fears and to promote their cooperation. Children's fears and lack of understanding of hospitals make the care of their pain, meeting their pre- and post-operative needs and the administration of medicines a particularly challenging part of nursing children and this module looks at these issues. It also considers how the differing structure and function of children's bodies from adults is particularly relevant when assessing sick children and providing nutrition and maintaining fluid balance. Much of the nurse's role for sick children in hospital and at home is working with parents to adapt usual family routines and including specific nursing care, and the module examines this surrogate role in hospital and in the community. As more children are being cared for at home, the module explores the provision of children's community nursing and the development of this role. Finally the module looks at the physical and psychological needs of the dying child.

1 CREATING AN APPROPRIATE HOSPITAL ENVIRONMENT FOR CHILDREN

INTRODUCTION

Cross reference

Hospitalisation and illness – page 209

In 1859 Florence Nightingale believed that hospitals should do the sick no harm. Although she was primarily concerned with nursing adults, she was stressing the importance of meeting the physiological and psychological needs of patients to avoid them physical or mental stress. This belief is still the concern of nurses over a century later and is a particular issue for nurses caring for hospitalised children.

Children in hospital have different needs from adult patients because their physical and emotional development is still ongoing and they are still dependent on their parents. Jolly (1981) describes the uniqueness of children's nursing as caring not only for children's physical problems but also responding to their thoughts, feelings and the need for their families. It has been accepted for some time that the physical well-being of children must be assured if they are to reach the maximum potential as adults (Illingworth, 1975). However, it is only comparatively recently that the importance of attending to children's psychological needs in hospital has been recognised as being of equal value. Robertson and Robertson (1952) clearly identified the severe psychological disturbances that occur during the hospitalisation of young children. Such bad experiences can slow children's recovery and impair their psychosocial development to such an extent as to affect adulthood behaviour (Audit Commission, 1993). Do hospitals in the 1990s take children's needs into account and do them no harm?

The Audit Commission (1993) recommended that the care of children in hospital should be based on six principles:

- Child- and family-centred care
- Specially skilled staff
- Separate facilities
- Effective treatments
- Appropriate hospitalisation
- Strategic commissioning

These six principles have been recognised since the Platt Report (1959) which was based on the work of Bowlby (1953) and Robertson (1958) and recognised the psychological trauma caused by hospitalisation (Nichols, 1993).

CHILD- AND FAMILY-CENTRED CARE

Even before these findings it was suggested that parents should be involved in the care of children in hospital (Spence, 1947). Most children's wards nowadays do recommend parental presence throughout the child's stay in hospital but the degree of acceptance by staff is still variable. NAWCH (1986) found that while 67% of parents were welcomed by staff, 24% were only accepted and 9% were tolerated. Many wards also practice family-centred care but 32% of parents consider that their involvement in care is a substitution for the lack of staff. Care must be negotiated with parents for them to appreciate that their involvement is important, otherwise they may well feel abused and frightened. These feelings may then be transmitted to the child. The importance of parental presence and involvement in care is often not recognised in other hospital units/department (Audit Commission, 1993). Family-centred care can pose difficulties for some staff who may fear loss of control (Bishop, 1988). Children's nurses may need to be more active in communicating the advantages of family-centred care to staff throughout the hospital if the concept is to be accepted more widely and psychological harm to the children is to be minimised.

Activity

Take time out to analyse the degree by which child- and family-centred care is practised in your own hospital. Investigate the views of staff, children and parents in all areas of the hospital where children are nursed.

SPECIALLY SKILLED STAFF

Specially skilled staff who can provide specific care for children and their families are necessary in every part of the hospital which provides health care for children. According to the British Paediatric Association (BPA, 1991a) 16% of district general hospitals have no junior doctors with sufficient paediatric experience and 15% of anaesthetists care for fewer than 20 children per year. Although there is no research to substantiate this, it may be that these anaesthetists are those who cause unnecessary psychological trauma to children by continuing to prescribe intramuscular pre-medication and do not encourage parental presence in the anaesthetic room.

Medical staff who have insufficient experience in caring for children often do not have the special skill necessary to treat children with the less common childhood illnesses. Stiller (1988) has shown that survival rates of children with cancer are significantly higher when they are treated in a paediatric oncology centre. This may also be true for children treated in paediatric intensive care units as opposed to a general

Family-centred care – Parents' views

Families of children with chronic health problems often feel:
- their role on the ward is unclear
- uninvolved in decisions about their child's care
- their experience in caring for their child was often ignored
- their role is to substitute for lack of staff
- unsure of the staff's attitude towards their participation in care
- their role is to provide support and reassurance for their child
- they provide continuity of care for their child in a frightening situation

Cross reference

Family centred care – page 612

Surgeons' and anaesthetists' practice with children

The Audit Commission (1993) found that many surgeons and anaesthetists had little experience with children. Each year:
- over 50% of surgeons perform less than 10 operations on babies under 6 months
- only 30% of surgeons performed over 50 operations per year on children aged 3–10 years
- over 90% of surgeons perform less than 50 operations per year on children between 6 months and 2 years
- only 10% of anaesthetists deal with more than 50 babies under 6 months each year
- less than 75% of anaesthetists annually deal with more than 50 children aged between 6 months and 2 years
- 45% of anaesthetists deal with less than 50 children aged 3–10 years each year

- Entrants to child nursing should have at least a record of sickness from their most recent place of employment
- Candidates with a history of major personality disorder should not be employed in children's nursing
- Consideration should be given to how GPs might certify that a candidate, for employment in the NHS, has no excluding medical history
- Consideration should be given to making a candidate's sickness records available to occupational health departments
- All nurses should undergo formal health screening before their first appointment after registration
- Procedures for management referrals to occupational health departments should clarify the criteria which trigger such referrals
- Coroners should send copies of post-mortem reports to every consultant involved in the patient's care
- The provision of paediatric pathology services should be available whenever a child's death is unexpected or unaccountable
- The DoH should take steps to ensure that the recommendations of Welfare for Children and Young People in Hospital are more closely observed
- When alarms on monitoring equipment fail, an untoward incident report should be completed and the equipment serviced before it is used again
- Reports of serious untoward incidents should be made, in writing, to District and Regional Health Authorities through a single channel
- That the Allitt disaster heightens awareness of the possibility of malevolent interventions as a cause of unexplained clinical events

(Clothier, 1994)

258

intensive care unit. The psychological stress of these children and their families must be less in a specialised unit with known successful outcomes. Parents also gain much psychological support from meeting other parents in similar stressful situations (Ramsay, 1990). Unfortunately, the Audit Commission (1993) found that referral to specialist centres is decreasing as hospitals try to lower costs and expand services.

The Audit Commission (1993) found that even paediatric units lacked sufficient numbers of registered sick children's nurses (RSCNs). (See also page 350.) Hutt (1983) identified that one reason for this was that general managers did not perceive a need for RSCNs. Since the Platt Report (1959) it has been accepted that RSCNs/RNs(child) have specialist knowledge, skills and attitudes. In 1991 the DoH set a target standard for 1995 of:

> ... two registered sick children's nurses – or nurses who have completed the child branch of Project 2000 – on duty 24 hours a day in all hospital children's departments and wards ... and a RSCN on duty 24 hours a day to advise on the nursing of children in other departments ...
> (See Figure 9.1 – page 350)

The Allitt inquiry (Clothier, 1994) recommends that these standards are more closely monitored. It is interesting to note that there were significant shortcomings in the RSCN staffing levels at the time of the Allitt murders. Although this was obviously an exceptional situation, it is certainly an instance of where a hospital did harm the patient. Another issue of concern raised by the Allitt inquiry is the supervision of non-RSCNs. Tucker (1989) questions the ethics of exposing general students to caring for children. This question becomes even more pertinent when it becomes apparent that such students do not always have the supervision of registered children's nurses. An appropriately qualified children's nurse at management level may help to ensure that sufficient attention is given to recruiting and retaining appropriate numbers of such nurses (Audit Commission, 1993). At this level a RSCN/RN(child) can also ensure good practices in the care of children throughout the hospital.

Activity

Look at the staffing in your own hospital in all the areas where children are nursed. How far does it meet the DoH guidelines? Is there a named children's nurse to provide advice about the care of children outside the children's ward?

Marriott (1990) states that it is essential for children's nurses to be part of clinical directorates to put forward the special needs of children.

Without this representation at directorate level it appears that hospital managers also do not recognise the importance of play and education for children in hospital. Thirty per cent of wards surveyed by the Audit Commission (1993) had less than 50% whole time equivalent trained play staff. If play in hospital enables children to restore normality, relieve anxieties and aid understanding (Muller *et al.*, 1992), hospitals may be harming children by not facilitating such diversion.

The 1944 Education Act stated that all children had the right to receive education which was appropriate to their age, ability and aptitude. It also enabled children to receive education in areas other than school. Schooling in hospital provides children with diversion and also provides continuity of the child's usual home routine. It is therefore an important aspect of hospital life for children but it requires appropriate facilities and the appointment of a flexible teacher who can meet the needs of different age-groups and abilities. Hospital teachers often only cater for younger children and are not usually available outside children's wards.

SEPARATE FACILITIES

Children in hospital also need separate facilities which are attractive, bright and age-related (Muller *et al.*, 1992). Such surroundings reassure children and parents and minimise the trauma of hospitalisation (Rodin, 1983). A separate area for play also helps to minimise the stress of hospitalisation and provides a secure place for children to act out their fears. A separate treatment room where clinical procedures can be carried out enables the child to keep the bed and play area as secure places. Most children's wards have these facilities and are bright and cheerful, but they do tend to only attract the younger children. Appropriate facilities for adolescents are largely lacking (NAWCH, 1986). Some hospitals have no policy for adolescents in hospital who are consequently sometimes admitted to adult wards where they can feel anxious and isolated (Miller, 1991). Even when they are admitted to children's wards they can still feel out of place and concerned about the lack of privacy in a mixed sex ward.

Activity

Take a critical look at how your hospital defines children. What is the hospital policy with regard to admitting adolescents to adult or children's wards?

In an English National Board (ENB) study in 1992, over 25% of hospitals did not use separate facilities for any children admitted for ophthalmic, ear, nose or throat surgery because of consultants' preferences. Many hospitals also have no separate out-patient or Accident and Emergency facilities for children (ENB, 1992). These areas

Functions of play in hospital
- Provides diversion from pain and fear
- Enables relaxation
- Helps to reduce the stress of hospitalisation
- Provides a link with normal home routines
- Enables expression of feelings
- Encourages interaction with others
- Allows the child some control over the environment
- Encourages creativity
- Helps to prepare and teach about hospital and related procedures

Cross reference

Play and education – page 94

Functions of education in hospital
- Links with home and usual school
- Stimulation and motivation to learn
- Continuity of education
- Therapeutic learning activities which also promote overall development
- Opportunities for acting out fears and anxieties
- Career advice, especially for disabled children

may be children's first contact with hospital and these initial impressions are important influences on any subsequent reaction to hospital.

Apart from the unsuitability of adult wards and departments for children, these areas also lack facilities for parents. Parents require time, provision and support for their needs if they are to be fully involved in the care of their child. If parents are anxious, tired or uneasy, children will sense this and also become alarmed (Muller *et al.*, 1992). In contrast, 60% of paediatric units usually provide parents with facilities for sleeping, washing, eating and drinking, and relaxing which are close to their child (Audit Commission, 1993) (Figure 1.1).

Figure 1.1

Parents' facilities in children's wards (Audit Commission, 1993). N = 41 wards in five hospitals.

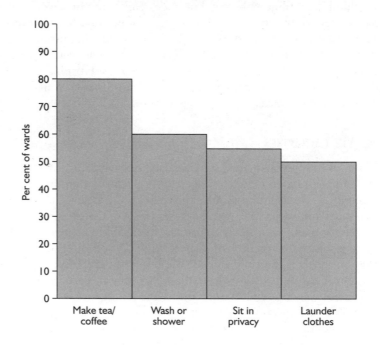

Activity

Analyse the separate facilities for children and their families in your own hospital. Consider how far these facilities meet the needs of different age-groups as well as the needs of parents.

Facilities for children in hospital also have to take into account children's special needs for safety. In 1992 the Child Accident Prevention Trust and the Royal College of Nursing discovered that accidents to children in hospital were largely preventable (CAPT, 1992). The children's area itself should be safe with high door handles or child-proof catches to prevent toddlers wandering away. Windows, lifts and stairs should be secure and all electrical points should be covered. Furniture in a children's ward should be sturdy and of an appropriate

Cross reference

Developmental factors and associated accidents – page 153

size to minimise the danger of falls. Beds should be lowered and cot sides kept raised at all times when children are unattended. Falls from cots mostly occur when cot sides have not been raised (Banco and Powers, 1988). Safety straps for seats should be used for small children.

Stock lotions, cleaning fluids and medicines should be kept in a securely locked cupboard or trolley, and medicines should never be left at the bedside. Treatment rooms, sluices and kitchens should be kept securely fastened when not in use. Electrical equipment should be regularly serviced and there should be a clear policy for the identification of out-of-order apparatus (Clothier, 1994). Special care should be taken with equipment used at the bedside; infusion pumps should have a child-locking device, plugs and fans should be placed out of reach and any tubing carefully secured so that it cannot pose any danger to the child.

Toys should be unbreakable, non-allergic and washable, and appropriate for the child's age and condition. Small toys can be swallowed by small children and can cause pressure sores when left in the beds of paralysed or immobile children.

Children also have special needs for safety in relation to infection control. Infants under 6 months have little natural immunity from infection and need to be nursed in protective isolation. Older children may need to be protected from children admitted with an infectious illness. Bathrooms should provide appropriate sized facilities to promote good hygiene after toileting.

Activity

Take a critical look at a children's ward and identify any areas where the children's safety may be compromised.

EFFECTIVE TREATMENTS

In the present climate of cost-effective care hospitals may find it difficult to rationalise expenditure on separate facilities. However, this money may be gained by savings on inappropriate or ineffective treatments. Black *et al.* (1990) found that 34% of myringotomies performed for the insertion of grommets were unnecessary. The Audit Commission (1993) suggests that the effects of the very expensive intensive care of newborn babies may not always be appropriate and should be monitored. Although such care has significantly reduced the mortality rate in low birth weight babies, the infants who survive are often disabled. This can cause great psychological trauma to the growing child and the family. Monitoring the treatment of such infants would enable staff and parents to make informed decisions about the suitability of such intensive care. Glasper (1993) stresses the need for children's nurses to become involved in practice-based research to enhance child

Cross reference

Ear surgery – page 464

and family care. Perhaps this is one area which would benefit from this type of investigation.

APPROPRIATE HOSPITALISATION

In addition to the evaluation of treatments it may also be useful to study whether hospitalisation is always necessary. NAWCH (1986) found a considerable expansion in day care surgery for children but the Audit Commission (1993) identified that some children were still experiencing an excessive stay in hospital due to administrative or organisational inefficiency. Earlier discharge from hospital may help to reduce the harmful effects of separation and hospitalisation for children and their families.

Activity

Find out the average length of stay for children in your hospital. Consider the appropriateness of the reasons why some children stay longer than average. Has the hospital made sufficient arrangements for day or short-stay care to meet local need?

Cross reference

Children's Charter – page 694

Effective and efficient hospital services for children rely on clear hospital policies and standards based on children's needs. Since 1991 District Health Authorities have been commissioning services. Few of these authorities identify children's services separately from those of adults or show any evidence of the specific health needs of children within their district (Audit Commission, 1993). Consequently, strategic plans rarely identify precise developments to meet the needs of children in hospital or provide examples of child-specific quality monitoring. This is another area where children's nurses could be more active in research to clearly identify children's needs and to pinpoint areas which need development and evaluation.

Activity

Obtain a copy of your hospital's business plans for the next year. Assess how much these plans take children's needs into account.

In the future it should be possible to see a more active interest in the development of services for children. In 1995 the Government produced a draft children's charter for discussion. This document listed some of the rights expected by children in hospital.

SUMMARY

Since the 1950s there have been many innovations and changes to provide appropriate care for children in hospital. However, it would appear that hospitals are still potentially causing the patient harm in relation to the needs of the child. Children's nurses should be more assertive and active in trying to establish and maintain recommended standards of care for children. They need to promote their specialist knowledge and skills so that they can be accepted as the specialists in child care. Swanwick and Barlow (1993) have begun to investigate the uniqueness of this branch of nursing. More research is needed in this area to strengthen the rationale for the need for more RSCNs/RNs (child). This research needs to be related to the benefits of meeting needs. Possibly the evidence that the lack of psychological care causes harm has lost its impact over time. It may be that now there is a need to show that such care reduces parental complaints and enables earlier discharge as parents who have been fully involved in their child's care are happy to take the child home knowing that they have access to specialised help and support. Such research would also help to provide research-based standards which relate to the specialist care of children. These could then form the basis of audits and quality assurance programmes which could be applied specifically to paediatrics. In these ways an argument can be put forward for the cost effectiveness of providing psychological care, enabling future league tables of hospital performance to include some measurement of this and thus improving the present situation so that the hospital really does do the patient no harm.

➤ *Key points*

1. Hospitals still do not always meet the psychological needs of children in hospital.
2. Children's nurses are necessary to promote these needs in all areas of the hospital.
3. More research is needed to strengthen the importance of the role of the children's nurse.
4. The importance of psychological care should be part of any evaluation of hospital performance.
5. Patients' charters should include the rights of the child in relation to health care.

2 PREPARATION FOR HOSPITAL AND PROCEDURES

INTRODUCTION

One of the unique roles of the children's nurse is the preparation of the child for hospitalisation or procedures. Children find illness and hospitalisation extremely stressful and frightening, and if these feelings are not allayed the child is at risk from developing behavioural changes and a long-term fear of hospital and medical intervention.

Any preparation has to be adjusted to suit the individual child whose personality and past experiences may all influence the reaction to hospital and understanding of procedures. Carson *et al.* (1992) believe that the child's conception of illness and hospital is the most important factor in determining how well the child will adjust. Other studies have discovered further factors influencing adjustment to illness and hospitalisation. Gillis (1990) found that children from rural areas responded less well to hospital than those in urban areas, perhaps because children in urban areas have more day-to-day contact with the local hospital. However, it appears that intimate knowledge of hospital and procedures is not helpful. Hart and Bossert (1994) discovered that prior experience and familiarity with hospital did not reduce children's fears. They suggest that fear of the unknown is replaced by fear of reality.

One of the most important strategies children use for coping with stress is play. In 1991 the DoH issued guidelines on the welfare of children in hospital and stated that play: ' ... can help them to resolve stressful situations like admission to hospital where they have to undergo painful procedures ... '. Using play to prepare children for the unknown not only decreases their fears but enables them to develop a feeling of control over the event, thus helping them to cope better. There are many types of play materials which can be used to prepare children and studies have not shown any method to be more effective than another. Becker (1972) even suggests that some of these methods may actually increase stress and anxiety. However, the age of the child does appear to influence which method is most effective. Bates and Broome (1986) found that small children reacted better to involvement in active play whilst older children preferred age-appropriate videos. Broome and Lillis (1989) discovered that the main benefit of preparation was increased cooperation from the child, but they also found a significant reduction in the amount of pain the children reported and in their heart and respiratory rates.

Parents need preparation too. Parents do not always know what to do or how best to support their child during hospitalisation or procedures. Children readily sense parental anxiety and this can increase their fears and resistance to the event. Some parents may be undecided

Children's reactions to hospital – influencing factors
- Personality – ability to cope with stress
- Conception of illness and hospital
- Age (especially preschool age)
- Intelligence
- Parental reactions
- Type and length of illness

about staying with their child during hospitalisation or a specific procedure and will need help and support from the nurse to make this decision.

PREPARING CHILDREN FOR HOSPITAL

The preparation for children having a planned admission to hospital is often well organised. Several hospital run pre-admission clubs for children on the waiting list. These clubs usually provide children with an opportunity to visit the ward, meet some of the staff and play with equipment. These clubs tend to be arranged to primarily meet the needs of younger children. There is some justification in this, as this is the age group known to be most traumatised by hospitalisation. However, this does not mean that older children do not also require information. The Children's Charter produced in 1996 (DoH, 1996) recognised this and recommended that adolescents have the chance to visit adult and children's wards, and be able to make a choice about where they are nursed. Parents also require information and while accompanying their child to a pre-admission club will provide them with increased knowledge it will not tell them about the normal and expected behavioural responses of children to hospital. Vulcan and Nikulich-Barrett (1988) found that parents who were told about such behaviour were less anxious and managed it better. Parents also need advice about the hospital routine and their role. Although many children's units claim to believe in the partnership with parents' philosophy, few of them explain to parents what this means (Audit Commission, 1993; Darbyshire, 1994).

Activity

Ask some parents and children in hospital about their preparation and consider how useful it was in meeting their needs.

Siblings often get missed in the preparation of a child for hospital. Siblings can feel neglected by the absence of parents or fear that they too may have to be admitted to hospital. At times they may feel guilt that they are somehow responsible for the hospitalisation. As a result, they often demonstrate feelings of anger and resentment towards the ill child or their parents. Even when these feelings are not exhibited the repressed emotion may result in other types of problem behaviour. Morgan (1990) found that even siblings of children admitted to hospital for short periods demonstrated behavioural changes when the hospitalised child returned home. It is obviously difficult to meet all the needs of children of various ages, their siblings and parents in terms of preparing them for hospitalisation. The efficacy of pre-admission clubs depends upon their ability to respond to these varying needs.

Cross reference

Pre- and post-operative care – pages 378–379

Principles of preparing children for procedures

- Assess the child's present level of understanding
- Find out parental wishes about presence and involvement
- Prepare the teaching and visual aids
- Use concrete terms and familiar words
- Explain any unfamiliar terminology
- Emphasise body parts and functions not involved
- Be honest
- Explain how the child will feel
- Demonstrate and practise any coping mechanisms
- Include negative information carefully
- Emphasise the positive aspects
- Evaluate learning and allow time for questions

Principles of preparing parents for their child's hospitalisation

- Show around ward
- Indicate parent's facilities
- Explain ward philosophy
- Outline ward routine and staffing
- Explain children's physical and psychological reactions to hospital and illness
- Warn of siblings' reactions
- Clarify nurses' role in providing care, support and teaching
- Provide opportunity to discuss issues, ask questions
- Consolidate verbal information with a written account

Think about how you could plan a pre-admission facility to meet the needs of siblings.

It is important not to overload the family with information at the pre-admission visit. However, it is unlikely that everything will be remembered. For this reason it is useful to have the information in a written format which can then act as consolidation to the advice given on the day. This written information could also address the needs of the different members of the family. Parents can also be given a resource list of books and play items useful for preparing children for hospital. Adams *et al.* (1991) found that a preparation booklet not only reduced children's anxieties on admission but also reduced the number of behavioural problems occurring after discharge and increased parental satisfaction when compared with verbal preparation alone. Hall (1996) describes how story telling prior to hospitalisation helps children gain confidence about going to hospital.

Activity

Visit your local children's library and see what books are available to prepare children of different ages for admission to hospital. Take a critical look at these books and consider how useful they are.

Children on the waiting list for planned admission are usually well catered for in terms of preparation but can the same be said for children entering hospital as an emergency? Every year, 25% of children in the UK between the ages of 0 and 16 years will visit an Accident and Emergency (A&E) unit and the majority of these will be preschool children (Campbell and Glasper, 1995). This visit is likely to be the child's first contact with hospital and can affect their future response to any further contact. A&E departments can be frightening and children taken there are often already stressed because of pain and fear. Although much can be done to alleviate the stress of the A&E department it would be much better if the child could become familiar with the environment before they needed to use the facility. Hospital tours alone are known to be ineffective in relieving anxiety (Peterson *et al.*, 1990) but in the 1990s a group of hospitals in Northern Ireland set up a Well Teddy Clinic to decrease children's anxiety about A&E. Children bring their teddies to hospital for a checkup and through play become familiar with the equipment used in hospital. Evaluations of this facility have been very positive (Burton, 1994). Other innovations to prepare children for emergency admission to hospital are visits by ambulance staff to nurseries and infant classes, providing the children a chance to see inside an ambulance and handle some of the equipment.

Cross reference

A&E – page 295

Activity

Investigate what strategies are used in your area to prepare children for emergency admission to hospital.

PREPARING CHILDREN FOR PROCEDURES

Children of any age need preparation for any procedure. They need to know what is going to happen and what they will need to do. Parents also need information about the procedure and their role. Care must be taken to give the information at an optimum time to reduce rather than heighten anxiety. Generally, small children can best deal with this sort of information as close as possible to the event. Older children manage better if given time between the preparation and the implementation of the procedure to allow them to absorb the information and ask questions. The preparation needs to take into account the child's age, stage of development, temperament, previous experiences and coping strategies, and the individual's need to know. Like adults, children vary in the amount of information they want to know (Peterson and Toler, 1986) and the nurse can be guided by the parents and the child's reaction to the preparation. The actual procedure is best carried out away from the bed area. Even babies can associate objects or places with painful experiences and protest when meeting them again. For all children, it is useful to have prepared the necessary equipment prior to the procedure so there is no added distress for the child by having to wait and watch this happen.

A child who has a distressing experience during a procedure will develop a long-lasting fear of the procedure and is likely to become more and more resistant to it. To prevent this negative cycle of events it is important to try and ensure that the child receives the optimum psychological and physical preparation.

PSYCHOLOGICAL PREPARATION

The nurse preparing the child for the procedure ideally needs to be someone who has had time to build up a rapport with the child and family. The child needs to be able to trust the nurse to have confidence in what is said. Babies are usually wary of strangers and have a strong attachment to their parents. They are too young for an explanation of the procedure but can be helped by parental presence during the procedure. If parents are unable to be present a familiar object may also help. Infancy is the period of sensori-motor learning and, although most babies are likely to actively withdraw from pain and need to be effectively restrained during procedures, the nurse or parent can still provide comfort by gentle massage, talking or singing quietly or providing a dummy.

Role of the nurse in caring for children before, during and after procedures

- *Be confident.* Even babies can sense anxiety in adults and will react by resisting

- *Provide realistic choices.* Allow children some control over events by offering choices, but only offer realistic choices. Children may not have any control over the timing of the procedure but they may be able to choose a toy to cuddle

- *Allow participation.* Providing children with something to do during the procedure will also help them to feel in control. They may like to hold the sticking plaster and help to apply it after the procedure

- *Help with coping strategies.* Remind the child of methods practised before the procedure. Join in breathing or singing

- *Accept child's response.* Small children usually react to stress by crying, shouting or hitting out. Older children may cry or swear. They should not be punished for reacting in this way to procedures

- *Give praise.* Help children's self-image by praising their coping skills whatever the outcome. They need to know that their reactions were acceptable in the circumstances and not to feel that they have failed. Rewards for bravery provide evidence of their ability to cope with the situation and may help to boost confidence

- *Provide comfort.* Give hugs and cuddles during and after the procedure

Toddlers are egocentric with limited communication skills. They attribute lifelike behaviour to inanimate objects and often believe that thoughts can cause events. They enjoy imitating adult behaviour but can also be very negative as they try to develop some autonomy. They need to be told in very simple terms what they will experience during the procedure and have time to play with equipment so they are not frightened of it. They should be given some opportunity for autonomy, perhaps by having a choice of toy to accompany them, so that they do not feel totally out of control. Toddlers also need very careful restraint but may be reassured by distraction, story telling or singing.

The preschool child is still egocentric but has developed more communication skills. At this age children are very conscious of their bodies and worry about the effect of any injury. Having now developed an independent personality, these children now try to take further control of situations by using their initiative. They can now understand that pain is not a punishment and the nurse can use simple terms to explain the reason and the effects of the procedure. They should be allowed to take part in the procedure, perhaps by holding equipment.

The school-age child is beginning to develop concrete thinking skills and is described by Erikson as having a sense of industry. In other words these children have an interest in learning and are keen to use their increased language and thinking skills to gain a greater understanding of the world. They need to have the reasons for procedures clearly explained and to understand the purpose and effect of the equipment involved. At this age children can relate to their peers and may be able to help each other prepare for a procedure. Their developmental need for industry should be satisfied by allowing some participation in the procedure and an active coping strategy.

The adolescent is concerned with developing his/her autonomy as an individual and is capable of abstract thought. Adolescents need to know the reason and consequences of the procedure and any effects it may have on their appearance. Their need for autonomy can be helped by enabling them some choice in the timing and place for the procedure. Peer groups are important to this age group and they may gain more benefit from preparation from another adolescent. The nurse may need to accept that the adolescent may refuse to consider a specific coping strategy and may resort to more childish ways of coping.

Use of play

Dolls can be used to explain exactly what the procedure entails. Some children may like to act out procedures on the doll which also provides them with an opportunity to handle the equipment. Dressing up as nurses or doctors enables children to act out feelings towards these people and may help them to come to terms with medical interventions. Drawing or colouring in pictures of the event may also help children to talk about any fears. Photographs or videos of other hospital departments and equipment will help to remove the fear of the

Cross reference

Functions of play in hospital – page 259

unknown and play equipment can then be used to give children some appreciation of procedures such as X-rays or scans (a rigid play tunnel can make a realistic scanner).

Older children may prefer to read about the procedure. There are children's books which provide information about medical procedures (Table 2.1) and, in addition, some hospitals provide information leaflets for children about specific investigations.

Annie West (1993) *Brinkworth Bear goes to Hospital* Blackie Children's Books	Age: 3 years+ the story of Brinkworth Bear who goes to hospital after falling out of a tree	
Diana Kimpton (1994) *The Hospital Highway Code* Peter Piper Publishers	Age: 8–12 years humorous book about hospital but also teaches about X-rays, pain, having a broken limb, tonsils removed, etc.	
Caroline Bucknall (1993) *One Bear in Hospital* Pan MacMillan Children's Books	Age: 3 years+ Ted falls off his bike and has to go to hospital	
Jean and Gareth Adamson *Topsy and Tim go to Hospital* Puffin Books	Age: 2–7 years a story of Topsy and Tim's stay in hospital	
Francine Pascal (1992) *The Twins go to Hospital* Bantam	Age: 7–11 years the Wakefield twins have their tonsils out	
H. A. and Margaret Rey (1995) *Curious George Goes to Hospital* Houghton Mifflin Juvenile Books	Age: 4–8 years an adventure with Curious George on a trip to hospital	
Magdelen Nabb (1993) *Josie Smith Goes to Hospital* Harper Collins	Age: 6–9 years spend the night with Josie in hospital when she has her tonsils out	

Table 2.1

Books available for preparing children for hospital

Activity

Visit some departments in your hospital where children undergo investigations and explore what specific preparatory information is available for them. Consider what additional information may be useful.

Coping strategies

Teaching coping strategies before a procedure helps to give children some control of the event. When procedures are to be repeated, successful strategies, such as relaxation instructions or favourite music, can be put on tape as a reminder of the technique. The most effective strategies are based on behavioural therapies and produce feelings of calmness and relaxation in situations which would otherwise provoke stress and maladaptive behaviour. This new behaviour weakens the connection between anxiety and its stimulus. The most appropriate strategy for the individual depends upon choice and the discomfort of the procedure. Children experiencing severe discomfort may not be able to concentrate wholly on a complicated coping strategy. Most children will benefit best by being able to choose the method most appealing to them.

During the last 20 years, hypnosis has been developed to deal with children's psychological problems. Hypnotherapy is often successful in children because their high imaginative skills make them easily susceptible candidates. Self-hypnosis can be taught to individuals so that the technique can be used independently. Cohen *et al.* (1984) suggest that children as young as 3 years can use this technique and it is particularly useful for adolescents and for children who require repeated painful procedures. Its success appears to relate to the child's control and mastery of the situation.

Relaxation and guided imagery (page 271) are techniques similar to hypnosis and are also well accepted by children with good imagination skills. Even small children can be helped to relax by rocking and quiet soothing words. Older children can be helped to relax by controlled breathing and progressive relaxation of different parts of the body. This can be combined with a discussion of an enjoyable event which can be enhanced by music or pictures of the event. Some children may cope better by being more active and controlled breathing may be used as a way of pretending to blow the pain away. Singing or even shouting can help children distract themselves from the reality of the procedure. Distraction can also be provided by story telling or a favourite video. The child usually needs help to use these methods and parents who have also been taught the strategy can often provide this support.

Children who are very uncooperative may benefit from some kind of positive reinforcement. Stars or tokens or a bravery certificate can be offered for cooperation. In addition, praise for coping well will provide the child with intrinsic reinforcement.

Physical preparation

Consideration should be given to the most appropriate means of physical preparation prior to distressing procedures. Sedation, analgesia or local anaesthetic may help to make the procedure more bearable but may need to be given 1–2 hours before the procedure. Whenever possible, injections should be avoided as most children regard these as painful procedures and their fear may actually be increased. Sometimes it is useful to give heavy sedation for the first of several procedures to enable to child to realise that the procedure is not to be feared. Once the child is more relaxed it may be possible to gradually reduce the medication.

SUMMARY

One of the unique roles of the children's nurse is the preparation of children for hospital and procedures. Children cannot be expected to

---

Relaxation exercise for children

Ensure that the child is lying or sitting down in a comfortable position and in a quiet, even voice say the following:

- put your hands on your tummy so that the tips of your fingers are just touching
- feel your finger tips moving apart as you breathe
- see how your tummy goes up and down as you breathe

Allow the child to experience this for 10–20 breaths. Then say:

- put one hand on your chest
- feel your hand going up and down as you breathe

Allow the child time to recognise this feeling and then say to the child:

- put one hand on your tummy and one hand on your chest and feel your tummy and chest going up and down. When I say 'down' let your tummy and chest go down and when I say 'up', let your chest and tummy lift up

Keep your voice quiet and even, giving your instructions at a suitable pace to ensure a deep, relaxing breathing rate with a slightly longer exhalation period. Remember that the child's respiratory rate is likely to be faster than your own passively accept strange interventions and children who are unprepared will not only be unable to cooperate but are likely to become progressively more upset and scared with subsequent contacts with health care. Children's nurses working with healthy children should consider how their patient group can be introduced to the hospital environment before they have a need to use these facilities. Children's nurses working with sick children should be able to use a range of techniques to prepare children of different ages and experiences for a variety of interventions. They should make themselves aware of the different interventions performed on children and the different departments in which these are performed so they can give truthful and informed preparation. Nursing assessment should include an assessment of the child and family's previous experiences and their individual need for information and preparation.

> ➤ **Key points**

1. Children who are exposed to unresolved stress and fear in hospital are likely to undergo long-term behavioural problems as a result of this experience.

2. Preparation for hospital or procedures should suit the individual child's age, stage of development, temperament and previous experience.

3. Parents and siblings should also be given information about the ill child's treatment and their supportive role.

4. Children need preparation for emergency admission as well as planned hospitalisation.

5. Behavioural therapies are useful strategies for helping children to cope with the discomfort of procedures.

Guided imagery for children

Guided imagery attempts to help children to concentrate on another image other than the one which is disturbing to them. It can also be used as an aid to relaxation by helping the children to imagine they are elsewhere. Children tend to have good imaginations and usually respond well to this technique. Individuals all have their own idea of pleasure and the imagery needs to be negotiated with them first. The following is only an example which will only be successful if the child is able to associate this scenario with relaxation

As with any strategy for relaxation the child should be in a comfortable and relaxed position. Spend a short time ensuring that the child is relaxed and breathing evenly – you could commence by using the breathing exercise described above. Then commence your description in a quiet and even tone:

Imagine you are lying on the beach. The sun is hot and the sand is warm. You can feel the sun on your skin making you warm and sleepy. The sand is so soft and warm that it is as if you were lying in bed. As you gently move your feet and hands you can feel the warm grains of sand between your toes and fingers. You can smell mummy's perfume and you can hear her turning the pages of her book as she sits beside you reading. In the distance you can hear the sound of the sea as it gently moves up to the beach and away again. You feel too tired to move and your arms and legs feel very, very heavy. It is difficult to keep awake so you make yourself more comfortable on the sand and listen to the sounds of the sea. You count the gentle waves as they come into the shore … 1 … 2 … 3 … 4 … 5. Think about the warmth of the sun … the feel of the sand … the smell of mummy's perfume … how heavy your legs and arms feel … and the sound of the sea …

Continue with the description with pauses to enable the child to really imagine the scenario

When the procedure is finished, gradually talk the child into a more wakeful situation

3 Assessment of the sick child

Introduction

Assessment of the child involves a knowledge and appreciation of usual child growth, development and behaviour as well as the skills of communication and observation. Assessment should be an ongoing process but is particularly important during the admission of the child to hospital. At this time assessment performs a number of functions. It primarily enables the nurse to make a systematic collection of information about the child to identify the child and family's individual needs for nursing care. However, it also provides an opportunity for the nurse to form a therapeutic relationship with the child and family and to develop a partnership with them in providing the care.

During the nursing assessment, the nurse will interview the child and family to discover their:

* usual home routines to help promote a more familiar environment in hospital;
* previous experience of illness or hospital and understanding of this admission;
* needs and concerns.

During the interview, observation skills will enable the nurse to identify physical and psychological problems. Measurement of vital signs and information from other health professionals will provide more detail.

The use of an appropriate nursing model for the care of children will provide structure for the assessment and ensure that all areas are explored in a holistic way.

Cross reference

Models of children's nursing – page 602

Preparation for assessment

First impressions are often very important on admission to hospital when children and families may be very anxious. Their first need is often to feel more at ease and preparing for the admission assessment may help to provide that reassurance. Arriving on a busy ward and being left alone will not help to relieve the anxieties of the child or family.

Activity

Consider how you might prepare for an admission assessment to provide a welcoming and reassuring atmosphere.

Even when nurses are busy, it is possible to provide a friendly and reassuring atmosphere. If possible, the child should welcomed by name and the nurse should introduce him/herself and find out the names of the family present. If the nurse is too busy to interview the parents at that moment, the child and family should either be taken to the bed area which has been prepared with a few suitable toys or shown to the playroom. The child and family can be introduced to other families or the play therapist and the nurse can promise to return.

Ideally, the admission assessment should be undertaken in a quiet, private area which is free from distractions. If an interview room is not available, an empty side room may be used for this purpose. Otherwise, curtains round the bed area may provide some psychological privacy. The area should be prepared with suitable toys to occupy the child with the nursing charts and equipment kept to a minimum to avoid making the assessment seem too clinical.

In most settings the nurse undertaking the assessment will be the child and family's named nurse for that admission. The nurse should explain the relevance of this concept as well as the purpose of the assessment. The child and family should understand that the assessment is as much for them to find out information as it for the nurse to collect data. Parents and older children may also be reassured by an assurance of confidentiality.

The child and family need time to adjust to their surroundings and an interview which commences with probing questions is unlikely to be successful. Similarly, an assessment which commences with a physical examination of the child is likely to end in tears. The nurse needs to build up a rapport with the child and family before trying to make in-depth investigations. This rapport is probably best developed by casual conversation, giving the child and family time to assess and be confident with the nurse.

FAMILY ROUTINES

Activity

What will you need to ask the child and family to find out as much as possible about their usual home routines?

Family routines can be ascertained by asking the child or family to complete a 24 hour diary of usual home events (Figure 3.1). This information can then be built upon by asking specific questions relevant to the child's age and condition.

Health problems

The nurse needs to be aware of any health problem for which the child is currently receiving treatment. This may be a long-term problem, such as asthma, which may be unrelated to this admission, or a new problem

Figure 3.1

Assessment of the child –
24 hour diary.

Please complete this diary with as much information as you can about your child's normal daily activities. This will help us to try and keep to this same routine while your child is in hospital			
Time	**Meals**	**Activity**	**Parental care**
01:00			
02:00			
03:00			
04:00			
05:00			
06:00			
07:00			
08:00			
09:00			
10:00			
11:00			
12:00			
13:00			
14:00			
15:00			
16:00			
17:00			
18:00			
19:00			
20:00			
21:00			
22:00			
23:00			
24:00			

which initiated the admission. The usual routine for medication and any other treatment should be ascertained.

Eating and drinking

It is important to know about the child's usual nutrition, meal and snack times, and appetite so that appropriate food and drink can be offered in hospital. Information about any special cups, bowls or cutlery and help required can also be used to help the child maintain usual nutrition.

Elimination

Information about the child's usual bowel and bladder habits will help the nurse to identify any changes and any problems the family may have. To avoid confusion it is also useful to know small children's stage of potty training and the family words used for toilet habits. The stress of hospitalisation can disturb menstruation so it is important to ask older girls about their periods and what sanitary protection they use.

Rest and activity

Individual children have very different patterns of rest and activity and the nurse needs to be aware of these to be able to identify what is normal for that child. The nurse needs to discover the child's usual bed-time and time of waking. If the child wakes in the night how do the family react? Special routines before bed such as a bed-time story, favourite toy or comforter, or nightlight are particularly important to know if the parents cannot be resident. Smaller children's nap times need to be known if this routine is to be continued in hospital.

An outline of the child's usual level of activity can be gained from the diary, the nurse can then ask about favourite pastimes or TV programmes which may help to relieve boredom in hospital.

Washing and dressing

The nurse needs to know how much help the child requires with washing and dressing as well as their usual routines. What is the family schedule for washing and is the child used to a bath or shower? If there is any aspect, such as hair washing which the child finds distressing, the nurse needs to discover how the family deals with this. If the child has a skin problem there may be special bathing creams or lotions which the nurse needs to know about.

Communication

To communicate with the child it is useful for the nurse to know who is important to the child at home. This information may include pets', teachers' and aunts' and uncles' names as well as friends. It is also useful for the nurse to have an appreciation of the child's usual temperament so any changes can be quickly identified. For instance, is the child usually quiet and shy or very active and talkative? What tends to upset the child and what does the child do when tired or upset? What comforting methods work best?

Religion

The nurse needs to appreciate the importance of religion to the child and family as there may be religious practices which they would like to be continued in hospital. Parents may also wish to discuss baptism if this has not been performed before admission.

IDENTIFICATION OF NEEDS AND PROBLEMS

Once the nurse has gained an idea of the usual home routine, the needs and problems of this admission should be identified. Actual needs and problems can be discovered by asking how the reason for this admission has affected or changed the child's usual behaviour. The knowledge and experience of the nurse will help the identification of potential needs and problems. The child and parents' understanding of the health problem can be gained at this time when the nurse should also be able to identify any learning needs the child or family have in relation to the hospitalisation.

For example, a child who has been newly diagnosed with asthma may report that exercise is a problem due to breathlessness. The parents may express sorrow that the child will probably need to give up sports. The nurse will recognise that one of the child's problems is being unable to play sport without becoming breathless and that the parents need teaching about asthma and exercise. If the nurse does not recognise these concerns, acceptance of the condition and compliance with treatment could become a potential problem. See the case history in Table 3.1.

Table 3.1

Assessment of a child's needs and problems

Jamie is an 8 year old who was diagnosed with asthma when he was 2 years old. He has been admitted with an acute attack. On admission he is very wheezy and cyanosed. He is also very scared as he has been in hospital many times before and hates it. He misses his two brothers, especially at night as he shares a room with them, and dislikes the 'pins' in his arm and the oxygen mask. During his assessment the needs and problems shown below were identified.

Activity	Needs	Problems
Breathing	Provide oxygen Avoid over-excitement	Unable to breathe with wheeze and cough
Eating and drinking	Maintenance of fluids and encouragement to return to normal after the asthmatic attack	Unable to eat or drink
Play	Provide reassurance (Teddy Edward is his special toy) Provision of more active play when able	Unable to get out of bed to play
Rest and sleep	Reassurance and company	Exhausted but too frightened to sleep
Hygiene	Help with washing while breathless	Unable to meet own hygiene needs
Elimination	Record all output	Has not passed urine for 7 hours – may be dehydrated
Concerns	Reassurance re needles and oxygen masks – use EMLA cream and nasal cannulae	Fear of IV and oxygen mask
Communication	Anticipate needs with help from parents	Too breathless to talk

It is important to identify needs and problems in negotiation with the child and family. A solution to a problem which is not shared by the child and family will never be found! Sometimes the parent may identify a problem which the nurse cannot appreciate. The nurse should gently probe to find the reason for the problem so that appropriate care can be given to overcome it. On occasions the nurse will identify a problem that the parent denies. In these situations the nurse may need to seek help from another colleague or approach the problem at a later time.

Reasons for potential problems should be explained so that the child and family fully understand their care and treatment and feel part of the assessment process.

INTERVIEW TECHNIQUE

It is apparent that the nurse needs to ascertain a great deal of information and without careful attention to a good interview technique the assessment process may become more like an interrogation.

Activity

What communication techniques can the nurse use to ensure that the assessment interview does not intimidate the child and family and encourages them to talk?

Communication can be transmitted by non-verbal means and the nurse should make sure that her posture or facial expression does not reveal disinterest, superiority, authority or insensitivity. A relaxed but alert sitting position facing the parents will facilitate communication. Writing down everything the child or parents say can prevent a dialogue and hinders listening as the writer cannot pay close attention to the speaker's words or behaviour. In Western cultures eye contact is a sign of interest and paying attention, but in other cultures this direct approach may be considered rude and hinder communication.

The nurse should address each family member by their name to convey interest and respect for them as individuals. Parents should be addressed as Mr/Mrs/Miss/Ms, as they prefer, until such time as they request to be called by their first names. The nurse should also be careful not to use jargon or medical terminology which the child or family do not understand, and the use of open-ended questions provides a non-threatening way of gaining more information than the use of direct questions. Ley and Llewellyn (1995) report that health care professionals often use vocabulary with which they presume patients are familiar. The nurse should include the child whenever possible and be alert when older children may want to share information without their parents' presence.

Active listening can also encourage others to talk. The nurse, although providing information, does not want to monopolise the conversation. Parents who are hesitant to talk may be helped by the accepting behaviour of the nurse, indicated by nodding or a murmur of assent. Sometimes the child or parent may be silent while they consider the best way to express what is possibly a difficult area for them. The nurse should allow this period of silence, as a rush to continue the discussion may destroy the moment at which a crucial problem was to be revealed.

COMMUNICATING WITH THE CHILD

Whatever their age the assessment interview should be directed at the child and their parents. However, at the end of the interview the nurse needs to examine the child and by this time it is helpful for the child to feel comfortable with the nurse. Children generally need time to evaluate strangers and do not respond well to rapid advances of friendship. They are also very sensitive to non-verbal communication and soon become anxious if they sense fear, hesitancy and concern in others. Many parents will exhibit just these emotions when bringing their child into hospital and the nurse needs to be able to dispel these attitudes and gain their confidence if the child is to be approached easily. A knowledge of the development of children's communication and thought processes can aid this approach.

Activity

Consider how communication can be facilitated between the nurse and an infant, toddler, schoolchild and adolescent.

Pre-verbal children rely on non-verbal communication both to make their needs known and to understand others' behaviour. They readily respond to their parents' anxiety, often transmitted by a change in voice or the way in which they are held. They can be reassured if their parents show signs of relaxing and by a quiet, calm voice and gentle, but firm, handling. Older infants who have begun to recognise the individual characteristics of their parents are best held in a position where they can still see them.

Preschool children only see events from their own perspective and can only understand things explained in concrete terms. Children at this age tend to give lifelike qualities to inanimate objects. This animism can cause them to be very fearful of medical equipment which they can believe is capable of causing them pain because of their naughtiness. However, Flavell (1985) has shown that animism usually occurs when the child has no information about the characteristics of the object. If the nurse can allow the child to play with the equipment and explains in simple terms how the equipment is used, the child's fears may be overcome. Any explanation also needs to include how the individual child will be affected. Because this age group has limited understanding and cannot differentiate between fact and fantasy they are very fearful of the unknown. Parents are still important to preschool children and in times of stress they still need the physical presence and comfort of their parents. Harris (1993) suggests that the best way of managing these children's fears is to provide the child with parental support. Thus, communication with these children can often be facilitated by first gaining the acceptance and trust of the parents and talking to the child in their presence.

The schoolchild has begun to explore the environment and is

Cross reference

Language development – page 77

Communicating with children

Infants

- handle firmly but gently
- avoid sudden movements and loud noises
- allow the parents to remain in sight
- discover the infant's preferred position

Toddlers

- position yourself at the child's level
- focus on the child
- use simple language and short sentences
- use only concrete terms

School-age children

- allow time for questions, give honest answers
- facilitate expression of fears
- explain everything
- use previous experiences

Adolescents

- expect mood changes
- treat as autonomous individuals
- accept hostility, anger, non-cooperation
- provide privacy, reassure about confidentiality
- be non-judgemental
- do not pry
- avoid giving advice unless asked

interested in finding out the reasons for everything around them. Giving them opportunity to question events before they happen helps them to communicate. They can interpret the meaning of words and are quicker to acknowledge when they do not understand. They are able to express their concerns and feelings about hospitalisation but need encouragement to do so. As schoolchildren grow older parents become less important to them but they still need parental support, comfort and advice in a strange environment. If the nurse includes school-aged children in the interview, they will feel accepted as an active participant and be more able to express their own thoughts.

Erikson describes adolescence as a phase of 'identity versus role confusion'. Adolescents find themselves changing physically and psychologically from children to adults, and this can be a difficult phase for them. They want to have autonomy but at the same time want help and support at times of stress. They tend to reject others' beliefs and values because of their need to make their own decisions. They can avoid conversation if they feel insecure or sense disapproval. The nurse probably needs to interview adolescents and parents separately, making clear that any information will be treated confidentially. Talking to the adolescent first may help to demonstrate the importance of that individual and keeping to casual conversation initially may help to give the adolescent a sense of security. The nurse needs to show respect, interest and acceptance by avoiding any indication of surprise, judgement or disapproval and by not offering advice unless asked.

Cross reference

Erikson – page 85

USING INTERPRETERS

Activity

Consider the disadvantages of using interpreters for the assessment interview.

On occasions it may be necessary to use an interpreter to carry out an assessment of a child and family. This can pose communication, cultural, ethical and legal difficulties. It is difficult for the nurse to show respect, concern and empathy when communicating via an interpreter, and it is not always easy to know if certain Western expressions can be translated directly into another language. The child and family may have difficulty talking to an interpreter, who may be a stranger of another class or gender, particularly if the questions are of a personal and confidential nature. This may be partly overcome by allowing the family time to meet the interpreter before the assessment interview (Slater, 1993). Legal and ethical issues arise when the nurse cannot be certain that all the necessary information has been given or understood to enable the child and family to make informed choices about care and treatment. The nurse can watch the non-verbal behaviour of the family in response to questions to try to assess understanding but if such direct observation is seen as threatening, this is not an easy or foolproof way of determining concern.

PHYSICAL ASSESSMENT

It is preferable to be able to talk to the child and family and gain their trust and acceptance before trying to make any assessment of the child's physical state. If the nurse makes an immediate move to examine the child before doing anything else, it is likely that the child will cry or refuse to cooperate, making this assessment impossible. However, during the interview phase the nurse can learn much about the child's physical condition by just observing the child.

Activity

Take time out to observe a child and consider how much you can learn about their condition by just looking and listening.

Cross reference

Growth – page 67

Although first impressions of a child and family must be used with caution, it is likely that at the first meeting the nurse will gain an immediate idea about the child's development and hygiene. An experienced nurse will be able to see if the child's weight, height and head circumference is within the normal range for that age. Obvious neglect of hygiene will also be immediately apparent. The child's colour will give information about fever, shock, jaundice or cardiac problems (Table 3.2). Difficulty in breathing can be seen from flared or blocked nostrils or sweating. Rashes, cuts, bruises or swellings will also be obvious as will any infected areas of the skin. The child's mobility, posture and behaviour will give some clue about the severity of the child's condition and the degree of anxiety. Dehydration may be apparent by the dryness of the mouth and, in babies, sunken fontanelle. Swollen fontanelle may indicate raised intracranial pressure. The characteristics of any vomit or sputum will also provide clues about the child's condition (Table 3.3).

Listening will give the nurse even more information. Respiratory problems can be heard by grunting, stridor, wheeze or cough (Table

Table 3.2

Observing the sick child: looking at skin colour

Observation	Significance
Pallor	Shock, anaemia or cold
Flushed	Possible pyrexia
Cyanosis	Cardiac or respiratory problem
Jaundice	Physiological or hepatic infection or obstruction
Bruising	Accidental or non-accidental injury or clotting disorder
Diaphoresis	Cardio-respiratory distress
Rash	Infectious disease or allergy

Excreta	Observation	Significance
Vomit	Undigested food/milk	Over indulgence, feeding too fast, gastric irritant
	Bile stained	Stomach is empty
	Blood stained	Following swallowed blood (dental extraction, epistaxis, tonsillectomy), oesophageal varices or stress gastric ulcer
	Projectile	Pyloric stenosis
Sputum	Mucous	Respiratory tract inflammation
	Yellow/green	Respiratory tract infection
	Blood stained	Trauma of coughing
Urine	Polyuria	Drinking heavily or diabetes mellitus/insipidus
	Oliguria	Dehydration, renal problem
	Dark coloured	Dehydration or biliary obstruction
	Pale coloured	Drinking heavily
	Blood stained	Urinary tract infection/trauma or renal problem
	Cloudy	Urinary tract infection
Faeces	Soft and yellow	Normal infant stool
	Watery	Gastro-enteritis
	Soft and green/brown	Gastro-enteritis
	Hard and green/brown	Hunger or constipation
	Mucous or blood	Inflammation of the bowel
	Black	Meconium of newborn or digested blood
	Undigested food	Intestinal hurry
	Pale and bulky	Undigested fat

Table 3.3

Observing the sick child: looking at excreta

	Observation	Significance
Rate	Tachyopnoea	
	Dyspnoea	Cardiac or respiratory problem
Movements	Nasal flaring	Respiratory distress
	Sternal retraction	Respiratory distress
	Intercostal recession	Respiratory distress
	Tracheal tug	Respiratory distress
Noise	Sighing, yawning	Shock, blood loss
	Stertorous	Altered conscious level
	Wheeze	Inflamed and narrow lower airway
	Cough/whoop	Irritation of upper respiratory tract
	Bark	Inflamed & narrow upper airway
	Stridor	Obstruction of upper airway
	Grunting	Respiratory distress (infants)

Table 3.4

Observing the sick child: looking and listening to respirations

3.4). The child's cry may reveal fear, hunger, exhaustion, pain or cerebral irritation.

Once the initial information has been gained by interview and observation, the nurse should be able to examine the child (Table 3.5). The less invasive techniques should be used first to avoid alarming the child and to enable the nurse to continue to gain the child's trust and

Cross reference

Urine testing – pages 477–481

Table 3.5

Observing the sick child: listening and looking at the child's behaviour

	Observation	Significance
Cry	Shrill/high pitched	Cerebral irritation
	Whimpering	Pain and/or fear
	Lusty	Anger or hunger
Position	Limp/flaccid	Toxicity
	Head/neck retraction	Cerebral irritation
	Knees drawn up	Abdominal pain
Behaviour	Unresponsive	Neurological deficit
	Lethargy or irritability	Toxicity
Relationship with others	Watchful	Pain/fear

confidence. The child should be involved in the examination process by being able to chose to sit on a parent's lap or on the bed and by handling the equipment.

The measurement of growth in children is one of the most important areas in the assessment of their health. Weight (Figure 3.2), height or length (Figure 3.3), and head circumference (Figure 3.4) should be measured and recorded on an appropriate percentile chart for all admissions. The percentile charts used in the UK use the 3rd and 97th percentile to indicate those children who are outside the normal growth parameters. However, such evaluations should be made with caution as small or large size may be genetic and the charts do not take into account the growth of children from different ethnic backgrounds.

Children under 36 months of age should have their length and head circumference recorded. A paper or metal tape measure should be used as false small recordings may be made with a stretchy cloth tape.

Young child have difficulty maintaining body temperature and this is a useful measurement to assess the child's condition. However, there has been much controversy about the optimum route and most accurate

Weighing babies and children (Figure 3.2)

Infants

- clean scales before each use
- weigh nude
- hold hand above baby to prevent falls

Children

- weigh in light clothing
- if weighing daily, weigh at same time of day in same clothing
- stand close to small children to prevent falls

Weight gain trends in childhood

0–6 months	=	140–200 g/week
6–12 months	=	double birth weight at 6 months
	=	85–140 g/week
	=	triple birth weight at 12 months
1–10 years	=	2–3 kg/year
10–16 years	=	1–5 kg/year

Note: In an emergency, a child's weight can be estimated by using the following formula:
$2 \times (4 + \text{child's age}) = $ approx weight (kg)

Figure 3.2

Weighing babies and children.

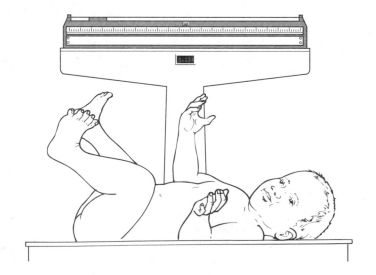

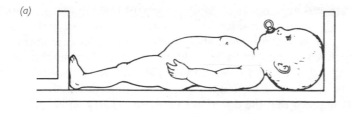

(a)

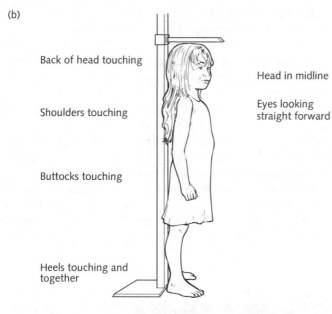

(b)

Back of head touching

Shoulders touching

Buttocks touching

Heels touching and together

Head in midline

Eyes looking straight forward

Figure 3.3

(a) Measuring length.
(b) Measuring height.

Recording children's height (Figure 3.3)
Children aged 0–2 years
- measure child's length when child is in the supine position
- place the head in midline
- hold the knees together and push gently until the legs are fully extended
- ensure head and feet are firmly against the ends of the measuring board

Older children
- measure when the child is upright
- remove child's shoes
- ensure child stands up tall and straight and looks straight ahead
- ensure child's shoulders, buttocks and heels touch the measure
- ensure child's feet are together

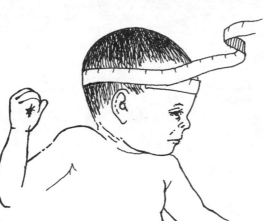

Figure 3.4

Measuring head circumference.

Measuring head circumference (Figure 3.4)
- Measure head circumference in babies 0–18 months or in any child whose head size appears abnormal
- Measure at the greatest circumference, slightly above the eyebrows and the tip of the ears and around the occipital prominence
- Use a metal or paper measure to avoid inaccurate results from a well-used tape which has become stretched
- Head circumference growth trends
  at birth = 33–35 cm
  0–6 months = 1.50 cm/month
  6–12 months = 0.5 cm/month

method of obtaining this recording. In the UK the digital thermometer or the tempadot are mostly used for an initial temperature recording as both methods have the advantage of measuring temperature quickly without invading either the mouth or rectum. Morley *et al.* (1992) found that these axillary measurements tended to underestimate core temperature and be easily affected by the environmental temperature, but they are probably useful for an initial determination of body temperature. This measurement also brings into question the normal temperature. Once thought to be 37°C, the mean body temperature is now recognised to be 36.8°C with a variable fluctuation between individuals of 0.5°C (Mackowiak *et al.*, 1992). In addition, Pontious *et al.* (1994) suggests that the difference between axillary and oral temperature is considerably less than the traditionally assumed 1.0°C.

An accurate pulse should be measured for a full minute and should be measured using a stethoscope placed over the apex of the heart in children under 2 years. Respiratory rates in young children should also be measured over a full minute and can be gained by watching abdominal movements as their respirations are diaphragmatic.

Blood pressure (BP) should be measured routinely in children to identify essential hypertension (Portman and Yetman, 1994). BP can be measured manually or with an electronic device, but either method can be inaccurate if not used correctly (Tables 3.6 and 3.7). The most important factor in accurate BP recording is the correct size cuff. Cuffs which are too narrow or too wide produce inaccurate measurements. De Swiet *et al.* (1989) recommend a cuff width equal to two-thirds limb length. Accuracy is further aided by positioning the limb at the level of the heart and holding it in position. Careful preparation and reassurance will help to minimise the child's anxiety which will produce an elevated BP.

Table 3.6

Recording children's blood pressure

Method	Rationale
Wrap the cuff snugly round the limb	A loose cuff will give false high recordings; a cuff which is too tight will also record inaccurately
Ensure that the lower edge of the cuff is 2–3 cm above the artery to be palpated; place the tubes superiorly	To prevent interference with auscultation
Place the sphygmomanometer at eye level on a flat surface	To facilitate accurate pressures
Palpate the chosen artery and inflate the cuff until pulsation disappears	To estimate systolic pressure; auscultatory gaps in phase I sounds can cause underestimation of systolic pressure unless already determined in this way
Place the stethoscope gently over the artery at the point of maximum pulsation.	If the stethoscope is pressed too firmly or touches the cuff, the diastolic pressure may be underestimated
Inflate the bladder to 30 mmHg above the estimated systolic pressure. Reduce the pressure by about 2 mmHg/second	Releasing the pressure too quickly will underestimate systolic pressure
Note the point at which repetitive clear tapping sounds first appear for at least two beats	This is the systolic pressure
Continue to gradually reduce the pressure and note the point at which the repetitive sounds become muffled	Releasing the pressure too quickly will overestimate the diastolic pressure; the point of muffled sounds is taken to be the diastolic blood pressure in children

Age	Systolic blood pressure (mmHg)	Diastolic blood pressure (mmHg)
0–1 month	65–85	53–55
1–3 months	85–90	50–53
6–12 months	90–92	53–56
1–5 years	90–95	54–56
6–10 years	96–102	56–62
11–16 years	101–115	62–67

Note: Blood pressure for children over 1 year may be approximated as follows: Systolic pressure (50th percentile) = 90 mmHg + (age in years × 2)

Table 3.7

Blood pressure norms in children

SUMMARY

The assessment process is one in which the nurse aims to develop a rapport with the child and family which will facilitate data collection by communication and observation. The nurse needs to have communication skills which not only encourage the parents to share information, but also enable children of different ages to express themselves and lose their anxieties about the strange hospital environment. This will enable the nurse to establish an appreciation of the family's usual homelife, identify the child's and family's needs and problems, and formulate a care plan. The nurse's observation skills enable an overall impression of the child's physical condition, state of nutrition, behaviour, and stage of development. Accurate measurements of growth and vital signs provide more objective assessments of the child's condition and provide a baseline for future observations.

➤ **Key points**

1. Assessment of a sick child enables the nurse to develop a relationship with the child and family whilst identifying the child's nursing problems.

2. A successful assessment requires careful preparation, a welcoming environment, time and privacy.

3. An assessment of usual home routines enables the nurse to adhere to these as far as possible, thus minimising the disturbance of hospitalisation for child and family.

4. Good communication skills are vital for an accurate assessment. These should be adapted according to the individual child and family's needs.

5. The needs and problems of the child should be identified in negotiation with the child and family.

6. Much of the assessment of a sick child can be gained by looking and listening to the child.

4 DAY CARE

INTRODUCTION

The Platt Report (1959) first recognised the value of minimising the stress of hospitalisation for children by shortening the amount of time they spent as in-patients. Gradually the concept of day care arose to provide essential medical interventions for the child whilst eliminating the need for an overnight stay in hospital. Apart from reducing the stress of a stay in hospital, day care also has the advantages of decreasing the chance of a hospital acquired infection, being a less expensive way of providing medical care and enabling a reduction in waiting list time (Campbell and Glasper, 1995). However, it can also have disadvantages and it is important to recognise that it might not be suitable for all children or beneficial for all families.

ADVANTAGES AND DISADVANTAGES

Activity

Jamie, aged 3, is to be admitted for circumcision as a day case. His father, a single parent, is self-employed. Jamie usually goes to a nursery during the day. Consider the disadvantages of day care for Jamie and his father.

When a child is admitted for day care a member of the family needs to be able to take them into hospital and be available for the discharge later in the day. In many instances, the parent then has to take on the role of carer at home. Some parents may feel unable or unwilling to do this. Providing care for the child during this period may necessitate taking time off work. Depending on the employer this may have to be unpaid leave which may lead to financial difficulties or even the loss of the job.

Day care also has the disadvantage that the nurse does not have the time to develop a relationship with the child and provide individualised care. Many day care units also use core care – plans which can impede individualised care. Children being admitted for surgery are often admitted early in the morning, for an operation 1–2 hours later, giving the nurse little time to get to know them.

PRE-ADMISSION INFORMATION

This short assessment time may be partially overcome by inviting the child to a pre-admission club (Figure 4.1). At this time the child and parents have an opportunity to visit the ward, meet the staff and have an outline of the day case routine explained to them. This means of

---

Cases suitable for day surgery

- Hernia repair: epigastric, femoral inguinal, umbilical
- Hydrocoele/varicoele: repairs or ligation
- Orchipodexy: unilateral >5 years
- Circumcision: meatotomy, separation of preputial adhesions
- Minor hypospadias
- Cystoscopy
- Division of tongue tie
- Proctoscopy, sigmoidoscopy, sphincter stretch
- Examination under anaesthetic
- Excision of skin lesions
- Lymph node biopsy
- Brachial sinus
- Thyroglossal cyst
- Correction of prominent ears
- Excision of superficial accessory auricules
- Minor orthopaedic surgery: manipulations, plaster change, release of trigger thumb, excision of ganglion, arthoscopy
- Dental surgery: extractions, excision or biopsy of oral lesions and cysts
- ENT surgery: EUA of ears, post nasal space, removal of FB, myringotomies, grommets, reduction of nasal fracture
- Sub-mucosal diathermy, electro-cautery of epistaxis, antrum wash-outs
- Ophthalmic surgery: correction of strabismus, EUA

(Royal College of Surgeons of England, 1992)

Figure 4.1

Invite to club.

> ## INVITATION TO THE PRE-ADMISSION CLUB
>
> Woodlands Children's Unit
> St. Someone's Hospital
> Anywhere, County.
>
> Dear
>
> Please come to our special club meeting on . . . .
>
> at . . . .
>
> You will be able to find out all about the hospital and what will happen when you have your operation next week. You will be able to see:
>
> - the ward where your bed will be
> - a video about your operation day
> - the theatre where your operation will take place
> - our playroom and toys
> - the nurses who will be helping mummy or daddy to look after you
>
> Please bring mummy or daddy with you. Brothers, sisters and toys can come too if you would like them to. Please ring and tell us if you can come.
>
> From all the nurses

preparation relies on a member of the family being available to accompany the child. Pre-admission clubs are usually held during the week prior to the child's admission but this may be too long for the younger child who may forget or misinterpret the information before admission.

These disadvantages can be overcome by sending the parents and child clear information with the date of admission. This can be in the form of a puzzle or colouring book for the child. Parents can also be advised of other useful resources to help prepare them and their child which are often available from children's libraries.

Before admission it is important that the parents are aware of any possibility that the child may have to stay in overnight, so they can make provisional arrangements for this before the day of admission. They also need advice about taking the child home so they do not have unrealistic plans to go home by public transport.

Whilst all this information can be given at the pre-admission visit it

Advice about transport
- Private transport or taxi
- An adult, other than the driver, should be available to sit with the child
- Have a pillow and blanket in case the child wishes to lie down
- Take a bowl in case of vomiting
- Do not make precise arrangements about timing – these may change

needs to be consolidated into some means of written communication. The written explanation also helps those who are unable to attend a pre-admission session.

Activity

Consider ways of encouraging parents and children to attend a pre-admission club.

Day care often has the disadvantage of expecting parents to make arrangements to visit the hospital on three occasions. The initial out-patient appointment, followed by a pre-admission session and then the actual day of admission. An eye catching, multilingual poster or display in the out-patient department would provide the means of explaining the purpose and function of the pre-admission club and could be supported by leaflets for parents to take home (Figure 4.2). Parents need to be aware of the dates and contents for these visits, and to realise the benefits to them and their child (James, 1995).

DAY CARE ADMISSION ASSESSMENT

One of the other disadvantages of day care is that the nurse has little time to develop a relationship with the child and parents. As a result of this the admission assessment is particularly important in day care.

Activity

Amy, aged 5, has been admitted as a day case for an adenoidectomy. What would you need to know from Amy and her mother on admission?

Firstly, the nurse needs to be aware of what the child and parents already know about the proposed surgery and the ward. If the child and parents have the pre-admission club this is an opportunity to check their understanding and consolidate information. If not, the nurse may need to begin preparation by showing them around the ward. Assessing previous knowledge is useful to correct misbeliefs. Jolly (1981) recalls a 5 year old who, in spite of careful preparation for his tonsillectomy, believed his throat would be cut during the operation.

The aim of any pre-operative care is to ensure the child is not only prepared psychologically, but also physically. Some children have been fasted at home prior to admission; the nurse needs to check the parents have understood this instruction and that the child has obeyed it. It is not always easy for parents to comply exactly with the hospital's requirements. For instance, they may have been told that the child may have nothing to eat or drink for at least 4 hours prior to the operation. If the child goes to bed after an evening meal at 19:30, is woken at

Is your child booked for surgery?

Not sure what to expect or how to answer questions?

**Help to reassure your child and yourself
and come to the:**

CHILDREN'S PRE-ADMISSION CLUB

- Held every Saturday morning 10–11 am
- Run by children's nurses and play staff
- Includes a tour, video and question time
- You and your child will have the opportunity to find out what the operation day entails

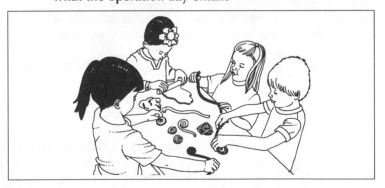

Figure 4.2

Poster for club. (Picture reproduced from Beaver et al., 1994)

07:00 and arrives at the hospital at 07:30 for an operation at 09:00, then the actual period of fasting has been for a period of over 12 hours and on admission the nurse may find the child is dehydrated. Alternatively, the nurse may discover that the child has been given a drink of water because the parents thought clear fluids were acceptable.

On admission the nurse needs to check that the child has no actual or potential health problems which could be exacerbated by surgery. Recording the child's vital signs not only gives the nurse an indication of the child's current health status, it also gives the child an opportunity to become familiar with these procedures.

The admission assessment is also an opportunity for the nurse to discover the family's usual home routine. Being aware of the child's likes and dislikes in relation to fluids and diet may help to encourage the child to return to normal eating and drinking habits after an anaesthetic. A knowledge of the child's behaviour and comforters will enable the nurse to recognise and respond appropriately to any signs of distress at an early stage. James (1995) suggests that much of the information required at the admission assessment can be gained by asking the parents to complete a pre-admission questionnaire (Figure 4.3).

PRE-PROCEDURAL CARE

Activity

Once the admission assessments have been completed, consider how the child's preparation for the day care procedure should continue.

When the initial assessment is complete the nurse should ensure the final preparations for the child's procedure are made. Simultaneous preparation of a favourite toy may be appreciated by some children. James (1995) advocates that children should be able to choose what they wear, arguing that theatre gowns are not always necessary. The removal of underwear is often the most distressing and bewildering for children, and should not be necessary except for procedures involving the genital area. In these cases cotton underwear may be an acceptable alternative.

If cannulation is required local anaesthetic cream can be applied to the selected site 1–2 hours before the procedure. Children who have been adequately prepared should not need pre-medication (James, 1995), but the nurse should assess each child's need for such medication, recognising that the aim of pre-medication is to allay anxiety, facilitate induction of anaesthetic and provide an analgesic effect. If a pre-medication is required it should be given in an oral form as most children's anxiety will only be heightened by an intramuscular injection.

Your child may go to theatre soon after admission which may not give us much time to get to know you. You can help us by completing the following questionnaire so that we can learn about your child and help you to look after your child in the same way as you do at home.

Previous experience of hospital/illness
Has your child been in hospital before? . . . . When? . . . .
What was the reason for this? . . . .
How did s/he react to this? . . . .
How have you explained the reason for this admission? . . . .
. . . .
Please tell us about any special worries your child has . . . .
. . . .
How does your child react to pain? . . . .
What method do you find best relieves their pain? . . . .
. . . .
If your child is taking any medicines please state what these are and the reasons for their use . . . .
. . . .
. . . .

Eating and drinking
What does your child use for drinking? bottle/cup/trainer beaker
What does s/he prefer to drink? . . . .
We usually offer toast or biscuits as the first solids after the anaesthetic.
Does your child have any preferences for these? . . . .

Toileting
What help does your child need to go to the toilet? . . . .
Does your child ever wet or soil her/himself . . . .
Toddlers: When does your child wear nappies? . . . .
           What words does s/he use to indicate the need for the
           toilet? . . . .
Teenage girls: Has your daughter started menstruating? . . . .
           When is her next period due? . . . .
           Does she use pads or tampons? . . . .

Play and comfort
Please tell us about any special toy/comforter your child has with them
. . . .
If your child is bored before or after surgery, what quiet forms of play would interest them? . . . .
. . . .

*Please use the back of this form to tell us anything else you think is important

Figure 4.3

Pre-admission questionnaire.

ANAESTHESIA

The child should also be able to choose the mode of transport if the procedure is to be carried out away from the day care ward. Small children often prefer being carried by a parent or to use a pedal car or bike. In recent years, there has been much discussion about the presence of parents in the anaesthetic room. The nurse should be aware of the benefit and drawbacks of parental presence at this time so that parents can be given appropriate advice.

Activity

What are the benefits and drawbacks of having parents present in the anaesthetic room?

Gauderer *et al.* (1989) found that most parents, although anxious, were grateful to have been able to provide support for their child during induction. Most children also expressed a need for parental presence at this time. However, Vessey *et al.* (1990) discovered that a few parents became obviously distressed at the induction procedure and were unable to support their child or the health care professionals. Understandably, it is these latter reactions which concern the anaesthetic team whose aim is to ensure a smooth and effective induction. Therefore, although most authors (Coulston, 1988; Glasper, 1990) found that the advantages of the presence of a parent in the anaesthetic room outweigh the disadvantages it is important that this issue is fully discussed with parents. If they feel that they would not be able to remain calm, they should not be made to feel guilty. Instead, they may accompany their child to the door of the anaesthetic room and the child's named nurse provide the necessary psychological support during induction.

RECOVERY FROM ANAESTHESIA

Parents should also be given the opportunity to be with their child in the recovery area following the procedure. Again, they should be well prepared for this and know their child's likely condition as well as their role in this situation. Staff in recovery areas have found that children who woke to a parent's presence were far less disturbed than those who woke alone in a strange environment. Distressed children tend to cry and this can often result in increased pain or post-operative bleeding.

If there are no specific contra-indications, as soon as the child is awake and able to swallow he/she should be able to drink and eat. Diet and fluids should usually be encouraged 1–2 hours following the procedure to reduce the risk of dehydration and hypoglycaemia.

Appropriate analgesia should be prescribed to enable the child to remobilise without fear of pain. Ibuprofen syrup or paracetamol suspension are appropriate oral analgesics, and are usually well accepted by children who have undergone minor procedures. Alternatives may be paracetamol suppositories or a local anaesthetic gel.

DISCHARGE HOME

Activity

What criteria would you use to determine a child's suitability for discharge after day surgery?

All day case children should meet given criteria before being discharged home. They should be able to eat and drink without vomiting, walk unaided and have passed urine without difficulty. Their pain should be controlled with an appropriate analgesic and be apyrexial. Any unexpected or excessive bleeding is reason enough for an overnight stay. Parents need general and specific advice about their child after day care procedures. They need to have these details explained to them and to have time in which to consider any questions. Written instructions will help them to remember what they have been told. These written instructions should be expressed in simple language and be available in a bilingual form. Ley and Llewellyn (1995) cite many studies showing that written instructions for patients were too difficult for them to understand and comply with. Written discharge information should have been distributed at the pre-admission visit to give them time to assimilate and question the information. Before the child goes home this information should be re-iterated. Any other specific advice such as wound care and/or medication should be carefully explained.

PAEDIATRIC COMMUNITY SUPPORT

In some areas the children's community nurse (CCN) will continue the child's care after discharge. In these instances it is ideal if the CCN can meet the child and family before discharge. Where a CCN is not available it is useful if the day care nurse can telephone at a pre-arranged time to check on the child's progress. This support has been shown to be welcome by parents who often just want reassurance that they are caring for their child correctly (James, 1995). It has also been shown to increase compliance with discharge advice (Spicher and Yund, 1989).

SUMMARY

In 1991, it was suggested that the health care of children could be improved by following a comprehensive set of standards for pre-admission and discharge care (Thornes, 1991). This report, titled 'Just

Discharge criteria

Before discharge all day case children should:

- be apyrexial
- not have experienced any unexpected complications or excessive bleeding
- be able to eat and drink without vomiting
- have passed urine
- be able to walk unaided
- have their pain controlled

Cross reference

Community nursing – pages 371–377

Discharge advice

Questions most commonly asked by parents:

- when to remove the dressing?
- are there stitches to come out?
- when can the child have a bath?
- when can the child return to nursery/school?
- should activity be restricted in any way?
- what can be given to eat and drink?
- what should be given for pain?
- Is there a review appointment?

(Norris, 1992)

Cases unsuitable for day surgery

- Operations > I hour
- Uncontrolled asthma, epilepsy, blood disorders
- Under 46 weeks' gestational age (gestation + age)
- Ex-premature infants <6 months
- Infants <5 kg
- Respiratory tract infection in last 2 weeks
- Cardiac, hepatic, renal or endocrine insufficiency

(Bradshaw and Davenport, 1989)

for the Day', has formed the basis of the operational policy of the many day care units.

In 1992, the Royal College of Surgeons published guidelines to facilitate more day care surgery. These guidelines do not take into account that surgery on children is not always undertaken by surgeons and anaesthetists who are experienced in paediatric surgery (Audit Commission, 1993). Markovitch (1991) found that children having day care surgery were often seen as a lower priority by inexperienced medical staff. Nevertheless, the number of day care units continues to increase, and their success is determined by the degree of preparation and planning which occurs before admission. These pre-admission arrangements should take into account the multicultural needs of the population to ensure that all children are treated equally. With careful preparation and planning the potential risks and disadvantages can usually be overcome.

Key points ➤

1. The individual child and family's suitability for day care should be assessed as it is not always beneficial.
2. Children having day care need to have fears allayed by careful pre-admission preparation.
3. Fasting times, pre-medication and anaesthesia should be adjusted to meet the individual child's needs.
4. Parents need careful preparation for the discharge of their child to enable them to continue care with confidence and recognise and react to complications.
5. Children should meet given criteria before discharge to minimise the possibility of complications.
6. Parents benefit from support in the community after their child has been discharged.

EMERGENCY CARE   5

INTRODUCTION

In the UK approximately 25% of all patients seen in the Accident and Emergency (A&E) department each year will be children (DoH, 1991a). This effectively means that about one in four children under the age of 16 years will attend an A&E department at some time in their childhood. A high proportion of these children will be under the age of 5 years and about 65% of them will have sustained some kind of trauma (Figure 5.1).

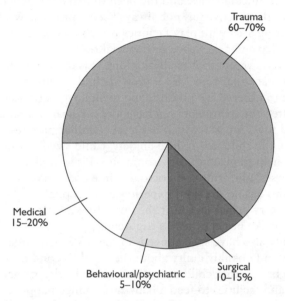

Figure 5.1

A&E attendance of children. (Adapted from Bentley, 1995.)

Most of these children will be seen in a busy adult A&E department as there are less than 10 dedicated paediatric A&E departments in this country (Morton *et al.*, 1994). Collins (1995) suggests that the two disciplines of children's nursing and A&E nursing have opposing philosophies, and that these differing beliefs add to the unsuitability of general A&E departments for the care of children.

The need for children to be treated in a different way began to be recognised in the 1980s and in 1988 the British Paediatric Association (BPA), British Association of Paediatric Surgeons (BAPS) and Casualty Surgeons Association (CSA) produced a joint statement which identified the optimum requirements for the care of children in A&E (Morton and Phillips, 1992). Whilst these indicators of good practice have not been universally adopted (Audit Commission, 1993) there are many exciting developments and innovations in the field of paediatric emergency care in relation to preparing children for admission to A&E, staffing the unit appropriately and the triage of children in a specific area of the department.

Minimum requirements for children in A&E

- A consultant paediatrician with specific responsibility for liaison with the A&E consultant regarding the care of children
- Nursing establishment to include at least one registered children's nurse
- A liaison health visitor to provide a link between hospital and community services
- Separate waiting area from adult area with facilities for play
- Separate child-friendly treatment area with appropriate equipment
- Private room available for distressed family

(Morton and Phillips, 1992)

THE A&E ENVIRONMENT

Activity

Imagine the busy A&E department of your local general hospital. Consider what a small child's reaction to this environment might be.

The A&E department is most children's first contact with hospital so it is important that this first experience is made as reassuring as possible. The A&E environment has traditionally been designed to provide fast and effective immediate care and the need to make the department welcoming and attractive has not always been a priority. Whilst a separate waiting area with play facilities is recommended, many A&E departments have not the space or financial resources to develop such an area. However, even with these limitations, it is important to ensure that the admission area has some decoration at child height and that children do not have to observe the physical and mental stress of other acutely ill patients. Often the treatment area has more medical equipment than pictures and toys. An area which has a few familiar pictures and toys can help to relax the child and reduce anxiety. Child sized trolleys and seating also help to make the environment safer as well as more friendly. Even the nurses' uniforms and doctors' white coats may be threatening to a child who has no previous experience of hospital (McMenamin, 1995). A nursery print tabard for the nurse looking after the children may help to make her appear less frightening.

The family also have special needs in the A&E department. They will feel anxious and possibly guilty about their child's condition and may have had to bring other children with them to the department. They need space and facilities to feed a baby, and change nappies. A push chair to soothe a fractious toddler or to lay a baby down is a useful addition.

THE A&E STAFF

Meeting the needs of the family and the child is the basis of children's nurse education and this is the reason why it is recommended that every A&E department has at least one RSCN or RN(child) on its staff (DoH, 1991a). Children have physiological and psychological needs which are different to those of the adult patient, and an appropriately qualified and experienced nurse is required to assess and meet these needs in a stressful situation. Recruiting an experienced children's nurse who also has A&E experience is not easy. To overcome this shortage of appropriate staff, some units have made the most of flexible rostering to ensure that their RSCN/RN(child) is on duty during their recognised peak periods for children attending the department. At other times a named nurse is identified from the paediatric unit to provide specialist advice.

A play leader or nursery nurse is also a useful addition to an A&E department. The use of therapeutic play to prepare children for procedures will decrease anxiety as well as making the wait for treatment less stressful.

Thornes (1993) suggests that the A&E department is no longer merely the provider of emergency health care but has to respond to the changing provision of health care by also providing primary and secondary health care. The children's nurse in the department can be actively involved in health promotion and provide display material and advice for parents, but there needs to be a formal means of communication between the hospital and the community staff if continuing care is to be effective. It is suggested that a liaison health visitor can provide this continuity.

A&E medical staff need to have experience of the emergency care of children and be able to handle them and their families when they are frightened and distressed. Currently, it is not essential for A&E staff to have such experience (Morton *et al.*, 1994). The first consultant in paediatric A&E medicine was appointed in 1971 although it was not until 1988 that this was recognised as a unique speciality. Morton and Phillips (1992) recommend that every A&E department has a paediatric A&E consultant. To gain such a post applicants must have had experience in general and A&E paediatrics as well as paediatric anaesthesia, orthopaedics, surgery and intensive care and are best able to manage paediatric medicine, surgery and trauma.

Activity

Consider whether children should only be seen in purpose built paediatric A&E departments.

The advantage of children being seen only in specific paediatric A&E units would be that the environment would be child oriented and that all the staff would be experienced in assessing and treating children. However, the disadvantage could be that specialist services are not readily available 24 hours a day. In addition, staff would not necessarily gain the wide experience in trauma available in a large general A&E department and injured families would have to be separated. The optimum arrangements for children may therefore be integrated or adjacent children's departments within the general A&E complex.

TRIAGE

Triage means assessing and prioritising patients according to their medical needs. The use of triage in A&E departments has enabled staff to meet Standard 5 of the Patient's Charter (DoH, 1991b) which states that patients in A&E departments should be seen and assessed within

Cross reference

Maturation – page 65

**Rapid cardiopulmonary
assessment**

A = Airway patency
   Able to maintain independently
   Requires assistance to maintain

B = Breathing
   Rate
   Mechanics
      retractions
      grunting
      accessory muscles
      nasal flaring
   Air entry
      chest expansion
      breath sounds
      stridor
      wheezing
      paradoxical chest
      movements
   Colour

C = Circulation
   Heart rate
   Blood pressure
      volume/strength
   Peripheral pulses
      present/absent
      volume/strength
   Skin perfusion
      capillary refill time
      temperature
      colour
      mottling
   CNS perfusion
      responsiveness
      recognises parents
      muscle tone
      pupil size
      posturing
(American Academy of Pediatrics,
1994)

5 minutes of admission. This immediate assessment is even more important for children who should be seen as a priority because of their age. Children need continuous supervision as their clinical condition can deteriorate much quicker than that of an adult. Action for Sick Children supports DoH guidelines (1991a) which state that A&E departments should have effective procedures to prioritise waiting children and ensure that they are seen promptly. In spite of these recommendations, Bentley (1995) found that only 20% of A&E departments in England had formal triage arrangements for children. Ten per cent of departments gave no priority to children and the remaining 70% mostly left triage decisions to the discretion of the individual nurse.

The nurse involved in the triage of children needs to understand the developmental differences in the anatomy and physiology of the 0–16 age group.

Activity

How would you make an immediate assessment of any child entering the A&E department? What specific differences need to be taken into account when making an immediate assessment of children?

The ABC criteria for the assessment of a patient are useful in any circumstance (Lloyd-Thomas, 1990).

A = airway

Children's airways are much more easily compromised than that of the adult. They have a comparatively large tongue and their airways are much narrower, shorter and straighter than those of an adult. As a result, upper respiratory tract infections soon affect the lower airways where a small amount of mucus or swelling can easily cause obstruction.

B = breathing

Unless the child has a congenital cardiac problem, breathing problems are likely before circulatory problems. The small child has a soft cartilaginous thorax and the intercostal muscles are underdeveloped, causing the chest to retract inwards when lung compliance is decreased by a respiratory obstruction. Nasal flaring, intercostal or substernal retractions are signs of respiratory distress. In addition, noisy respirations will be heard; wheezing and grunting are signs of lower respiratory obstruction, stridor indicates upper respiratory tract obstruction. Children have a high metabolic rate and therefore a comparatively high oxygen need; if this is compromised they easily become hypoxic resulting in agitation and bradycardia.

Cyanosis is a late sign in children who are more likely to become pale.

Age	Range	Average
Neonate	30–50	35
1–11 months	25–40	30
1–3 years	20–30	25
4–5 years	20–30	23
6–7 years	18–25	21
8–9 years	18–25	20
10–13 years	16–24	19
14–16 years	12–20	18

Table 5.1

Respiratory rates in childhood

C = circulation

Children naturally have a comparatively high pulse and a pulse of 60 or less in an infant is sufficient reason to commence cardiac arrest procedures as this pulse rate is insufficient to provide an adequate circulation. Circulation is affected by the volume of circulating fluid. Children's fluid balance, in comparison to that of an adult, has been likened to a kettle with a large spout and a small lid! In other words, their ability to lose fluid is much higher than their ability to gain it because of their large surface area to volume ratio. They can rapidly become hypovolaemic due to diarrhoea, vomiting or inability to drink. A small blood loss can also be catastrophic for an infant who may only have 240–300 ml of circulating blood volume (Figure 5.2). Colour, capillary refill, and skin turgor are quick ways of making a cardio-vascular assessment.

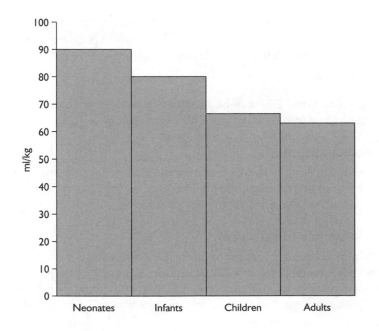

Figure 5.2

Circulating blood volumes.

Table 5.2

Pulse rates in childhood

Age	Range	Average
Neonates	100–180	140
1–11 months	100–160	120
1–3 years	80–130	100
4–5 years	80–120	95
6–7 years	75–115	90
8–9 years	70–110	85
10–13 years	70–110	80
14–16 years	60–100	72

Cross reference

Neurological assessment – page 502

C can also stand for conscious level. Small children's neurological status is never easy to assess and an adapted form of the Glasgow Coma scale is needed for pre-verbal children (Figure 5.3). The following is usually used to make a rapid initial assessment of the level of consciousness:

A awake

V non-verbal, quiet, calm, opens eyes to voice

P only responds to pain

U unresponsive

For children, the Glasgow Coma scale scores (Figure 5.3) are usually interpreted as:

Cross reference

See Module 6

13–15 mild neurological deficit

9–12 moderate neurological damage

<8 severe neurological damage

Activity

Once these immediate assessments have been carried out, what other observations may be useful to determine the severity of the child's illness?

The mnemonic DEF can be a useful way of determining the other useful observations to make of a child during triage.

D = diet and fluids

A clear history of the child's recent intake may help to determine the possibility of dehydration, the likelihood of an infective type of gastro-enteritis or the possibility of an allergic reaction.

E = evidence of infection

Children can quickly become severely ill due to infection and in children under 5 years temperature control is poor. Any small child presenting with a pyrexia over 38°C should be given an antipyretic as soon as possible to prevent a febrile convulsion. The history from the parents

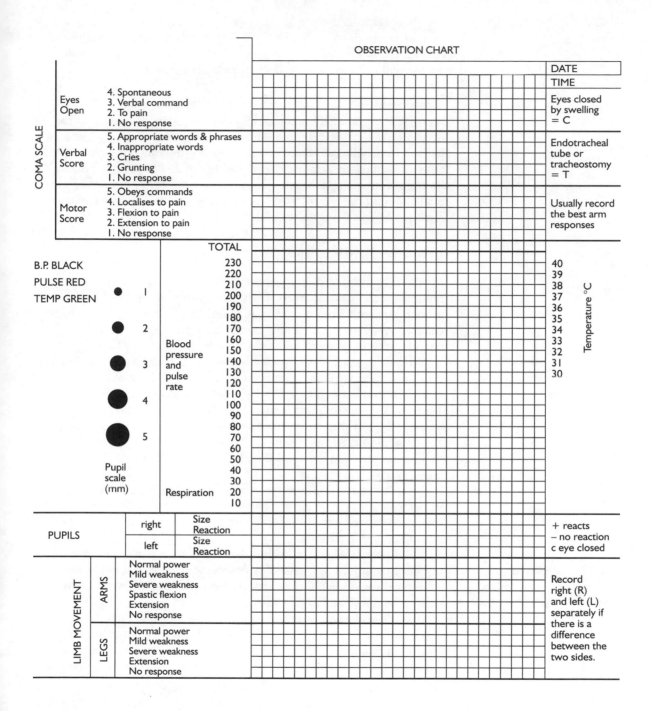

Figure 5.3

Child neuro chart (L & D), 2–5 years.

may give a clue to the site of infection by revealing that the child has been loathe to drink or has been rubbing the ears, but there may be no obvious clues. Always look for skin rashes, a child with an infectious disease will need to be kept away from other patients.

F = fontanelle

Looking at an infant's fontanelle may provide some indication of the diagnosis. In dehydration, the fontanelle become depressed while a bulging fontanelle is an indication of raised intercranial pressure. The anterior fontanelle usually closes at the age of 2–3 months while the posterior fontanelle does not close until 18 months. These closures are not solid until the age of 10–12 years and it may still be possible to identify changes in an older child.

RESUSCITATION OF CHILDREN

In infants and children, prevention is the recognised management of respiratory and cardiac arrest. Early recognition of the child at risk may prevent an arrest from occurring (Collins, 1994). Survival is low for children who suffer a cardiopulmonary arrest and the risk of neurological impairment for survivors is high (Simpson, 1994a).

Whilst the principles of basic life support for adults and children are the same, there are some important differences because of certain variations in the anatomy and physiology of children (Simpson, 1994a). There is evidence to indicate that these differences are not always appreciated and that nurses have poor knowledge and understanding about paediatric arrests (Collins, 1994).

Cardiac arrest in the child is rarely a primary event. The child is likely to have a cardiac arrest secondary to hypoxia and respiratory acidosis. If there is no response from a child and cardiac arrest is suspected a quick assessment of airway, breathing and circulation (ABC) should be carried out. An infant's responsiveness is best checked by flicking or gentle shaking.

Respiratory movement in children 0–6 years is mainly abdominal so respirations should be assessed by observing the rise and fall of the abdominal region. As respirations are likely to be shallow the child will need to be undressed to do this accurately.

Infant's necks are short and chubby so the brachial pulse is used to check circulation. A pulse rate of 5 beats or less in 5 seconds is an indication to commence cardiac massage as an infant's normal pulse rate is 150–160 per minute. Sixty beats or less indicates that circulation is severely compromised.

Airway management

Obstruction by the relaxed tongue is common in children as their tongues are relatively large. In addition, because infants' upper airways

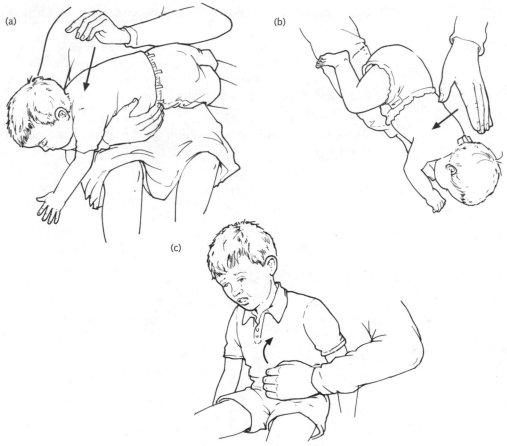

(a)

(b)

(c)

Figure 5.4

*Management of choking.
(a) Child back blows. (b) Infant
back blows. (c) Heimlich
manoeuvre.*

are relatively narrow and short, extending the neck will obstruct the
airway. To open the airway the infant's head and chin should be tilted to
the 'sniffing position' (Figure 5.5a). The airway should only be cleared
manually if the obstruction can be observed. Use the little finger to hook
it out. Finger sweeping can cause damage to the delicate childhood soft
palate. In infants it can also push the obstruction further down as their
pharynx is funnel-shaped.

Breathing

Infant artificial respiration is given by small breaths or puff from the
cheeks at a rate to inflate the lungs every 3 seconds. Such low pressure
breaths minimise the risk of gastric distension. If resistance is felt during
artificial respiration, it is most likely that the airway position is incorrect
If a change of position is unsuccessful, the airway may be blocked by a
foreign body which is one of the main causes of arrest in children
(Woodward, 1994).

If an infant's airway is occluded:

• Support the baby in the prone position over the forearm.

- Give five back blows (Figure 5.4b) between the shoulder blades with the heel of the hand.
- If this fails, turn the baby over and administer five chest thrusts (place two fingers on the sternum, one finger breadth below the nipple line, and push upwards). Never administer abdominal thrusts to a baby as the stomach and liver lie below the rib region.

If a child's airway is occluded:

- Perform back blows with the child over the lap (Figure 5.4a), in the upright position

or

- Perform the Heimlich manoeuvre (Figure 5.4c).

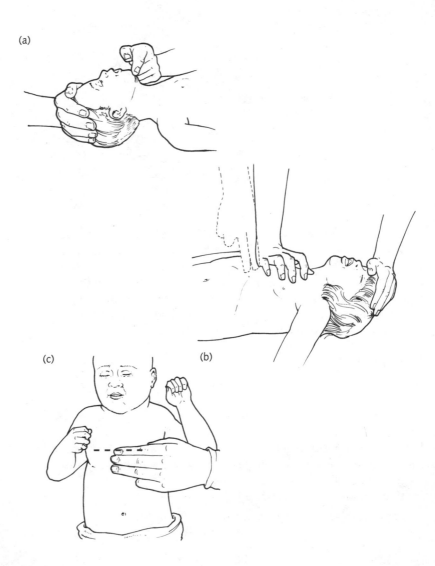

Figure 5.5

Infant and child resuscitation. (a) The sniffing position. (b) Child compressions. (c) Infant compressions.

Circulation

In an infant, draw an imaginary line between the nipples, and place two fingers on the sternum, one finger's breadth below this line. Compress the sternum 1.3–2.5 cm at a rate of at least 100 compressions/min (Figure 5.5c).

In a child, locate the site of compressions as in an adult and use the heel of one hand to compress the sternum 2.5–3.8 cm at a rate of 80/min (Figure 5.5b).

In any paediatric resuscitation the ratio of respirations to cardiac massage should be 1:5 whether or not the rescuer is accompanied.

Advanced life support

Cardiac arrest in children does not follow a prescribed pattern and is dictated by the individual child. Once basic resuscitation techniques have commenced, electrocardiogram (ECG) leads should be positioned to aid further diagnosis and treatment. The *British Medical Journal* (1993) set out algorithms to guide advanced resuscitation.

Asystole is the commonest arrest situation in children and is treated initially by ventilation and intubation followed by adrenaline 10 mcg/kg (Figure 5.6). Electro-mechanical dissociation, which is the absence of a palpable pulse while the ECG monitor shows acceptable complexes, is

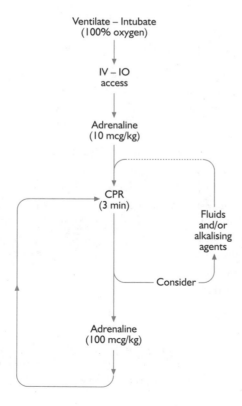

Figure 5.6

Cardiac arrest: asystole.

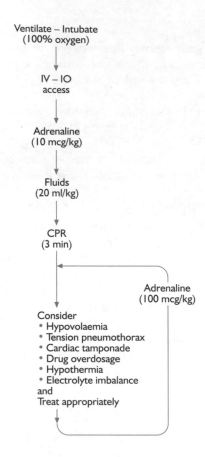

Figure 5.7

Cardiac arrest: electro-mechanical dissociation.

commonly caused by severe shock. It is also treated initially with ventilation, intubation and adrenaline (10 mcg/kg). This is followed by a rapid infusion of 20 ml/kg crystalloid or 10 ml/kg plasma (Figure 5.7).

Ventricular fibrillation (VF) is seen in fewer than 10% of paediatric arrests (Somes, 1991). If VF is seen developing, a precordial thump can be given (using two fingers). Otherwise it is treated by defibrillation (using infant paddles for babies under 10 kg) at 2–4 J/kg. Acidosis is corrected by sodium bicarbonate 8.4% (4.2% for neonates) 1 ml/kg (Figure 5.8).

Access for drugs during advanced resuscitation can be:

- intravenous (IV)
- intraosseous (IO)
- via an endotracheal tube

As children quickly become peripherally constricted IV access may be impossible. In such cases an intraosseous (IO) line can be inserted into the tibial or femoral medullary cavity (Lawrence, 1980).

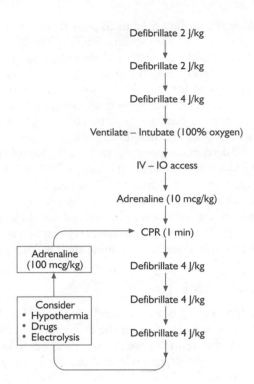

Figure 5.8

Cardiac arrest: ventricular fibril-lation.

Unless the child is hypothermic or has had an overdose of a cerebral depressant drug, the Advanced Life Support Group (1993) recommends that resuscitation attempts should stop after 30 minutes with no evidence of cerebral activity or cardiac output.

PROBLEMS IN PAEDIATRIC RESUSCITATION

There is little research evidence to indicate the success or failure of particular ways of managing paediatric cardiac arrest situations (Cole, 1995). However, there is evidence to indicate that there are three main factors which hinder paediatric arrests:

- Drugs and fluids have to be given to children according to their body weight and surface area. These precise measurements are often not known in an emergency.
- The equipment used for paediatric arrests varies in size. Staff must be able to identify the correct sized equipment and know how to use it
- A&E staff are largely inexperienced in the management of paediatric emergencies (Hughes, 1990) and Collins (1994) showed that many RSCNs were unable to demonstrate competence in resuscitation.

Cole (1995) suggests that some of these problems may be overcome by the use of the Broselow paediatric resuscitation system. The Broselow tape measure, designed in the US, aims to provide information about the correct sized equipment and appropriate drug dosage for individual children. It is laid alongside the child and the colour segment which corresponds with the child's length gives the necessary information. The correctly sized equipment for that child is stored in a colour-coded pack. Research into the accuracy of the Broselow system shows that it greatly facilitates decision making but care must be taken when using it for obese or emaciated children (Coles, 1995)

UK methods of determining appropriate sized equipment and drug dosages are the BMA reference chart (Oakley, 1988) and the modified paediatric resuscitation chart (Burke and Bowden, 1993) (Figures 5.9 and 5.10). Burke and Bowden modified the BMA reference chart after they found it to be of dubious benefit because of the time and complexity of its use. However, these charts rely on age-specific weights and no research has been done to determine their accuracy.

SUDDEN DEATH IN A&E

Further reading

RANDLE, H. (1998) What happens now? Information for parents whose child has died in A&E. *Paediatric Nursing*, **10** (4) 22–23.

The sudden death of a child is an overwhelming event for the family. They need time to come to terms with the event, express their grief and ask questions. Even children who are already dead on arrival to A&E should be brought into the department and the family shown to a private room. To avoid false hope, they need to have the death confirmed as soon as possible in an honest but sensitive way. Some professionals try to avoid the term death but sometimes by using euphemisms the family do not appreciate exactly what has occurred.

Parents' reactions will vary according to their personality, culture, previous experience and the circumstances surrounding the death. The nurse will need to accept their reactions and demonstrate empathy and support. Parents will need to ask questions about the death and the nurse should be prepared for these. Once the child has been made presentable, parents should be given the chance to see and hold their child, but they also need to know that they can inform the hospital mortuary at any time should they want to return to do this. They may also wish to be involved in washing their child. Some A&E departments will take a Polaroid photograph of the child or take hand or foot prints. These may be appreciated by the parents, especially if the child is very young.

Parents also need advice about what will happen next. They need to be advised of the coroner's role in sudden or unexplained death without being made to feel that they are suspected of some crime. A post-mortem is often requested in these cases and they need to understand this procedure and the reasons for it. The nurse will need to appreciate that some religions do not permit post-mortems. Practical advice about funeral arrangements, the death certificate and registration of the death should be discussed before the family leave the department. Written information booklets, such as those available from the DoH, provide a

Paediatric resuscitation chart

Endotracheal tube

Length (cm)	Internal diameter (mm)	
18.21	7.5–8.0	
18	7.0	
17	6.0	
16	6.5	
15	5.5	
14	5.0	
13	4.5	18 m
12	4.0	9 m
11	3.5	6 m
10	3.0–3.5	3 m

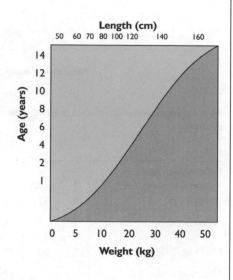

Drug						
Adrenaline (ml of 1/1000) intravenous or endotracheal	0.5	1	2	3	4	5
Atropine (mg) intravenous or endotracheal	0.1	0.2	0.4	0.6	0.6	0.6
Bicarbonate (ml of 8.4%) intravenous	5	10	20	30	40	50
Calcium chloride (mmol)* intravenous	1	2	4	6	8	10
Diazepam (mg) intravenous	1.25	2.5	5	7.5	10	10
per rectum	2.5	5	10	–	–	–
Glucose (ml of 50%) intravenous	10	20	40	60	80	100
Lignocaine (mg) intravenous or endotracheal	5	10	40	60	80	100
Salbutamol (µg) intravenous	25	50	100	150	200	250
Initial DC defibrillation (J)	10	20	40	60	80	100
Initial fluid infusion hypovolaemic shock (ml)	50	100	200	300	400	500

* One millilitre calcium chloride 1 mmol/m = 1.5 ml calcium chloride 10% + 4.5 calcium gluconate 10%

Figure 5.9

The BMA paediatric resuscitation reference chart (Oakley, 1985).

Figure 5.10

Modified resuscitation chart (Burke and Bowden, 1993).

Paediatric resuscitation chart

All doses are expressed as volumes (ml) and to be given intravenously unless stated otherwise.

Endotracheal tube								
• internal diameter (mm)	3	3.5	4	5	5.5	6.5	7.5	8
• length (cm)	10	12	13	14	15	17	18	21
Maximum age	2	6	1	3.5	6	10	13	14
	⊢ Months ⊣		⊢————— Years —————⊣					
Maximum length (cm)	55	70	75	90	115	135	155	160
Maximum weight (kg)	5	7.5	10	15	20	30	40	50
Adrenaline (1/10 000)*	0.5	0.75	1	1.5	2	3	4	5
Atropine (600 µg/ml)*	0.2	0.25	0.3	0.5	0.7	1	1	1
Bicarbonate (8.4%)	5	7.5	10	15	20	30	40	50
Calcium chloride (1 mmol/ml)	1	1.5	2	3	4	6	8	10
Diazepam (5 mg/ml)								
• intravenously	0.25	0.4	0.5	0.75	1	1.5	2	2
• per rectum	0.5	0.75	1	1.5	2	–	–	–
Glucose (50%)	5	7.5	10	15	20	30	40	50
Lignocaine (1% = 10 mg/ml)*	0.5	0.75	1	1.5	2	3	4	5
Salbutamol (50 µg/ml)	0.5	0.75	1	1.5	2	3	4	5
Initial fluid bolus (ml)								
• colloid	50	75	100	150	200	300	400	500
• crystalloid	100	150	200	300	400	600	800	1000
Initial DC defibrillation (J)	10	15	20	30	40	60	80	100

All intravenous drugs may be given intraosseously at the same dose.
* May be given by the endotracheal route at the same dose.

useful resource to shocked parents who will not remember all that they have been told. Liaison with the family GP or health visitor will enable continued advice and support on their return home.

THE FUTURE

Whilst advances have been made in the care of children in A&E departments, there is still scope for further developments. In Nottingham, an emergency children's nurse practitioner post has been in operation since 1991 and is able to take total responsibility for the assessment and treatment of about 5% of children seen in the department (Kobran and Pearce, 1993). As nurses continue to develop their roles, as prescribers for instance, this type of emergency practitioner may become more common with a greater scope of practice.

Another recent development in A&E nursing practice is telephone triage. Many parents call A&E departments for advice about their child's symptoms (Campbell and Glasper, 1995) and Burton's 1989 study revealed that some parents attend A&E for reassurance rather than treatment. Areas which have developed a formal telephone triage system have found this to be a cost-effective system which helps to reduce the number of inappropriate visits to the A&E department. This formal system needs to be one with an experienced and suitably qualified children's nurse which is available 24 hours a day. Calls need to be well documented in case of further problems as well as providing a means of referral and auditing the effectiveness of the service.

> **Key points**

1. A significant number of children are seen in accident and emergency departments in the UK yet few departments have dedicated facilities for them.

2. Many accident and emergency departments do not have nurses or medical staff who have specific qualifications in the care of children.

3. Specific differences in paediatric anatomy and physiology need to be taken into account when undertaking an initial ABC assessment.

4. In infants and children, the recognised management of cardiac arrest is prevention of the two main causes: hypoxia and respiratory acidosis.

5. Specific differences in paediatric anatomy and physiology give rise to important variations in basic life support between adults and children.

6. The management of paediatric arrests is hindered by the need for varied dosages of fluid and medication and different sized equipment according to the size and weight of the child.

6 ADMINISTRATION OF MEDICINES

INTRODUCTION

The administration of medicines has always been an integral part of nursing care, but when caring for children it involves several problem areas. The responsibility of the children's nurse in ensuring that the correct medication is safely and appropriately administered to the correct child is a huge undertaking which requires many different skills.

Children are at particular risk from medication for a number of reasons. Their immature body systems make them less able to absorb, metabolise and excrete drugs (Figure 6.1). Their age, weight and surface area varies widely making standardised dosages impossible. In addition, many children dislike taking medication, so the nurse has to be able to find an acceptable method of administration for each individual child to promote compliance. This may be further aided by the nurse's knowledge of alternative preparations available for each medication.

Figure 6.1

Immaturity affecting the metabolism and excretion of medication.

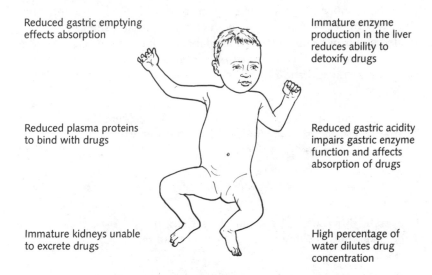

Reduced gastric emptying effects absorption

Immature enzyme production in the liver reduces ability to detoxify drugs

Reduced plasma proteins to bind with drugs

Reduced gastric acidity impairs gastric enzyme function and affects absorption of drugs

Immature kidneys unable to excrete drugs

High percentage of water dilutes drug concentration

Although it is mostly the doctor's responsibility to prescribe appropriate medication, the nurse who will be administering the prescription should have an understanding of the appropriate dosage, route of administration, desired action, possible side effects and contra-indications of each medication to be given (UKCC, 1989). The nurse will also need to be able to explain most of these aspects to the child and family to ensure continued acceptance of the regime.

The nurse has a professional responsibility to question any drug prescription which appears inappropriate and may be justified in refusing to administer a medication when there are clear contra-indications to any part of the prescription.

ABSORPTION, METABOLISM AND EXCRETION OF DRUGS

Babies and children not only need a different dose of drugs than adults because of their comparatively low body weight, but also because of the differences in the distribution of body fluids and in the developmental stage of their body organs. These latter differences are complex and mean that a child cannot just be given a smaller proportion of the adult dose.

Water is the largest constituent of the body, but the actual percentage varies according to age and the amount of body fat (Figure 6.2). About 85% of a premature baby's weight consists of water compared with an adult whose water content averages 55% of body weight. In an infant water is about 70% of the body weight.

Cross reference

Body water – page 67

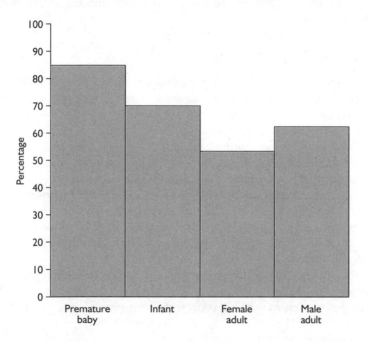

Figure 6.2

Percentage of water to total body weight.

This means that certain drugs which are water soluble are less concentrated in a small baby than they would be if taken by an adult. Consequently, higher doses relative to the baby's weight may need to be given initially.

Children under 3 years of age have a round stomach which is slow to empty. The secretion of gastric acid is also reduced, which is believed to impair the function of the gastric enzymes and alter the absorption rate of oral medications.

The mature liver can detoxify or excrete into bile certain drugs such as antibiotics. It can also chemically alter or excrete steroids. However, these functions are not fully developed in infancy and, as a result, some drugs could reach a dangerous concentration unless prescribed in a very reduced dosage. In older children, the opposite applies as the liver becomes relatively large in comparison with body size.

Complete maturity of the renal system does not occur until the child is about 3 years old. Before this age the glomerular filtration rate is much reduced resulting in an inability to excrete drugs as efficiently as the older child and adult. This may lead to the accumulation of high concentrations of drugs in the bloodstream and the dosage of certain drugs therefore needs to be comparatively low.

Nurses also need to be aware of these differences when breast-feeding mothers have been prescribed medication. Small molecules of drugs can pass from the bloodstream into the milk-producing cells of the breast causing the breastfed baby to also receive a small dose of the drug. Drugs which are fat soluble pass across in greater concentrations than other drugs and are more likely to produce unwanted effects in the baby.

Cross reference

Maturation of renal system – page 65

SAFETY OF THE DRUG

Apart from the differences in drug dosages because of the different and immature body systems of the small child, some drugs are contra-indicated for children because there is some evidence that they are harmful when used during childhood.

Aspirin or salicylate-containing medication, is contra-indicated in children under 12 years because it was thought to have some role in the development of Reye syndrome. Although this link is now being questioned (Casteels-Van Daele, 1993) aspirin is still not advised for children. Reye syndrome is a degenerative condition characterised by cerebral oedema and liver dysfunction and has also been linked with the administration of anti-emetics to children during viral illnesses (Whaley and Wong, 1995).

Trimeprazine, an antihistamine which may also be used as a pre-medication for children, because of its sedative action, is not advised for infants under 6 months as it has been shown to have a possible link with cot death (Ellis, 1995).

Some drugs are only licensed for use for adults because there is insufficient evidence about their therapeutic use for children. When the prescribed drug is unfamiliar, the nurse should always check the drug data sheet, a paediatric formulary or their pharmacologist.

THE EFFECTS OF MEDICATION

Medication is obviously prescribed to achieve a positive result but most drugs also have other effects in addition to the beneficial effects. Before administering any medication, the nurse should be aware of the desired effects as well as the possible side effects and adverse effects.

Side effects are the frequently experienced, expected reactions to a drug. It is almost inevitable that a drug taken for its beneficial effect on one part of the body, will have other effects on other organs. For instance, salbutamol given to reduce bronchospasm, has the common side effect of tachycardia. Antibiotics often affect the normal flora in the rest of the body and may lead to oral thrush or diarrhoea. Side effects can be trivial or so serious that they require the cessation of treatment, but their severity is usually determined by the individual child's condition.

Adverse effects are unusual and unexpected reactions to a drug. They can be predictable or unpredictable. Predictable adverse effects are often due to a child's known medical history. For example, propanalol, a beta blocker which can be prescribed for migraine to dilate cerebral blood vessels, also dilates bronchioles and can trigger an asthmatic attack in known asthmatics. It also suppresses the body's response to hypoglycaemia which is a potential danger to a diabetic child. Unpredictable adverse effects are abnormal allergic reactions which can occur at any time during the administration of the drug and can range from skin rashes, urticaria, wheezing, or tachycardia to anaphylactic shock.

The effects of any medication may be altered if it is taken in combination with certain other drugs, food or drink. Some of these interactions may be desirable, but others may be unwanted and harmful. Two or more drugs which depress the central nervous system, such as codeine and an antihistamine should not be given in combination as they will cause dangerous over-sedation. Theophylline and salbutamol can cause cardiac arrhythmias when given in combination. Tetracycline and iron combine in the intestine to make a non-chelated mixture which is not readily absorbed, reducing the effect of both drugs. In a similar way, milk also reduces the effect of some drugs and this should be considered with any medication prescribed for infants.

Sometimes an interaction can be beneficial. Naxalone, when given with morphine, blocks the receptors used by narcotics to reduce respirations and is thus used as an antagonist for morphine over dosage. Antibiotics are given in combination so that a smaller dose of each may be prescribed, not only reducing side effects but lessening the risk of bacterial resistance.

MONITORING THE EFFECT OF DRUGS

Drug administration includes the observation of the child for any effect of the prescribed medication. Evaluation of the response to drug therapy is not always easy, especially in very young children, and a knowledge of the child's usual behaviour is vital. Parents should be encouraged to share any changes they have noticed.

To accurately monitor the effect of any drug the nurse needs to appreciate its reaction and duration time. Whereas salbutamol can take effect within 5–15 minutes and be effective for up to 6 hours, metronidazole starts to work within an hour of administration but beneficial effects may not be apparent for 24–48 hours. Parents need to be advised of reaction times as this may affect their compliance.

Observations of vital signs may also help to indicate the effects of the medication. Monitoring the temperature of a child being treated with an antipyretic and checking the peak flow readings before and after administration of a bronchodilator will help to determine the efficacy of these drugs. Checking the pulse rate of a child taking frequent doses of salbutamol or regular doses of digoxin will help to ensure that they are not receiving too much of the drug. Certain drugs such as gentamycin and sodium valproate are very toxic when they reach a certain concentration in the blood stream. Gentamycin is nephrotoxic and sodium valproate can cause liver damage so blood levels are checked periodically to ensure that safe concentrations are maintained.

CALCULATING DRUG DOSAGES

The dosage of any medication must be carefully calculated to ensure that the required site of action receives the drug at the appropriate concentration to achieve a therapeutic effect. The appropriate dose for an individual child can be calculated by age, weight or body surface.

The use of age to determine drug dosage is not to be recommended except in an emergency as there is a huge range of normal for children's body weight at any age. The most commonly used method in the UK is by weight, with most drugs for children giving a recommended dose per kilogram body weight. In the USA, the most

Figure 6.3

Nomogram (Whaley and Wong, 1991). Surface area (SA) is calculated by drawing a straight line to connect the child's height and weight. Surface area is given at the point where this line crosses the SA column. If a child is thought to be an average size, weight alone may be used to calculate SA (second column).

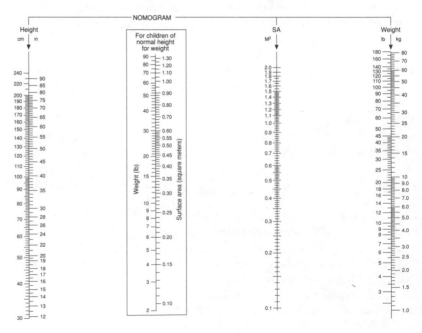

commonly used method involves the calculation of the child's body surface area (BSA) which is estimated by the child's weight and height using the West normogram (Figure 6.3). The drug dosage is then determined by:

$$\text{child's BSA (m}^2) \times \text{dose/m}^2 = \text{child's dose}$$

At present, this method is only used in the UK when the margin between the therapeutic and the toxic dose is very small, e.g. with cytotoxic agents.

Before administering any medication the nurse should be aware of the correct range of dosage for the specific child. Each child is likely to require a different dose corresponding to their individual weight. Because most drugs are prepared and packaged in adult-dosage strengths, the ability to calculate fractional drug dosages from larger amounts is essential to the children's nurse. Such calculations may also involve the conversion of grams (g) to milligrams (mg) or micrograms (mcg).

Activity

Consider the following prescriptions and determine the correct amount to be given.
(a) Stock drug contains 30 mg/5 ml. The child has been prescribed 21 mg.
(b) Stock drug contains 1 g/2 ml. The prescription asks for 375 mg to be administered.
(c) A child has been prescribed 4 mcg of a drug which is available as 0.006 mg/ml.
Answers overleaf.

Although some nurses may be able to use mental arithmetic or calculators to determine the answers, to justify the answer it is necessary to be able to demonstrate the calculation used. Brains and calculators are not infallible! A rough idea of the correct answer is an additional check of accuracy. For instance in problem (a) in the 'Activity' above, it can easily be seen that 21 mg is over half of 30 mg and that the required dose will be more than 2.5 ml. The calculation which should be used is:

dose required ÷ dose available × dilution = amount to be given

Calculations of dosages are further complicated if reconstituting drugs for injection. Many of these are prepared in powder form and have to be reconstituted with sterile water which often causes a displacement value which must be taken into account if only part of the reconstituted solution is to be used. The calculation in these situations is:

dose required ÷ dose available × dilution + displacement value = amount

Metric conversions
Metric units of mass
- 1 kilogram (kg) = 1000 g
- 1 gram (g) = 1000 mg
- 1 milligram (mg) = 1000 mcg

Conversions
- kilograms to grams = multiply by 1000
- grams to milligrams = multiply by 1000
- milligrams to grams = divide by 1000
- grams to kilograms = divide by 1000

Calculations
1 Bobby is prescribed 0.6 mg Atropine. The ampoule of Atropine states that it contains 600 mcg/ml. How much does Bobby need?
   0.6 mg × 1000 = 600 mcg (decimal point moved three places to right)
   Bobby needs 1 ml of Atropine
2 Jane is prescribed 250 mcg Lanoxin. The stock elixir is 0.25 mg/ml. How much does Jane need?
   250 mcg ÷ 1000 = 0.25 mg (decimal point moved three places to left)
   Jane needs 1 ml of Lanoxin

Now try the following:
- Convert 300 g to kg
- Convert 5 kg to g
- Convert 0.3 mg to mcg
- Convert 20 mcg to mg
(Answers overleaf)

Drug calculations

How to calculate the amount needed

- What you want ÷ what you have × the dilution = the amount needed

(a) Tom is prescribed 42 mg Vallergan. The stock bottle contains Vallergan 30 mg per 5 ml. How much should you give Tom?

$$\text{what you want} = 42 \text{ mg}$$
$$\text{what you have} = 30 \text{ mg}$$
$$\text{dilution} = 5 \text{ ml}$$
$$\tfrac{42}{30} \times 5 = \tfrac{42}{6}$$
$$= 7 \text{ ml}$$

(b) Emma is prescribed 64 mg of Gentamycin. The stock ampoule contains 80 mg in 2 ml. How much should you give?

$$\tfrac{64}{80} \times 2 = \tfrac{64}{40}$$
$$= \tfrac{16}{10}$$
$$= 1.6 \text{ ml}$$

Answers to calculations in Activity on p. 317

(a) $\tfrac{21}{30} \times 5 = \tfrac{7}{10} \times 5$
$$= \tfrac{35}{10}$$
$$= 3.5 \text{ ml}$$

(b) 1 g = 1000 mg
$$\tfrac{375}{1000} \times 2 = \tfrac{750}{1000}$$
$$= \tfrac{3}{4}$$
$$= 0.75 \text{ ml}$$

(c) 0.006 mg = 6 mcg
$$\tfrac{4}{6} \times 1 = \tfrac{2}{3}$$
$$= 0.66 \text{ ml}$$

The drug data sheet or your pharmacy department will be able to give advice about specific displacement values.

ROUTES OF ADMINISTRATION

Oral administration

The preferred route of administering drugs to children is by mouth. Most paediatric medications are dispensed in palatable and colourful preparations to make them attractive and acceptable for children. However, this may not be the most appropriate route and it does have some disadvantages. The absorption of oral drugs is variable, there may be a risk of gastric irritation, small children can aspirate oral medication given too quickly and discoloration or destruction of tooth enamel can be caused by very sugary solutions.

The most accurate method for administering oral drugs to children is the plastic disposable syringe. Measured plastic cups and spoons are less accurate as some of the liquid tends to adhere to these devices. The child should always be prepared for medicine. Forcing a crying child to take medicine may result in aspiration and the child is likely to resist further doses (Figure 6.4). Orenstein et al. (1988) suggests that swallowing can be induced in infants by blowing a small puff of air into their face.

Oral medicines should not be added to drinks as there is no guarantee that the child will finish the drink and any change in the taste may then cause the child to refuse drinks. However, it is acceptable to offer the child a favourite drink or foodstuff once the medication has been taken. It is often useful for the nurse to sample a small amount of the medication and therefore appreciate when its taste needs to be camouflaged.

Most young children have difficulty swallowing tablets and preparations which are not available in liquid form may need to be crushed. Some tablets have a protective coating to facilitate slow release so it is always advisable to check that breaking or crushing the tablet does not affect the action of the drug.

Rectal

The rectal administration of medication, usually in the form of suppositories, can be a very effective route for children, especially if they are nauseated or cannot have anything orally. Sedatives, analgesics and antiemetics can be given in this way, but the absorption and action of the drug can be slowed or impaired by a rectum loaded with faeces. To ensure acceptance of the drug the suppository needs to be placed beyond both rectal sphincters and held in place until the danger of reflex expulsion has passed. Abd-El-Maeboud et al. (1991) suggest that insertion of the suppository blunt end first reduces the risk of expulsion

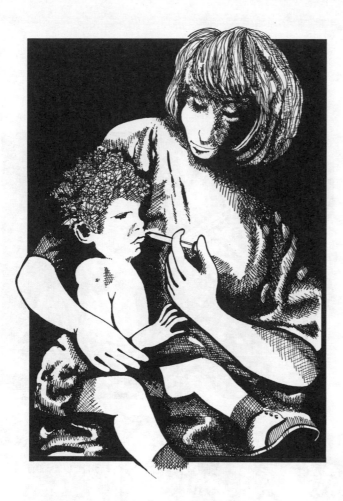

Figure 6.4

Infant restraint – oral drug.

but no study is available to determine if the discomfort of insertion is affected by this method.

Inhalation

Bronchodilators, steroids and antibiotics, suspended in particulate form, can be inhaled directly into the airway using a nebuliser or a metered dose inhaler. Nebulisers can be used with air or oxygen and metered dose inhalers are available in a range of different formats. Children and parents need to be prepared for the use of inhalants to ensure the maximum effect is gained from the drug. The noise of the nebuliser can be frightening for the unprepared child who may be further scared by the mask. Metered dose inhalers can be used successfully by children over 5 years but they need to be able to coordinate their breathing with the administration of the drug and to hold their breath for about 10 seconds after inhalation. A spacer device makes inhalation techniques easier for younger children but again careful preparation will facilitate

Figure 6.5

(a) Spacer device. (b) Inhaler.

(a)

(b)

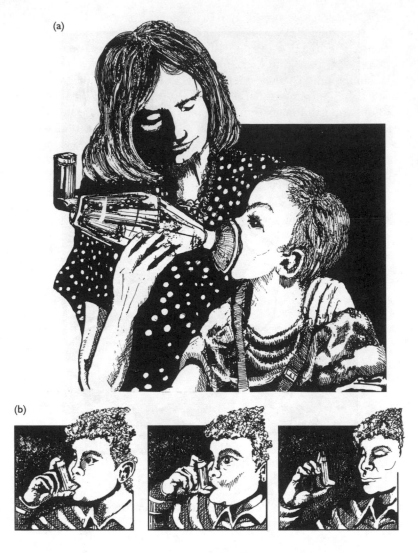

acceptance of the mask and device which can otherwise appear alarming. See Figure 6.5.

Topical

Topical medications are used for their local effect and can be applied to the skin, eyes, ears or nose. Although this route minimises systemic side effects of the drug, it should be remembered that such effects can occur if the drug is given over a long period of time.

To ensure cooperation, children need preparation for topical administration but all discomfort can be eliminated by careful technique. A small child will need to be restrained to avoid sudden movements. To prevent the child from being able to taste eye drops apply gentle pressure to the lacrimal punctum for 1 minute after administration to

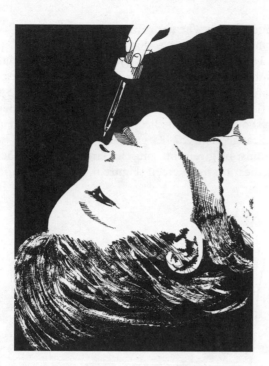

Figure 6.6

Position for administration of nose drops.

prevent the medication from draining into the nasopharynx. Ear drops should be allowed to warm to room temperature before being instilled to prevent the discomfort and shock of cold fluid in the ear. The unpleasant sensation of nose drops trickling into the throat can be avoided by placing the child in a head downwards position (Figure 6.6).

Subcutaneous and intradermal injections

Insulin and hormone replacements are the drugs commonly given subcutaneously. These injections can be given wherever there is subcutaneous tissue, and the injection given with a short needle at an angle of 90° to avoid giving an intradermal injection. Pain is reduced by not injecting more than 0.5 ml fluid.

Intradermal injections are commonly used for local anaesthetics, or tuberculin or allergy testing. The preferred site is the forearm but the medial aspect should be avoided as this is the most sensitive. The needle should be 3/8–1/2 inches long and inserted at an angle of 10–15°.

Intramuscular injections

Most children are frightened of injections which can often be painful. The use of intramuscular (IM) injections should be avoided in children and only given when their is no alternative route.

The discomfort of IM injections can be minimised by selecting the most appropriate equipment and injection site. The needle length can be estimated by pinching a fold of lateralis or deltoid muscle between the thumb and index finger. The appropriate needle length is half the length between the finger and thumb in this position. Hicks *et al.* (1989) have shown that a 1 inch needle is necessary to penetrate the muscle in infants 4 months old and Whaley and Wong (1995) suggest that 0.5–1 inch needles are necessary for most IM injections, with 1.5 inch needles used for injections into the gluteus maximus muscle in older children. Needle gauge should be the smallest which will deliver the drug safely, with the usual range being 22–25 gauge.

Injections must be given into muscles large enough to accept the amount of medication to be given (Figure 6.7). There is no research to

Figure 6.7

IM injection sites. (a) Vastus lateralis. Upper third of distance between greater trochanter and knee joint. (b) Gluteus maximus. Upper outer quadrant of buttock. (c) Gluteus medius. Centre of 'V' formed by index and middle finger when palm placed over greater trochanter. (d) Deltoid. Upper third of muscle which begins two finger breadths below acromion process.

(a)

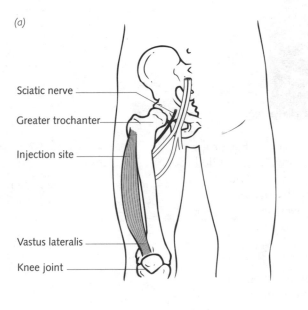

(b)

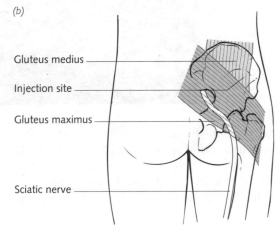

(c)

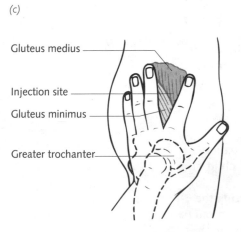

(d)

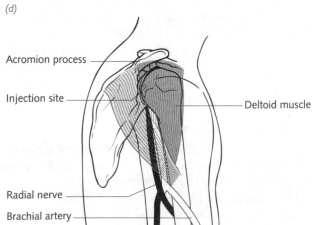

identify the optimum IM injection site for children but it is recommended that the gluteus maximus muscle is not used until the child has been walking for at least a year, since this muscle only develops with locomotion. The preferred site for infants is usually the vastus lateralis but Beecroft and Reddick (1990) recommend the use of the gluteus medius muscle for all ages of child as it is a safe, easily accessible site and injections here are less painful than those given into the vastus lateralis muscle. This muscle can be located by placing the palm over the greater trochanter, the index finger over the anterior superior iliac spine and the middle finger over the posterior iliac crest. The gluteus medius muscle is then between the V formed by the fingers. The deltoid muscle is also easily accessible and a relatively painless injection site and has the added advantage that medications injected here have a faster absorption rate. However, as it is a small muscle, only small volumes of fluid (0.5–1.0 ml) can be given.

IM injections can cause complications. Injections close to the sciatic nerve can cause permanent disability and repeated use of a site may result in fibrosis and contracture of the affected muscle. In addition, unless the child is held securely, sudden movement once the injection is in progress can cause the needle shaft to break. Preparation for IM injections should be given briefly and immediately before the event. One nurse should hold the child gently but securely so that no movement of the chosen area is possible and reduce discomfort by giving the child some distraction.

Intravenous injections

If a rapid action is required the intravenous (IV) route will be chosen. The drug enters the bloodstream directly and a higher serum concentration is possible allowing for a constant therapeutic effect if the drug is given regularly. However, there is a higher risk of complications for drugs administered by this route. There is a higher risk of toxicity, allergic reactions and, because the normal body protective systems are bypassed, infection. Mixing more than one drug in a syringe or infusion can lead to instability and precipitation, especially if those drugs or fluids contain calcium or magnesium or have very different pH values (e.g. Gentamycin and penicillin). Saline flushes should be given between two IV drugs and should also be used prior to IV administration to ensure venous access and following the procedure to flush the cannula.

Drugs can be given IV by bolus, intermittent or continuous infusion. Bolus injections should generally be given over 2–3 minutes but some drugs (e.g. Tazocin) require a specific rate. If the drug is to be given by intermittent infusion it is diluted in a specific volume of a specific fluid and infused over a given time using a syringe or infusion pump. A continuous infusion may be necessary if the drug has a short life in the body or when the clinical effect needs careful control by adjusting the infusion rate.

Cross references

Uses, risks, principles of care and advantages and disadvantages of central venous devices – pages 345–347

IV drugs are mostly given for a short period via an intravenous cannula but for a few children, who need venous access for a period of time, other devices may be more appropriate. If IV drugs are required for a week or more, a long line inserted into a major vein, usually the subclavian, is more appropriate than a short cannula inserted into a peripheral vein which tends to become dislodged after 48–72 hours of use. Long lines are kept patent with the use of heparin after each episode of drug administration. Children with chronic health problems (cystic fibrosis, leukaemia) who need long-term IV drug therapy usually have either an indwelling central venous catheter (Broviac or Hickman, see Figure 6.8) or an implanted infusion port (Mediport, Port-a-cath, see Figure 6.9). Special care must be taken when administering drugs by these routes to avoid infection and clotting.

Figure 6.8

Hickman line.

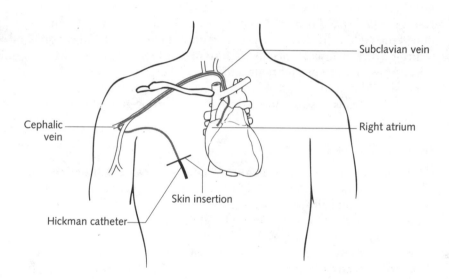

Activity

What would be the most appropriate route of drug administration for the following children?
* Tom, aged 4, who is vomiting post-operatively after repair of an inguinal hernia and is complaining of pain.
* Lucy, aged 6, who has cystic fibrosis, needs to achieve long-term control of her repeated chest infections.

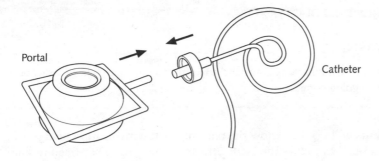

Portal

Catheter

Figure 6.9

Port-a-cath. Portal is placed under the skin and sutured to the chest wall. The catheter is tunnelled as the Hickman line with the tip resting within a major vein or right atrium.

CHECKING DRUGS

Before checking the drug to be administered, the nurse should ensure that the appropriate drug has been prescribed correctly.

Activity

What should the nurse check to ensure that the prescription is correct?

The prescription should be legible and written in a way which compiles with local policy. The nurse should check that the drug is suitable for the individual child's age and condition, and that the dosage and the route is appropriate

Activity

Having decided that the prescription is correct, what precautions should the nurse now take to ensure the administration is carried out safely?

The nurse is responsible for ensuring that the correct child receives the correct dose of the correct medication at the correct time and by the correct route. Most hospital drug policies state that two nurses must check and administer all drugs to children, but in certain circumstances it may be permissible for named nurses to give specified drugs on their own. Before dispensing the drug, the details of the prescription should be double-checked against the details of the bottle or vial. The expiry date of the drug should be checked as well as any special instructions (e.g. to be given with food). Finally the child's identity should be checked by comparing the hospital identification band with the prescription chart. The child may prefer a parent to give the medication, but the nurse is responsible for ensuring that the drug is taken.

PARENTAL EDUCATION

Activity

Consider what parents may need to know about their child's medication before going home.

Parents will need to know the reasons for the medication being prescribed as well as the likely effects of the drug. They need to know the amount, frequency and length of time of the drug's administration. They may need to know how to measure up the drug and how best to give it to their child. They may need help to organise a schedule which best fits into their home routine. This advice and teaching is ideally performed before discharge to give parents time to assimilate the information and practise new skills.

SUMMARY

Drug administration is not a role to be taken lightly. The children's nurse needs to have a wide understanding of drugs to be able to administer them safely and accurately. Doctors outside the paediatric team often have little experience of prescribing drugs for children and the nurse should be alert to recognise any prescriptions which appear inaccurate. For this reason, drugs should be given by qualified children's nurses with appropriate knowledge and experience, whenever possible. The administration of IV drugs is usually considered to be outside the usual scope of nursing practice, and nurses should ensure that they gain the additional knowledge and skills required for this role before accepting accountability and responsibility for this additional role.

Key points ➤

1. Children's immature body systems and wide variations in age, weight and body surface cause them to be at risk from medication.
2. Children's nurses need to be skilled at promoting compliance for each individual child.
3. Children's nurses have a professional responsibility to be aware of the appropriate medication and dosage for each child for whom they are caring.
4. Some drugs, used commonly in the treatment of adults, are contra-indicated for use in children.
5. Children's nurses should be aware of the different routes for medication and be able to identify the most appropriate route for the children in their care.
6. Children's nurses need to be able to explain the purpose and the administration of any medication both to the child and the family if compliance is to be maintained.

PROVIDING NUTRITION 7

INTRODUCTION

Childhood diseases can often be complicated by poor nutrition. Babies with respiratory problems may find it difficult to suck; ill toddlers and small children often suffer from accompanying anorexia. Older children may be fussy eaters and this fussiness may be exacerbated by illness. In addition the actual disease process may prevent adequate nutrition. As a result of any of these situations the child is unable to consume, absorb or utilise sufficient energy and nutrients to grow.

Providing adequate nutrition for sick children is a challenge for children's nurses. Recent surveys appear to suggest that this challenge is not always recognised or responded to. These studies reveal that children can actually suffer from malnutrition whilst in hospital (Moy *et al.*, 1990; Cross *et al.*, 1995). Protein and energy malnutrition has serious effects for children who are still growing and developing.

Activity

Consider the reasons why children may not be able to consume, absorb or utilise energy and nutrients.

Mechanical problems which prevent normal sucking, chewing and swallowing prevent children from being able to consume sufficient energy and nutrients. An adequate intake is also impaired by respiratory and cardiac problems as the child is unable to breathe and eat simultaneously. Anorexia, which may be the result of chronic illness or a psychological problem will also prevent an adequate intake.

Metabolic disorders prevent the absorption and utilisation of nutrients as do problems of the digestive tract resulting in protracted vomiting or chronic diarrhoea. Some children have increased metabolism and require increased energy and nutrients. In such cases nutritional support may be implemented to meet these additional needs. When children are unable to maintain an adequate oral intake of oral energy and nutrients support must be provided enterally or parenterally.

Booth (1991) recommends careful evaluation of the need for enteral or parenteral nutrition as an alternative to oral feeding, because resistance to normal feeding results from any long-term feeding method which bypasses the mouth. This evaluation should consider if the child is:

- unable to consume high energy supplements to maintain an adequate energy intake;
- demonstrating severe and worsening effects of protein and energy malnutrition;
- exhibiting a downward growth deviation.

Effects of protein and energy malnutrition for children
- Growth deviations
- Development delay
- Mental retardation (infants)
- Muscle atrophy
- Gastrointestinal disturbances
- Reduced resistance to infection
- Behavioural changes (irritability, apathy, lethargy)
- Delayed puberty

Reasons why children cannot maintain an adequate oral intake of energy and nutrients
REDUCED INTAKE
Mechanical problems
- gastro-oesophageal reflux
- mental retardation/unconsciousness
- oro-facial injuries/malformation
- tracheo-oesophageal fistula
Breathlessness on feeding
- respiratory problems
- cardiac failure
REDUCED ABSORPTION
- chronic diarrhoea
- glycogen storage disorder
- short bowel syndrome
FAILURE OF UTILISATION
Increased requirements
- cystic fibrosis
- metabolic disorders
- chronic infection
Food intolerance
- reduced appetite
- chronic illness
- malignancy
- anorexia nervosa

Enteral feeding can be defined as any method of providing nutrition using the gastro-intestinal tract. It includes the oral route as well as the alternative methods of naso-gastric, gastrostomy and jejunostomy feeding.

Parenteral nutrition is also known as intravenous (IV) alimentation or hyperalimentation involving IV infusion of highly concentrated solutions of protein, glucose and other nutrients. It is used to maintain the nutritional needs of those children in whom it is impossible to use the gastro-intestinal route.

ORAL FEEDING

Once a child has been identified as having a poor nutrition it is useful to obtain a full dietary history.

Activity

Consider the information you would need to obtain a detailed picture of the child's dietary and feeding routines.

Careful questioning of the family is required to establish a child's dietary and feeding routines. It does not just involve information about the child's exact intake. It is also important to discover times and places of meals and snacks and the family's involvement in these feeding routines. Failure to meet nutritional needs may not be related to an organic cause. Psychosocial factors may be the only reason for poor nutritional intake and should be excluded before investigations for organic problems.

Activity

Think about the psychological factors which could lead to a child having inadequate nutrition.

When the dietary history is completed it is possible to analyse the child's nutritional intake with dietary reference values and estimated average requirements for age and sex. The history will also provide information about the family's beliefs and routines in relation to food.

Janes (1996) believes that in the majority of situations the problem may be overcome by adapting the child's usual diet to include high energy and nutritious versions. In addition, snacks between meals will provide extra calories. It is important that families understand the rationale for such interventions which contradict usual healthy eating advice.

If such interventions do not enable sufficient increase in energy requirements additional dietary supplements may be used. As far as

Poor nutritional intake – psychosocial factors

Poverty
- insufficient food
- cheap foodstuffs, low in nutrients

Health beliefs
- fad diets
- excessive concern with health

Nutritional ignorance
- cultural confusion
- lack of parental dietary knowledge
- immature, inexperienced parents

Psychological stress
- emotional deprivation
- family dysfunction
- maternal depression
- school, peer pressures
- need for attention

Lack of feeding pattern
- inconsistent meals, snack routines
- inconsistent carers

possible the child should always be enabled to maintain the usual feeding routine so that this normality is not lost. To ensure that the normal routines can be maintained supplements should be given at a time when the appetite for a meal is not suppressed, e.g. bedtime.

In some situations, parents may also require advice about the management of their child's eating habits. When a child's eating habits become the focus of attention the child can use this to manipulate the situation. The child then becomes in control and will only eat certain foods at chosen times.

Activity

Think about your own meal times. What factors may help or hinder a child's eating habits?

ENTERAL FEEDING

Naso-gastric feeding

Infants and children can be fed by naso-gastric tube for years (Holden *et al.*, 1996). A polyvinyl, silicone or polyurethane tube is passed into the stomach via the nose. It can be left in place after feeding or removed and re-inserted before each feed. The main disadvantages of this route of feeding are psychological. The insertion of the tube is usually very distressing for the child and family as well as the nurse. When the tube is left *in situ* the child and family can become upset by the attention it attracts in others.

Naso-gastric tubes are chosen according to the child and the frequency and length of time required for an alternative method of feeding. Polyvinyl tubes quickly lose their flexibility when in contact with gastric secretions and need to be changed at least weekly. Polyurethane and silicone tubes do not harden, but their softness and flexibility make them more difficult to insert and easier for the child to dislodge. Their small lumen also makes them unsuitable for use with thick feeds.

The length of tube is usually estimated by measuring from the nose to the bottom of the earlobe and then to the end of the xiphoid process. Ellet *et al.* (1992) suggests that using the child's height is a more reliable way to judge the distance from nose to stomach.

Activity

Consider how you could check the correct placement of a naso-gastric tube and check your local procedure for the recommended method in your area of work.

Care must be taken when inserting a naso-gastric tube to ensure it passes into the oesophagus and stomach and not into the bronchial tree.

Additional dietary supplements

Glucose polymer
    Amount of nutrient: 15 g carbohydrate per 100 ml
    EXAMPLES: MAXIJUL. POLYCAL and CALOREEN
    USE: Add to soups, drinks and desserts
    Available on prescription: YES

Glucose drinks
    Amount of nutrient: 30 g glucose per 100 ml
    EXAMPLES: HYCAL and LIQUID MAXIJUL
    USE: Dilute with water or squash
    Available on prescription: YES

Milk shake drinks
1   Amount of nutrient: 1 kcal/ml
    EXAMPLES: 200 ml CARTONS: FRESUBIN
    USE: Ready made drinks in various flavours
    Available on prescription: YES
2   Amount of nutrient: 1.5 kcal/ml
    EXAMPLES: 200 ml CARTONS: FORTISIP and ENSURE PLUS
    USE: Ready made drinks in various flavours
    Available on prescription: YES

Fortified juice drinks
    Amount of nutrient: 1.25 kcal/ml
    EXAMPLES: 200 ml CARTONS: PROVIDE and FORTIJUCE
    USE: Ready made drinks in various flavours
    Available on prescription: YES

Fortified puddings
    Amount of nutrient: 250 kcal/142 g
    EXAMPLES: FORMANCE and FORTIPUDDING
    USE: Ready made mousse style pudding
    Available on prescription: YES

Milk shake products
    Amount of nutrient: 4.5–5.0 kcal/mg
    EXAMPLES: BUILD UP and COMPLAN
    USE: Added to milk
    Available on prescription: NO

Table 7.1	Principle	Rationale
Principles of tube feeding	Check placement of tube and flush with sterile water	To ensure tube is in stomach
	Warm feed to room temperature	To prevent discomfort and maintain body temperature
	Allow feed to flow into stomach by gravity at a rate of 5 ml/5 minutes for infants and 10 ml/1 minute for children	To prevent nausea, ingestion and regurgitation
	Replace aspirate in infants	To prevent electrolyte imbalance
	Flush the tube with sterile water	To clear the tube and encourage patency

Behavioural management of nutritional problems

- Establish regular meal times
- Offer snacks only as a complement to meals
- Make meal times a social, family event
- Praise eating successes, ignore poor eating
- Ensure meal times are free of distractions
- Maintain calm and peaceful environment for meals
- Avoid force-feeding

Disadvantages of indwelling naso-gastric tubes

- Aspiration
- Gastric perforation
- Nasal airway obstruction
- Ulceration/irritation of mucous membranes
- Epistaxis
- Displacement into bronchial tree
- Embarrassment about appearance

Naso-gastric tubes can also become displaced after insertion. For this reason it is essential to check the placement of the tube before and after each feed. The methods for checking the correct placement of the tube have recently been called into question.

Aspiration of gastric contents has been accepted as a safe method checking tube placement, but Metheny (1988) suggests that stomach contents can be mistaken for respiratory secretions. However, Metheny *et al.* (1989) found that respiratory, gastric and intestinal secretions all had different pH values and that pH testing of aspirate correctly identified the whereabouts of the tube in about 80% of cases.

When there is no aspirate it is difficult to ascertain whether the tube is displaced or the stomach is empty. A small amount of air injected into the tube results in gurgling on ausculation. However, it is possible to hear this when the tube is sitting at the cardiac sphincter of the stomach. In addition, copious respiratory secretions can transmit sound to the epigastric area.

If doubt exists on the correct placement of the tube X-rays should be taken. This is obviously not practical before each feed or when naso-gastric feeding occurs at home. Nurses need to be aware of the shortcomings of existing methods of checking tube position which poses a significant disadvantage of this method of feeding.

Naso-jejunal feeding

For some children naso-jejunal feeding is more appropriate than the naso-gastric route. The tube is passed via the nose into the stomach and time is allowed for gastric emptying to enable it to pass through the pylorus. This can be aided by positioning the child on the right side or by medication which increases gastric emptying.

The position of the tube is then checked by radiography by performing abdominal postero-anterio and lateral X-rays. Naso-jujunal tubes can return spontaneously to the stomach and before feeding the position must be confirmed by checking the pH of the alkaline aspirate.

The naso-jujunal route minimises the aspiration risk of naso-gastric feeding but many of the other disadvantages of naso-gastric tube feeding still apply. In addition, abdominal pain and diarrhoea can occur with bolus feeding because the stomach's natural reservoir and anti-infective properties are bypassed.

Gastrostomy feeding

Feeding via a gastrostomy tube is used for children who require a long-term means of complementary feeding to increase energy and nutrient intake (e.g. children with cystic fibrosis) or whose anatomy does not allow the passage of a tube through the mouth, pharynx or oesophagus (e.g. children with oesophageal atresia). A contra-indication to gastrostomy feeding is gastro-oesophageal reflux which may be exacerbated by feeding directly into the stomach.

A gastrostomy tube is inserted surgically or percutaneously into an opening through the abdominal wall giving direct access into the stomach. Both these procedures are carried out under general anaesthetic for children. There are many different types of tube for gastrostomy feeding but the main types are balloon catheters and button devices. Balloon catheters have a balloon at the distal end which is inflated with a prescribed amount of water and pulled up against the wall of the stomach thus maintaining its position as well as preventing the leakage of gastric contents into the peritoneum. The sterile water in the balloon should be changed weekly checking that no leakage has occurred and that the balloon is still patent. Some of these catheters have a securing device which lies flush against the skin to prevent excessive traction on the tube causing soreness and widening of the opening. If such a device is absent the tube should be taped securely onto the surface of the abdomen. Button devices can be inserted via percutaneous endoscope gastrostomy (PEG), usually after an established tract has been created. Button devices are better in appearance than balloon catheters as the button is positioned at skin level and no tubing is visible but they are more expensive than balloon catheters. These devices incorporate a one-way valve at the proximal end which prevents the leakage of gastric juices when the button is open. However, if displacement occurs they require a general anaesthetic for replacement whilst balloon catheters can be replaced immediately.

Method	Rationale
Loosen securing device	To free catheter
Stabilise site and gently pull catheter out	To minimise trauma to the stoma
Clean and dry site	To avoid entry of bacteria
Lubricate tip of replacement tube	To facilitate entry
Guide tube through stoma to a depth of 1–1.5 inches	To ensure tube reaches stomach
Inflate balloon with sterile water (amount prescribed by manufacturer) and pull up until resistance is felt	To ensure balloon fits snugly against stomach opening to prevent leakage of gastric contents
Slide locking disc down tube until snug against abdominal wall	To prevent undue friction of tube

Table 7.2

Gastrostomy tube replacement (balloon catheters)

331

Because of the danger of displacement of the tube, its position should be checked before feeding. Gastric fluid should be easily aspirated and its acidity can be checked with litmus paper. Displacement into the peritoneum or duodenum will make the tube difficult to aspirate and will cause abdominal pain, vomiting and diarrhoea. Gastrostomy tubes can be accidentally removed and should be replaced within 4–6 hours or spontaneous closure of the stoma will occur. Blockage of the tube can be avoided or overcome by flushing the tube with lemonade or inserting a pancreatic enzyme solution. Any artificial material inserted into the body can cause irritation and inflammation. Localised infection can occur around the gastrostomy site unless it is kept clean and dry. Granulation of tissue around the stoma can also lead to infection.

Jejunostomy feeding

Jejunal feeds are administered via a jejunostomy (surgical incision through the abdominal wall into the jejunum). Such feeding is necessary for children with severe reflux, in whom other methods of enteral feeding would carry a significant risk of reflux and aspiration. However, because this method of feeding bypasses the reservoir and anti-infective functions of the stomach, there is always a risk of gastro-intestinal infection and an aseptic technique and sterile feeds should always be used. The lack of a reservoir function of the jejunum means that feeds should be given continuously, as bolus feeds by this route can cause abdominal distension and diarrhoea. In addition, the tube should be flushed 4 hourly to prevent blockage, stasis and infection. As with other methods of enteral feeding the tube can become dislodged and its position should be checked prior to feeding by using blue litmus paper to verify the alkalinity of the aspirate.

PARENTERAL FEEDING

Total parenteral feeding (TPN)

TPN is usually administered via an established central venous or long line into a central vein with a high blood flow. It is used to maintain nutrition for children who are unable to use their gastro-intestinal tract to ingest and/or absorb their nutritional needs. It can be used as a long-term treatment for children with structural gastro-intestinal anomalies, such as short bowel syndrome, or as a temporary measure to allow an inflamed or diseased gastro-intestinal tract to rest and heal (necrotising enterocolitis, Crohn's disease)

Parenteral nutrition solutions mainly consist of glucose and amino acids. Electrolytes, vitamins, minerals and trace elements can be added according to individual need. Lipids may also be given as a separate solution. The exact amount of nutrients will be calculated according to the individual child's growth pattern, health problem and age (Table 7.3). High concentrations of glucose (over 12.5%) are very irritating to

Amino acids	1.5–3.0 g/kg
Glucose	20–30 g/kg
Lipids	20–30 g/kg
Potassium	2–4 mEq/kg
Sodium	3–8 mEq/kg

Table 7.3

Guidelines for providing daily TPN for children

vessels and therefore need to be infused into wide-diameter veins which have sufficient blood volume and pressure to enable rapid dilution and absorption. However, it is possible to use lipids as the main source of calories and these together with dilute glucose and amino acid solutions can be infused into peripheral veins. In principle the care of children undergoing TPN is the same as the care of any intravenous therapy but the result of any complication is potentially more severe because major vessels are being used. Major problems can result from displacement of the central catheter or long line. Central catheters can migrate into the right ventricle causing cardiac dysrhythmias, and haemothorax or pneumothorax can be caused by migration of a subclavian catheter.

There are also potential problems caused by the content of the infusate. The high concentration of glucose in TPN solutions makes it an excellent medium for bacterial growth. In addition, this high level of glucose can cause hyperglycaemia, and the rate of the infusion must be gradually increased to allow the child's natural production of insulin to accommodate this change in glucose load. Sudden changes in the rate of infusion can cause hypoglycaemia or hypoglycaemia and the child should be observed for features of these conditions. Acidosis can occur in vulnerable children if immature or diseased kidneys cannot excrete all the ammonia created by the breakdown of amino acids. Trace element deficiencies are common in neonates or children receiving long-term TPN. The infusion of lipids creates the risk of fat emboli when prolonged contact with the amino-acid solution causes emulsification. To minimise this risk lipid solutions are usually joined to the amino-acid infusion at the nearest point to the infusion entry site.

Some children develop reactions to lipid infusions and complain of breathlessness, nausea, headache, dizziness, chest or back pain. Lipids bind with albumin to displace bilurubin and cannot be given to children with known liver disease. Cholestatic jaundice is a common complication of long-term TPN and raises ethical issues about using TPN to maintain nutrition in children with no functional gastro-intestinal tract, although at present the alternative of gastro-intestinal tract transplant is not yet widely available or successful. Increased serum conjugated bilurubin results in bile duct proliferation and bile stasis eventually causing liver failure.

Complications of TPN
- Infection
- Hepatic dysfunction
- Hyperglycaemia
- Hypoglycaemia
- Hypomagnesaemia
- Hyperlipidaemia
- Acidosis
- Trace element deficiencies
- Cardiac dysrhythmias
- Air or fat emboli
- Phlebitis
- Tissue necrosis
- Liver failure
- Migration of central catheter/long line

Activity

From the information given above, draw up a plan of care for a child receiving TPN.

Care of children requiring TPN

Prevention of infection

- aseptic technique for: preparation of solutions, changing bags and giving sets, and changing occlusive dressing site
- infuse solutions via micropore filter
- change bags and giving sets every 24 hours
- perform routine blood cultures
- observe infusion site for erythema or exudate
- record 4 hourly TPR

Prevention of vascular injury

- monitor site hourly for extravasation, phlebitis
- infuse using electronic pump to enable constant rate of infusion
- monitor rate hourly
- do not increase rate if infusion behind time
- avoid air embolus or haemorrhage by ensuring connections are secure
- maintain line patency with Heparin if intermittent TPN

Prevention of electrolyte and glucose imbalance

- check solutions with daily prescription before administration
- measure blood glucose 2–4 hourly
- test urinary glucose, ketones, protein and pH 4 hourly
- do not stop infusion suddenly
- monitor for hypoglycaemia if TPN stopped
- weekly checks of serum magnesium, phosphate and calcium
- weigh daily
- record strict intake and output chart

PRINCIPLES OF PROVIDING ENTERAL OR PARENTERAL NUTRITION

There are certain common principles of care when providing enteral or parenteral nutrition. Whatever the feeding route the aims of care are to:

- facilitate adequate nutrition;
- enable desired growth and development;
- maintain the child's safety during the period of alternative feeding;
- maximise normal lifestyle;
- enable the child and family to manage the feeding.

The dietician should be involved in planning feeds which provide the correct amount of energy and nutrients to ensure that the child can reach and maintain average growth parameters (Table 7.4). Regular developmental assessments should be performed to monitor development; Booth (1991) found that gross motor and language skills are most likely to be delayed in children undergoing alternative methods of feeding. If oral feeding is not possible, babies should be given a dummy to enable them to associate sucking with feeding and encourage oro-motor skills. Holden *et al.* (1996) advocate the use of oral feeds whenever possible to enable the development of chewing and swallowing. The speech therapist and physiotherapist will advise on facial movements to develop the muscles involved with chewing and speech.

The nurse and family should be aware of the likely problems and complications of the chosen method of feeding and how to deal with and recognise these. Bacterial contamination of enteral feeds prepared at home is common (Anderton *et al.*, 1993) and parents need to be taught how to avoid this. Bags of feed should not be allowed to hang for more than 6 hours and pre-prepared feeds should be kept refrigerated for no more than 24 hours. If children are having enteral feeds overnight, they should be positioned in bed with the head end raised to encourage gastric emptying and minimise the risk of aspiration. To minimise their different lifestyle children having bolus feeds should have feeds at family meal times and be allowed to sit at the table with the family. They should be involved with normal family activities as much as possible.

Table 7.4

Nutrient requirements of normal children. (Adapted from DoH, 1991b)

Age	Energy (kcal/kg/day)	Protein (g/kg/day)
0–6 months	115	2.2
6–12 months	95	2.0
1–3 years	95	1.8
4–6 years	90	1.5
7–10 years	75	1.2
11–14 years	55–65	1.0
15–18 years	40–60	0.8

School-age children can often attend school as usual with the school nurse or family member administering a bolus feed at lunchtime. If oral feeding is continued the child should be involved in the choice of complementary foods and/or drinks. Children unable to have an oral intake should be encouraged to brush their teeth and rinse their mouths regularly to avoid infection of the oral mucous membranes caused by lack of saliva. TPN further dries mucous membranes because of the hyperosmolarity of the infusate.

Cross reference

Dental hygiene – page 184

FAMILY TEACHING AND HOME CARE

When alternative feeding is required for a long period of time the family may wish to learn the necessary techniques to enable them to continue care at home. The decision to continue treatment at home should be a joint decision between parents and nursing, medical and dietetic staff.

Activity

Consider what criteria you would use to determine the appropriateness of any family for managing enteral or parenteral feeding at home.

Casey (1988a) describes the role of the children's nurse as one who provides family care as well as nursing care, and also acts as a teacher, supporter and resource person. In the preparation for home feeding the nurse will use all these roles. The nurse can show the family how to adapt usual family care and routines to incorporate the chosen method of feeding as well as demonstrating the specific nursing care required. The family will need teaching about the specific feeding method and its complications, and will require support to come to terms with providing such care at home. Planned support should be available from community or hospital staff with written advice available for schools. The family will also be grateful for advice about other resources available to them. A social worker may be able to help with financial allowances and a list of parenteral support groups such as 'Half PINNT', a sub-group of 'Patients receiving Intravenous and Naso-gastric Nutrition Therapy (PINNT)'.

Activity

Compare one child's nutritional intake for 24 hours whilst in hospital and at home. Compare your findings with Table 7.4 to assess whether these intakes meet recommended energy and protein requirements.

Figure 7.1

Home enteral feeding learning goals.

HOME ENTERAL FEEDING LEARNING GOALS

Patient name .... Hosp No .... Ward ....

Named nurse .... Dietitian ....

Goal	Demo/ Discuss (date)	Comments	Sign
When discharged from hospital the patient or carer will know:			
• The principles of normal gastrointestinal tract function and how this has changed for the individual patient			
• The principles of enteral nutrition			
• How to set up a feed using an enteral infusion pump*			
• How to manage a pump and its alarms*			
• Negotiate approriate equipment for home with dietitian and Nutrition Nurse Specialist			
• Ayliffe's handwashing technique			
• Aseptic preparation of feed			
• Correct hang time for feed			
• Correct use of enteral feed sets, adaptors and syringes			
• Prevention, recognition and action to take in the event of: - infection of the gastrointestinal tract - infection of the stoma site - chest infection (aspiration of feed) - occlusion of tube - misplacement of tube - malfunction of tube			
• How to irrigate a blocked tube			
• How to change or repair the tube as appropriate			
• How to store enteral feeds and equipment and how they will be delivered			
• The names and telephone numbers of health care professionals available to provide advice 24 hours a day			

Goal	Demo/ Discuss	Comments	
• Of the existence (including name, telephone number) of a patient support group eg PINNT or the paediatric subgroup of PINNT (half PINNT)			
• The follow-up arrangements - dietitian NNS consultant			
• The social security benefits to which he/she may be entitled (refer to Medical Social Worker if appropriate)			
The patient/carer (eg parent or guardian in the case of a child) will be able to:		*Practice under Supervision*	*Practice unprompted*
• Check the tube position			
• Secure the tube adequately			
• Prepare the feed ready for administration			
• Connect the feed to the feeding tube			
• Programme the feeding pump for continuous feeding*			
• Administer a bolus feed down the tube*			
• Administer medications down the tube			
• Disconnect the feed and flush water down the tube			
• Contact the appropriate health professional when necessary			
* delete as necessary			
The patient or carer will state or indicate that he/she feels:	*Discuss*	*Comments*	
• Confident in his/her ability to self-care or in the ability of a carer			
• That expression of physical, emotional or social discomfort, when shared with the hospital staff, will be treated with respect and an appropriate intervention			
• Trust in his/her General Practitioner's knowledge of HETF			
• That he/she is one of many patients receiving HETF in the United Kingdom			

Key points ➤

1. Sick children do not always receive adequate nutrition in hospital.

2. Inadequate intake of nutrition and energy causes mental and physical problems for growing children.

3. Careful evaluation should be made before commencing alternative methods of feeding.

4. The advantages and disadvantages of the different methods of enteral feeding should be explained to the child and/or family before any choice is made.

5. The chosen alternative method of feeding should enable the child to carry out as normal a lifestyle as possible.

6. The use of TPN as a long-term method of feeding involves ethical decision making.

7. Home enteral or parenteral feeding needs careful preparation and teaching.

MAINTAINING FLUID BALANCE 8

INTRODUCTION

Fluid balance is the term used to mean that the various body compartments contain the required amount of water for the body's needs. Because electrolytes are dissolved in body fluids it is impossible to separate fluid balance from electrolyte balance.

Water is the largest single constituent of the body, the actual percentage of total body weight varying with the age and fat content of the body. An infant has the highest proportion of water compared with body weight. This fact, together with the inability of the small child's physiological immaturity to react to changes in fluid intake and output, make the maintenance of fluid balance crucial in the care of children.

The main sources of fluid intake are ingested fluids and food and that produced by energy released from chemical reactions within the body. The main routes of fluid output are the skin and the renal, gastro-intestinal, and respiratory systems. Dehydration resulting in sensations of thirst controls fluid intake, whilst fluid output is mostly under hormonal control.

Cross reference
Body water – page 67

Daily fluid requirements
Adults
    2500 ml/day
Children

1–10 kg	100 ml/kg
11–20 kg	1000 ml + 50 ml/kg per kg over 10 kg
>20 kg	1500 ml + 20 ml/kg per kg over 20 kg

Activity

Infants and small children have a greater need for water and are more vulnerable than adults to fluid and electrolyte imbalances. Consider why this is so.

Insensible fluid losses are controlled by heat, humidity, body temperature and respiratory rate. An immature hypothalamus makes children unable to regulate body temperature until about 5 years of age. Until this age body temperature responds readily to changes in environmental temperature and increases with any activity. Infections cause a more rapid and higher increase in temperature than in adults. For each degree of temperature above the norm, the basal metabolic rate increases by 10% with a corresponding increase in the need for extra fluid.

Whaley and Wong (1995) estimate that the surface area of the premature neonate is five times greater than that of an adult and that the newborn has a surface area two to three times greater. This allows a greater proportion of fluid to be lost by insensible means. In addition, infants lose a greater proportion of fluid via the gastro-intestinal tract which is proportionally longer than in the adult. The larger surface area of the growing child results in a high metabolic rate which creates a greater amount of waste for excretion by the kidneys. Unfortunately, these organs are not fully efficient in childhood and cannot concentrate or dilute urine according to the body's need for water.

Dehydration is a common problem in babies and small children and occurs whenever the total output of fluid exceeds the total intake. This can occur as a result of a decreased intake or an increased output. Such disturbances occur more often and more rapidly than in adults and small children are not able to adapt to these changes as readily as adults. Therefore one of the most important aspects of caring for sick children is maintaining an accurate record of fluid balance.

MEASURING FLUID BALANCE

Activity

List the situations when it would be important to record fluid balance for a sick child.

If an accurate fluid balance record is to be kept it is important to measure all intake and output. This may not be easy with children who have not learnt to control any elimination. Urine collection bags can be used but frequent application and removal may cause excoriation of the skin. Nappies can be weighed before and after use and the amount of urine passed estimated by the difference in weight. (The volume of fluid in millilitres is equal to the weight in milligrams.) However, this method has disadvantages. If stool is mixed with urine it is impossible to be accurate about the type of loss and additional losses may occur because of evaporation and/or leakage. Any other form of output (vomit, wound drainage, naso-gastric aspirate) must also be measured and recorded. If a child's only intake is fluid this can be easily measured but it is not easy to estimate the amount of fluid in a mixed diet. Because of the difficulties in ensuring the accuracies of all intake and output measurements a daily weight is often the preferred method of determining fluid balance. This also has potential problems. To ensure accuracy, the scales should be regularly serviced and the child weighed at the same time of day in the same clothing.

Older children may like to help in the recording of fluid balance and may enjoy recording details or drawing pictures of their intake. They and their parents should be reminded of the importance of saving all excreta for measurement. Parents may be happy to keep records of intake and output.

Cross reference

Weighing children and babies – page 282

RESTRICTED INTAKE

Children with renal problems or following surgery to the gastro-intestinal tract may need a restricted intake. Children having surgery or certain investigations may need a period of time with no intake. Such restrictions pose a challenge for the children's nurse as many children may be too young to appreciate the reasons for the restrictions or may simply forget that they have been told not to have anything to eat or drink. Periods of starvation before surgery or investigations should be kept to a minimum. Children can easily become dehydrated or hypoglycaemic if left for too long without fluid or food but many studies show that children are sometimes starved for unnecessary lengths of time (Welborn *et al.*, 1986; While and Crawford, 1992a). Most research indicates that the maximum starvation period for food or milk is 6 hours but that juice or glucose drinks can be given up to 2 hours before a general anaesthetic (Meakin *et al.*, 1987; Splinter and Schaeffer, 1990).

Activity

Look at your hospital policy for the pre-operative fasting of children and critically evaluate it in relation to the above research findings.

To inform others about restrictions a notice needs to be attached to the child and many children enjoy wearing a special badge. Drinks and sweets should be removed from the bedside to help the child avoid temptation. Small children need close attention as their thirst may cause them to drink straight from the tap or to take another child's drink. Children who are starved for a longer period post-operatively will have intravenous fluids to overcome dehydration and hypoglycaemia but this will not prevent the discomfort of being unable to eat or drink. In these situations the mouth should be kept clean and moist and lip salve applied to prevent the lips from cracking. A dry mouth may also pose a problem for children on restricted intake. These children have the additional difficulty of trying to eke out their allotted amount of fluid throughout the day and often need help to do this and not drink the whole amount in the morning leaving nothing for later.

Activity

Think out a strategy to help a 5-year-old child maintain a restriction of 500 ml fluid/day without becoming too distressed or uncomfortable.

INTRAVENOUS FLUID THERAPY

Children with problems maintaining fluid and electrolyte balance are often given intravenous (IV) fluids. Livesley (1993) suggests that specific guidelines are needed for the management of IV fluids in the treatment of children because of the unique problems. To maintain the child's safety during IV therapy the nurse should be aware of all the associated risks and their prevention.

Calculation of IV fluid rates

Replacement of fluid is essential if 10% of the child's total body weight is lost

Bobby is 4 years old and has been vomiting for 24 hours. His normal weight is 17 kg. He is unable to take anything orally at present and it is estimated that he is 10% dehydrated

- calculate his daily fluid requirement
- add 10% to overcome his dehydration
- calculate the hourly rate of his infusion

SITE AND EQUIPMENT

In most children the IV cannula of choice is a 22–24 gauge over-the-needle catheter. The insertion site should be chosen with the child's age and development in mind (Figure 8.1). Using a non-dominant arm allows the older child to be able to continue most of their normal activities with the minimum of help. Avoiding the use of a vein at a joint prevents accidental dislodgement as the child tries to use the limb as normal. A scalp vein can be used in babies under 9 months as, at this age, these veins are prominent and easily accessible. They also do not interfere with the baby's movement. However, they do require part of the head to be shaved which may distress the parents.

Figure 8.1

Cannulation sites for children.

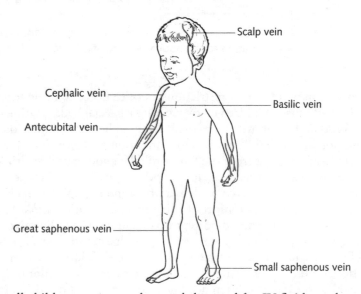

Small children cannot understand the need for IV fluids or the need to keep the site relatively still. The cannula should be secured in such a way that the insertion site is easily visible and the cannula is stable. The cannula site is an open wound and should be managed aseptically and therefore sterile dressing or tape should be used to protect the site. Cannula-related sepsis is associated with the proliferation of skin flora at the insertion site so any sterile transparent dressings used should allow the escape of moisture from the skin to prevent this occurrence. To ensure that the insertion site remains visible splints and bandages are not usually used for adults but these items are usually necessary for children to prevent interference and to provide extra stability for the insertion site. Splints should be washable and padded to avoid the risk of pressure sores over bony prominences. Stickers can be applied to make them more acceptable to children. A plastic gallipot can be cut to shape to provide protection for a scalp vein site.

An infusion pump is nearly always used in the care of children to reduce the risk of circulatory overload and speed shock. The nurse should not presume the accuracy of the pump. Any electronic device depends upon the competency of the operator. The nurse should check that the prescribed rate is appropriate for the child before setting the pump. The pump should then be checked every 1–2 hours to ensure the fluid is running as programmed. Most infusion pumps will alarm when the infusion stops for whatever reason but it is possible for pressure to build up if the rate exceeds the capacity of a small vein. Hecker (1988) suggests that a build up of pressure can cause hyperplasia of the vein lining which can lead to phlebitis. Many pumps also have a tamper-proof facility to prevent mischievous children from interfering with the device.

PREVENTION OF INFECTION

Phebitis or inflammation of the vein can result from sepsis, chemicals or mechanical trauma (Table 8.1). It can often be misdiagnosed (Griffiths-Jones, 1990), but it should be noted and reported quickly as, if untreated, it can lead to septicaemia. Its may be recognised by erythema, pain, swelling or inflammation around the insertion site. Septic phlebitis is associated with contaminated cannulae or infusates. The insertion of cannulae should be a speedy, aseptic procedure preceded by effective skin cleansing. The infusate should be checked for signs of contamination before administration and any breakage of the infusion line to change infusates or administer drugs should include disinfection at the point of insertion. In long-term infusions, IV tubing and solutions should be changed daily to prevent bacterial growth. In adult nursing the rotation of cannula sites every 48–72 hours is recommended but this is a debatable practice in children's nursing where it is known that children and their families experience a great fear of cannulation. In addition, there is now evidence to suggest that after 72 hours there is actually less risk of complications in children with peripheral IVs (Garland *et al.*, 1987). The risk of septic phlebitis is also reduced if a closed infusion system can be maintained. Weinbaum (1987) identified that three-way taps provided a reservoir for micro-organisms. Removal of the IV cannula should be performed with an aseptic procedure. The cannula should be removed gently and firm pressure applied to the site immediately to prevent haematoma formation and potential infection. Once the bleeding has ceased a sterile dressing can be applied.

Chemical phlebitis is related to IV fluids which have a high osmolarity and low pH and some IV medications. IV medication such as potassium chloride and antibiotics should always be diluted according to manufacturers' instructions and their compatibility with the IV fluids checked.

Mechanical phlebitis is caused by the presence of a foreign body in the vein. This problem is exacerbated if there is movement of the cannula within the vein. It can be prevented by careful fixation of the cannula and the infusion giving set. Effective methods of securing the

Table 8.1

The prevention of complications of IV therapy

Complication	Prevention
Phlebitis	Aseptic technique for all associated procedures Inspection of infusates for contamination Secure cannula to prevent movement Inspect insertion site 1–2 hourly for inflammation, erythema and pain Dilute additives as per manufacturers' instructions Change infusates and lines every 24 hours Maintain a closed infusion system
Extravasation	Secure cannula Inspect insertion site for local oedema, leakage of infusate
Circulatory overload/ under-infusion	Check prescribed rate Monitor rate of infusion 1–2 hourly Monitor intake and output hourly Report any dyspnoea, cough
Allergic reaction	Check allergy history Report any rashes, itching, dyspnoea
Air embolism	Clear all air from infusion set when commencing infusion Do not allow infusion to run dry – ensure rate does not exceed amount of fluid Check all connections are air-tight Maintain a closed infusion system
Occlusion of IV line	Maintain limb in optimum position Ensure line not kinked or compressed Ensure line is free of air Maintain flow of infusate to prevent fibrin formation Treat fibrin formation with saline flush
Venous spasm	Keep affected limb warm Do not administer refrigerated medication until at room temperature

line also help to prevent the cannula from becoming dislodged from the vein and slipping into the surrounding tissues (extravasation). Extravasation of some infusates can cause necrosis of surrounding tissues and can result in severe injuries and long-lasting consequences (Wehbe and Moore, 1985). The increased subcutaneous fat found in children tends to make infiltration difficult to identify. The site and nearby dependent areas (palms, soles, behind the ears) should be examined for coolness, hardness and swelling and the infusion stopped if these features are found.

PREVENTION OF MECHANICAL PROBLEMS

Mechanical problems can also cause serious problems. Air in any part of the infusion set may result in an air embolism. The child will become cyanosed, tachycardic and shocked. If this occurs the infusion should be stopped, a doctor informed and the child should be laid in a head down position on the left side to prevent the air from entering the pulmonary artery. Most infusion pumps are programmed to detect air but air can enter below the detection chamber when connections are broken. All connections should be checked when the nurse checks the infusion site.

CARE OF THE CHILD

The reason for the IV therapy and the need to protect the site can be explained to most older children whose mobility need not be impaired. If these children feel well they should be allowed to walk around and join in play as far as possible. Small children can only be allowed to mobilise with supervision as they will not understand or remember the need to care for their IV infusion. When children are confined to bed their personal belongings should be placed within easy reach on the side without the infusion so they do not dislodge the cannula by stretching. They will also require help with most of their activities of daily living. The type of play should be chosen with care to maintain the integrity of the infusion. To prevent accidental damage water play and the use of scissors are probably contra-indicated.

Activity

Consider what help will be required by an adolescent with an IV infusion sited in the non-dominant hand. Try putting your own non-dominant hand in your pocket and seeing what can be done single handed.

Activity

Plan suitable play for a 5 year old with an IV infusion sited in his left (non-dominant) arm.

CENTRAL VENOUS DEVICES

Peripheral cannulae have a relatively short lifespan and children are easily distressed by repeated cannulation. When long-term venous access is required to maintain fluid and electrolyte balance, an indwelling central venous catheter or implanted infusion port may be sited within the superior or inferior vena cava or right atrium via a large vein (Figure 8.2). There are a range of devices for central venous use which all have their advantages and disadvantages. The choice depends on the age of the child, the reason for the device and the amount of available access.

There are many complications associated with the insertion of a central venous catheter and for this reason, the insertion is usually performed in a clean environment under heavy sedation or a general anaesthetic. Implantable ports carry fewer risks but do require surgery and a general anaesthetic for their insertion. Correct placement requires radiological confirmation. Hickman, Broviac or Groshung catheters are made of clear, radiopaque, flexible silicone and designed to remain in place indefinitely. They are tunnelled subcutaneously for a short way before entering a large vein thus reducing the risk of infection of having long-term access directly into a main vein. Implanted ports are metal or

Cross references

Hickman line – page 324
Port-a-cath – page 325

Figure 8.2

Sites for central venous devices.

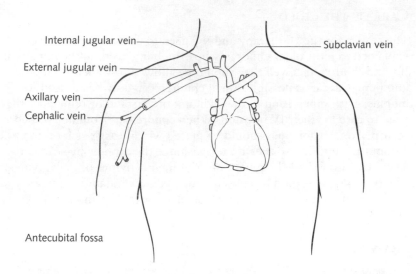

Internal jugular vein

External jugular vein

Axillary vein

Cephalic vein

Subclavian vein

Antecubital fossa

Uses of central venous catheterisation

1 To monitor central venous pressure in acutely ill children
2 To replace large amounts of IV fluids or blood in cases of severe shock and/or haemorrhage
3 To provide long-term venous access for:
- fluid and electrolyte maintenance
- long-term IV cytotoxic therapy
- long-term IV antibiotic treatment
- regular blood tests
4 To administer total parenteral nutrition

Risks of central venous catheterisation

- Sepsis
- Haemorrhage
- Thrombosis
- Cardiac dysrhythmias
- Haemothorax
- Hydrothorax
- Pneumothorax
- Cardiac tamponade
- Air embolism
- Catheter embolism
- Misplacement
- Brachial plexus injury
- Thoracic duct injury

plastic devices which lie under the skin and are sutured to the chest wall. The port is attached to a silicone catheter which is tunnelled subcutaneously into a large vein. All catheters which are tunnelled into place have a Dacron cuff sited part way along their length which promotes tissue in-growth and prevents bacterial migration. Although these tunnelled catheters have a reduced risk of infection that risk is still present and exit site infections can result in septicaemia and removal of the device. At present no study has been able to clearly identify a strategy for managing the exit site to reduce the incidence of such infection. Lucas and Attard-Montalto (1996) found that dressing the site actually increased the incidence of infection, although they recognise the limitations of their small study. These long-term devices were introduced primarily to allow patients having long-term treatment to return home between treatments. To ensure the child's safety, the family should have the opportunity to learn, practise and feel confident in the care of the device before discharge.

An alternative to the above devices is the safer and cheaper peripherally inserted central (PIC) catheter or long line which is a central venous catheter usually sited within the axillary or subclavian vein via the antecubital vein (Rountree, 1991). These lines have their entry point directly into a vein and therefore are not usually suitable for care at home. They are usually used for medium-term access (7–10 days).

One disadvantage of intermittent access to central venous catheters is occlusion of the line as a result of clot formation. Groshung catheters have a two-way valve to minimise this problem but still require weekly saline flushes to ensure patency between uses. Other catheters should be flushed with 2.5–5 ml heparinised saline between uses and weekly when the device is not in use. If occlusion does occur gentle flushing and aspiration with saline should dislodge the clot. Silicone catheters expand

Device	Advantages	Disadvantages
Hickman/Broviac	Dacron cuff reduces risk of bacterial migration Self-administration easy	Exit site must remain dry Must be clamped Protrudes outside body Heavy activity restricted Daily Heparin flushes May affect body image Difficult to repair
Groshung	Low maintenance two-way valve: • no clamping • backflow unlikely • air entry unlikely Easy to repair Self-administration easy Dacron cuff reduces risk of bacterial migration	Weekly saline flush Exit site must remain dry Heavy activity restricted Protrudes outside body May affect body image
Implanted ports (Port-a-cath, Infus-a-port)	Low infection risk Lies under skin Activity less restricted No dressing required Monthly Heparin flush Body image less affected	Port accessed by injection Difficult to self-administer Special equipment needed to access port

Table 8.2

Advantages and disadvantages of long-term central venous access devices

on pressure and will allow the saline to pass around the clot and dislodge it. If a larger thrombus has formed it may be necessary to administer prescribed urokinase or streptokinase. Excessive pressure to dislodge an occlusion is not recommended as silicone is prone to cracking and splitting (Marcoux *et al.*, 1991).

> **Key points**

1. Differences in children's physiology make the maintenance of fluid balance one of the most important aspects in the care of the sick child.

2. Children and their families can be involved in the measurement and recording of intake and output.

3. Periods of fasting should be kept to a minimum and the child carefully monitored to ensure dehydration does not occur.

4. Children receiving IV therapy have unique problems and require specific care.

5. The use of central venous access devices enable the child to go home between long-term treatments but the family need careful teaching about the care of the device to avoid complications.

Principles of care for central venous catheter devices

Prevention of infection
- strict aseptic technique for all procedures
- observe exit site for erythema, discharge or swelling
- apply dressing after insertion until sutures removed

Prevention of haemorrhage or air embolism
- maintain a closed system
- use luer locks for all equipment
- clamp lines securely

Prevention of clot formation and occlusion
- flush catheter when not in use
- flush catheter between medications to prevent precipitate formation
- ensure line does not become kinked or compressed by clothing
- retain fluid in the catheter by using a positive pressure injection technique

Prevention of damage to the catheter
- avoid the use of sharp-edged forceps/clamps
- use no smaller than 10 ml syringes to access the line
- only allow the child to play with scissors under close supervision

9 CARING FOR CHILDREN IN PAIN

INTRODUCTION

All children have a fundamental right to have their expressions of pain recognised, believed and managed appropriately. Unfortunately, the difficulties inherent in responding to children in pain in this way represents a major challenge to children's nursing practice.

Pain is not a topic which is easy for any health care professionals to understand. As McCaffery (1983) rightly stated '*Pain is what the patient says it is and exists when he says it does*'. Pain is unique to the individual and it is impossible for the nurse to be able to recognise the experience for any one else. Consequently, nurses need to be able to appreciate the various factors which affect the individual's perception and reaction to pain. They also have to be able to identify the varied manifestations of pain, especially when children are too ill, too young or too frightened to verbalise their pain. It is important that the nurse does not dismiss such communications. Finally, it is crucial that the nurse is able to offer pain management strategies which take into account the impact pain is having on the child's physical and psychological state.

FACTORS AFFECTING PAIN

Sociological factors

The word pain is derived from the Latin *poena* meaning penalty. Historically the experience of pain was thought to be beneficial to the individual as it helped to strengthen the character. This belief is still held by some cultures, particularly in relation to the male sex.

Children learn by others' behaviours and will soon recognise the accepted response to pain. Depending upon their childhood experiences they learn to bear pain with stoicism or to display overt expressions of distress. Bond (1979) reports frequent complaints from children whose home environment is stressful. Budd (1984) dealt with more frequent complaints of pain among children from large families whose parents argued and used physical abuse, or whose siblings exhibited pain as part of a neurotic behaviour pattern. Children from Italian and Jewish families may learn to respond openly and emotionally to pain, while British children may believe it should be borne quietly (Bond, 1979).

Pfefferbaum *et al.* (1990) support this idea that cultural factors affect responses to pain but warn that this influence is probably minimal.

Activity

Think about your own childhood and what you learnt about the expression of pain. Consider what effect this may have had on your nursing care.

Cross reference

Neonatal pain – page 549

Definitions of pain

- Suffering or distress of body (from injury or disease) or mind (*Concise Oxford Dictionary*)
- Range of unpleasant bodily sensations (*Oxford English Dictionary*)
- An unpleasant sensation, occurring in various degrees of severity, especially as a consequence of injury, disease or emotional disorder.
- Suffering or distress (*Readers Digest Universal Dictionary*)
- Hurt, distress, discomfort, anguish, misery, agony, suffering, ordeal, torment, torture (*Rogets Thesaurus*)

Most adult values and beliefs about pain have originated from their childhood experiences. Nurses who as children were expected not to make a fuss about their pain, probably still manage their own pain quietly and without reliance on others. Such nurses probably find it more difficult to respond to a child who screams loudly at any discomfort than the nurse who was brought up to vocalise pain.

Political factors

The United Nations (UN) Convention on the Rights of the Child (1989) provides minimum standards for the care and treatment of children. It recognises that children are still discriminated against because of their immaturity, and recognises that children have a right to the highest attainable standards of health care (Newell, 1991). Although the UN cannot enforce the convention, governments that ratified the convention are required to submit a progress report.

In spite of repeated government and pressure group reports recommending improvements in child care the UK is still struggling to ensure that these rights are met. Platt (1959) realised that children in hospital have special needs which are best met by nurses and other health care professionals who have had specific training and education. This is particularly true in the care of children in pain. Other reports (Court, 1976; NAWCH, 1986; DoH, 1991a) reiterate this point and the most recent Audit Commission inquiry (1993) into the care of children in hospital revealed that there is still a concerning lack of specialist nurses in children's wards (Figure 9.1).

Such reports, as mentioned above, also recognise the important contribution that parents make to a sick child's care. Parents are able to recognise when their child's behaviour is different, they often know their child's way of expressing pain and they also understand the best comforting measures for their child. In partnership with the nurse they can help to provide the optimum pain management. However, many hospitals still do not cater well for parents who are sometimes still left to feel 'in the way' or 'interfering' and are at the best 'tolerated' (Audit Commission, 1993). Instead of being able to help care for their child's pain, many parents become helpless witnesses and feel as anxious and fearful as their child (Carter, 1995).

Government initiatives to improve standards of care such as the skill mix review and the named nurse concept may have been designed to help these problems. Using one nurse skilled in pain management to supervise others giving care to children could prove useful. In addition, if each child and family had a named nurse accountable for their care, that nurse could appreciate their individual reactions to pain. However, in reality, these initiatives have been slow to develop. Nurses want to be able to give individualised, holistic care but the separation of nursing into specialist skills can appear a retrograde step and a return to task allocation. At the same time, the lack of appropriately qualified children's nurses makes it difficult to provide children and families with

Cross reference

UN Convention on the Rights of the Child (1989) – page 691

Parents' view of partnership and pain control

- Parents are usually familiar with their own child's responses to stress but nurses rarely use this expertise (O'Brien and Konsler, 1988)
- Parents are able to recognise their own child's non-verbal cues of pain (Elander et al., 1991)
- Parents prefer to remain with their child during painful procedures (Dearmun, 1992)
- When given appropriate information, parents can help their child cope with pain (Schepp, 1991)
- Parents can feel powerless if their child is in pain and they do not know how to cope (Wyckoff and Erickson, 1987)
- Parents find that the central part of their child's anxiety in the first 3 post-operative days is the management of their pain (While and Crawford, 1992b).
- Parents believe that nurses tend not to prepare children for post-operative pain (Gillies et al., 1995)

Figure 9.1

*Number of registered children's
nurses on duty. (Adapted from
Audit Commission, 1993).
(a) Day duty. (b) Night duty.
N = 31 wards in seven
hospitals.*

(a)

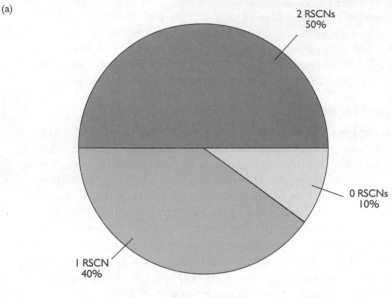

2 RSCNs
50%

0 RSCNs
10%

1 RSCN
40%

(b)

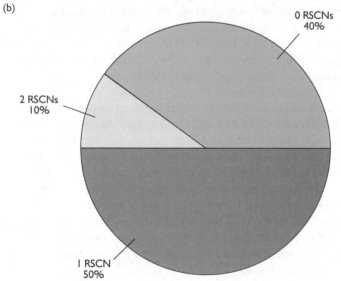

0 RSCNs
40%

2 RSCNs
10%

1 RSCN
50%

an individual named nurse. Often the named nurse is the senior nurse
on duty who provides little clinical care.

Economic factors

Health provision nowadays is based on consumerism and the market
economy (Langdon, 1995) and as a result quality assurance is
emphasised. Written polices and measurable standards of care to ensure
a high quality of care for children in hospital were recommended by the
Audit Commission (1973) but have been slow to develop. Llewelyn

(1991) suggests that pain is one area where a written standard would be invaluable to ensuring children's needs are met in a knowledgeable and consistent way; perhaps because of the subjective and individual nature of pain such standards are rare.

The market place approach to health care may also provide nurses with a moral dilemma in relation to pain control. It may be difficult for them to offer a wide range of pain control methods if constrained by cost. The way in which nursing care is organised in the UK relates to the political and economic factors. In spite of the introduction of Project 2000 (UKCC, 1986) student nurses still provide much of the direct care to children in hospital. Student nurses are less aware of the influences of pain assessment and so may be more susceptible to the myths about children's pain. Their lack of experience also means that they are less likely to detect certain pain behaviours (Read, 1994).

Direct care is also often provided by nurses who are not qualified children's nurses and lack the special skills needed to assess children in pain.

Many authors advocate that the initial nursing assessment of any child coming into hospital should include an assessment of the child's perceptions and experience of pain (Hester, 1979). Such specific areas are not usually investigated which may also be due to the fact that this initial assessment is allocated to the less qualified members of the ward team.

CHILDREN'S PERCEPTIONS OF PAIN

In addition to family and cultural influences, children's individual perceptions of pain are also affected by their age, cognitive and lingual ability, neurological development, experience, personality and family and cultural beliefs. Assessing pain in pre-verbal children is difficult, especially in the neonatal period, and evaluation is thus based on behavioural and physiological changes such as crying, diffuse body movements, facial expressions and increased heart rate. However, these are not exact indicators, as an infant who is lying still with his/her eyes closed may still be experiencing pain (Shapiro, 1989). Communicating with toddlers (1–3 year olds) is also difficult; their language is largely imitative and they are egocentric, often believing doctors and nurses deliberately set out to hurt them (Perry, 1994). School-age children can consider viewpoints other than their own but still think mostly in concrete terms and can believe that pain is a punishment for their misdeeds. They cannot understand words such as 'pain' and 'anxiety', and may deny pain for the fear of the consequences, such as having an injection or staying in hospital. Adolescents are capable of fairly mature reasoning but their lack of experience of pain may make it difficult for them to cope with it. McCaffery and Beebe (1989) report a 17 year old in pain saying: 'Tell the nurses we're younger than adults and more scared, so we need more attention'.

Cross references

Children's perceptions of health – page 144

Children's perceptions of illness – page 214

Activity

Question some children of different age groups who have never been in hospital about the meaning of pain and anxiety. Consider carefully some the reasons for their answers.

Experience of pain alters infants' and children's perception of it. A study of behavioural responses in infants during subsequent visits to an immunisation clinic showed that a significant number cried in anticipation (Levy, 1960). Older children who have had previous experiences of illness and pain may become stoic in painful situations, while others with no experience may become terrified when they first feel a significant amount of pain (Eland, 1985). Fear and anxiety heighten pain (Alder, 1991), and Bond (1979) suggests that children with an emotional personality report greater levels of pain than more placid individuals. First born and only children seem to be more anxious about pain, possibly because they have not been able to observe siblings (Eland, 1985). The context of pain also affects perception (McGrath, 1990): children who have been distracted from their pain often report less discomfort, while those who have seen a cannula during insertion or blood spillage generally complain of more pain (Johnson *et al.*, 1993).

Activity

Now question some children who have had painful procedures about the meaning of pain and anxiety. Are their answers significantly different from those children of similar ages whom you questioned earlier?

NURSES' PERCEPTION OF PAIN

Nurses are as vulnerable as their patients to the psychological and sociocultural factors which influence the perception of pain. Bradshaw and Zeanah (1986) suggest that health professionals have additional biases from working with patients in pain. Their study indicated that many nurses still rely on intuitions, assumptions, personal beliefs and knowledge about pain related to specific diagnoses to assess children's pain. Nethercott (1994) found that nurses still rely on physiological measurements and verbal expressions as indicators of pain although it has been consistently shown that these are not reliable indicators. I once saw a teenage boy who had received no analgesia during his first 12 hours following a splenectomy because he did not appear in pain or ask for pain relief. In reality, he was frightened of any intervention and was lying rigid to avoid further pain. In another situation, a neonate with intercerebral haemorrhage following a traumatic delivery, whimpered whenever handled, yet received no analgesia for 24 hours, 'because he was not pyrexial'.

Read (1994) found that more experienced nurses had a higher perception of children's pain. Gadish *et al.* (1988) suggested that nurses who were mothers themselves often provided better pain measurement. They also found that graduate nurses had a better understanding of the assessment and management of pain than those nurses with a basic nurse education.

Nurses are also affected by the misconception about the effects of analgesia on children. Controversy still exists over the safety of pharmacological interventions and children's ability to feel pain. In addition, it has been noted that nurses give less priority to relieving pain than to more measurable nursing duties (Baillie, 1993). To enable nurses to identify their own beliefs and values about pain which may interfere with their ability to make a subjective assessment, Whaley and Wong (1995) advise nurses to reflect on their answers to a series of questions about children's pain.

Activity

Answer the questions in the box overleaf 'Reflection about views regarding children's pain' and consider the reasons why you have made your responses.

PAIN ASSESSMENT

Pain assessment aims to identify all the factors that affect a child's perception of pain (Pritchard and Davis, 1990). Since pain is both a sensory and emotional experience, a multidimensional approach to assessment is preferable. One such approach is QUESTT (Baker and Wong, 1987):

- Question the child.
- Use pain rating scales.
- Evaluate behaviour and physiological changes.
- Secure the parents' involvement.
- Take the cause of pain into consideration.
- Take action and evaluate results.

Where it is possible to communicate with children, verbal statements and descriptions of pain are vital sources of information.

Question the child

On admission or pre-operatively when the child is able to communicate, questions such as in the box at the foot of page 354 may help to ascertain the child's understanding of pain. Children under the age of 6 may not understand the word pain (Eland and Anderson, 1977) and may be more familiar with terms such as hurt or sore.

Myths and misconceptions about children's pain

- Infants do not feel pain
- Infants do not expect pain
- Children tolerate pain better than adults
- Children cannot accurately locate their pain
- Children become used to repeated pain
- Children are always truthful about their pain
- Children's behaviour accurately determines the degree of their pain
- Children are more susceptible than adults to the side effects of narcotics

---

The use of narcotics for children

- The administration of narcotics for pain is no more dangerous for children than it is for adults (Burrows and Berde, 1993)
- Respiratory depression as a side effect of opiates is rare in children (Paice, 1992)
- Addiction to opiates used to treat children's pain is extremely rare in children (Morrison, 1997)
- By 3–6 months of age children can metabolise narcotics in the same way as adults (Koren et al., 1985)
- Increased doses of opiates for increased pain do not increase the side effects (Paice, 1992)
- Continuous infusions of opiates provide more constant analgesia for post-operative children (Dilworth and MacKellar, 1987)

Use of pain rating scales

Pain rating scales (Table 9.1) should ideally be selected with this prior knowledge about the individual child, who should be shown how to use the scale before any pain occurs. However, few reliable tools are available for assessing children's pain Jackson (1995) and Ellis (1988) believe that pain measurement should be based on behaviour, physiological measurements and the child's own report. However, self-assessment of pain in children relies on children's participation and upon their communication, numerical or drawing skills.

Table 9.1

Pain rating scales

Rating scale	Principles	Age of use
FACES pain rating scale (Nix et al., 1994)	Facial expressions to represent degrees of pain	3 years+
Oucher (Beyer, 1989)	Photographs of children's faces showing degrees of pain	3–13 years
Numeric scale	Straight line marked 0 (no pain) to 10 (worst pain)	5 years+
Poker chip tool	Four counters given to child to represent 'pieces of hurt'	4 years+
Word graphic scale	Horizontal line marked at intervals with descriptions of pain intensity	8 years+
Color tool (Eland, 1993)	Child constructs own colour tool choosing different colours to represent degrees of pain	4 years+
Liverpool Infant Distress Score (LIDS) (Hogan et al., 1996)	Eight behavioural categories each with a 0–5 score enable carer to calculate pain score	Neonates
Pain Assessment Tool for Children (PATCh) (Quershi and Buckingham, 1994)	Combines face scale, body outline and numeric scale with descriptions of pain and behavioural changes	All ages

Evaluating behaviour and physiological changes

Buckingham (1993) has designed a pain scale for pre-verbal toddlers that combines assessment of physiological changes with changes in behaviour and body language. This could be adapted for use in neonates. The faces scale (Wong and Baker, 1988) can be used for children as young as three; studies show it is one of the most accurate pain assessment tools for children and is well received by them (Wong and Baker, 1988). Older children can usually use a numerical scale, which may range from 1 (no pain) to 10 (worse pain); some children can relate to the intensity of their pain better if these numbers appear on a vertical line (Beyer and Ardine, 1988). The Eland colour scale seems to be the most accurate assessment tool for the location of pain. The child locates the pain on a body outline and represents its severity with different colours (Eland, 1985). The Hester poker chip scale can be used with children as young as 4. The child is given four or five counters (chips) and asked to display none or all of them to represent the amount of pain felt (Hester, 1979). McCaffery and Beebe (1989) gave a selection of assessment questions and tools that can be duplicated for use in practice. There is, however, a lack of research about the reliability of these scales and many authors have criticised their use (Wilson, 1993), so it is advisable to combine the use of pain scales with an objective form of measurement.

Activity

Use a variety of these assessment tools with children of different ages. Consider their ease of use and effectiveness.

Secure parental involvement

When children are unable to communicate, parental involvement is crucial. They can be questioned on admission to ascertain the child's knowledge of pain and reaction to it. It is also useful to question parents wherever possible about the child's usual patterns of behaviour *before* any pain occurs; parents often find it difficult to make a subjective assessment of their child when he/she is distressed, as their own distress, anxiety and sometimes guilt interferes with their ability to judge behaviour (McCaffery and Beebe, 1989). It is also important to discuss the parents' role in pain assessment with them if they are to be partners in their child's care. Parents are, too often, unaware of their role when the child is in hospital (Audit Commission, 1993). If they are helped to work in partnership with the nurse they will be alert to manifestations of pain and can help in controlling the pain. In a similar way, they can help an older child to express pain and make a choice about its management.

Activity

Talk to some parents about their child's pain. How does their information add to your knowledge and care of the child?

Taking the cause of the pain into account

The cause of potential pain should not be forgotten. Children may deny pain because of a lack of understanding or fear of intervention. Eland (1985) describes a teenager with chronic pain who denied any discomfort because he had forgotten what it was like to be pain-free. A knowledge of disease pathology offers a clue to the type of pain being experienced. Whaley and Wong (1995) suggest that nurses should accept that whatever is painful to an adult is painful to an infant or child unless proved otherwise. This is particularly pertinent to A&E work, where it is not always possible to undertake a detailed assessment of the child's and family's previous experience of pain. Children in A&E departments often present in pain which can be heightened by the fear and anxiety caused by the strange and stressful situation, while painful and frightening procedures are undertaken to aid diagnosis and treatment. Gay (1992) and Read (1994) found that nurses tended to underestimate actual and potential pain in these situations. Gay (1992) also found that preparatory information about procedures and equipment alleviated children's stress and pain. Nurses may need to give more consideration to finding out about procedures in order to prepare children in a more realistic way.

Taking action and evaluating results

The aim of caring for a child in pain should be to provide total pain relief. This may be done using a variety of methods suitable for each individual child's pain. Both pharmaceutical and non-pharmaceutical interventions can be used. If the nurse is familiar with a range of such interventions, the child and/or parents can select the one which seems most suitable.

The most suitable method for relieving pain often depends on the child's personality and participation. It also relies upon a therapeutic relationship between the child, parents and the nurse. The child and parents need to be able to trust the nurse to believe their concerns about the pain and to react accordingly. Whatever the method used, the nurse should teach the child and family about the pain whilst trying to avoid words which may describe the type of pain. In the same way, the nurse should prepare the child and family for painful procedures. If the nurse is not evaluative about the type of pain experienced, the child does not anticipate pain and may be able to give a clearer description of it as an individual experience. Parents who are well prepared can often lessen a child's anxiety and therefore pain by their presence. They can also be taught non-pharmacological techniques and can help the child in their use.

Non-pharmacological methods of pain relief are best taught to the child and family *before* the child actually experiences pain. Some techniques can be put on audio or video tapes and used again at a later date. Cleeland (1986) suggest that this type of pain control is best used for children with pain which they describe as being mid-range. Children with severe pain often cannot relax sufficiently to make best use of these methods and children with little pain may not be motivated to learn the technique.

When nurses are first taught about the administration of medicines, they learn that it is the responsibility of the nurse to ensure that the patient receives the *right drug* in the *right dose* at the *right time* and by the *right route*.

Whilst the nurse is not responsible for the prescription of medicines, a knowledge of these principles in relation to the pharmacological

Sidebar

- *Non-pharmacological* – relating to the use of strategies to minimise the perception of pain which do not involve the administration of drugs; these strategies should not be seen as an alternative to drugs but as a means of enhancing the effectiveness of pharmacological interventions
- *Pharmacological* – relating to the use of medicinal drugs

Non-pharmacological interventions

General strategies
- reassurance
- parental presence
- explain reason for pain
- emphasise positive information

Distraction
- play
- singing or shouting
- stories

Relaxation
- rocking
- deep breathing
- muscle relaxation

Guided imagery

Use of heat or cold or massage

management of pain enables the optimum pain relief to be used. In discussion with medical colleagues the nurse can advise the most suitable intervention for each individual child.

Ensuring that a child receives the right drug is dependent on an accurate assessment of the pain. Non-opioids and non-steroidal anti-inflammatory opioids (NSAIDS) are suitable for mild to moderate pain (Table 9.2). Opiates are needed for moderate to severe pain (Table 9.3). The 'analgesic' ladder is a useful way to determine the right medication as the child and parents may lose confidence in the nurse if the wrong medicine is prescribed. If the chosen drug is too mild the child may refuse further doses because it is not having any effect. If the chosen drug is too strong, the child may suffer severe side effects and again refuse further doses.

Drug	Recommended dose	Precautions
Ibuprofen	5–10 mg/kg 6–8 hourly	Can cause gastric irritation if given on an empty stomach
Aspirin	300–2600 mg 4 hourly	Not recommended for under 12s
Naproxen	5 mg/kg 12 hourly	Children older than 2
Diclofenac sodium	0.5–1 mg/kg 8–12 hourly (orally or rectally)	Maximum dose 3 mg/kg/day (enteric coated – do not crush)

Table 9.2

Non-steroidal anti-inflammatory drugs

Drug	Route	Recommended dose
Morphine	Oral	0.2–0.4 mg/kg 3–4 hourly
	Sustained release	200–800 mcg/kg 12 hourly
	Intramuscular	0.1–0.2 mg/kg 3–4 hourly
	Continuous IV infusion	Loading dose 50–100 mcg/kg Hourly dose 10–30 mcg/kg
	Patient controlled IVI	Loading dose 50–100 mcg/kg Background infusion 2–8 mcg/kg Bolus dose 10–20 mcg/kg/5–15 minutes
Pethidine	IV or IM injection	500 mcg–2 mg/kg/dose
	IV infusion	Loading dose 1 mg/kg Background 100–400 mcg/kg/hour
Codeine phosphate	Oral (1–12 years)	3 mg/kg/day, doses every 4 hours
	IM injection	1 mg/kg/dose every 4–6 hours

Table 9.3

Use of opioids for children

Distressing side effects of inadequate pain control may also occur if the dosage of the drug is wrong or if it is given at an inappropriate time. Dosages should be carefully calculated according to the age, height and weight of the child. In chronic pain analgesia should be given regularly to ensure continuous pain relief. Mild analgesics given regularly can often be more effective than infrequent doses of strong opioids.

Once the right dosage and frequency of the medicine has been decided the most appropriate route must be chosen (Table 9.4). Although the oral route is often the first choice it is not always the most appropriate for frightened toddlers and children who are nauseated. Intramuscular injections are not well tolerated by most children and many children will deny pain if they think an injection will follow.

Table 9.4

Routes of administration for analgesia

Route	Advantages	Disadvantages
Local	Ease of administration Usually well accepted	Slow onset of action Cannot be used under 6 months of age
Oral	Ease of administration Usually well accepted	Inappropriate in the post-operative period Absorption and action may be slow Gastric irritation Danger of aspiration for infants Discoloration of tooth enamel
Rectal	Useful if child is vomiting or unable to swallow	Social acceptability? Ineffective in loaded rectum
IM	Rapid onset of action	Disliked by children: 'The worst hurt ever'
IV	Rapid onset of action Continuous action if infusion	Discomfort of IV cannula Potential hazards of IV therapy
Inhalation (Entonox)	Child can self-administer	Needs careful preparation Child needs to understand use

Patient controlled analgesia

Definition

Patient controlled analgesia (PCA) is a technique which was developed in the 1970s to enable adult patients to have some control over the dose and frequency of their analgesia. Its use began to be extended to children in the 1980s

Variations

The PCA pump can be programmed to deliver an opioid analgesia in three different ways:

- *bolus dose* – the child can press a button to deliver a bolus pre-programmed dose of analgesia as required. A lock-out device prevents this dose from being repeated so often that the child receives an overdosage. However, the pump records every request for analgesia so that the nurse can assess how often the child is requiring analgesia and adjust the dose if necessary. The nurse or parent can use this method on the child's behalf

- *continuous background infusion* – delivers a continuous pre-programmed dose of analgesia.

- *continuous background infusion and bolus doses* – a combination of the above, allowing the child to receive an extra dose of analgesia as required.

All children receiving a form of PCA should be regularly observed for the side effects of opioids and have their respiratory rate, depth and pattern monitored to detect any complications

Infusions are a more effective way of providing continuous pain relief and if the child and parents are prepared well, they can be given some control over the dosage and frequency. Llewelyn (1991) found that children as young as 3 could use patient controlled analgesia (PCA) well. Morphine at 1 mg/ml is the choice of drug for PCA as it is considered to provide significantly more pain relief and fewer side effects than other opioids (Vetter, 1992).

Morphine, in conjunction with a long-acting anaesthetic is also the choice of drug for the epidural route. It can be given continuously or intermittently via an infusion and acts directly upon opiate receptors in the spinal cord. This lessens the risk of sedation and respiratory depression which can occur from the effect of opioids on the brain.

Prior to potentially painful procedures involving punctures of the skin a topical local anaesthetic cream can be used. EMLA (eutectic mixture of local anaesthetic) is approved for children over 1 year in age. It takes 60–90 minutes to numb an area of intact skin for up to 4 hours after application (see overleaf). AMETOP gel can be used for children over 6 months. It takes 30–45 minutes to act and its effect can last for 4–6 hours. Whilst EMLA cream can cause constriction of blood vessels, AMETOP dilates them. However, AMETOP can cause blistering or skin discoloration if left in position for longer than 45 minutes (Hewitt, 1988). The use of patient controlled inhalation devices such as Entonox, which due to the advantage of its almost immediate effect can be useful prior to more invasive painful procedures.

All medicines have undesired as well as desired side effects and the nurse needs to be aware of these so that a careful evaluation of the medication can be made. This evaluation of the medication needs to also include the child's and the parents' views of the efficiency of the method used. Evaluation of care is not understood or undertaken well by nurses and more consideration needs to be given into incorporating this aspect of care into care plans.

Activity

Compile your own list of analgesia for children, finding out the dose range, method of action, use, side effects and variety of routes for each medication listed.

SUMMARY

Primary nursing may be a way of providing more individualised and effective pain control. One nurse acting as a key figure for a child throughout the hospital stay will be able to establish a close therapeutic relationship with the child and family (Binnie *et al.*, 1988). Providing care in this way calls for good interpersonal skills, and one of the crucial elements of such a nurse–patient relationship is self-awareness – being honest about personal thoughts and emotions. It also requires the nurse to evaluate the relationship and care given. As yet this type of nursing is not widely practised in the UK, but now the focus of nurse education has changed, it may be possible to provide individualised pain management within such a therapeutic relationship.

The introduction of a systematic method of pain assessment such as that suggested by Baker and Wong (1987) could also improve pain management, especially if introduced before the pain occurs. The use of such methodology would give the nurse more experience on which to base the assessment of children admitted in acute pain. However, further research is required on the validity and reliability of pain scales to ensure that children are able to define their pain in meaningful ways.

Children continue to suffer unnecessary and treatable pain (Action for Sick Children, 1993). Nurses need increased education about pain, while improved methods of assessing pain are crucial to identifying and managing pain effectively. Nurses should consider how best to incorporate specific pain assessment tools into their care and how children's care can best be organised to enable consistency of care and an individualised approach. Further research into the accuracy of children's pain assessment will also help to improve this area of practice.

Side effects of opioids

- *Depresses central nervous system* – sedation, drowsiness, mental clouding
- *Action on the respiratory centre in the brain stem* – respiratory depression
- *Stimulation of the chemoreceptor trigger zone which activates the vomiting centre* – nausea and vomiting
- *Release of histamine* – pruritus, flushing and sweating
- *Increase of smooth muscle tone* – urinary urgency or retention
- *Decrease of peristalsis and intestinal secretions* – constipation

Administration of AMETOP cream

Used to numb pain from the following procedures:

- lumbar puncture
- finger or heel pricks
- arterial or venous access
- implanted port access
- superficial skin biopsies
- removal of chest tubes
- bone marrow biopsy
- SC or IM injections

Procedure

- not recommended for children under 1 year
- use on intact skin
- apply thickly to area 1 hour before procedure (90 minutes for dark skin when absorption is slower, 2 hours for deep procedures)
- apply occlusive dressing
- pallor or erythema indicates local anaesthetic effect
- wipe off remaining cream 5 minutes before procedure to allow vaso-constrictive effect to reverse

Key points ➤

1. Nurses need more education about pain assessment in children.

2. Children's perceptions of pain are influenced by many factors.

3. It is important to be aware of one's own beliefs and values about pain to prevent them from interfering with one's professional judgement.

4. Wherever possible, it is advisable to question children and their families about pain before it occurs.

5. The organisation of care may need to change to enable the effective assessment of children's pain.

6. The use of both pharmacological and non-pharmacological interventions will enhance pain control.

THE ROLE OF THE NURSE AS A SURROGATE 10

INTRODUCTION

Peplau's (1952) model of nursing, created initially to define mental health nursing, describes six roles of the nurse. One of these roles is described as the surrogate role. Peplau defines this role as helping the patient to become aware of the nurse as an individual and thus promoting an interpersonal relationship between them to enable the nurse to take over roles which the patient is unable at present to fulfil. If the term 'patient' is seen as the child and family, this role becomes the development of the partnership relationship with the child and family.

Whilst the children's nurse does not want to take over the role of the parent when caring for children, there is sometimes a need for the nurse to take on aspects of care which the parents would usually provide. Casey (1988b) describes this as family care, in contrast to nursing care which relates to the technical care the nurse provides because of the child's health problem. The nurse adopts the role of surrogate carer when the parents are unable to perform their usual role.

Parents may be unable to perform their usual role because they are unable to be resident in hospital with their child. Although most children's wards encourage parents to stay with their child in hospital it is not always possible for all parents to do so. Parents who have other children, are self-employed or are single parents and have no close family near-by may be unable to be resident. Other parents may stay with their child but, for a number of reasons, may find it difficult to carry out their child's usual care. As one parent of a 6 year old admitted for revision of a hypospadias repair, said: 'I want to be with Richard to support him, but please do not ask me to help with his care because I am too squeamish'. Parents who are unable to carry out family care should not be made to feel guilty but supported in their decision and enabled to take their chosen responsibility. Ahmann (1994) suggests that parents should be reassured that they have an essential role in the care of their child in hospital, but such reassurance can cause stress to parents who cannot provide that care.

Parents who are resident and take on most of their child's care are often abandoned by the nursing staff. These parents are often anxious about this responsibility and feel obligated to stay with their child for fear that no care will be given in their absence. They become exhausted with lack of adequate nutrition, rest and sleep. The nurse should not let this situation develop and should be available to take on the family care to give parents a respite.

Ideally, a named nurse is assigned to each child and family. This nurse can provide family and nursing care as necessary to meet the needs of the child and family. This surrogate role requires a detailed knowledge of the child as an individual as well as the family's usual daily routine.

Cross references

Peplau's model of nursing – page 607

Casey's partnership model – page 608

FAMILY CARE

Family care for the child in hospital should be as similar as possible to the care that the family would give their child at home. Times of waking, eating and resting should be adhered to as closely as possible. Hospitalisation is not an appropriate time to try and change family routines which do not meet with the nurses' approval unless these are putting the child in danger. However, helping with family care can give the nurse an opportunity to advise the family about health education.

Washing and dressing

Bath time is often also playtime for younger children. The nurse should recognise this and spend time playing with the child as well as ensuring cleanliness. To avoid frightening the child the big bath should only be used if this is what the child normally uses. All children should be supervised in the bath, but some children may need help with aspects of washing.

Any specific lotions or creams should be used as at home. The stress of the hospital environment can be minimised by encouraging the child to wear clothes from home. Help should be given according to the child's level of independence. The under 8s usually require help with teeth cleaning. Hair should be cared for as at home which may include shampooing.

Eating and drinking

Children often react to illness or hospitalisation by loss of appetite and the named nurse needs to appreciate the child's usual likes and dislikes to encourage eating and drinking. Bottles, teacher beakers and toddler cutlery should be available as at home. If possible, a normal family meal time can be simulated by having the child eat at the table with others. The times and content of meals should correspond to the home routine as far as possible, with cooked meals provided at midday or evening according to the family's usual practice.

Play

Play is an important part of a child's usual home routine and should not be forgotten when the child is in hospital. The nurse providing surrogate care should provide for play as the parents would do at home. Favourite toys or stories brought from home can be included. Story time may be an important part of the child's day at home; time for a cuddle on mother's lap or a quiet time before sleep. Letting the child play in the playroom with other children cannot replace this and the named nurse should organise to spend one-to-one time with the child so that this special time is not lost.

Cross reference

Nutrition – page 177

Encouraging the ill child to eat and drink

- Use attractive eating utensils – bowls and plates with familiar characters on the surface, coloured mugs, curly straws
- Arrange the food attractively on the plate [make a picture of a face or garden with the food, cut sandwiches into shapes (boat, teddy, star, etc.)]
- Serve small portions – an overloaded plate can be off-putting
- Provide the child's favourites – bring from home if necessary
- Serve the food imaginatively, e.g. in a paper bag for a picnic, use straws as skewers to eat sausages, etc., by hand
- Make meal times into social events by gathering children together
- Involve the child, e.g. filling in food/fluid chart, choosing from a menu, etc.

Cross reference

Play – page 94

Elimination

Children in hospital can find it difficult to maintain their usual elimination patterns in hospital because of their anxieties, the strange environment and lack of privacy. The nurse can help by ensuring that the child is given the opportunity to go to the toilet in the same way as parents will usually ask small children to go to the toilet, for instance, on waking, after breakfast and before going to school. This routine may help to avoid constipation or urinary tract infections caused by ignoring the desire to eliminate. The nurse should provide the same amount of help as the parents usually provide. A knowledge of the child's usual bowel habits will help to alert the nurse of any problems.

Usually toddlers begin toilet training at around 2 years. Some parents will sit the younger child on the potty at set times to familiarise the child with the pot. Although children often regress in hospital, the surrogate nurse should keep to home potty routines so that training is not interrupted and can continue on discharge.

Mobility

Children who are ill rarely want to be as active as usual. However, as they recover they will regain this and it is useful to know the child's usual level of activity to be able to cater for this. The surrogate nurse needs to be aware if the 1 year old can walk unaided or if the child with special needs requires assistance to mobilise. This knowledge will also help to maintain children's safety as they become more active.

Rest and sleep

Often children sleep more when they are feeling unwell, but they need to feel safe in order to relax and rest. If parents are unavailable the nurse should ensure that home routines are maintained. This will require careful organisation of work to ensure that the nurse is able to settle the child for a nap or for bed at the usual time. Any special routines like drawn curtains, nightlight, cuddly toy or blanket or night-time drink should be followed.

Cross reference

Sleep – page 41

Communication

Infants' communication is largely non-verbal by touch and tone of voice. Even with such limited communication an infant is usually aware of strangers. The surrogate carer cannot explain this temporary role and can only provide security for this age group by following home routines. As children's vocabulary and understanding increases it is important that the named nurse has an idea of the common words and expressions used. To prevent accidents it is particularly important to understand the words used by the child to communicate elimination needs. A knowledge of the family and those close to the child, including pets, enables the nurse to talk with the child about home.

Communication may also include the need for prayer. Family

Cross reference

Language development – page 77

routines in relation to this should be noted and respected so that the child may be given time and, if necessary, privacy to pray.

If the nurse is to identify stress in hospital it is also important to know the child's usual personality. Is the child normally talkative and friendly or shy and uncommunicative? The surrogate carer needs to know how the child usually reacts to stress and the most comforting way to respond as the parents would. For example, Alex, a 3 year old is best comforted by having his feet stroked. Fergus, aged 6, prefers to hide behind the door and to be left alone to talk to his teddy.

Providing family care is not always easy in a hospital environment and the nurse may have to be flexible and imaginative and use skills of advocacy to enable children to follow home routines.

Activity

Compare the usual routine of a children's ward with the usual home routine of a child known to you. Consider how the hospital day might be adjusted to meet your child's usual routines. Identify any areas of difficulty and consider how you might be able to change these.

CARE OF THE CHILD CONFINED TO BED

On occasions family care has to be adapted because of the child's condition. The named nurse has a carer/surrogate role in this situation in helping the family to adjust their routines to meet these changed circumstances. The nurse can also offer advice to parents caring for children at home who are temporarily confined to bed.

Activity

Consider the aspects of family care which will need adaptation for the child who is confined to bed.

Washing and dressing

The child confined to be bed should be bathed at the usual times for washing at home. If the bed linen and any wound dressings are protected with plastic, bed baths can still provide an opportunity for play, boats or ducks can swim in the washing bowl and the child can splash the water around. It is important to ensure that teeth, nails and hair still receive attention. Hair may become very matted and difficult to brush if the child is unable to move and this problem will only worsen if brushing is neglected. Shampooing should be considered if the child is confined to bed for longer than a week.

Eating and drinking

The child confined to bed may find it difficult to eat and drink because the recumbent position hinders normal digestion. This position also impairs elimination and can result in constipation due to sluggish peristalsis and urinary tract infections because of inadequate bladder emptying. It is therefore particularly important to encourage fluids. Favourite fluids should be offered at regular intervals and the use of bendy straws or dolls' teacups may promote cooperation. Food should be easily digestible and provided in small and attractive servings, making full use of the child's likes. Food from home may be more acceptable than that provided by the hospital.

Activity

Consider ways in which you could encourage the child confined to bed to eat and drink.

Play

Play is still important for the child in bed but will have to be adapted to meet the child's altered abilities, medical equipment and their position. Generally, children who feel unwell will have reduced levels of concentration. As a result, a range of different types of play must be organised to respond to this. For example, allowing a child with a plaster of Paris to play with water may be hazardous! Equally, unsupervised cutting out with scissors may be risky for any age of child with an intravenous infusion or traction, who may, by accident or design, cut through their equipment. Children who have to lie flat will need particular attention. Travel games which can be played on a magnetic board are useful as is a slanting easel for drawing, painting or just supporting reading books.

Elimination

It is difficult to maintain a home routine for toileting when the child is confined to bed and potty training may have to be delayed until this period of immobility has ceased. However, because of the complications of constipation and urinary tract infection associated with immobility, it is important to retain some semblance of routine. If a child defecates at a specific time of day bedpans should be offered at this time. If a child is used to going to the toilet at set times in the day (on waking, before school, midday) this routine should continue. In the hospital setting privacy for toileting must be ensured as some children may be very self-conscious about such activity. Small children may wet the bed during illness because they are less aware of the need to urinate, are scared of using bedpans or because of an urinary tract infection. It is important not to punish them but to analyse why it happened and try and prevent a reoccurrence.

Extrinsic causes of pressure sores

- *Pressure.* The blood pressure at the arterial end of capillaries is approximately 32 mmHg. At the venous end this pressure is about 12 mmHg. The mean capillary blood pressure is around 20 mm Hg and any external pressure higher than this will cause capillary obstruction. Tissues usually served by these capillaries will be deprived of their blood supply and will eventually die from ischaemia
- *Shearing forces.* When the child slips down the bed or is dragged into a new position, the skeleton moves over the underlying tissues and the circulation of these damaged tissues is destroyed
- *Friction.* Friction and stripping of the upper layer of the epidermis also occurs when children slip down the bed or are dragged. This results in a superficial break in the skin rendering it more prone to further damage

Mobility

Children who are immobile are at risk from pressure sores, stiff joints, wasted muscles and joint deformities. Changes of position and physiotherapy are required to minimise the risk of these complications. Although the incidence of pressure sores in children is less than in adults because children tend to have healthier skin and a vigorous circulation, immobile children are at risk and preventive care should be taken. Pressure sores can develop when the pressure on the skin and underlying tissues is greater than the pressure within the underlying capillaries. If this degree of pressure is maintained, the capillaries collapse, the underlying tissues become ischaemic and eventually necrose. The primary causes of pressure sores are direct pressure, friction, and shearing forces. The immobile child should be positioned carefully to ensure that bony prominences are not under pressure from other limbs or medical equipment. Change of position is the most effective way of preventing pressure sores but care should be taken to ensure that the child is moved without causing friction or shearing. Pressure relieving devices should be used for children who are at risk from pressure sores. Although there are several well researched tools for assessing adults' risk of pressure sores, this is a poorly explored area of children's nursing. Risk-assessment tools need to take into account all the secondary factors which predispose to pressure sores. These factors are those which make the skin less healthy and more liable to the effects of pressure.

Table 10.1

Preventing the complications of immobility

Complication	Nursing care
Pressure sores	Encourage movement of mobile limbs Encourage change of position Observe pressure areas for redness Avoid pressure, shear or friction
Circulation problems (deep vein thrombosis, pulmonary embolus)	Encourage movement as able Encourage deep breathing exercises to aid venous return Note complaints of calf or chest pain
Chest infection	Encourage deep breathing Record temperature and respirations Note chestiness, cough, pyrexia
Elimination problems (constipation, urinary tract infection)	Encourage good fluid intake Enable usual routine and privacy for toileting Monitor urine output and bowel action
Anorexia	Encourage appetite
Boredom and depression	Provide daily programme of activity Encourage family and friends to visit
Joint stiffness/deformity/muscle weakness	Encourage active exercises for mobile limbs Provide passive exercises for immobile limbs
Difficulty in resting and sleeping	Provide daily programme of activity Keep to home bed-time routines

Further reading

WATERLOW, J. (1998) Pressure sores in children – risk assessment. *Paediatric Nursing,* **10** (4), 22.

Activity

Consider which secondary factors would cause a child to be more at risk from pressure sores.

Joint stiffness, muscle wastage and joint deformities may be prevented by exercise and position. Depending on the child's condition these may be passive or active exercises. All limbs should be put through a range of movements at least twice a day. Active exercises can be incorporated into play. Immobile children should have their limbs placed in a natural position which maintains body alignment.

Activity

Make up a list of games which would enable a child on traction to exercise the unrestricted limbs.

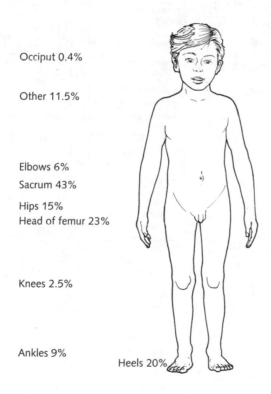

Occiput 0.4%

Other 11.5%

Elbows 6%

Sacrum 43%

Hips 15%
Head of femur 23%

Knees 2.5%

Ankles 9%

Heels 20%

Figure 10.1

Pressure areas at risk. Torrance (1983) revealed those areas of the body most at risk from the effects of pressure. A sample of 1000 people found the percentage risk to be as shown. It also discovered that when in the sitting position, the pressure on the ischial tuberosities was 300 mmHg and when supine, the pressure on the buttocks was 70 mmHg.

Prevention of pressure sores

- *Assessment.* All children should have a risk assessment calculated on admission and this should be updated regularly as their condition changes significantly
- *Plan of care.* Care plans should incorporate specific measures to combat pressure sores according to child's degree of risk
- *Careful positioning.* Children should be positioned to avoid pressure. Care should be taken that all traction equipment and infusion, feeding, oxygen, or urinary or wound drainage tubing is not causing pressure. The use of bean bags rather than angled bed rests reduces friction and shearing forces
- *Good bed making.* Beds should made with taut bottom sheets to prevent pressure from creases. Crumbs and small toys are also risks for small children who are immobile
- *Hygiene.* Pressure areas should be kept clean and dry. The affected area should not be rubbed as this action macerates the subcutaneous skin which degenerates
- *Nutrition.* The child should receive a nutritious diet and adequate fluids to prevent excessive weight loss or gain and dehydration whilst promoting a healthy skin. Vitamins A and C and zinc are especially useful for maintaining healthy skin
- *Patient lifting and handling.* The most effective treatment and prevention of pressure sores is the relief of pressure. If a child is unable to move and change position the nurse must help. Nurses should have short finger nails and no rings which may damage the child's skin during repositioning. Incorrect lifting will result in the child being dragged up the bed causing damage to underlying tissues
- *Pressure relieving devices.* A wide variety of pressure relieving devices are available but their efficacy is not always research based. Nurses should be aware of their use, function, disadvantages and advantages and base their choice according to the specific child's needs
- *Patient/family education.* The older child and family should be told about the risk of pressure sores and how to prevent their occurrence so that they can cooperate with the care prescribed

Figure 10.2

Pressure sore risk assessment chart for children (Bedi, 1993).

Date			
Weight			
Average according to age	0	0	0
Below birth weight	2	2	2
Below weight according to age	3	3	3
Overweight	3	3	3
Continence			
Continent	0	0	0
Catheterised	1	1	1
Incontinent for children >4 years	2	2	2
Nappies	2	2	2
Nappy rash	3	3	3
Enuretic	3	3	3

Date			
Skin types			
Dark	0	0	0
Fair	1	1	1
Sensitive	2	2	2
Broken/spot	3	3	3
Mobility			
Fully	0	0	0
Restless/fidgety	1	1	1
Sedated/non-walker restricted	2	2	2
Paralysed	4	4	4
Appetite			
Average/good	0	0	0
Poor	1	1	1
NG tube			
Fluids only	2	2	2
Malabsorption	3	3	3
Failure to thrive	3	3	3
Nil by mouth dehydrated	3	3	3

Date			
Age			
Neonates	3	3	3
Infant	1	1	1
Toddler	1	1	1
Pre-school (2–5)	1	1	1
12 years plus	1	1	1
General assessment			
Severe cyanosis and clubbing	5	5	5
Moderate cyanosis	3	3	3
Mild cyanosis	1	1	1
Asymptomatic	0	0	0

Date			
Special risks			
Tissue malnutrition e.g. terminal cachexia	8	8	8
Circulatory/vascular disease	5	5	5
Diabetes	4	4	4
Hypoxaemia	5	5	5
Inotropic support	3	3	3
Known infection, e.g. MRSA, *Pseudomonas*	2	2	2
Neurological deficit			
Unconsciousness	5	5	5
Developmentally delayed	2	2	2
Normal milestone achieved	0	0	0
Major surgery/trauma			
On table > 2 hours	5	5	5
On table > 5 hours	7	7	7
Medication			
Antibiotic induced diarrhoea/thrush/rashes	3	3	3

Total score at end of each assessment

Significant event	Date	Score	Name of nurse
Admission			

Score classification	10+ At risk	15+ High risk	20+ Very high risk

Rest and sleep

Rest and sleep is often difficult for children confined to bed as their usual mobility is severely curtailed. This is a particular problem for children on traction who do not feel ill but are forced to be immobile for long periods of time. Such children need to have their days planned carefully to ensure that they are as mentally and physically active as possible during the day with a planned routine of events just as they would have at home. These activities should be as close as possible to the normal home routine. For instance, if a boy plays football after school, a game of blow football may take its place. In this way the nurse can endeavour to ensure that the child is tired by bed-time and will sleep as well as usual.

Activity

Rashid, aged 8, is being nursed on traction for a fractured femur. Plan a day's activity for him for a Friday and a Saturday.

Communication

Because children are normally so active, a period of forced immobility is particularly frustrating. If clear explanations are not given to rationalise the need for immobility small children can believe that it is a punishment for bad behaviour. Immobilisation alters the number of environmental stimuli that the active child receives and affects their growing need for autonomy and independence, leading to feelings of boredom, frustration, depression and isolation. Children of varying ages and personality will respond differently, but young children tend to become more attention seeking and may regress to earlier behaviour such as thumb sucking or bed wetting. Older children may become aggressive, irritable, argumentative or uncooperative in an attempt to assert some control over the situation. Boredom tends to decrease communication, concentration and problem-solving skills. These types of behaviour are not usually acceptable but in difficult situations such as immobility children need to be able to express their anger without fear of further punishment. They need to be helped to act-out this anger appropriately in play and given a full and varied programme of activity to avoid boredom and its consequential maladaptive behaviour changes.

Activity

Check your answer to the previous activity and assess whether you have enabled Rashid to overcome his frustration and boredom.

Breathing and circulation

Immobility can lead to a sluggish circulation and clotting problems as well as stasis of respiratory secretions and chest infections. Chest physiotherapy should be included in the day's planned activities to improve venous return and breathing and avoid these complications. Chest physiotherapy, which consists of deep breathing exercises can be incorporated into play.

Activity

Consider what play to use for an immobile child which would also provide chest physiotherapy.

Intrinsic causes of pressure sores

- *Weight*. Reduced subcutaneous fat causes an increased localised pressure over bony prominences. Extra subcutaneous fat does not combat the increased pressure caused by the extra weight of the obesity (Waterlow, 1988)
- *Temperature*. An increase in temperature causes a rise in basal metabolic rate and a greater need for oxygen to maintain healthy tissues. It also causes sweating
- *Moisture*. Moisture increases the risk of pressure sores by 5%. Perspiration, wound drainage and incontinence result in waterlogged skin which is softer and weaker than healthy skin. Faecal incontinence further damages this fragile skin by exposing it to bacteria and toxins (Wyngaarden and Smith, 1988)
- *Nutrition*. Oedematous and adipose areas are poorly vascularised causing the skin to become thin and fragile. Dehydration leads to dry, wrinkled and withered skin which breaks down relatively easily (Waterlow, 1988)
- *Mobility*. Lack of mobility impairs the ability to change position, thus relieving pressure and improving the circulation to the tissues (National Pressure Ulcer Advisory Panel, 1989)
- *Circulation*. Low diastolic blood pressure (BP) (below 60 mml lg) indicates poor peripheral circulation and therefore poor tissue perfusion
- *Neurological factors*. Sensory loss due to paralysis, coma, sedation or analgesia decreases or prevents the awareness of pressure and the ability to react to it (Waterlow, 1988)
- *Age*. Increasing age causes a decrease in tissue elasticity, texture and cell replacement. The healthy skin of a baby or young child helps to counteract many of the intrinsic causes of pressure sores but care should be taken to protect it from damage as pressure sores can still occur (National Pressure Ulcer Advisory Panel, 1989)
- *Emotional stress*. Raised glucocorticoids produced by stress result in derased collagen formation. Stressed individuals may also have a low self-concept and neglect to take care of their skin

Maintaining body temperature

Ill children may have a pyrexia which interferes with their usual ability to be alert and active. Pyrexia can be relieved simply by pharmacologic intervention or cooling measures such as minimal clothing and reducing the circulating air temperature. Cooling measures should not induce shivering as this is the body's compensatory mechanism and will increase metabolic requirements even further. Antipyretic drugs include paracetamol and non-steroidal anti-inflammatories such as ibuprofen. The child's temperature should be checked approximately half an hour after the administration of an antipyretic. Pyrexias are thought to be incidental in enhancing immunity and recovery from infection so treatment should be aimed at reducing the child's discomfort rather than the fever itself. Traditional methods of reducing fever such as tepid baths are now known to be infective and generally add to the child's discomfort (Newman, 1985).

Key points ➤

1. The children's nurse has to take on the role of surrogate carer when parents are unable to give their child the usual family care due to other commitments, the nature of the child's illness or the need for a break from the demanding hospital routine.

2. Providing family care as a surrogate carer requires the nurse to have an intimate knowledge of usual family routines.

3. The child's usual activities of normal living may need adaptation to be continued in hospital and to fit the child's altered abilities.

4. Children confined to bed are at risk from complications of immobility and their care needs to take the prevention of these into consideration.

COMMUNITY NURSING 11

INTRODUCTION

Nursing children at home is not a new concept. Before the industrial revolution sick children were cared for at home by their mothers or siblings and rich families employed a physician or nurse to care for the child in the home. It is only since the development of scientific medicine, and the emergence of the National Health Service (NHS) in 1948, that hospital care has become the accepted place for the sick. This shift to institutional care occurred in spite of evidence from psychologists and government recommendations that children may become traumatised by hospitalisation and are best nursed at home. It is only within the last 25 years that schemes have emerged to provide care and support in the community for ill children to avoid hospital admission or to shorten their hospital stay. However, the type and degree of specialist services to assist children to be nursed at home vary considerably throughout the country.

Activity

Find out what facilities there are in your area for nursing children at home.

BACKGROUND

It appears that in some areas of the UK, children's community care does not have a high priority in spite of the recognition by the government that children should be nursed at home whenever possible (RCN, 1994). This recognition largely developed from the work of psychologists who were able to demonstrate the adverse effects of hospitalisation for children. However, it must not be forgotten that long before this some doctors and nurses were aware that hospitalisation was inappropriate for some children. In 1909, Nichol reported on a day surgery scheme in Glasgow and suggested 'that with a mother of average intelligence and assisted by advice from the hospital sister, the child will fare better at home than in the hospital'. The following year, Boge recognised that the value of children's nurses in the community had not been fully realised and that some nurses could help 'people to keep crippled children at home'. However, wider recognition of the need to minimise hospitalisation for children did not occur until 1950s. In 1951, Bowlby identified that after admission to hospital young children suffered 'maternal deprivation' and as a result became depressed, withdrawn and failed to thrive. His findings were supported by Robertson and Robertson (1958). These findings initiated the Platt Committee's report (MoH, 1959) which recommended the creation of a specialist community nursing service for the home care of ill children to prevent or minimise the need for admission to hospital. Very few Health Authorities responded to this recommendation but specialist services were introduced in Rotherham (Gillet, 1954), Paddington (Lightwood, 1956), and Birmingham (Smellie, 1956). The children's community nurses (CCNs) involved mostly cared for children with infectious diseases (Whiting, 1994). This poor response needs to be considered alongside children's services generally in the 1950s. Most general hospitals did not have any registered sick children's nurses (RSCNs) and the concept of involving the family in care was largely unknown. Many of the hospitalised children at this time were admitted with complications following infectious diseases such as measles, chicken pox, whooping cough or tuberculosis (Conisbee, 1982), and parents were only allowed to visit twice weekly for 1 hour because of the fear of the spread of infection (Currie, 1982). Therefore, it is not surprising that many Health Authorities did not respond to the Platt Report.

From the 1960s the government began to emphasise the importance of community care generally (MoH, 1962). In 1971 they again specifically investigated children's community services and found them lacking. Further emphasis was placed on the importance of caring for children in their own homes (MoH, 1971). In 1976, the Court Report recommended the development of nursing advice and support for sick children in the community by child health nurses (DHSS, 1976a). Children were identified as a priority group and it was suggested that an increase in the provision of community and preventive care for children would reduce spending on acute and institutional care areas (DHSS, 1976b). However, major re-organisation of the Health Service was occurring at this time and was repeated in 1982. These changes in Health Service management resulted in Health Authorities being no longer obliged to have a senior nurse and medical officer responsible for child health (Graham, 1987). Some areas showed a decline in child care services because of the loss of such posts and the consequent lack of commitment to the care of children from the Health Authority. Children continued to be mainly nursed in hospital by general nurses.

CHILDREN'S COMMUNITY NURSING IN THE 1990s

In the 1990s government reports and policies continued to stress that children should only be admitted to hospital if their needs cannot be met at home or on a day care basis (DoH, 1991a; Audit Commission, 1993). In addition pressure groups campaigned for the expansion of children's community nursing services so that children could be nursed in their own homes (British Paediatric Association, 1991b; Caring for Children in the Health Service, 1993; Action for Sick Children, 1993).

None of these seem to have had much impact on the provision for community care for children in many areas. Some NHS Trusts employ a liaison health visitor who takes responsibility for informing the

The role of the children's community nurse

Neonatal care
- care of babies with home oxygen
- management of babies with physiological jaundice

Care of children with acute problems
- respiratory tract infections
- gastro-enteritis
- constipation

Post-operative care
- ear, nose and throat surgery
- wound dressings
- circumcisions
- hernia repairs

Follow-up and support following trauma
- fractures stabilised in plaster of Paris
- children discharged on traction

Support and teaching for families of children with long-term health problems
- chronic respiratory problems (asthma, cystic fibrosis)
- skin disorders (eczema, psoriasis)
- haemoglobinopathies (including administration of blood)
- alternative methods of feeding
- taking blood/administering IV medication from established lines
- peritoneal/haemo-dialysis

Care and support for families of terminally ill children
- cytotoxic therapy
- palliative care

community nurses and/or health visitors of all children discharged from hospital, all new births and all children seen in the Accident and Emergency unit. In these areas, any nursing care required at home is often performed by community nurses who are not RSCNs/RNs(child). Their job descriptions state that they will 'provide care for patients of all ages'. As Muller *et al.* (1992) indicate, the competence of these staff is not in question, but the inability to provide care by registered children's nurses does not give those children receiving care at home the same rights and specialist care that they can receive in hospital. It also does not meet the Court Report (1976) recommendations that paediatric skills and knowledge be applied in the care of all children whatever their age or disability and wherever they live. Fradd (1990) recognises that most general trained district nurses are not experienced in the care of sick children, are inappropriately equipped and may be frightened by this involvement. The Audit Commission (1993) discovered that many children have a prolonged period of hospitalisation if there is no specialised community care available. Certainly, children with asthma, diabetes and fractures, conditions which the Commission suggest could be mainly cared for at home with appropriate support, tend to stay in hospital for at least seven days in areas where there are no specialist community children's nurses (Kitchener, 1993).

In other areas there may only be one CCN who liaises directly with the wards and neonatal unit as well as receiving referrals from other clinical areas. These post-holders find it impossible to take on the responsibility of actual nursing care for a large number of acutely ill children and can only provide a Monday to Friday office hours service. Instead they teach the family and/or district nurses the necessary care and provide them with specialist support. They also provide liaison with school nurses and teachers. Patel (1990) agrees that one of the advantages of community care to the child is the ability to continue school. When Fradd (1990) set up a CCN service in Nottingham she quickly realised that one nurse could not cope with the workload but even this minimum service meets the needs of mothers as identified by McDonald (1988). Although a small study, this research discovered that over 50% of parents whose child had been discharged from hospital would have appreciated more support and information for care continuing at home. The Audit Commission (1993, page 54) reports similar responses; for instance, one parent in their survey stated: 'I was terrified of doing something wrong and could never have come out of hospital without the paediatric nurse'. A single CCN can enable children with asthma and fractures to go home earlier than similar children in areas where there is no CCN service.

Activity

Find out about the service for diabetic children in your area. Does it have the support and advice of a children's nurse?

It is interesting in view of the guidelines produced by the DoH (1991b) (supported by the Clothier Report, 1994) and the Audit Commission (1993), that the care of children should be by appropriately qualified staff, that the responsibility for the care of diabetic children is often passed to a general trained diabetic team who also do not have the resources to manage these children at home. Yet it is accepted that newly diagnosed diabetes is best managed in the child's home with sufficient help in the community (Swift *et al.*, 1993). It is important that these children are helped to 'develop as secure and stable young adults' without feeling that their diabetes will impair this. Thus help is best provided by a children's nurse (McEvilly, 1993).

THE ADVANTAGES AND DISADVANTAGES OF NURSING CHILDREN AT HOME

Activity

Is nursing children at home always beneficial? Consider if there are any disadvantages to this service and whether these drawbacks outweigh the benefits.

It should be appreciated that home care may cause problems for some children and their families (Table 11.1). Although children who have day care avoid the traumatic effects of hospitalisation (Visintainer and Wolfer, 1975), they can become fearful at home if their parents are anxious about home care and are not confident in their own caring abilities (Glasper *et al.*, 1989). There is evidence that parents can cope better with children's impending death if they can care for them at home, but not all parents feel able to take on this responsibility (Sidey, 1990). Siblings of children cared for at home sometimes suffer as a result of reduced attention to their needs (Bluebond-Langer, 1989). Although these problems cannot be ignored, they can be overcome by the careful assessment of families before discharge by an experienced

Table 11.1

Advantages and disadvantages of home care

Advantages	Disadvantages
Child feels safe in familiar environment	May associate parts of home with painful procedures
Reduced risk of cross infection in own home	Home may not be suitable for aseptic procedures
Parents may feel more in control	Nurse must respect family values
Nurse has fewer distractions than in a busy ward	Parents may feel unsupported when nurse not there
Nurse able to know child and family better as individuals	Nurse may find the closer relationship stressful
Increased bed availability in hospital	Increased patient dependency in hospital wards
Nurse has more autonomy in care	Nurse may feel unsupported by colleagues

children's nurse. A CCN, who will be used to working in partnership with parents, can also be alert for signs that home care is becoming too stressful for the family.

Although there is little research to show the benefits of a CCN service, Stein and Jessop (1984) found that home care for children with chronic illness was effective in improving the satisfaction of the family with care and the child's psychological adjustment. It also reduced maternal stress. However, this was an American study which may not compare with health care in this country. The researchers also used lay interviewers who may have unknowingly confounded the results. In 1985, Atwell and Gow found that the CCN service in Southampton reduced patient stay by 3.2 days, increased patient turnover, reduced waiting lists and saved 215 000 a year. However, Catchpole (1986) and Whiting (1989) found that the majority of districts without a CCN service cited finance as the main reason for this. This is perhaps more likely to be overcome as chief executives are now striving to gain contracts and meet the aims of the patients charter.

THE ROLE OF THE COMMUNITY CHILDREN'S NURSE

The aims of many community children's services include parental support, and the avoidance of hospitalisation for children by preventing admission or enabling early discharge. The early services were set up to provide community care for children with acute illnesses who would otherwise be admitted to hospital. However, the number of children now being discharged from hospital with long-term needs is increasing, and their care and support is beginning to form a considerable portion of the CCN's caseload. As a result the care of acutely ill children at home is decreasing. In 1954, the first recorded RSCNs were appointed to care for children in the community and the Paddington Home Care Unit was established. At this time GP referrals formed 60% of the caseload. In 1994, this proportion had decreased to six referrals per year. In response to this trend, Hospital at Home schemes have developed. These schemes provide an integrated service between hospital and home. Nurses rotate from ward to community, enabling them to transfer their skills in acute care to the child's home whilst helping them to appreciate discharge planning when working in the ward area. The child and family are visited by the nurse whilst still in hospital and they remain in the care of this nurse and the hospital consultant until discharged from the scheme.

Since the growth of the children's community nursing service the question of specific preparation for CCNs has arisen. Whilst all CCNs are registered children's nurses many of them do not have a specific children's community nursing qualification. Some services make the community nursing course an essential pre-requisite for applicants. The validity of this course as a means of preparation for a CCN has been debated, as the theory and practice relate mostly to adult nursing with the emphasis on the care of the elderly (Godman, 1994). However, at present, there are still very few courses specifically designed for the CCN. As the present RN(child) course prepares the nurse to work in hospital and community settings, it may be argued that such preparation is not necessary.

THE FUTURE?

Cross reference

The future of children's nursing – page 635

Campbell (1987) suggests that the reason that community services for children vary across the country is that local services develop to meet local need. This does not appear so in some areas where there is such a large child population and a known increase in childhood diabetes, asthma and accidents (Kitchener, 1993). This may be because the needs of children in such regions have not been specifically identified. There may be no senior nurse to provide a focus for children's services as recommended by the Audit Commission (1993) and, apart from childhood accidents, public health reports often do not relate to children specifically. This is in spite of the opening statement of the Court Report: 'We want to see a child and family-centred service'. This omission may be because the local health plans are based on the government's *Health for All* targets which also do not specifically relate to children. It may be that children's nurses have not been proactive enough to promote the advantages of their unique skills and to actively support these recommendations.

Activity

Take time to discuss with others the possible reasons government policies such as this do not recognise previous recommendations.

In 1996, the government began to discuss increasing GP services and the re-introduction of GP-led 'cottage' hospitals where GPs would care for patients with short-term problems and perform minor surgery. This could result in further changes in the admission of children to hospital and the role of the CCN.

SUMMARY

It seems likely that nursing children in the community will continue to be a developing service. It not only meets parents' and children's wishes but relieves the pressure on hospital beds. However, as more children are nursed at home there is a great need for more specialised support for the parents. They need specialised nursing support as well as a respite service to enable them to spend uninterrupted time with the rest of the family. To meet this need more community nursing programmes are required for children's nurses and all community nurses need to emphasise the importance of having the specific community nursing preparation for caring for their own client group. In this way these nurses can recognise and act as advocates for their client group in urging for other forms of support in the community.

1. The provision of community children's care in many areas is still poor. There has been little recognition of government reports which recommend such services and there is no senior children's nurse to promote the development of the services.

2. The type of service available to provide care for children at home is very variable across the UK.

3. The role of the CCN is varied and has changed over time to meet the changing health needs of the population.

4. There needs to be more research into the benefits and drawbacks of home care for children.

5. Children's nurses need to be more assertive and active in trying to establish and maintain recommended standards of care for children. They need to promote their specialist knowledge and skills so that they are accepted as the specialists in child care.

12 PRE- AND POST-OPERATIVE CARE
Tina Moules

INTRODUCTION

Caring for children undergoing surgery requires expertise to ensure that the experience is as positive as it can be. Hospitalisation can be traumatic for any child but the added stress of surgery may cause considerable anxiety for the child and his carers. Personal experience has shown that even minor surgery can be distressing to a parent who for a period of time has no control at all over what happens to their child. It is vital, therefore, that the surgical experience is managed effectively and with a degree of empathy in order to achieve a successful outcome.

Activity

Critically reflect on experiences that you may have had – perhaps you had surgery as a child – perhaps you have a child who has required surgery at some time. Were the experiences positive ones? What were the negative aspects (if any)?

The nurse's role before and after surgery is to ensure that:
- the child and family are helped to cope with the experience in a positive manner;
- the child is adequately prepared physically;
- the child's safety is not compromised;
- the likelihood of post-operative complications is minimised and the child's recovery is uneventful;
- the child and family are adequately prepared for discharge home.

Surgical interventions can be divided into two groups:
- *Planned or elective procedures.* In this case surgery can take place when the child is in the best possible condition physically. Much of the preparation can take place before admission and the child and his carers can be given opportunity to come to terms with the forthcoming surgery. Children can be admitted in good time to allow physical preparation to be carried out. Admission to hospital can sometimes be arranged on a day care basis so that the effects of hospital are minimised. However, even planned short-stay surgery can cause distress and anxiety and so care must be implemented accordingly.
- *Emergency or unplanned procedures.* Emergency surgery is carried out when the severity of the child's condition may be life threatening

Examples of procedures which may be done on an elective basis
- Adenotonsillectomy
- Insertion of grommets
- Correction of squint
- Circumcision
- Correction of orthopaedic deformities
- Some heart surgery
- Orcidopexy
- Dental extractions

Cross reference

Day care – page 286

or disabling. In these cases preparation time is much reduced for the child and his carers who have to cope not only with sudden illness or trauma but also the uncertainty of emergency surgery. It is important therefore to ensure that all essential preparation is done and that the child and carers are given sufficient information on which to base any decisions. This can be a difficult time and decisions may have to be taken quickly. You should ensure that carers are given support and someone to talk to especially while the child is in theatre.

Activity

Try to put yourself in the following situation (if possible try role playing it with some colleagues – use any experiences that you have had to help you). Make a list of all the feelings you might have and consider what support you would like. You are the young parent of a 4-year-old daughter, Sarah, who has been admitted following a road traffic accident in which she was knocked over by a speeding car. The driver of the car is suspected of being under the influence of alcohol. Sarah is your only child and she requires emergency life-saving surgery within the next 2 hours. Your partner is working away from home and will not be with you until the next day.

Whether surgery is planned or not, you must endeavour to ensure that the child and family are helped to cope with the experience of surgery in the best way possible. Activities to achieve this may include the following:

- Arrange to talk to groups of young children in a variety of settings (e.g. play groups and schools) about hospital and surgery. Preparing children in this way can promote understanding of hospitals and help to dispel misconceptions. Rodin (1983) found that children who had this sort of preparation and who were subsequently admitted to hospital were less anxious and more cooperative than other children.

- Ensure that preparation is geared towards the child's cognitive and emotional level. Using inappropriate words can cause more distress than they are meant to alleviate. Young children think literally and those under 7 may take analogies literally.

Activity

Consider how a young child might interpret the following – in each case think of a more appropriate way to explain: (a) 'I am just going to suck out your mouth to take away all the spit', (b) 'I am going to take your blood pressure', (c) 'Your lungs are like balloons' and (d) 'Your heart is like a pump'.

- Organise 'Saturday Clubs' or pre-admission sessions – many wards and units have set these up as a way of preparing groups of children for planned surgery.

Examples of procedures which may be done on an emergency basis

Appendicectomy

Some neurosurgery

Hernias

Pyloric stenosis

Stabilisation of fractures

Surgery for abdominal trauma

Cross references

Language development – page 77

Preparation for procedures – page 267

Day care – page 286

Further reading
OSTER, G. D. and GOULD, P.
(1987) *Using Drawings in Assessment and Therapy*. New York: Brunner/Mazel.

Factors influencing body image
These factors include:
- social class
- skin colour
- culture
- physical attractiveness
- weight and height
- speech
- puberty
- congenital abnormalities
- learning disability
- life-limiting illness
- chronic illness
- physical disability

(White, 1995)

Cross references
Anaesthesia – page 292

Weighing babies and children – page 282

- Encourage children to draw in the pre-operative period. O'Malley and McNamara (1993; see also Oster and Gould, 1987) describe the use of drawing as a means of assessing children's understanding of forthcoming surgery and of highlighting their fears and anxieties. Drawing allows children to express feelings and ideas. Artwork can reveal concerns such as loss of control, body changes and mutilation. Personal use of this technique demonstrated how effective this can be. A young boy had been admitted to my ward for tonsillectomy. His mother was unable to stay and after she left he became withdrawn and displayed signs of extreme anxiety. He would talk to no one and concerns about his psychological state prompted the Sister to ask for help from the psychologist. She asked the boy to draw a picture of himself after surgery – his picture showed himself with only one leg. On further investigation it was discovered that the boy's uncle had recently been in hospital for amputation of his leg. The boy was under the misconception that his surgery would be the same – his fears were allayed.

Activity

Try this technique out on some children waiting for surgery. What do their pictures tell you?

- Consider the possible effect surgery may have on the child's body image (for example plastic surgery, stoma formation, limb surgery). Art therapy may highlight any fears that the child may have. Many factors influence a child's perception of their body image. A concern with appearance is part of physical development (particularly during adolescence) and therefore the implications of surgery need to be discussed. Often a child's fears can be allayed through detailed explanation. Where physical deformity is a likely outcome of surgery time must be made to ensure counselling from specialist nurses (e.g. the stoma nurse).
- Encourage the presence of parents in the anaesthetic and recovery rooms where appropriate.

PREPARING CHILDREN PHYSICALLY FOR SURGERY

The aim of pre-operative preparation is to ensure that the child is well enough for surgery and to obtain relevant information in order to plan and implement care appropriately. A general assessment should be done and the following specific interventions carried out:

- Accurate weight – the dosage of anaesthetic drugs are generally calculated according to the child's weight. The importance of this cannot be stressed enough. The child should be weighed wearing the minimum of clothing and in some units the weight must be checked by two people (check your hospital policy on weighing children). The weight should be prominently displayed on the relevant documentation.

- Urine test – a routine urine analysis should be carried out on all children having surgery. Testing the urine will identify children who may have undiagnosed renal disease or diabetes.

- A discussion about pain control – prior to surgery it is useful to discuss pain with the child and his carers.

- Ensure that consent for surgery has been given and that the consent form is attached to the child's notes. Whilst this is the responsibility of the surgeon the nurse should check that the parents and child have been fully informed and that all relevant information regarding surgery has been explained. Where possible it is advisable for a nurse to be present when consent is gained to ensure misconceptions are avoided.

- Implement pre-operative fasting – children who are 'nil by mouth' must be clearly identified.

- Administration of pre-medication – prior to giving the pre-med it is useful to encourage the child to visit the toilet to pass urine. This enables the last passage of urine prior to surgery to be noted and reduces the need for the sedated child to be disturbed.

Cross references

Urine testing – pages 477–478

Caring for children in pain – page 348

Informed consent – pages 651–660

Restricted intake – page 340

Pre-medication – page 290

Activity

Investigate the pre-medication protocol in your children's surgical unit. Discuss with the anaesthetist.

- Children from certain ethnic groups (Asian, North African, Mediterranean and Afro-Caribbean origins) will require assessment of sickle cell or thalassaemia status. Surgery on a child with an undiagnosed abnormality may provoke a crisis.

Cross reference

Sickle cell crisis – page 421

SAFETY OF THE CHILD

To ensure that the child's safety is not compromised you should take the following actions:

- Check all notes and other relevant documentation are in order.
- Ensure that the child is wearing a correct identification band.
- Ensure that the child removes all jewellery – diathermy is used to cauterise blood vessels during surgery and any contact with metal objects can cause diathermy burns.
- Ensure that the child is not wearing any make up or nail varnish – this is so that the child's skin and nailbeds can be monitored for signs of hypoxia during surgery.
- Check for loose teeth and make appropriate note on child's records. Loose teeth can become dislodged during intubation.

- Ensure that the child is transferred safely to and from theatre.
- Ensure that the child's condition is stable before leaving the recovery area. It is the anaesthetist's responsibility to ensure that full recovery is assured (Simpson, 1977). This responsibility can be delegated to the nurse in recovery providing that proper training has been given. It is therefore important that the nurse collecting the child from theatre checks all aspects of the child's surgery and recovery before taking the responsibility of escorting the child back to the ward. If you are in doubt you should ask for the child to be checked by the anaesthetist.
- Prepare for the child's return to the ward – prepare the bed area – oxygen and suction equipment should be close by along with any other specific equipment.
- Implement post-operative care

POST-OPERATIVE CARE

The purpose of care during this period is to monitor the child's recovery and detect signs of any complications. The frequency of observations will depend on the child's general condition and will be decreased or increased accordingly. The observations made post-operatively can help to detect complications.

Potential hypoventilation and asphyxia

Hypoventilation is common in the immediate post-operative period and can lead to serious respiratory complications (hypoxaemia, hypercarbia, collapsed segment of the lung, pneumonia). Hypoventilation can occur as a result of (Watson, 1979):

- central nervous depression by anaesthetic agents;
- respiratory muscle depression by muscle relaxant;
- partial airway obstruction by tongue or lower jaw;
- laryngeal oedema following endotracheal intubation.

Observe the child for signs of hypoventilation which include: abnormally slow or shallow respirations, excessive secretions, wheezing; restlessness, cyanosis and rapid pulse rate.

Asphyxia can occur if the relaxed tongue and lower jaw 'fall back' blocking the pharynx or following aspiration of mucus and vomit which can occur due to loss of the swallowing reflex. Measures should be taken to promote adequate ventilation as follows:

- The child should be nursed in the lateral or semi-prone position until a gag reflex is well established. If necessary the position can be maintained by the use of pillows.
- Remove excessive secretions as necessary using pharyngeal suction.
- Administer oxygen by nasal cannulae or mask as directed.

- Once recovered encourage deep breathing and coughing to remove secretions and expand lungs and assist to the sitting position. Small children will assume the most comfortable position for themselves which often means lying flat. In this instance therapy from the physiotherapist may be required.

Shock

Shock is defined as circulatory failure which leads to inadequate perfusion of body tissues and organs. It can develop immediately after surgery or slowly becoming evident several hours after surgery. It is important that signs of shock are identified early so that treatment can be implemented. One of the most important observations to make is that of the general appearance of the child. Often a child will 'look bad' before there are any measurable changes in vital signs. A child who is in shock will have pale mucus membranes, mottled cold extremities, irritability then lethargy. Other signs include weak thready rapid pulse (bradycardia is a dangerous sign and should be reported immediately), tachypnoea and temperature instability. Hypotension is a late sign of shock in children. Report any signs of shock promptly. Support a child who is shocked by keeping the surroundings calm, treat pain (which reduces the demand for oxygen), keep the child warm and administer oxygen as needed.

Types of shock

- *Hypovolaemic* – 'a compromise in systemic perfusion resulting from inadequate intravascular volume relative to the vascular space'.
- *Cardiogenic* – caused by impaired myocardial function which compromises cardiac output.
- *Septic* – that which occurs 'when an infectious organism triggers a host response which compromises cardiovascular function, systemic perfusion and oxygen delivery and use'.

(Hazinski, 1992).

Haemorrhage

Haemorrhage following surgery (reactionary) may occur as a result of a slipped ligature or an increase in blood pressure which dislodges a clot that plugged a severed vessel. Haemorrhage may be visible at the wound site or may be internal in which case it can only be recognised by a change in vital signs. These include rapid thready pulse, fall in blood pressure (a late sign in children), rapid respirations, pallor, apprehension, restlessness and weakness. Report any suspicion of haemorrhage promptly. Secondary haemorrhage can occur several days or weeks after surgery and parents should always be warned of this and given information as to what action to take.

Nausea and vomiting

Post-operative nausea and vomiting (PONV) is an important complication of surgery in children. Many of the common surgical procedures in childhood are associated with a high incidence of PONV (Patel *et al.*, 1995). The highest incidence occurs in the 5–12 age group. Factors affecting the degree of PONV include the type of surgery, history of motion sickness, excessive pre-operative fasting, anaesthetic technique used, too rapid mobilisation after surgery (stimulates the vestibular system which may have been desensitised by opioids – White *et al.*, 1988) and early oral intake after surgery. Nursing actions should therefore be implemented to take account of these factors. Any nausea or vomiting should be reported immediately so that treatment with an anti-emetic can be implemented.

Urine retention

Urine output may be reduced due to the effects of anaesthetic gases. This can be complicated by the stress response to surgery which increases ADH from the anterior pituitary which in turn acts on renal tubules increasing permeability and reducing/preventing the excretion of water. The child's urine output must be monitored and the first passage of urine following surgery noted. Normal excretion is considered to be 0.5–1.0 ml/kg/hour. Anything less than this should be reported. Anxiety, fear of pain and/or recumbent position can all contribute to urine retention. Therefore actions can be taken to reduce all of these to encourage the child to pass urine. One favourite trick is to take the child to the bathroom and run the tap – try it yourself!

Wound complications – infection, dehiscence

Surgical wounds in children rarely become infected (Foale, 1989) and are commonly closed using dissolvable sutures. However, it is important to be vigilant for signs of wound infection which include redness, swelling, pain at site and, oozing. Any suspicion of infection should be reported and a wound swab taken. Dressings, where they are used, need to be changed using aseptic technique to avoid introducing infection. When changing dressings the nurse may have to utilise distractive techniques to avoid the child interfering with the procedure. The use of play and music is useful as is the assistance of another person. Where possible encourage children not to explore underneath the dressing. This can be made harder to do if the dressing is taped all round with appropriate tape. A variety of dressings and cleansing agents are available and their use will depend on the type of wound and local policy.

Activity

Critically explore your local policy on wound care and the use of particular types of dressing.

It is common for many surgical wounds to be left uncovered after the first 48 hours. The use of leeches is becoming more common, particularly in the management of reconstructive surgical wounds and in plastic surgery. Godfrey (1997) suggests that children take to the use of leeches quite readily whilst the parents need a little more persuasion.

Wound breakdown (dehiscence) can occur as a result of infection, excessive coughing and general debilitation. Immediate action should be taken and the wound covered with a sterile pad. Resuturing is usually carried out.

Pain

The child should be monitored using an appropriate pain assessment tool and nursing actions implemented accordingly.

Stages of wound healing

- *Inflammatory stage* – initial bleeding when incision made stops after diathermy and during the clotting phase. Vasodilation and oedema result

- *Destructive stage* – polymorphs and macrophages clear dead tissue and debris. The formation of fibroblasts stimulates angiogenesis. This stage can be delayed by vitamin C, iron or oxygen deficiency

- *Proliferative stage* – fibroblasts produce collagen to promote tensile strength of the wound

- *Maturation stage* – wound contracts, collagen fibres reorganised, tensile strength gradually returns

(Galvani, 1997)

Wound cleansing agents

- Tap water (Angeras et al., 1992)
- Saline
- Antiseptics

Cross references

Caring for children in pain – page 348

Relieving pain – pages 356–359

Other

Other care which may need to be considered includes:

* management of fluid balance;
* mobilisation/physiotherapy.

Activity

Critically reflect on a child you have nursed following surgery. Which of any of the above complications occurred? What actions were taken ? Do the same activity with children of differing age groups. Make notes of any research-based care which was implemented.

PLANNING FOR DISCHARGE

The aim of care is for the child to be discharged home as soon as possible following surgery. This has implications for the family and any decisions must be made with their full cooperation.

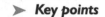

> **Key points**

1. The role of the nurse before and after surgery is vital to ensure optimum recovery.
2. Care of the child and family must be adapted to suit the needs of children undergoing planned or emergency procedures.
3. The safety of the child must not be compromised.
4. The nurse must understand the potential complications of surgery and the management, therefore, to promote uneventful recovery.

Dressings

According to Turner (1985) dressings should have the following characteristics to promote optimum healing – they should:

* maintain a high humidity between the wound and the dressing
* remove excess exudate and toxic compounds
* allow gaseous exchange
* provide thermal insulation to wound surface
* be impermeable to bacteria
* be free from particles and toxic wound contaminants
* allow removal without causing trauma

Cross references

Discharge home – page 293

Management of fluid balance – page 339

Leeches

Leeches are parasites that feed on the blood of mammals. The leech breaks the skin by sawing through it with minute teeth and then attaches itself with a sucker. The leech secretes a local anaesthetic (to avoid detection by the host) and an anticoagulant (to keep blood running freely so that it can feed efficiently). The blood sucking power of the leech is used to relieve venous congestion which can cause delicate tissues to die.

(Godfrey, 1997)

13 ASPECTS OF PAEDIATRIC INTENSIVE CARE

INTRODUCTION

Because of the relatively small number of paediatric intensive care beds in the UK many critically ill children undergo treatment in general intensive care units which cater predominately for adults. In these units children may be nursed in an open area alongside adults undergoing intensive care. Alternatively, critically ill children may be nursed in part of a general children's ward. Neither arrangement is satisfactory and both have serious disadvantages. Firstly, staff involved in the care of these children may not have sufficient experience or education of paediatric intensive care, and this cannot merely be extrapolated from the knowledge of the care of critically ill adults or the care of less acutely ill children. Secondly, equipment for monitoring and treating children may be inadequate, and because children's wards are often located some distance from the main hospital facilities, specialist assistance in an emergency may not be immediately available. Thirdly, critically ill children need unrestricted access and visiting from their family and this may not be possible or appropriate in an adult intensive care unit.

In 1991 the British Paediatric Association (BPA) set up a working party to conduct a national survey into hospital in-patient and intensive care services for children in the UK. The BPA drew attention to the lack of available information on the numbers of critically ill children, referral patterns, illness severity measures and outcomes, but concluded that the:

- great majority of adult intensive care units were clearly neither staffed nor equipped to care adequately for critically ill children;
- availability and staffing of facilities for children's intensive care were severely deficient;
- provision of paediatric intensive care varied widely between regions;
- area of major deficiency was the provision of facilities to transport sick children;
- provision of intensive care on children's wards was a most unsatisfactory standard of care.

As a result of the survey the BPA recommended that:

- virtually all critically ill children should be cared for in a designated paediatric intensive care unit (PICU);
- there should be regional networks of PICUs with adequate facilities for the safe transfer of critically ill children;
- a national initiative should develop PICU services;
- a national mechanism be established to collect information about the need for and the provision of PICU beds.

THE DEMAND FOR PAEDIATRIC INTENSIVE CARE

The BPA (1993) estimated the need for PICU beds as 1:48 000 children but it also recognised that seasonal variations may increase this demand in the winter months to 1:26 000 children. In 1993 it estimated that the national shortfall was at least 72 beds.

Activity

Find out the child population in your own county and use this figure to calculate the county's need for PICU beds.

Activity

Take a critical look at your local provision for the care of acutely ill children and consider if it is sufficient and whether it meets the BPA (1993) recommendations.

In the winter of 1996/7 the media highlighted a number of disturbing cases of severely ill children being transported long distances in the search for a PICU bed. As a result of this growing problem, government ministers agreed to provide additional funds of some £5 million to help maintain momentum on improvements to PIC in 1997/8. These funds were designated according to the main priorities:

- recruitment and training of nurses with specialist PIC skills;
- recruitment and training of medical staff with specialist PIC skills;
- enhancing retrieval services;
- opening new beds in lead centres to allow care to be moved out of inappropriate areas (e.g. general children's wards).

However, 1997 research appears to indicate that other factors are involved in the lack of PICU beds. Fraser *et al.* (1997) questioned all PICUs in England and Scotland and discovered that children requiring long-term ventilation were occupying 12% of the available beds. During the 3 month period of the study 267 critically ill children were refused admission to these units because no beds were free and the authors estimate that an additional 273 beds could have been available if these children could have been cared for more appropriately. They suggest that prioritisation be given to:

- enabling children requiring long-term ventilation to be cared for at home or at their local hospital;
- providing community rehabilitation centres or hospital long-term ventilation units for children;
- clarification about which authority has the financial responsibility for

Definitions of levels of high dependency and intensive care

- *High dependency care (Level 1).* Those children needing close monitoring and observation, but not requiring assistance form life-support machines. For example, the recently extubated child; the child undergoing close post-operative supervision with ECG, oxygen saturation or respiratory monitoring and who may be receiving supplementary oxygen and intravenous fluids or parenteral nutrition. *This level of care requires a nurse to child ratio of at least 0.5:1*
- *Intensive care (Level 2).* The child requiring continuous nursing supervision who is intubated and is undergoing intermittent positive pressure ventilation or continuous positive airways pressure. Some non-intubated children may also fall into this category if their airway is unstable. For example, the child with acute upper airway obstruction requiring nebulised adrenaline. *Requires a nurse to child ratio of at least 1:1*
- *Intensive care (Level 3).* The child who needs intensive supervision at all times requiring additional complex and regular nursing and therapeutic procedures. This would include ventilated children undergoing peritoneal dialysis or receiving intravenous infusions of vaso-active drugs or inotropes, and children with multiple organ failure. *Requires a nurse to child ratio of at least 1.5:1*

(BPA, 1993)

Cross reference
Resources and rationing – page 679

such children, thus enabling funds for alternative care arrangements to be readily available.

INTERHOSPITAL TRANSFERS

One of the BPA's 1993 recommendations was that the care of critically ill children should be centred around designated PICUs. The NHS criticised the BPA for basing their recommendations on opinion rather than evidence but two independent reviews commissioned by them agreed on the need for severely ill children to be cared for in dedicated PICUs (De Courcey-Golder, 1996). The centralisation of PICUs increases the need for acutely ill children to be transported long distances to access these services.

Barry and Ralston (1994) indicated the dangers of non-specialised transfers of critically ill children between hospitals. Their study, undertaken at Birmingham Children's Hospital, indicated that almost 75% children who were transferred suffered serious complications, with nearly 25% of these adverse events defined as life threatening. On arrival at the referral unit 11% of children needed immediate intubation and 9% were hypotensive. In most of these children monitoring of vital signs was not possible during transfer. Kanter and Tompkins (1993) estimated that at least 10% of episodes of physiological deterioration and adverse events were related to the lack of monitoring equipment during transportation.

In 1991 about 33% of PICUs provided specialised retrieval services (BPA, 1993). A study by Britto et al. (1995) of 51 critically ill children transferred from hospitals in and around the London area to a PICU at a tertiary centre concluded that a specialist retrieval team could rapidly deliver intensive care to children awaiting transfer. They can also transfer these children to PICU with minimal morbidity and mortality. This opinion is supported by Edge et al. (1994) and Logan (1995), although Logan (1995) recommends careful costing and evaluation of newly established retrieval teams to ensure a more evidence-based approach for future developments.

The provision of an effective retrieval team relies upon the availability of appropriate transport to transfer the PICU team to the referring hospital as well as returning the team and the child. It also requires a specifically trained transport team which usually consists of a senior registrar and senior intensive care nurse. Kelly et al. (1996) emphasise the importance of communication between the referral hospital, PICU and the retrieval team and recommend the use of a portable telephone to enable the retrieval team to remain in contact with the referring hospital and PICU throughout the transfer. A dedicated retrieval team requires preparation and training. After the initial training an in-house education programme can continue to train and update staff and provide opportunities for other staff to accompany the team to gain supervised experience.

THE PICU ENVIRONMENT

Children over 4 weeks requiring intensive care in a general hospital are often admitted to adult intensive care units (Audit Commission, 1993). Although there is no evidence from UK studies about the efficacy of such care, studies from the USA suggest that survival rates may be four times higher in a tertiary unit (Pollack *et al.*, 1991). This, with other evidence discussed above, seems likely to perpetuate the concept of centralisation of PICUs. Although centralisation has disadvantages of cost and travel it is probably the most realistic option given the limited specialist resources available. Centralisation also meets the needs of the two key principles in the care of children endorsed by government guidelines (DoH, 1991b, 1995):

- infants, children and young adults have a right to safe and competent care, especially when they are critically ill and requiring intensive care;
- sick children have a right to be cared for by appropriately qualified nurses.

Who can provide safe and competent nursing care for children requiring intensive care? Atkinson *et al.* (1996) argue that critically ill children are not just biophysical beings requiring a high degree of technical care. They believe that registered children's nurses are essential for the care of these children who, more than ever, need their carers to recognise their unique developmental needs as children. The Audit Commission (1993) highlighted the importance of the play therapist who can help the child to overcome the stresses of hospitalisation. The play therapist is therefore of particular importance in the PICU. Children who are in adult intensive units often do not have children's nurses or play staff available to them.

PICUs are busy, clinical environments which are stressful for the children, and their families. Parents often find their altered parental role as well as their children's behavioural and emotional responses the most stressful aspects (Miles and Manthes, 1991). Children's stressors in the PICU environment vary according to their developmental age but a high level of parental anxiety will lead to a high level of anxiety in the child, whatever their age group. Hughes *et al.* (1995) advocates asking parents what they find most stressful and then helping them to cope with these specific stressors rather than presuming all parents have the same perceptions.

When a stay in PICU is anticipated, such as after major surgery, the parents and child can be prepared for the experience.

Activity

Arrange to visit your local intensive care unit and consider the impression such a unit might make upon parents who have never visited such an area. How could you prepare them for the unfamiliar sights and sounds? Consider if the area is child friendly and the possible changes you could make to enhance this aspect.

The PICU provides a physical environment of constant noise, light and activity (Redman, 1994). Weibley (1989) compares noise in a intensive care unit from rubbish bins, monitor alarms, telephones and staff voices with that of road traffic and industrial machinery. My personal recollection of my first 2 days working in a PICU is hearing monitor alarms constantly, even when off duty! Extensive and continuous monitoring makes it difficult to differentiate between day and night. As a result, the child's usual waking and sleeping routine is destroyed by constant noise, light and/or stimulation. Movement and positioning are likely to cause pain and discomfort to children attached to ventilator circuits and multiple lines. Such intensive care is known to cause pain in adults (Calne, 1994) and, as suggested by Whaley and Wong (1995, page 1088) 'what causes pain to adults will cause pain to children unless proven otherwise'. Whilst frequent handling of critically ill children can increase stress and cause abrupt changes in arterial blood pressure, therapeutic touch can aid relaxation. Weibley (1989) advocates the use of stroking, cuddling and gentle touch which also provides the most fundamental form of communication.

Lack of meaningful stimuli causes sensory deprivation and enhances the stress of an intensive care environment. Psychological stress can lead to physiological complications and impair growth and development (Mann *et al.*, 1986). In addition, constant light for infants in an intensive care environment may disturb the development of circadian rhythms and result in poor nocturnal sleep patterns in childhood.

Supporting the family

- Provide encouragement to continue their important role in the child's life
- Assist them to participate in their child's care
- Encourage them to teach the staff about their child's individual needs and behaviour
- Share all information
- Ensure explanations are consistent and recognise the need to repeat these
- Stress the importance to their child of a familiar touch and voice
- Help them to understand the important issues necessary to make informed decisions
- Recognise signs of stress and exhaustion
- Help them to feel able to take a break and remind them of their need for food, drink and rest

Activity

Consider how these PICU stimuli can be reduced and the child's usual routine enhanced whilst maintaining the child's safety and care.

In recognising the adverse effects of PICU, Weibley (1989) identified factors which would provide a 'growth enhancing critical care unit'. White (1997) introduced the use of snoezelen as a relaxation technique within the PICU environment. Snoezelen incorporates the use of sight, hearing, touch and smell to provide gentle stimulation which leads to relaxation. White (1997) suggests that this technique can involve the whole family and enable them to relax, reduce feelings of helplessness and humanise intensive care.

FAMILY SUPPORT

Parents can feel confused, anxious and bewildered about what is happening to their child in PICU. It is vital that staff recognise this and help them to interact and care for their child. If parents do not have this opportunity, problems such as inadequate parenting and family breakdown can occur (Shellabarger and Thompson, 1993). Continuity of carers is useful for parents who are then able to gain confidence and trust in a consistent approach. Weibley (1989) suggests that primary nursing is crucial in optimising individualised family care in a critical care environment.

Parents should be encouraged to stay with their child in the PICU to provide the child with the comfort and security of their presence. Despite this beneficial effect, the nurse should not forget the stresses of the critical care environment and the constant anxiety that parents feel when their child is critically ill. Sometimes parents become exhausted by their constant vigil and the sensitive nurse needs to recognise this and suggest periodic respites. Darbyshire (1994, page 99) describes this vigil as a way of parents 'dwelling attentively and receptively with their child' which gives some indication of the fatigue caused by such watchfulness.

Siblings should not be forgotten. Siblings provide each other with companionship and emotional support and the loss of these can make hospitalisation for a critical illness particularly stressful for the well sibling. Simon (1993) advocates early visiting by siblings to prevent the well sibling from imagining and magnifying fears. However, Morrison (1997) found that siblings who visited most frequently demonstrated the most stress. It would appear that this issue is best discussed and explained carefully to siblings and parents to enable them to make an informed decision. Then the timing and length of sibling visits can be well prepared and planned in advance.

The family and child can experience further stress when the time comes for transfer back to the general ward. They have gained confidence and trust in the close monitoring strategy within the PICU environment and the 1:1 nursing they have received. The sudden loss of this intensive care can make them feel very insecure. Transfers should be carefully planned to ensure that they continue to feel that their child is receiving appropriate care for this next stage of the health problem.

Activity

Prepare a plan to transfer a school-aged child and family from a central PICU back to the general paediatric ward of their local hospital.

SUPPORTING THE STAFF

Staff in an intensive care environment are subject to many stresses which can be overcome by a supportive relationship with other staff members. Foxall *et al.* (1990) found that intensive care nurses were most likely to be stressed by death and dying than the work-overload stress of nurses working in general wards. Benner and Wrubel (1989) recognise the temporary benefit of laughter and detachment for ICU staff in overcoming their stress but suggest that acknowledgement of the stress

The growth-enhancing critical care unit

The PICU which avoids stress and enhances the growth of the children is that in which staff:

- provide care, concern and gentleness
- give psychological care the same priority as physical care
- make the unique needs of children and families the focus of attention
- organise care and procedures with consideration of the child's needs
- address the child and family by name
- are constantly alert for features of distress and provide relief
- comfort and reassure the children with touch and positive contact to counterbalance the unpleasant treatments
- teach and help the child to use positive coping strategies
- acknowledge the child as an individual and include the child in age-appropriate conversation
- make full use of toys and play and encourage parents to bring in the child's favourite objects from home
- make parents welcome and rarely ask them to leave their child's bedside
- never leave a dying child alone

(Weibley, 1989)

Providing play in PICUs

- Low volume, low pitch music is relaxing
- Make use of familiar toys and comforters from home
- Audio cassettes of familiar voices or songs can be comforting and provide security
- Make use of all the senses to stimulate play – rotating mirrors, familiar perfumes, different fabrics
- Allot a specific time for play
- Use the expertise of hospital play therapists to create a plan of play
- As the child improves encourage them to initiate play

Stresses for PICU nurses

Ethical dilemmas

- withdrawal of life support
- use of technology for severely injured children
- conflicts between family and staff values
- scarcity of resources

Death and dying

- supporting the family
- organ donation
- personal feelings

Interpersonal relationships

- conflict with medical opinion
- lack of positive feedback from senior staff
- difficulty in relationships with parents

and support from one's colleagues are a much more effective long-term strategy. Support groups can help this sharing of feelings and encourage communication between the multidisciplinary team.

➤ Key points

1. Critically ill children should be nursed by registered children's nurses in a designated PICU.
2. More evidence is required about the national need and provision of PIC.
3. Transfers of children from general hospitals to designated PICUs are more safely undertaken by specialist retrieval teams.
4. The role of the PICU nurse is to allay parental anxiety and provide a growth-enhancing environment for the critically ill child.
5. The whole family can benefit from careful preparation for the admission, stay and discharge from the PICU.

CARING FOR THE DYING CHILD 14

AND THE FAMILY

INTRODUCTION

The child is not a small adult and this concept is especially true when caring for the dying child. More than ever in this situation should the nurse be able to recognise children's different levels of understanding according to their individual ages and experiences. This appreciation will enable the nurse to be able to talk to the child about death and dying in a meaningful way and be able to identify physical and psychological needs. A knowledge of how children respond to their illness will aid the planning and implementation of specific care to meet these needs.

Family-centred care provides the children's nurse with the additional roles of educator and support person for the parents as they help to care for their child. The nurse has to be able to appreciate and respond to the various emotions displayed by the parents whose child is dying. The situation will also have a psychological impact on the affected child's healthy siblings and they will need help and support to cope with this trauma. Often families in such severe turmoil have difficulty in recognising and dealing with each other's grief and the nurse may be the person who can help them communicate and share their thoughts and worries. Last, but not least, the nurse needs to be able to recognise that providing such support for the whole family is not easy, to be aware of personal values and beliefs concerning death and to have a strategy for releasing their stress.

MEETING PSYCHOLOGICAL NEEDS

Children's perceptions of death

Most children have some ideas about death. Their games often involve death, usually in an violent way, probably as a result of television and cartoons. Some children have also had some experience of the reality of death because of the death of a grandparent or family pet. These ideas about death will be different for every child because of their individual experiences but also according to their stage of cognitive development.

Activity

Consider your own experiences of death as a child. Have these had any effect on your adult views?

The work of Piaget demonstrates that children's understanding varies between different age groups and that this variation is largely

Cross reference
Death and the family – page 217

predictable. Several researchers have found that these development changes can also be seen in children's understanding of illness. Children's understanding of death has not been studied extensively, possibly because it is a more difficult topic to explore ethically with young children but the few studies which are available indicate that this understanding is also linked to age. These studies relate to children over the age of 2 years. It is difficult to know whether children under this age have any awareness or understanding of death. Preschool children (2–5 years) are described by Piaget as being at a pre-operational (or pre-logical) stage. During this stage children do not think logically and tend to view ideas from their own perspective. At this age they are unable to accept the irreversibility of death and can only relate it to their understanding of sleep which is only a temporary process. This may be partly due to the influence of cartoon characters who always return to normal after violent occurrences.

Activity

Watch a cartoon with a preschool child and discuss the violent episodes. Find out how this child perceives them.

These young children usually consider a dead person as being somewhere else (e.g. in heaven or under the ground). Often death is associated with darkness which may be connected with the child's experience of sleep which mostly occurs at night, in the dark. Vidovich (1980) reports that a 5 year old who was dying was heard to ask: 'When will it be dark? Will mummy be there when it gets dark?'.

The egocentricity of young children may cause them to feel responsible in some way for the death of a loved one. They consider it as a punishment for being naughty. They may have wished a sibling would go away because of jealousy or anger and when this becomes a reality they may see themselves as having caused it to happen. These feelings may be perpetuated if they find themselves neglected because the rest of the family are overcome by grief. They also find it difficult to perceive death as a normal event which happens to everyone including themselves.

Children between the ages of 5 and 8 are beginning to understand that death is a natural event. Lansdown and Benjamin (1985) found that 60% of children in this age group had realistic ideas about the finality of death although they were still largely unaware that it could happen to them during childhood. Although this reasoning is more sophisticated than that of the younger child, the cause of death is still generally seen as external and they may still be concerned about death being infectious, occurring at a certain age or after a specific event. Lucy, aged 7, was terrified of going to hospital after a leg injury and it was eventually ascertained that granny had died in hospital following a fractured femur and Lucy thought that everyone with an injured leg died in hospital. It is also difficult for a child at this age to perceive the future and therefore they do not have the ability to recognise gradual deterioration in themselves or others or to consider what may follow this deterioration.

During middle childhood, children acquire an even more realistic picture of death and recognise it as an inevitable and universal process. They are also able to gather information together and make reasoned judgements about that information. Thus, children who are terminally ill can come to realise that death is imminent. Piaget terms adolescence the formal operational stage of cognitive development. This is the age at which children can think beyond the present and conceptualise the future. They can imagine processes such as death, even if they have not directly experienced such events. They also appreciate that emotions can affect body functions. Because the adolescent is able to visualise the future and has goals and aspirations for adulthood, anger and resentment often occur because death has interfered with these.

COMMUNICATING WITH THE DYING CHILD

The use of Piaget's stages of cognitive development is a useful guide when caring for dying children but the nurse also needs to consider the individual child. Reilly *et al.* (1983) discovered that children who had had personal experience of death generally had an accelerated understanding of death. It is therefore important that the nurse knows as much about the child as an individual as possible so that she can communicate at an appropriate level. This understanding of the child as an individual will also help her to become aware of the child's willingness or otherwise to talk about dying.

Bluebond-Langer (1989) suggests that children often appreciate the seriousness even when they have not been told of their condition. They often choose not to discuss their fears of dying because they have learnt from others behaviour that death is not something that is talked about openly. Lansdown (1980) summarises the stages children pass through when recognising the inevitability of their own death:

* 'I am very sick'
* 'I have an illness that can kill people'
* 'I have an illness that can kill children'
* 'I may not get better'
* 'I am dying'

Thus the pretence that the child is not fatally ill and the unwillingness to pursue difficult questions about the nature of dying is an affront to children's intelligence. A tendency to avoid the issue may lead to the child loosing trust and confidence in the nurse. Communication with the dying child is discussed further elsewhere.

Cross reference

Jean Piaget – page 74

INVOLVING PARENTS IN CARE

When they have a child who is dying, parents may feel they are losing control and they may see the nurse as taking over that control. A supportive relationship with the parents should enable the nurse to help them maintain their role as decision makers and carers. All care should be negotiated and the nurse's and parents' roles clearly defined. At the same time the nurse should be alert to parental needs, abilities and stresses. Parental involvement can range from a presence at the bedside to total care of the child under supervision from the nurse (Evans, 1991). Parents may need support from the nurse to take time away from the dying child and not to feel guilty at the need for sleep, relaxation or time for home or work.

To provide the parents with both physical and psychological support the nurse needs to be available to answer questions, explain care and to respond to spoken and unspoken fears, anxieties, stresses and strains.

SUPPORT FOR THE FAMILY

Children's nursing is concerned with supporting the family as much as it is about caring for the child. This is particularly pertinent when caring for the dying child. Studies, as well as personal accounts, have shown that this support is often lacking for parents' whose children have died (Bennett, 1984). Davies (1979) voices parents' reactions very succinctly when she describes her feelings when her daughter Sarah was dying: 'You feel totally inadequate, lost, helpless and stupid'.

Other emotions experienced by parents caring for a dying child are shock, confusion, fear, anger and guilt. Parents are often so shocked at being told their child is dying, even if this is confirmation of their own suspicions, that they do not hear any further explanations. The nurse needs to give parents time to come to terms with this news and then provide opportunities to answer questions. Following the initial shock parents then feel confused about their parental role, they no longer feel able to care for their child and they do not know how to divide their time between the dying child and the other members of the family. Their lives have been completely altered by this event and they do not know how to cope. Mothers particularly experience a loss of control or mastery, perhaps because they tend to bear the burden of the caring role (Jennings, 1992). The nurse can help both parents rediscover their role, involve them in the care of their child and support them in making decisions about sharing their time and presence amongst other family members. Muller *et al.* (1992) suggests that this is best achieved by a primary nurse who can get to know the family's values, beliefs and relationships.

Confusion can also be due to fear. Many parents are frightened by their perceptions of the actual death and often visualise that this will be violent and painful for the child. They are also frightened that they will not be able to cope with the physical care or be able to control their emotions. Like nurses, they often have difficulty in communicating with their child about dying and they sometimes dread the questions that this child might ask, because they fear they will be unable to respond in an appropriate way. The nurse needs to be able to give the parents the time and opportunity to express these fears and provide them with simple guidelines on how to deal with the child's questions.

Anger may arise from their fear and confusion often as a result of their need to understand the situation and control it. This anger can be directed at the nurse. It is not easy for the nurse to accept such emotions but as Wright (1991) acknowledges, the verbal expression of anger can often aid catharsis. If the nurse can accept the anger and remain supportive, she can strengthen her relationship with the family. Often an angry outburst will cause the parents to feel guilty at causing distress to others. Guilt is a common reaction amongst parents of dying children, they may feel guilty because the illness is hereditary or because their behaviour (e.g. smoking) somehow triggered the illness. Even if there is no obvious cause, parents can always imagine that some action or omission on their part is the reason for their child's illness. The nurse should be alert to parental expressions of guilt or self-blame and assist parents to examine the validity of their apportion of blame. If necessary, this may also involve helping them to forgive themselves or others.

These emotional reactions to the dying child are not confined to the parents. Bluebond-Langer (1989) recognises that the destructive effects of terminal illnesses involve the whole family. In particular, siblings of the dying child may feel rejected and neglected as the sick child become the centre of attention (Collinge and Stewart, 1983). Healthy siblings may feel anxiety about their own health (Cairns *et al.*, 1979). In addition, jealousy and resentment may result from parental pre-occupational with the dying child. This, in turn may lead to feelings of guilt, as the siblings try to direct attention upon themselves (Burton, 1975). If these effects are not recognised and/or managed behavioural problems such as enuresis, school phobia, depression and abdominal pain may ensue. The nurse can help parents to recognise the needs of siblings and by her presence with the dying child, can enable them to spend time with the siblings. She can also help the parents to meet siblings' needs by accepting the siblings' involvement in the care of the sick child (Doyle, 1987). The parents may also need help to maintain as normal a family routine, including discipline, as possible for all members of the family. This helps the affected child and the siblings to feel secure (Cairns *et al.*, 1979; Cleary, 1986).

Such enormous responsibilities for parents in these situations may cause break-up of the family (Gonda and Ruark, 1984). Hill (1993) shows how the strain of a terminal illness of a child upon a marital relationship can be destructive. The stress involved in coming to terms with the varied emotions described above combined with the sheer physical exhaustion caused by trying to maintain normal work and family

Useful addresses

CRUSE
126 Sheen Road, Richmond, Surrey
TW9 1UR
Tel: 0181 940 4818

The Compassionate Friends
53 North Street, Bristol BS3 1EN
Tel: 01179 539 639

Parents' Lifeline
Station House, 63d Stapleton Hall
Road, London N4 3QF
Tel: 0171 263 2265

routines whilst caring for the dying child may often cause conflict. The nurse should be aware of these potential tensions and as far as possible help parents to spend time together and give them time to express feelings separately or together. Muller *et al.* (1992) suggests that the use of outside agencies such as social workers or 'CRUSE' may be helpful. Jennings (1992) suggests that mothers find it easier than fathers to express and work through their feelings. Nurses need to be alert to the possibility that this may be because mothers are more available, or that female emotions are easier for nurses to deal with. Consequently, it may be that fathers are given less opportunity to share their feeling especially if their feelings are hidden as they strive to demonstrate strength.

CARE OF THE NURSE

Caring for dying children is stressful. Vidovich (1980) found that the death of a child may cause the nurse to feel failure, guilt, anger or overwhelming sadness. Support for nurses caring for the dying child and family is essential if burnout is to be avoided. Siedel (1981) suggests that a systematic approach to death education in nurse training may partly help to prepare nurses for meeting the needs of the dying. She also proposes that such a programme allows nurses to come to terms with their own beliefs about dying so that they are better able to cope with their own emotional needs.

Muller *et al.* (1992) suggested regular support group meetings for nurses caring for dying children. This gives them the opportunity to acknowledge their feelings and discuss them with colleagues. It also allows them to discuss actions such as symptom control and talking with parents. Saunders (1982) suggests that for many nurses a support group provides encouragement that they are doing the right thing.

Nurses need to be informed of a child's death even when they have been off duty, they need to know what happened to cope with their own feelings and support the other children on the ward. Many nurses find it useful to be given time to attend the child's funeral to allow them to say their final goodbye.

Activity

Find out what facilities are available to you to help you come to terms with stressful events on the ward.

MEETING PHYSICAL NEEDS

Cross reference

Caring for children in pain – page 348

Pain relief

Pain is the most common feature of the dying and the feature which is most feared by the child and his parents. Eighty per cent of dying children will experience pain (Hill, 1993). If it is not managed well it can lower their morale and ability to cope. The first stage in relieving the dying child's pain is an accurate assessment of the severity, the type and the cause of the pain. Observing physiological changes can be a useful assessment of pain in infants who are less influenced by pain and stress. With toddlers, it is useful to listen to comments from parents who know their child well enough to recognise changes in behaviour which may indicate pain. In this way the nurse can begin to recognise for herself the subtle changes in a child which reveal his individual response to pain. Objective ways of assessing pain using the child's own viewpoint are invaluable in planning and evaluating pain relief.

The planning and implementation of pain relief should follow established models unless the child presents in severe pain. Generally the principle should be a gradual progression from a non-opioid analgesia to a weak opioid and finally a strong opioid (Hill, 1993). In her moving account of the care of a dying teenager Hunt (1990) describes the gradual progression from 30 mg dyhydrocodiene daily to 300 mg twice daily of morphine slow release tablets in the successful management of terminal pain. Unfortunately, there are still many myths about the use of opioids for children and the nurse may need to act as the patient's advocate to ensure that the dying child receives the appropriate analgesia at the correct strength for his pain. If this is not achieved, the resulting negative effects of insufficient or over-powerful analgesia will cause the child and family further distress.

Pain in terminal illness is usually constant and for this reason analgesia should be given regularly so that the child can maintain a continuous level of pain relief. To ensure this goal is met the adequacy of the relief should be re-assessed regularly. Oral analgesia is the route of choice for children, but is not necessarily accepted well by all children. The nurse may need to be imaginative in the use of play to ensure the acceptance of medicine on a regular basis. When nausea and vomiting do not allow oral medication subcutaneous analgesia can be given using a syringe pump. This method has the advantage of enabling the child to remain mobile. Hill (1993) suggests that pain-free mobility should be one of the goals for pain relief. She suggests that the primary goal is to enable relief from pain during sleep. Secondly the nurse should aim to provide sufficient analgesia to give the child relief from pain at rest, and finally the child should be able to move around without pain.

Psychological methods of pain relief may also provide a useful adjunct to medication. Hypnosis, distraction techniques and the use of imagery and relaxation can all be helpful in the management of children's pain. (Alder, 1990). They are relatively easy for children of all ages to use and have the advantage of giving them some control over their situation. The nurse should not forget the influence of fear upon pain and should aim to keep the child as relaxed as possible with explanations of treatment and reassurance. Simple measures such as

Cross reference

Assessment of pain – pages 353–356

Cross reference

Coping strategies – pages 269–270

touch, being settled into a more comfortable position, or the presence of a nurse or parent may help to relax a frightened child and reduce the intensity of the pain.

Nausea and vomiting

Nausea and vomiting is a common problem for children who are dying and can cause them much distress. The commonest causes are constipation, raised intracranial pressure or excessive pharyngeal excretions (Hill, 1993). Prescribed anti-emetics should act on the site of the cause. When the cause is uncertain a combination of anti-emetics which act on different sites may be useful. When oral medication cannot be used, anti-emetics can be given rectally or via a subcutaneous infusion.

Nausea and vomiting is sometimes seen as a side effect of opioids but is usually only troublesome initially. Hill (1993) estimates that 25–30% of children will experience nausea or vomiting when opioids are first used but generally these symptoms are overcome in 5–10 days. She does not recommend the regular use of prophylactic anti-emetics and suggests halipenidol (25–50 mg/kg) or cyclizine (up to 75 mg daily) only if vomiting occurs.

Anorexia

Pain and/or nausea and vomiting may cause anorexia which is often more a problem for the parents than the child himself. It may also be caused by offensive respiratory secretions or wounds. The child may be helped by small frequent snacks of favourite foods rather than two or three large meals a day. Parents may be reassured by understanding that the child's energy requirements are less because of his relative immobility. They may also feel that they are be able to help the problem by bringing in favourite foods or drinks from home.

Cross reference

Encouraging eating and drinking – page 362

Dyspnoea

Dyspnoea in the dying child may be caused by secondary lung tumours, pleural effusion or direct respiratory centre invasion in children with malignant disease. It may be due to the primary disease process as in cystic fibrosis or due to respiratory muscle dysfunction in children with degenerative disease. Often a chest infection will exacerbate the primary cause.

Treatment of dyspnoea is often empirical. Dyspnoea is frightening for the child and his parents, and their anxiety can often aggravate the problem. The nurse can often do much simply by providing a reassuring and calm atmosphere. Careful positioning of the child using a bean bag or elevating the head of his bed may increase his comfort. A frightened child can be helped by being supported in an upright position on a parent or a nurse's lap.

Excess secretions may be overcome by gentle physiotherapy or the administration of hyoscine. A dry cough which prevents rest and sleep can be overcome with simple linctus which is usually well accepted by children and will also act as a cough suppressant.

Constipation

Constipation is an inevitable consequence of opioid use and children who are prescribed strong opioids should also be given regular prophylactic laxatives. Constipation leads to abdominal distension, discomfort, nausea, vomiting and anorexia, and causes needless distress to the child and his parents.

Danthron (12.5–25 mg) is well accepted by children and can be given once at bed-time but it increases gut mobility and can cause abdominal cramps. It is not useful in children in nappies or those that have become incontinent as prolonged contact with the skin can cause discomfort and excoriation.

Lactulose (2.5–10 ml) acts by osmosis and softens stools by maintaining a volume of fluid in the bowel. It is a useful laxative when given regularly but children often dislike the taste and consistency and a twice daily dose is recommended.

The nurse should be aware of the child's usual bowel habits and be alert to any changes in them so that the discomfort and distress of constipation does not occur.

Cross reference

Lactulose – page 473

Anxiety

If the anxiety of the dying child and his family is not managed it will aggravate his physical symptoms. Rodin (1983) has clearly shown that the anxiety of a child is directly related to the anxiety of his parents. Harris' (1981) study showed that just having a child in hospital caused parents to become uncertain and frightened. It is easy to imagine how these feelings are magnified if the child has a terminal illness. Parental anxiety is reduced by having information about their child's treatment and the hospital routine and being able to discuss the future (Sadler, 1988). They may also be helped by reassurance that their feelings are neither unusual or silly (Muller et al., 1992).

Depression

Often, increasing physical deterioration in the child who is dying causes the child to become depressed. Children often demonstrate depression by psychological regression and they become very dependent and clingy to one parent. Depression may also cause a withdrawal and a loss of interest in normal activities such as play and watching television.

The nurse can help the child by encouraging him to express his feelings. Such expressions of feelings may be initiated by the nurse's acknowledgement of them. Judd (1993) suggests that 'I know you are feeling sad', 'This must be very hard for you', may be useful ways to open the discussion. The nurse may also help by enabling the child to achieve control over his daily routine. The dying child often feels powerless and this can sometimes increase feelings of despair and dependence. Encouragement to make decisions about care and any efforts towards independent behaviour should be encouraged.

HOME OR HOSPITAL CARE?

Goldman *et al.* (1990) considers that almost all children prefer to die at home in familiar surroundings. Caring for the dying child at home seems to reduce the long-term problem of guilt and depression experienced by bereaved parents and siblings (Lauer *et al.*, 1983). However, Bluebond-Langer (1989) disputes this and suggests that siblings can often feel confused, rejected and lonely when their home environment changes to care for the dying child. It would appear that there are both advantages and disadvantages of caring for a terminally ill child at home, and a positive outcome may relate to the amount of support available to the family.

Activity

Consider the factors involved in considering whether home or hospital is the most suitable place for a child to die.

If the child has been in hospital parents will need clear instructions and advice. It has been shown that this is not always forthcoming. McDonald (1988) studied the discharge information given to mothers and found that many mothers left hospital with unclear or insufficient explanations.

It must also be recognised that not all parents will feel able physically and psychologically to care for their dying child at home. These parents should not be made to feel guilty at such a decision. Harris (1988) found that care at home sometimes fails because of lack of family resources and/or community support. The decision to care for the dying child at home needs careful assessment of all the factors involved in negotiation with the parents, siblings and affected child. Provision should be made for alternatives if home care does fail so parents recognise that they can return to hospital care without feeling inadequate.

An alternative to hospital care is the hospice which will centre care entirely around the support of the family (Copsey, 1981). The nurse may be the person to discuss with the family the best option for them and their child.

SUMMARY

Caring for the dying child and family is probably one of the most challenging roles of the children's nurse. The nurse needs to be sensitive to the needs, fears and anxieties of all the family members, and to try to enable them to maintain a normal family life. The aim of nursing in this situation becomes not to aid a cure but to help the child and family face the reality of death, and to enable the child to die with peace and dignity. It may also be to continue to support the family after the child's death and to help them cope with their grief. Inevitably, such experiences are stressful to the nurses involved with the family and they too need to share their feelings.

➤ **Key points**

1. Children's perceptions of death vary according to their stage of cognitive development and their individual experiences.

2. Children are usually only able to discuss death with the nurse in a secure atmosphere of trust and confidence.

3. Nurses need to have explored and confronted their own feelings and beliefs about death before being able to provide effective help for dying children and their families.

4. When a child is dying the whole family is affected and the nurse has to handle a variety of emotions from fear, anxiety, and guilt to despair, confusion and anger.

5. When their child is dying parents often need help to identify how they can best help their child.

6. The nurse has to recognise that this type of nursing is stressful and has to be able to access strategies which will help to overcome the effects of stress.

References

ABD-EL-MAEBOUD, K., *et al.* (1991) Rectal suppository: common sense and mode of insertion. *Lancet*, 338 (8770), 798–800.

ACTION FOR SICK CHILDREN (1993) Planning paediatric home care. *At Home Newsletter*, 5.

ADAMS, J., *et al.* (1991) Reducing fear in hospital. *Nursing Times*, 87 (1) 62–64.

ADVANCED LIFE SUPPORT GROUP (1993) *Advanced Paediatric Life Support*. London: BMJ.

AHMANN, E. (1994) Family centred care: the time has come. *Pediatric Nursing*, 20 (1), 52–54.

ALDER, S. (1991) Taking children at their word: pain control in paediatrics. *Professional Nurse*, 5 (8), 398–402.

AMERICAN ACADEMY OF PEDIATRICS (1994) *Pediatric Advanced Life Support*. Dallas: American Heart Association.

ANDERTON, A., *et al.* (1993) A comparative study of the numbers of bacteria present in enteral feed preparation and administration in hospital and in the home. *Journal of Hospital Infection*, **23** (1), 43–49.

ANGERAS, M. H., BRANDBERG, A., FALK, A. and SEEMAN, T. (1992) Comparison between sterile saline and tap water for the cleaning of acute traumatic soft tissue. *European Journal of Surgery*, **158** (33), 347–350.

ATKINSON, B., GLASPER, E. and PURCELL, C. (1996) Very sick children need children's nurses too. *Paediatric Nursing*, **8** (10), 10–11.

ATWELL, J. and GOW, M. (1985) Paediatric trained district nurse in the community: expensive luxury or economic necessity? *British Medical Journal*, **291**, 227–278.

AUDIT COMMISSION (1993) *Children First: A Study of Hospital Services*. London: HMSO.

BAILLIE, L. (1993) A review of pain assessment tools. *Nursing Standard*, 7 (23), 25–29.

BAKER, C. and WONG, D. (1987) QUESTT: A process of pain assessment in children. *Orthopaedic Nurse*, **6** (1), 11–21.

BANCO, L. and POWERS, A. (1988) Hospitals; unsafe places for children. *Pediatrics*, **82** (5), 794.

BARRY, P. and RALSTON, C. (1994) Adverse events occurring during inter-hospital transfer of the critically ill. *Archives of Disease in Childhood*, **71**, 8–11.

BATES, T. and BROOME, M. (1986) Preparation of children for hospitalisation and surgery: a review of the literature. *Journal of Pediatric Nursing*, **1** (4), 230–234.

BEAVER, M. *et al.* (1994) *Babies and Young Children, Book 1. Development 0–7.* Cheltenham: Stanley Thornes (Publishers) Ltd.

BECKER, R. D. (1972) Therapeutic approaches to psychopathological reactions to hospitalisation. *International Journal of Child Psychology*, **1**, 65–67.

BEDI, A. (1993) A tool to fill the gap. *Professional Nurse*. November, 112–118.

BEECROFT, P. and REDICK, S. (1990) Intramuscular injection practices of pediatric nurses: site selection. *Nurse Education*, **15** (4), 23–28.

BENNER, P. and WRUBEL, J. (1989) *The Primacy of Caring: Stress and Coping in Health and Illness.* Addison-Wesley: Menlo Park.

BENNETT, P. (1984) A care team for terminally ill children. *Nursing Times*, **80** (10), 26–27.

BENTLEY, J. (1995) Triage of children in A&E: research shortfall addressed. *Nursing Times*, **91** (51), 38–39.

BEYER, J. (1989) *The Oucher: A User's Manual and Technical Report.* Denver: University of Colorado.

BEYER, J. and ARDINE, C. (1988) Content validity of an instrument to measure young children's intensity of pain. *Journal of Pediatric Nursing*, **1**, 386–394.

BINNIE *et al.* (1988) *A Systematic Approach to Nursing Care.* OUP: Milton Keynes.

BISHOP, J. (1998) Sharing the caring. *Nursing Times*, **84** (30), 60–61.

BLACK, N. A., SANDERSON, C. F., FREEELAND, A. P. and VESSEY, M. P. (1990) A randomised controlled trial of surgery for glue ear. *British Medical Journal*, **300**, 1551–1556.

BLUEBOND-LANGER, M. (1989) Worlds of dying children and their well siblings. *Death Studies*, **13**, 1–16.

BOGE, E. (1910) The nurse on district. *Nursing Times*, **vi** (288), 916.

BOND, M. (1979) *Pain: Its Nature, Analysis and Treatment.* Edinburgh: Churchill Livingstone.

BOOTH, I. W. (1991) Enteral nutrition in childhood. *British Journal of Hospital Medicine*, **46**, 111–113.

BOWLBY, J. (1953) *Child Care and the Growth of Love*. Harmondsworth: Penguin.

BRADSHAW, E. and DAVENPORT, H. (1989) *Day Care: Anaesthetics and Management*. London: Edward Arnold.

BRADSHAW, C. and ZEANAH, P. (1986) Paediatric nurse assessments of children in pain. *Journal of Paediatric Nursing*, 1, 314–22.

BRITISH PAEDIATRIC ASSOCIATION (1991a) *Paediatric Medical Staffing in the 1990s*. London: BPA.

BRITISH PAEDIATRIC ASSOCIATION (1991b) *Towards a Combined Child Health Service*. London: BPA.

BRITISH PAEDIATRIC ASSOCIATION (1993) *The Care of Critically Ill Children: Report of the Multidisciplinary Working Party on Paediatric Intensive Care*. London: BPA.

BRITISH PAEDIATRIC ASSOCIATION, BRITISH ASSOCIATION OF PAEDIATRIC SURGEONS, CASUALTY SURGEONS ASSOCIATION (1988) *Joint Statement of Children's Attendances at Accident and Emergency Departments*. London: BPS.

BRITTO, J., NADEL, S., MacCONOCHIE, I., LEVIN, M. and HABIBI, P. (1995) Morbidity and severity of illness during interhospital transfer: impact of a specialist retrieval team. *British Medical Journal*, 311, 836–839.

BROOME, M. and LILLIS, P. (1989) A descriptive analysis of pediatric pain management research. *Journal of Applied Nursing Research*, 2 (2), 74–81.

BUCKINGHAM, S. (1993) Pain scales for toddlers. *Nursing Standard*, 7 (25), 12–13.

BUDD, K. (1984) *Pain*, 2nd edn. London: Update Publications.

BURKE, D. and BOWDEN, D. (1993) Modified paediatric resuscitation chart. *British Medical Journal*, 306, 1096–1098.

BURROWS, F. and BERDE, C. (1993) Optimal pain relief in infants and children. *British Medical Journal*, 307, 815–816.

BURTON, L. (1975) *Family Life of Sick Children*. Boston: Routledge & Kegan Paul.

BURTON, R. (1989) Parental perceptions of Accident and Emergency. *Paediatric Nursing*, 1 (3), 19–20.

BURTON, R. (1994) How to bear the pain – a well teddy clinic as an educational tool. *Child Health*, 1 (6), 251–254.

CAIRNS, N., CLARK, G., SMITH, S. and LANSKY, S. (1979) Adaption of siblings to childhood cancer. *Journal of Paediatrics*, 95, 484–487.

CALNE, S. (1994) Dehumanisation in intensive care. *Nursing Times*, 90 (17), 31–33.

CAMPBELL, A. (1987) Children with ongoing health needs. *Nursing* (3rd series), 23.

CAMPBELL, S. and GLASPER, A. (eds) (1995) *Whaley and Wong's Children's Nursing*. London: Mosby.

CARING FOR THE CHILDREN IN THE HEALTH SERVICE (1993) *Bridging the Gaps*. London: CCHS.

CARSON, D., GRAVELY, J. and COUNCIL, J. (1992) Children's pre-hospitalisation conceptions of illness, cognitive development and personal adjustment. *Child Health Care*, 21 (2) 103–110.

CARTER, B. (1995) A fundamental duty and right. *Child Health*, 3 (1), 4.

CASEY, A. (1988a) A partnership with the child and family. *Senior Nurse*, 8 (4), 8–9.

CASEY, A. (1988b) Developing a model of paediatric nursing practice. In GLASPER, A. and TUCKER, A. (eds), *Advances in Child Nursing*. London: Scutari.

CASTEELS-VAN DAELE, M. (1993) Reduction of deaths after drug labelling for risk of Reyes syndrome. *Lancet*, 341, 118–119.

CATCHPOLE, A. (1986) *Community paediatric nursing services in England 1985.* Unpublished DN thesis.

CHILD ACCIDENT PREVENTION TRUST (1992) *Accidents to Children on Hospital Wards.* London: CAPT.

CLEARY, J., GRAY, O., HALL, D., ROWLANDSON, P., SAINSBURY, C. and DAVIES, M. (1986) Parental involvement in the lives of children in hospital. *Archives of Disease in Childhood*, **61**, 779–187.

CLEELAND, C. (1986) Behavioural control of symptoms. *Journal of Pain Symptom Management*, **1** (1), 36–38.

CLOTHIER, C. (1994) *The Allitt Inquiry.* London: HMSO.

COHEN, D., *et al.* (1984) The use of relaxation – mental imagery (self-hypnosis) in the management of 505 pediatric behavioural encounters. *Developmental and Behavioural Pediatrics*, **5** (10), 21–24.

COLE, R. (1995) When every second counts – reducing inaccuracy and delay in paediatric resuscitation. *Child Health*, **3** (2), 63–67.

COLLINGE, P. and STEWART, E. D. (1983) Dying children and their families. In ROBBINS, J. (ed.), *Caring for the Dying Child and the Family*, 1st edn. London: Harper & Row.

COLLINS, P. (1994) Knowledge and practice of CPR. *Paediatric Nursing*, **6** (2), 19–22.

COLLINS, P. (1995) Put the child first: paediatric attendance in A&E. *Child Health*, **2** (6), 225–228.

CONISBEE, L. (1982) *A Bedfordshire Bibliography.* Bedfordshire Historical Record Society.

COPSEY, M. K. (1981) Time to care. *Nursing Mirror*, **153** (22), 38–40.

COULSTON, D. (1988) A proper place for parents. *Nursing Times*, **84** (19), 26–28.

COURT, S. D. M. (1976) *Fit for the Future: Report of the Committee on Child Health Services*, vols 1 and 2. London: HMSO.

CROSS, J. H., *et al.* (1995) Clinical examination compared with anthropometry in evaluating nutritional status. *Archive of Disease of Childhood*, **72**, 60–61.

CURRIE, M. (1982) *Hospitals in Luton: An Illustrated History.* Hitchin: Powis.

DARBYSHIRE, P. (1994) *Living with a Sick Child in Hospital.* London: Chapman & Hall.

DAVIES, J. (1979) *Death of a Child.* London: Pitman Medical.

DEARMUN, A. (1992) Perceptions of parental participation. *Paediatric Nursing*, **4** (7), 6–10.

DE COURCEY-GOLDER, A. (1996) A strategy for development of paediatric intensive care within the United Kingdom. *Intensive and Critical Care Nursing*, **12**, 84–89.

DE SWIET, M., *et al.* (1989) Measurement of blood pressure in children. *British Medical Journal*, **299**, 497–498.

DoH (1991a) *Welfare of Children and Young People in Hospital.* London: HMSO.

DoH (1991b) *The Patient's Charter.* London: HMSO.

DoH (1991c) *Dietary Reference Values for Food, Energy and Nutrients for the UK.* Report on Health and Social Subjects no. 41. London: HMSO.

DoH (1995) *The Patient's Charter: Services for Children and Young People.* London: HMSO.

DoH (1996) *The Patient's Charter: Services for Children and Young People.* London: HMSO.

DHSS (1976a) *Fit for the Future (The Court Report).* London: HMSO.

DHSS (1976b) *Priorities for Health and Personal Social Services*. London: HMSO.

DILWORTH, N. and MacKELLAR, A. (1987) Pain relief for the pediatric surgical patient. *Journal of Pediatric Surgery*, **22**, 264–266.

DOYLE, B. (1987) I wish you were dead. *Nursing Times*, **83** (45), 44–46.

EDGE, W., KANTER, R., WEIGLE, C. and WALSH, R. (1994) Reduction of morbidity in inter-hospital transport by specialist pediatric staff. *Critical Care Medicine*, **22**, 1186–1191.

ELAND, J. (1985) Paediatrics. In CAREY, K. (ed.), *Nursing Now: Pain*. Pennsylvania, Springhouse.

ELAND, J. (1993) Children with pain. In JACKSON, O. and SAUNDERS, R. (eds), *Child Health Nursing*. Philadelphia: J. B. Lippincott.

ELAND, J. and ANDERSON, J. (1977) The experience of pain in children. In JACOX, A. K. (ed.), *Pain: A Source Book for Nurses and other Health Professionals*. Boston: Little Brown.

ELANDER, G., LINDBERG, T. and QUARNSTROM, B. (1991) Pain relief in infants after surgery: a descriptive study. *Journal of Paediatric Surgery*, **26** (2), 128–131.

ELLET, M., *et al.* (1992) Predicting the distance for gavage tube placement in children using regression on height. *Pediatric Nursing*, **18** (2), 119–121.

ELLIS, J. A. (1988) Using pain scales to prevent under medication. *American Journal of Maternal and Child Nursing*, **13**, 180–182.

ELLIS, J. A. (1995) Administering drugs. *Paediatric Nursing*, **7** (4), 32–39.

ENB (1992) *A Survey of Students Gaining Nursing Experience in Children's Wards*. London: ENB.

EUROPEAN RESUSCITATION COUNCIL (1994) Guidelines for paediatric support. *Resuscitation*, **27**, 91–105.

EVANS, M. (1991) Caring by parents. In GLASPER, A. (ed.), *Child Care – Some Nursing Perspectives*. London: Wolfe.

FLAVELL, J. H. (1985) *Cognitive Development*: Englewood Cliffs, NJ: Prentice-Hall.

FOALE, H. (1989) Healing the wound. *Paediatric Nursing*, **1** (5), 10–12.

FOXALL, M., ZIMMERMAN, S. and BENE, B. (1990) Comparison of frequency and sources of nursing job stress perceived by intensive care, hospice and medical-surgical nurses. *Journal of Advanced Nursing*, **12**, 281–290.

FRADD, E. (1990) Setting up a paediatric community nursing service. *Senior Nurse*, **10** (7), 4–5.

FRASER, J., MOK, Q. and TASKER, R. (1997) Survey of occupancy of paediatric intensive care units by children who are dependent on ventilators. *British Medical Journal*, **315**, 347–348.

GADISH, H. *et al.* (1988) Factors affecting nurses' decisions to administer paediatric pain medication post operatively. *Journal of Paediatric Nursing*, **3** (6), 383–390.

GALVANI, J. (1997) Not yet cut and dried. *Nursing Times*, **93** (16), 88–89.

GARLAND, J., *et al.* (1987) Infectious complications during peripheral IV therapy with Teflon catheters: a prospective study. *Paediatric Infectious Disease Journal*, **6** (10), 918–921.

GAUDERER, M., LORIG, J. and EASTWOOD, D. (1989) Is there a place for parents in the anaesthetic room? *Journal of Pediatric Surgery*, **24** (7), 705–707.

GAY, J. (1992) A painful experience. *Nursing Times*, **88** (25), 32–35.

GILLET, J. (1954) Domicillary treatment of sick children. *The Practitioner*, **172**, 281–283.

GILLIES, M., PARRY-JONES, W. and SMITH, L. (1995) Post-operative pain in children under five years. *Paediatric Nursing*, **3** (1), 31–34.

GILLIS, A. (1990) Hospital preparation: the children's story. *Child Health Care*, **19** (1), 19–27.

GLASPER, A. (1990) Accompanying children: parental presence during anaesthesia. *Nursing Standard*, **4** (24), 6.

GLASPER, A., GOW, M. and YERRELL, P. (1989) A family friend. *Nursing Times*, **85** (4), 63–5.

GLASPER, E. R. (1993) Telephone triage: extending practice. *Nursing Standard*, **7** (15), 34–36.

GODFREY, K. (1997) Uses of leeches and leech saliva in clinical practice. *Nursing Times*, **26** (9), 62–63.

GODMAN, L. (1994) Case history – paediatric nursing training. *Paediatric Nursing*, **6** (1).

GOLDMAN, A., BEARDSMORE, S. and HUNT, J. (1990) Palliatuse care for children with cancer – home, hospital or hospice. *Archives of Disease in Childhood*, **65**, 641–643.

GONDA, T. and RUARK, J. (1984) *Dying Dignified. The Health Professional's Guide to Care*. Menlo Park, CA: Addison-Wesley.

GRAHAM, P. (1987) *Child Health Ten Years after the Court Report*. London: NCB.

GRIFFITHS-JONES, A. (1990) Prevalence of IV devices. *Nursing Times*, **86** (1), 6–7.

HALL, C. (1996) The art of storytelling. *Paediatric Nursing*, **8** (1), 6–7.

HARRIS, A. C. (1993) *Child Development*, 2nd edn. Minneapolis: West.

HARRIS, P. (1981) How parents feel. *Nursing Times*, **77** (42), 1803–1804.

HART, R. and BOSSERT, E. (1994) Self reported fears of hospitalised school-age children. *Journal of Pediatric Nursing*, **9** (2), 83–90.

HAZINSKI, M. F. (1992) *Nursing Care of the Critically Ill Child*. St Louis: Mosby.

HECKER, J. (1988) Improved technique in intravenous therapy. *Nursing Times*, **84** (34), 28–33.

HESTER, N. (1979) The pre-operational child's reaction to immunisation. *Nursing Research*, **28** (4), 250–255.

HEWITT, T. (1988) Prolonged contact with topical anaesthetic cream: a case report. *Paediatric Nursing*, **10** (2), 22–23.

HICKS, J. F., *et al.* (1989) Optimum needle length for diptheria–tetanus–pertussis inoculation of infants. *Pediatric Nursing*, **84** (1), 136–137.

HILL, L. (1993) *Caring for Dying Children and Their Families*. London: Chapman & Hall.

HOLDEN, C., *et al.* (1996) Enteral nutrition. *Paediatric Nursing*, **8** (5), 29–33.

HORGAN, M., CHOONARA, I., *et al.* (1996) Measuring pain in neonates: an objective score. *Paediatric Nursing*, **8** (10), 24–27.

HUGHES, G. (1990) Tape measure to aid prescription in paediatric resuscitation. *Archives of Emergency Medicine*, **7**, 21–27.

HUGHES, M., *et al.* (1994) How parents cope with the experience of neonatal intensive care. *Child Health Care*, **23** (1), 1–14.

HUNT, J. (1990) Symptom care of the child with cancer. *Nursing Times*, **86** (10), 72–73.

HUTT, R. (1983) *Sick Children's Nurses. A Study for the DHSS of the Career Patterns of RSCNs*. Brighton: Institute of Manpower Studies.

ILLINGWORTH, R. (1975) *The Normal Child*, 6th edn. Edinburgh: Churchill Livingstone.

JACKSON, K. (1995) The state we're in. *Child Health*, **3** (1), 14–17.

JAMES, J. (1995) Day care admissions. *Paediatric Nursing*, **7** (1), 25–29.

JANES, S. (1996) Failure to thrive in children with chronic illness. *Paediatric Nursing*, 8 (3), 19–22.

JENNINGS, P. (1992) Coping strategies for mothers. *Paediatric Nursing*, 4 (9), 24–26.

JOHNSON, C., STEVENS, B. and ARBESS, G. (1993) The effect of the sight of blood and the use of decorative adhesive bandages on pain intensity ratings by pre-school children. *Journal of Pediatric Nursing*, 8 (3), 147–150.

JOLLY, T. (1981) *The Other Side of Paediatrics*. London: Macmillan.

JUDD, D. (1993) Communicating with dying children. In DICKENSON, D. and JOHNSON, M. (eds), *Death, Dying and Bereavement*. London: Sage.

KANTER, R. and TOMPKINS, J. (1989) Adverse events during interhospital transport: physiological deterioration associated with pretransport severity of illness. *Pediatrics*, 84, 43–48.

KELLY, M., FERGUSON-CLARK, L. and MARSH, M. (1996) A new retrieval service. *Paediatric Nursing*, 8 (6), 18–20.

KITCHENER, P. (1993) *Health in Bedfordshire*. Bedford: Bedfordshire Health Authority.

KOBRAN, M. and PEARCE, S. (1993) The paediatric nurse practitioner. *Paediatric Nursing*, 3 (5), 11.

KOREN, G. *et al.* (1985) Post-operative morphine infusion in newborn infants: assessment of disposition characteristics and safety. *Journal of Pediatrics*, 107 (6), 963–967.

LANGDON, J. (1995) Neglect of an essential right. *Child Health*, 3 (1), 10–13.

LANSDOWN, R. (1980) *More Than Sympathy*. London: Tavistock.

LANSDOWN, R. and BENJAMIN, G. (1985) The development of the concept of death in children aged 5–9 years. *Child Care and Development*, 11, 13–20.

LAUER, D., MULHERN, R., WALLSCOG, J. and CAMITTA, B. (1983) A comparison study of parental adaption following a child's death at home or in hospital. *Pediatrics*, 71 (1), 107–112.

LAWRENCE, A. (1993) Intraosseous infusion. *Nursing Standard*, 7 (4), 21–24.

LEVY, D. (1960) The infant's earliest memory of inoculation. *Journal of Genetic Psychology*, 96 (3), 46–50.

LEY, P. and LLEWELLYN, S. (1995) Improving patients' recall satisfaction and compliance. In BROOME, A. and LLEWELLYN, S. (eds), *Health Psychology: Processes and Applications*. London: Chapman & Hall.

LIGHTWOOD, R., BRIMBLECOMBE, F., REINHOLD, J., BURNARD, E. and DAVIS, J. (1956) A London trial of home care for sick children. *Lancet*, i 313–316.

LIVESLEY, J. (1993) Reducing the risks. Management of paediatric intravenous therapy. *Child Health*, 1 (2), 68–70.

LLEWELYN, M. (1991) A headache all over my body. *Paediatric Nursing*, 3 (7), 14–15.

LLOYD-THOMAS, A. R. (1990) ABC of major trauma: primary survey and resuscitation. *British Medical Journal*, 301, 334–336.

LOGAN, S. (1995) Commentary: evaluation of specialist paediatric retrieval teams. *British Medical Journal*, 311, 839.

LUCAS, H. and ATTARD-MONTALTO, S. (1996) Central line dressings: study of infection rates. *Paediatric Nursing*, 8 (6), 21–23.

McCAFFERY, M. and BEEBE, A. (1989) *Pain*. St Louis: Mosby.

McCAFFERY, P. (1983) *Nursing the Patient in Pain*. London: Harper & Row.

McDONALD, M. (1988) Children discharged from hospital – what mothers want to know. *Nursing Times*, **84** (16), 63.

McEVILLY, A. (1993) Childhood diabetes. *Paediatric Nursing*, **5** (9), 25–28.

McGRATH, P. (1990) *Pain in Children*. London: The Guildford Press.

McMENAMIN, C. (1995) Making A&E less traumatic for children. *Professional Nurse*, **2**, 310–313.

MACKOWIAK, P., WASSERMAN, S. and LEVINE, M. (1992) A critical appraisal of 98.6°F, the upper limit of normal body temperature. *Journal of the American Medical Association*, **286** (12), 1578–1580.

MANN, N. *et al.* (1986) Effect of night and day on pre-term infants. *British Medical Journal*, **293**, 1265–1267.

MARCOUX, C., *et al.* (1991) Central venous access devices in children. *Pediatric Nursing*, **16** (2), 123–133.

MARKOVITCH, H. (1991) Day case treatment for children. *Archives of Disease in Childhood*, **66**, 734–736.

MARRIOT, M. (1990) Parent powers. *Nursing Times*, **86** (34), 68.

MEAKIN, G., *et al.* (1987) The effects of fasting on oral pre-medication – pH and volume of gastric aspiration in children. *British Journal of Anaesthesia*, **59**, 687–682.

METHENY, N. (1998) Measures to test placement of naso-gastric and naso-intestinal feeding tubes: a review. *Nursing Research*, **37** (6), 324–329.

METHENY, N., *et al.* (1989) Effectiveness of pH measurements in predicting feeding tube placement. *Nursing Research*, **38** (5), 280–285.

MILES, M. and MANTHES, M. (1991) Preparation of parents for the ICU experience: what are we missing? *Child Health Care*, **20** (3), 132–137.

MILLER, S. (1991) Adolescents alone together. In GLASPER, A. (ed.), *Child Care: Some Nursing Perspectives*. London: Wolfe.

MoH (1959) *Welfare of Children in Hospital (The Platt Report)*. London: HMSO.

MoH (1962) *A Hospital Plan for England and Wales*. London: HMSO.

MoH (1971) *Hospital Facilities for Sick Children*. London: HMSO.

MORGAN, E. (1990) *Siblings reactions to short-term hospitalisation*. Unpublished dissertation, City University.

MORLEY, C., *et al.* (1992) Axillary and rectal temperature measurements in infants. *Archives of Disease in Childhood*, **67** (1), 122–125.

MORRISON, L. (1997) Stress and siblings. *Paediatric Nursing*, **9** (4), 26–27.

MORRISON, R. (1991) Update on sickle cell disease: incidence of addiction and choice of opioid in pain management. *Pediatric Nursing*, **17** (6), 503.

MORTON, R. J. and PHILLIPS, B. M. (1992) *Accidents and Emergencies in Children*. Oxford: Oxford University Press.

MORTON, R., TOUQUET, R. and FOTHERGILL, J. (1994) Children in the accident and emergency department. *Maternal and Child Health*, June, 176–182.

MOY, R. J., *et al.* (1990) Malnutrition in a UK children's hospital. *Journal of Human Nutrition and Dietetics*, **3**, 93–100.

NATIONAL PRESSURE ULCER ADVISORY PANEL (1989) Pressure ulcers: incidence, economics and risk assessment. *Care – Science and Practice*, **7** (4), 96–99.

NAWCH (1986) *NAWCH Update*, Autumn.

NETHERCOTT, S. (1994) The assessment and management of post-operative pain in children by RSCNs. *Journal of Clinical Nursing*, **3**, 109–113.

NEWELL, P. (1991) *The Convention of Children's Rights in the UK*. London: The Children's Bureau.

NEWMAN, J. (1985) Evaluation of sponging to reduce body temperature in febrile children. *Canadian Medical Association Journal*, **132**, 641–642.

NICHOL, J. (1909) The surgery of infancy. *British Medical Journal*, **2**, 753.

NICHOLS, K. (1993) *Psychological Care in Physical Illness*, 2nd edn. London: Chapman & Hall.

NIGHTINGALE, F. (1859) *Notes on Nursing*: London: Camelot Press.

NORRIS, E. (1992) Making the day bearable. *Paediatric Nursing*, **4** (3), 21–22.

O'BRIEN, S. and KONSLER, G. (1988) Alleviating children's post-operative pain. *Maternal & Child Nursing*, **13** (3), 183–86.

O'MALLEY, M. E. and McNAMARA, S. T. (1993) Children's drawings – a pre-operative assessment tool. *AORN Journal*, **57** (5), 1074–1089.

OAKLEY, P. (1988) Inaccuracy and delay in decision making in paediatric resuscitation. *British Medical Journal*, **97**, 1347–1351.

ORENSTEIN, S., *et al.* (1988) The Santmyer swallow – a new and useful infant reflex. *Lancet*, **i** (8581), 345–346.

OSTER, G. D. and GOULD, P. (1987) *Using Drawings in Assessment and Therapy*. New York: Brunner/Mazel.

PAICE, J. (1992) Pharmacologic management. In WATT-WATSON, J. and DONAVON, M. (eds), *Pain Management: Nursing Perspectives*. St Louis: Mosby.

PATEL, N. (1990) The child with cancer in the community. In THOMPSON, J. (ed.), *The Child with Cancer*. London: Scutari Press.

PATEL, R. I., *et al.* (1995) Complications following paediatric ambulatory surgery. *Ambulatory Surgery*, **3** (2), 83–86.

PEPLAU, H. (1952) *Interpersonal Relationships in Nursing*. New York: Putnam.

PERRY, S. (1994) Communicating with toddlers in hospital. *Paediatric Nursing*, **6** (5), 14–17.

PETERSON, L. and TOLER, S. (1986) An information seeking disposition in child surgery patients. *Health Psychology*, **5** (4), 343–358.

PETERSON, L., *et al.* (1990) Preparing children for hospitalisation and threatening medical procedures. In BELLACK, A. and HERSEN, M. (eds), *Handbook of Clinical Behavioural Problems*. New York: Plenum Press.

PFEFFERBAUM, B., ADAMS, J. and ACEVES, J. (1990) The influence of culture on pain in Anglo and Hispanic children with cancer. *Journal of the American Academy of Child and Adolescent Psychiatry*, **29** (4), 642–647.

PLATT, S. (1959) *The Welfare of Children in Hospital*. London: HMSO.

POLLACK, S., *et al.* (1991) Improved outcomes for tertiary center pediatric intensive care. *Critical Care Medicine*, **19** (2), 150–159.

PONTIOUS, S., *et al.* (1994) Accuracy and reliability of temperature measurement by instrument and site. *Journal of Pediatric Nursing*, **9** (2), 114–123.

PORTMAN, R. and YETMAN, R. (1994) Clinical uses of ambulatory blood pressure monitoring. *Paediatric Nephrology*, **8**, 367–376.

QUERSHI, J. and BUCKINGHAM, S. (1994) A pain assessment tool for all children. *Paediatric Nursing*, **6** (7), 11–13.

RAMSAY, J. (1990) *Parental knowledge and management of children with cystic fibrosis*. Unpublished MSc thesis.

READ, J. V. (1994) Perceptions of nurses and physicians regarding pain management of pediatric emergency room patients. *Pediatric Nursing*, **20** (3), 314–318.

REDMAN, C. (1994) Handling with care. *Child Health*, **1** (5), 177–180.

REILLY, T., HASAZI, J. and BOND, L. (1983) Children's conception of death and personal mortality. *Journal of Paediatric Psychology*, **8**, 21–31.

ROBERTSON, J. (1958) *Young Children in Hospital*. London: Tavistock.

ROBERTSON, J. and ROBERTSON, J. (1952) *A Two Year Old Goes to Hospital*. Ipswich: Concord Films.

RODIN, J. (1983) *Will This Hurt?* London: RCN.

ROUNTREE, D. (1991) The PIC catheter: a different approach. *American Journal of Nursing*, **91** (8), 22–26.

ROYAL COLLEGE OF NURSING (1994) *The Care of Sick Children*. London: RCN.

ROYAL COLLEGE OF SURGEONS OF ENGLAND (1992) *Guidelines for Day Case Surgery*. London: RCS.

SADLER, S. (1988) Being there. *Nursing Times*, **84** (34), 19.

SAUNDERS, B. (1982) Staff support. *Nursing*, **1** (34), 1498–1499.

SCHEPP, K. G. (1991) Factors influencing the coping effort of mothers of hospitalised children. *Nursing Research*, **40** (1), 42–46.

SHAPIRO, C. (1989) Pain in the neonate: assessment and intervention. *Neonatal Network*, **8** (1), 7–21.

SHELLABARGER, S. and THOMPSON, T. (1993) The critical times: meeting parental needs throughout the NICU. *Neonatal Network*, **12** (2), 39–44.

SHELLEY, P. (1991) *Children in A&E Departments*, Keypoints no. 17. London: Action for Sick Children.

SIDEY, A. (1990) Cooperation in care. *Paediatric Nursing*, **2** (3), 10–12.

SIEDEL, M. (1981) Death education a contravening process for nurses. *Topics in Clinical Nursing*, **3** (3), 87–89.

SIMON, K. (1993) Percieved stress of nonhospitalised children during the hospitalisation of a sibling. *Journal of Pediatric Nursing*, **8** (5), 298–304.

SIMPSON, K. (1977) Eighteenth John Snow Memorial Lecture: the anaesthetist and the law. *Anaesthesia*, **32**, 626.

SIMPSON, S. (1994a) Paediatric basic life support – an update. *Nursing Times*, **90** (21), 40–42.

SIMPSON, S. (1994b). Paediatric basic life support – an update. *Nursing Times*, **90** (27), 37–39.

SLATER, M. (1993) *Health for all Our Children: Achieving Appropriate Health Care for Black and Ethnic Minority Children and their Families*. London: Action for Sick Children.

SMELLIE, J. (1956) Domicillary nursing service for infants and children. *British Medical Journal*, **i**, 256.

SOMES, J. (1991) Ventricular fibrulation in a 2 month old infant. *Journal of Emergency Nursing*, **17** (4), 215–219.

SPENCE, J. (1947) The care of children in Hospital. *British Medical Journal*, **i**, 125–130.

SPICHER, C. and YUND, C. (1989) Effects on pre-admission preparation on compliance with home care instructions. *Journal of Pediatric Nursing*, **4** (4), 255–262.

SPLINTER, W. and SCHAEFFER, J. (1990) Clear fluids three hours before surgery do not affect gastric fluid contents. *Canadian Journal of Anaesthesia*, **37** (5), 498–501.

STEIN, R. and JESSOP, D. (1984) Does pediatric care make a difference for children with chronic illness? *Pediatrics*, **73** (6), 845–852.

STILLER, C. A. (1988) Centralisation of treatment and survival rates for cancer. *Archives of Disease in Childhood*, **63**, 23–30.

SWANWICK, M. and BARLOW, S. (1993) A caring definition: defining quality care. *Child Health*, **1** (4), 137–141.

SWIFT, P., *et al.* (1993) A decade of diabetes – keeping children out of hospital. *British Medical Journal*, 307, 96–98.

THORNES, R. (1991) *Just for the Day*. London: NAWCH.

THORNES, R. (1993) *Bridging the Gaps: An Explanatory Study of the Interfaces between Primary and Specialist Care for Children within the Health Services.* London: Action for Sick Children.

TORRANCE, C. (1983) *Pressure Sores: Aetiology, Treatment and Prevention.* London: Croom Helm.

TUCKER, A. (1989) Who cares for the child? *Nursing Times*, 85 (38), 34–35.

TURNER, T. (1985) Which dressing and why? In WESTABY, S. (ed.), *Wound Care.* Heinemann: London.

UNITED KINGDOM CENTRAL COUNCIL (1986) *Project 2000 – A New Preparation for Practice*. London: UKCC.

UNITED KINGDOM CENTRAL COUNCIL (1989) *Exercising Accountability*. London: UKCC.

VESSEY, J. A. (1990) Parental participation in paediatric induction. *Children's Health Care*, 19, 116–118.

VETTER, T. R. (1992) Pediatric patient controlled analgesia with morphine versus mepidine. *Journal of Pain Symptom Management*, 7 (4), 204.

VIDOVICH, M. (1980) Caring for kids – death in the ICU. *Australian Nurses Journal*, 9, 43–44.

VISINTAINER, M. and WOLFER, J. (1975) Psychological preparation for surgical patients – the effect on children and parents. *Pediatrics*, 56, 187–202.

VULCAN, B. and NIKULICH-BARRETT, M. (1988) The effect of selected information on mothers' anxiety levels during their children's hospitalisation. *Journal of Pediatric Nursing*, 3 (2), 97–102.

WATERLOW, J. (1988) Prevention is better than cure. *Nursing Times*, 84 (25), 69–70.

WATSON, J. E. (1979) *Medical–Surgical Nursing and Related Physiology*. London: W. B. Saunders.

WEHBE, M. and MOORE, J. (1985) Digital ischaemia in the neonate following IV therapy. *Paediatrics*, 76 (1), 99–103.

WEIBLEY, T. (1989) Inside the incubator. *Maternal & Child Nursing*, 14, 96–100.

WEINBAUM, D. (1987) Nosocomial bacterias. In FASER, B. (ed.), *Infection Control in Intensive Care*. New York: Churchill Livingstone.

WELBORN, L., *et al.* (1993) Peri-operative blood glucose concentrations in paediatric outpatients. *Anaesthesiology*, 65, 543–547.

WHALEY, L. and WONG, D. (1991) *Nursing Care of Infants and Children*. St Louis: Mosby.

WHILE, A. and CRAWFORD, J. (1992a) Paediatric day surgery. *Nursing Times*, 88 (39), 43–45.

WHILE, A. and CRAWFORD, J. (1992b) Day surgery: expediency or quality care. *Paediatric Nursing*, 4 (3), 18–21.

WHITE, C. (1995) Life crises for children and their families. In CARTER, B. and DEARMAN, A. K. (eds), *Child Health Care Nursing*. Oxford: Blackwell Scientific Publications.

WHITE, J. (1997) Creating a Snoezelen effect in PICU. *Paediatric Nursing*, 9 (5), 20–21.

WHITE, P., *et al.* (1988) Nausea and vomiting: causes and prophylaxis. *Seminars in Anaesthesia*, 6, 300–308.

WHITING, M. (1989) Home truths. *Nursing Times*, 85 (14), 74–75.

WHITING, M. (1994) Meeting needs – RSCNs in the community. *Paediatric Nursing*, 6 (1), 9–11.

WILSON, K. (1993) Management of paediatric pain. *British Journal of Nursing*, 2 (10), 524–6.

WONG, D. and BAKER, C. (1988) Pain in children: comparison of assessment scales. *Pediatric Nursing*, 14, 9–17.

WOODWARD, S. (1994) A guide to paediatric resuscitation. *Paediatric Nursing*, 6 (2), 16–18.

WRIGHT, B. (1991) *Sudden Death*. Edinburgh: Churchill Livingstone.

WYCKOFF, P. M. and ERICKSON, M. T. (1987) Meditating factors of stress on mothers of seriously ill hospitalised children. *Children's Health Care*, 16 (1), 4–12.

WYNGAARDEN, J. and SMITH, L. (1988) *Cecil Textbook of Medicine*, 18th edn. Philadelphia: Saunders.

ZIDEMAN, D. (1993) Paediatric resuscitation. In BASKETT, P. (ed.), *Resuscitation Handbook*. London: Wolfe/Mosby.

Further reading

OSTER, G. D. and GOULD, P. (1987) *Using Drawings in Assessment and Therapy*. New York: Brunner/Mazel.

SPECIFIC CARE OF
SICK CHILDREN

Joan Ramsay and Tina Moules

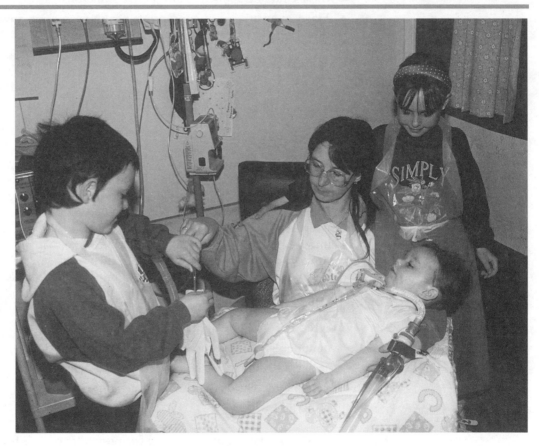

OBJECTIVES

The material contained within this module and the further reading/references should enable you to:

- Revise your knowledge and understanding of applied anatomy and physiology.
- Develop an understanding of the pathophysiology of common disorders and problems of childhood.
- Appreciate the significance of specific assessment for sick children and your role before, during and after medical investigations.
- Discuss some of the more common nursing interventions and how these could be applied to alternative situations.
- Have an awareness of appropriate health promotion advice for discharge.

INTRODUCTION

The purpose of this module is to enable you to explore the problems associated with the structure and function of the body. It does not give detailed information about every disorder found in children, but seeks to provide sufficient principles of care and to enable you to apply these to any given situation. You are encouraged to add your own material and information as you meet different problems so that you can build up a resource file which is individual to your own practice. In the same way in which we have used our experience of nursing children to write this book, we would like to think that you might reflect upon children you have nursed. Each part of the module is arranged in a similar way:

- revision of structure and function;
- common disorders with pathophysiology where relevant;
- specific assessment (including medical investigations);
- nursing interventions (including drug administration);
- discharge advice.

The module begins by examining the principles of care for a variety of disorders. There is no specific order in which this content has been arranged but you will find cross references to other modules. The latter part of the module explores mental health in children, neonatal care, and the care of children receiving cytotoxic treatment and radiotherapy.

PRINCIPLES OF CARE – CHILDREN WITH BLOOD DISORDERS 1

INTRODUCTION

Due to the central importance of blood within the body, its normal function can be affected by primary conditions and as a result of problems in other systems. Many of the primary abnormal conditions of the blood give rise to chronic problems for children. Although advances in understanding and management of these problems have improved the quality of life for children, repeated treatment and care can detract from normality. In order to understand the causes and consequences of blood disorders and implement appropriate care you need to have a working knowledge of the haematological system and its functions and the basis of genetics.

Activity

Test your knowledge of the structure and function of the blood (see box on right). Check your answers in an anatomy and physiology textbook. Read the section on genetics in Module 2 (pages 53–56) and Module 3 (page 131). If necessary renew your knowledge.

The most common disorders of the blood seen in children are bleeding disorders (Table 1.1) and anaemias (Table 1.2)

ASSESSMENT

Assessing the child with blood disorders requires the nurse to use her skills to examine a number of features alongside the general assessment process (Figure 1.1 – page 419).

Activity

A toddler is admitted to your ward and on examination you find a number of bruises on his body. How do you differentiate between old and new bruises? What information might you need to ascertain from the child and his mother in order to conclude that the bruises may be a result of haemolytic disease?

Activity

Pallor is a common sign of blood disorders. However, it is also associated with many other serious chronic conditions – find out which so that your assessment of the child with pallor can be more informed.

Test your knowledge
- List seven functions of the blood
- Plasma constitutes about ?% of the blood
- Apart from water what are the other constituents of plasma?
- Draw a diagram to show the life cycle of a red blood cell (RBC). What factors are essential for the formation of mature cells?
- What is the role of erythropoietin in the formation of RBCs?
- List the types of white cells in the blood and describe their function
- Identify the major steps in coagulation of the blood

Table 1.1

Bleeding disorders in children

Haemophilia	Sex-linked recessive disorder; deficiency of any of nine factors required for normal coagulation cascade; results in bleeding tendency – into joints, muscle and subcutaneous tissue
Haemophilia A (classic)	Deficiency of factor VIII (80% of cases)
Haemophilia B (Christmas disease)	Deficiency of factor IX (13% of cases)
Haemophilia C	Deficiency of factor XI (6% of cases)
Von Willibrand's disease	Hereditary disorder; basic defect in ability of platelets to aggregate in the presence of normal platelet count (accompanied by deficiency of factor VII) – leads to increased bleeding time and tendency towards purpura, epistaxis, ecchymosis, gastro-intestinal bleeding
Idiopathic thrombocytopenic purpura	Acquired of unknown aetiology; decreased production of platelets – leads to prolonged bleeding time and bleeding tendencies as above plus petchiae and superficial bruising
Henoch–Schönlein purpura	Acquired of unknown aetiology; inflammation of small blood vessels and vasculitis of dermal capillaries – leads to extravasation of red blood cells; petechial skin lesions

Pathology of a bleed into a synovial joint

- Hypertrophy of the synovial membrane due to reabsorption of blood and absorption of iron pigments
- Synovium becomes a thickened seaweed-like substance, and begins to invade the articular cartilage and grow over edge of joint surface
- At the same time chemical action of the blood in the joint damages the cartilage which eventually begins to peel off leaving exposed bone
- With repeated bleeds and no treatment the bone becomes soft and joint's surface develops cysts leading to collapse of the joint

Haemoglobin

Normal haemoglobin (HbA) consists of a red pigment haem and four polypeptide strands, two alpha chains and two beta chains. The difference between the two types of chains lies in the sequencing and kinds of amino acids which make up the strands. HbS is caused by the substitution of valine for glutamine at position 6 on the beta chain

(Groer and Shekleton, 1979)

Iron-deficiency anaemia	Infants' iron stores at birth are sufficient for about 3–4 months. After this additional iron is needed from diet. Insufficient nutrition iron leads to deficient haemoglobin formation – red cells hypochromic and microcytic
Megaloblastic anaemia	Folic acid and vitamin B12 essential for synthesis of nucleoproteins required for maturation of red blood cells; deficiences of either interferes with this synthesis; RBCs immature and larger than normal (megaloblastic and macrocytic); number of circulating blood cells decreased; total amount of haemoglobin reduced
Aplastic anaemia congenital	All formed blood elements simultaneously depressed. e.g. Fanconi – autosomal recessive condition.
acquired	Acquired type caused by overwhelming infection, irradiation, drugs (chemotherapeutic acquired agents), chemicals (benzene); can be idiopathic.
Haemolytic anaemia	Red blood cells have an abnormally short lifespan and are destroyed at an abnormally high rate – leads to increase in products of RBC breakdown; jaundice results when liver unable to clear resulting pigment; bone marrow increases production to attempt to compensate – becomes hypertrophied
Sickle cell anaemia	Abnormal Hb (HbS) has reduced solubility within the RBC under conditions of hypoxaemia and hyperthermia; leads to formation of sticky gel-like substance in the Hb molecule leading to unusual sickle shape of RBC; abnormally shaped cells stick together easily increasing blood viscosity; obstruction of blood flow; ischaemic tissue; pain (sickle cell crisis)
Thalassaemia	Deficiencies in the synthesis of beta globulin chains in Hb; defective synthesis of Hb; structurally impaired RBCs (large and immature) with a short lifespan; leads to compensatory bone marrow hyperplasia; produces overgrowth of facial and skull bones. Excess iron accumulates in tissues
Hereditary spherocytosis	Autosomal dominant condition; red cell membrane highly permeable to sodium; RBCs spherical in shape with increased osmotic fragility

Table 1.2

Anaemias in childhood

Note: in all instances the oxygen carrying capacity of the blood is reduced.

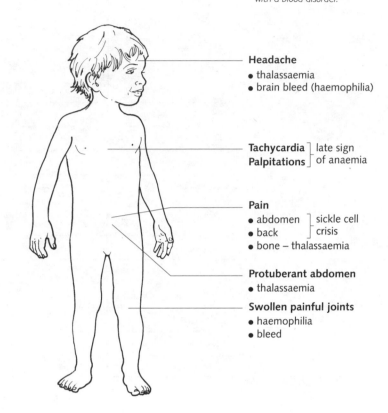

Figure 1.1

Specific assessment of the child with a blood disorder.

Tiredness, lethargy, listlessness
- early signs of anaemia

Weakness
- late sign of anaemia
- possible sickle cell crisis

Anorexia
- early sign of anaemia
- possible sickle crisis
- thalassaemia

Pallor
- early sign of anaemia
- sickle cell crisis
- progressive pallor-thalassaemia

Fever
- sickle cell crisis

Bruising
- bleeding disorder

Haematuria
- haemophilia
- bleed

Headache
- thalassaemia
- brain bleed (haemophilia)

Tachycardia ⎤ late sign
Palpitations ⎦ of anaemia

Pain
- abdomen ⎤ sickle cell
- back ⎦ crisis
- bone – thalassaemia

Protuberant abdomen
- thalassaemia

Swollen painful joints
- haemophilia
- bleed

In assessing the child with a blood disorder the nurse may be required to assist in the implementation and interpretation of medical investigations. Table 1.3 shows the various investigations which may be carried out. Also see Table 1.4.

Activity

Find out in what circumstances each one might be used, what it might show and what the role of the nurse should be. Make notes in the boxes in Table 1.3 for future reference.

NURSING INTERVENTIONS

When caring for a child with a blood disorder you may be required to implement specific interventions. For the purposes of this section the following interventions will be examined:

Table 1.3

Medical investigations (copyright is waived for the purpose of photocopying and enlarging this table.)

Investigation	When and what for?	Role of the nurse
Blood count RBCs WCC platelets differential WCC reticulocyte count		
Hb		
Red cell indices		
Serum bilirubin		
Coomb's test: direct indirect		
Hb electrophoresis		
Serum iron		
Bleeding time		
Coagulation time		
Bone marrow aspirate		
Chest X-ray		

Table 1.4

Normal blood values

	Infant	6–12 years	Adolescent
Haemoglobin (g/dl)	9–14	11.5–15.5	12–16
Haematocrit (volume fraction)	0.28–0.48	0.33–0.47	0.36–0.54
Red cell count	2.7–54	3.9–5.3	4.1–6.1
Platelet count (fl)	150–400	150–400	150–400
Red cell indices			
mean corpuscular volume (fl)	70–86	77–96	80–99
mean corpuscular Hb (fmol/cell)	0.39–0.48	0.39–0.54	0.39–0.54
mean corpuscular Hb concentration (mmol)	29–36	31–37	31–37
Reticulocyte count (%)	0.3–3.1	0.5–2.5	0.5–2.5
White blood count ($\times 10$/l)	5.0–17.5	4.5–13.5	4.5–11.0
Differential WCC (number fraction)			
neutrophils	0.23	0.31–0.61	0.54–0.75
lymphocytes	0.61	0.28–0.48	0.25–0.40
monocytes	0.05	0.04–0.045	0.02–0.08
Bleeding time (minutes)	1–6	1–6	1–6
Clotting time (minutes)	5–8	5–8	5–8

- management of a sickle cell crisis;
- iron chelation therapy;
- blood transfusion;
- diet.

Management of sickle cell crisis

The factors which can precipitate a sickle cell crisis include:

- infection;
- dehydration;
- hypothermia;
- stress;
- strenuous physical exercise;
- acid–base imbalance.

Children and their carers should be made aware of these factors so that they can take steps to avoid them wherever possible.

Activity

What advice could you give a child with sickle cell anaemia and her carers about how to avoid the factors which precipitate a crisis? Design a leaflet to back up your ideas.

The nursing interventions during a sickle cell crisis are aimed mainly at relieving pain, promoting hydration, and offering support and understanding to the child and family.

- The pain which accompanies a sickle cell crisis is classified as being either mild, moderate or severe. Severe episodes require urgent and effective treatment. Schecter *et al.* (1988) suggest that sickle cell pain is often under-treated due to lack of knowledge, inappropriate attitudes about children with sickle cell pain, concerns about addiction and lack of objective assessment criteria. As a result the child develops persistent pain with repeated requests for pain killers. This leads to the child being described as manipulative. It is therefore important to use an appropriate pain assessment tool before implementing treatment. Pain is usually controlled with opiates, often in large doses and administered by continuous infusion. Drugs reported to be effective include papavertum (Sartori *et al.*, 1990) and morphine (Morrison and Vedro, 1989). The use of oral opiates where possible is recommended by Shapiro (cited by Carter, 1994) who suggests that this will 'take the drama out of the crisis' and makes admission to hospital less likely. The use of patient controlled analgesia devices has been advocated as this enables the child to be in control. Non-pharmacological approaches to pain control should be considered alongside drug therapy. Children can be taught how to

Additional aspects of management of sickle cell crisis

- Administration of oxygen – helps to prevent sickling but will not reverse it
- Bed rest at child's discretion – reduces oxygen consumption
- Application of heat to affected areas (NOT cold as this enhances sickling and vaso-constriction)
- Antibiotics for infection

(Whaley and Wong, 1987)

Oxygen therapy

Oxygen therapy is considered not to be useful in vaso-occlusive episodes unless hypoxia is present (Charache *et al.*, cited by Whaley and Wong, 1995). It does not shorten the duration of pain or stop new pain (Zipursky *et al.*, 1992)

Cross reference

Assessment and management of pain – pages 348–359

Cross reference

Relaxation and imagery – pages 269–271

Complications of iron overload

- Cardiac complications – cardiomyopathy occurs as a result of iron deposition in the heart; arrhythmias and pericarditis may also occur
- Hepatic complications – hepatitis B, cirrhosis
- Endocrine complications – retarded growth due to growth hormone deficiency; hypothyroidism; hypoparathyroidism caused by low levels of parahormone as a result of iron deposition in the parathyroid glands; diabetes mellitus

Desferrioxamine

Subcutaneous 20–50 mg/kg/day plus

Vitamin C 2 mg/kg daily on infusion nights (increases iron excretion in response to desferrioxamine)

Cross reference

IV fluid therapy – page 341

use self-hypnosis and imagery. They need to be taught about pain control, so that they are informed when treatment becomes necessary. This will help to reduce fear and tension and will encourage the development of a trusting relationship with nurses and medical staff.

- Hydration therapy in the form of an intravenous (IV) infusion will be considered. This will help to dilute the viscous blood and reverse agglutination of sickled cells within the small blood vessels. At the same time oral fluids should be encouraged.

Iron chelation therapy

Children with thalassaemia require repeated blood transfusions every 3–4 weeks. Such frequent transfusions lead to an accumulation of iron which cannot be excreted or absorbed. Instead it is deposited in other body structures. To prevent the build up of serum ferritin, iron chelation therapy is usually administered about five to six times per week. The chelator of choice is desferrioxamine which is given subcutaneously via a syringe pump over 8–12 hours (usually at night) (Roberts *et al.*, 1996). The nurse must be aware of the complications of chelation therapy:

- local reactions – itching and rash – are common; poor hygiene can result in skin infection and abscesses;
- severe allergic reaction – the first dose must always be administered in hospital;
- too rapid infusion of IV desferrioxamine can cause vertigo, hypotension, erythema and generalised pruritis (Roberts *et al.*, 1996).

Where possible home chelation therapy is implemented with the support of the community children's nurse. In this instance a teaching programme must be instigated which ensures that carers and children understand the theoretical background to the treatment and its practical management.

Blood transfusion

It is likely that you will care for many children who require a blood transfusion for a variety of reasons. However, children with disorders of the blood are more likely to need this therapy and on a more regular basis. You therefore need to be familiar with the procedure and the role of the nurse in its administration:

- Concerns about the transmission of hepatitis and HIV may be voiced by the child and carers. They should be told that the risks are minimal and that this should be balanced against the effects of foregoing the transfusion. Information about how the blood has been collected and tested could help to reassure.
- The nurse should ensure safe administration of the correct blood. This requires careful checking of the blood and blood group against

the child's identity band and notes. Administration of the blood should commence within 30 minutes of its arrival from the blood bank. Unused blood should be returned to the blood bank.

- The nurse must be aware of the potential complications of a blood transfusion (Table 1.5) and monitor the child according to local policy.

Complication	Features	Nursing interventions
Haemolytic reaction – severe but rare reaction caused by incompatible blood	Fever, chills, shaking Pain at needle site and along venous tract Nausea/vomiting sensation of tightness in chest Red or black urine, headache, Flank pain Progressive signs of Shock and renal failure	Stop transfusion immediately in event of signs of reaction Notify doctor Monitor for shock
Febrile reaction – due to the presence of leukocyte, platelet or plasma protein antibodies	Fever and chills	Stop transfusion and notify doctor
Allergic reaction – recipient's blood reacts to allergens in donor blood	Urticarial rash, flushing Asthmatic wheezing Laryngeal oedema	Administer antihistamines as prescribed Stop transfusion immediately and seek help
Circulatory overload – due to too rapid transfusion or an excessive quantity of transfused blood	Precordial pain Dyspnoea Rales Cyanosis Distended neck veins	Take steps to ensure transfusion runs at the prescribed rate Stop transfusion immediately in event of signs of overload
Air emboli – due to blood transfused under pressure	Sudden difficulty in breathing Sharp pain in chest – apprehension	Ensure no air infiltration to administration set Stop infusion and seek help

Table 1.5

Complications of blood transfusions and related nursing interventions

Activity

Take an opportunity to donate blood. While you are there find out how donors are screened and what for.

Activity

Visit the blood bank to find out how the blood is stored and prepared ready for administration.

Activity

Find out what your local policy says about monitoring children during a blood transfusion.

The need for repeated transfusions can be very disruptive. The child will be required to spend the day on the ward perhaps missing school and all its attendant activities. Each child should therefore be allocated the same nurse (wherever possible) on each occasion so that a trusting relationship can be developed. The school teacher and play leader can be involved to encourage appropriate activities and help to reduce boredom.

Diet

According to the DoH (1994) iron deficiency is the most commonly reported nutritional disorder in early childhood in the UK. In a study by Gregory *et al.* (1997) 12% of children aged 1.5–2.5 years old and 65% of children aged 2.5–4.5 years old were described as being anaemic. Children who present with iron deficiency anaemia are managed by a combination of dietary modification and iron supplements. Carers need advice on:

- The sources of bioavailable iron. This describes the proportion of total iron in food which is absorbed and utilised for metabolism. Iron is most readily absorbed from foods rich in haem – liver, red meats, other meat (e.g. poultry) and meat products. Other sources of iron, although less well absorbed, include egg yolks, whole grains, fortified cereals and bread, legumes, green leafy vegetables, dried fruits and potatoes.
- Foods which enhance iron absorption – vitamin C.
- Foods which reduce absorption of iron – cereals, plums, green beans, spinach, tomatoes and tea.

When weaning infants, parents should be encouraged to avoid giving too much milk but should ensure that adequate amounts of solid food are given. Milk (especially cows' milk which is not advocated until after 12 months) is not a good source of iron.

HOME MANAGEMENT FOR CHILDREN WITH BLOOD DISORDERS

Prior to discharge the child and family must be familiar with all aspects of management of their particular problem. Table 1.6 highlights some of the important specific elements of care that must be taught to different children.

Activity

Contact some of the support agencies identified below. Ask for copies of information sheets and analyse the advice available for children and their carers at home.

- OSCAR (Organisation for Sickle Cell Anaemia Research), Sickle Cell Community Centre, Tiverton Road, Tottenham, London N15 6RT. Tel: 0181 802 3055/0944.

Disorder	Education for discharge
Sickle cell disease	Prevention of a crisis: • importance of maintaining hydration with a high fluid intake. Parents need to know how much to give per 24 hour period. They need to be aware of the signs of fluid loss – dry mucosa, weight loss, sunken fontanelle in the young baby; • prevention of infection – importance of adequate nutrition to enable the child to fight infection, hygiene and the avoidance where possible of sources of infection. Prompt medical care should be sought if signs of infection are evident Details of support agencies
Thalassaemia	Parents and children need psychological support to enable them to deal with this chronic life-threatening disorder. Education for home management of iron chelation therapy
Iron-deficiency anaemia	Dietary advice (see above). It may not be sufficient just to tell parents what foods are rich in iron. The nurse may need to help with suggestions for recipes and buying the right foods. Paediatric dietician should be involved in education of family. Correct administration of iron supplements – as an increased stomach acidity reduces absorption of iron, supplements should be taken in between meals with a drink of citrus fruit juice to enhance absorption. Warn parents of effect of iron on stools – can make them tarry green. Liquid iron can cause temporary staining of the teeth – advise giving through a straw and cleaning teeth after administration. Warn parents that ingestion of large amounts of iron is dangerous so all preparations must be stored safely out of the reach of children
Haemophilia	Advise about regular dental care and good dental hygiene. Child should wear Medic-Alert identification. Teach parents and child how to recognise early signs of a bleed so that prompt treatment can be implemented – early signs of bleeding into a joint include stiffness, tingling, ache and reduced movement. Signs of internal bleeding include headache, slurred speech, loss of consciousness (bleed in the brain), black tarry stools, haematemesis (intestinal bleeding). Teach administration of Factor VIII/IX

Table 1.6

Education for discharge

- Sickle Cell Society, 54 Station Road, Harlesden, London NW10 4UB. Tel: 0181 961 7795/8346.
- UK Thalassaemia Society, 107 Nightingale Lane, London N8 7QY. Tel: 0181 348 0437.
- Haemophilia Society, 123 Westminster Bridge Road, London SE1 7HR. Tel: 0171 928 2020.

Many of the procedures and treatments needed by children with blood disorders can now be implemented at home with support from community children's nurses and in ambulatory care settings such as outpatient clinics. In each case the child and carers need an individualised teaching plan to ensure that they have the necessary knowledge and skills to carry out the procedures safely and effectively. For example, the administration of home treatment for haemophilia has developed considerably over the last 10 years and has reduced hospital admissions. Children are encouraged to learn self-administration of Factor VIII/IX before they reach senior school. Some require regular therapy, others can manage with intermittent use of Factor VIII/IX.

Activity

Draw up a teaching plan to use with a 10-year-old boy with haemophilia to help him learn how to administer Factor VIII/IX. Give a rationale for your plan.

PRINCIPLES OF CARE – CHILDREN WITH PROBLEMS OF BONES, JOINTS AND MUSCLES

2

INTRODUCTION

Caring for children with problems of the bones and joints requires skill and patience. These problems can affect mobility, activity and almost every other activity of living to varying degrees. The child's appearance may be altered giving rise to problems with body image. Many of the problems require long-term management and treatment which can necessitate frequent visits to hospital and sometimes periods of immobility. It is important that you have an understanding of the structure and functions of the musculoskeletal system and its development and maturation during childhood. A degree of prior knowledge is assumed but you may need to refresh your memory.

Cross reference

Maturation – page 65

Activity

Revise the structure and function of bones and joints. In doing this ensure that you understand:
* osteoblasts, osteocytes, osteoclasts
* the periosteum
* the role of parathyroid hormone, vitamin D, calcitonin
* the difference between types of joints.

For the purpose of this text some of the problems likely to be faced by children are divided into congenital or genetic (Table 2.1) and acquired (Table 2.2).

ASSESSMENT

Some problems of bones, joints and muscles will be obvious to the eye (e.g. some fractures, congenital abnormalities). Others will require you to be able to assess movement and function of the musculoskeletal system.

Fractures

It is probable that you will have been made aware of a child's fracture before he reaches the ward. However, it is important that you know the features of fractures so that you can assess children in Accident and Emergency and at the scene of an accident if necessary. The main features are:
* *Pain* – may be throbbing or localised, aggravated by passive or active movement.

Further reading

CRAIG, C. (1995) Congenital talipes equinivarus. *Professional Nurse*, **11** (1), 30–32.

Table 2.1

Congenital/genetic problems of bones, joints and muscles

Problem	Pathophysiology
Talipes (Craig, 1995)	
equinivarus	Foot is plantar fixed, the heel is inverted, the mid- and forefoot adducted. Interrelationships between bone, ligaments and muscle are disrupted. Often accompanied by neurological problems
calcaneovalgus	Foot is dorsiflexed and everted. Underlying structural deformity less profound – foot more amenable to manipulation
Congenital dislocation of the hip (CDH)	
unstable ('clicky hip')	Head of femur can be moved in and out of the acetabulum through manipulation. Head of femur and acetabulum are normal or near normal in shape
subluxed	Head of femur only in partial contact with acetabulum. Lack of development shape of acetabulum
dislocated	Head of femur lies completely out of joint. Shape and size of head of femur and acetabulum are abnormal. Will deteriorate if left
Scoliosis	Caused by failure of vertebral formation and segmentation. Lateral flexion of the spine causes trunk to shift from the midline, altering centre of gravity and shortening the spine. Spine rotates on its longitudinal axis; vertebra become permanently wedge shaped; shape of rib cage alters
Marfan's syndrome	Autosomal dominant disease consisting of arachnodactyly, hypermobile joints, ocular abnormalities, high arched palate. Commonly associated deformities of spine and chest
Osteogenesis imperfecta (brittle bone disease)	Autosomal dominant (occasionally recessive). Underlying failure in collagen metabolism resulting in multiple fractures of fragile bones, lax joints and thin skin. Other features include blue sclera, scoliosis
Duchenne muscular dystrophy	Sex-linked recessive disease affecting male children. Progressive degeneration of groups of skeletal muscles and replacement of muscle by fibrous tissue leads to generalised wasting, kyphosis with thoracic deformity, hip and ankle contracture, inability to walk (usually apparent by 8–11 years), scoliosis and eventually cardiac muscle involvement. Gene has been mapped to p21 band and the X chromosome (Cree, 1997)

Congenital Dislocation of the hip

- Now commonly termed developmental dysplasia of the hip (DDH) as the defect may not be congenital and the hip is not always dislocated
- Several possible interconnecting influencing factors
- Degrees of dysplasia:
  - preluxation
  - subluxation
  - dislocation

Figure 2.1

Developmental dysplasia of the hip, possible history (after Watson 1990)

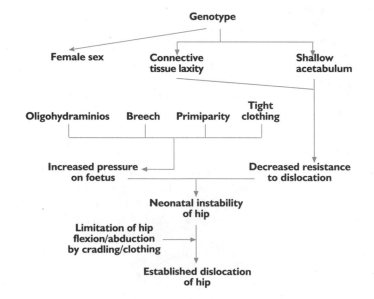

Problem	Pathophysiology
Juvenile rheumatoid arthritis	Inflammation in joints; initially localised in joint capsule; tissue becomes thickened from congestion and oedema. Inflammatory response follows which invades interior of the joint; inflammatory tissue extends into interior of the joint along surface of articular cartilage; deprives the cartilage of nutrients; articular cartilage slowly destroyed. Growth plates may fuse prematurely; inflammatory changes may occur in tendons and sheaths; inflammation of muscle may occur
Osteomyelitis	Infection in metaphysis of long bones caused by bacteria – mainly *Staphylococcus pyogenes*. Resulting inflammatory reaction causes tissue necrosis, thrombosis of vessels leading to bone ischaemia; pus forms and spreads towards diaphysis, extending through cortex of bones; subperiosteal abscess forms raising periosteum from bone. Will either heal or progress to chronic condition
Idiopathic adolescent scoliosis	Affects mainly girls 10–14 years. See Table 2.1 for pathophysiology
Perthes' disease	Aseptic necrosis of the femoral head. Three stages: • *Stage 1* – avascularity; spontaneous interruption of blood supply to upper femoral epiphysis. Bone ceases to grow, swelling of soft tissue round hip; • *Stage 2* – revascularisation; growth of new vessels – bone resorption and deposition take place; new bone is weak; • *Stage 3* – reossification; head of femur gradually reforms, dead bone is removed, replaced with new bone which gradually spreads to heal lesion
Slipped upper femoral epiphyses	Posterior slipping of epiphysis of femoral head in relation to its metaphysis; results in shearing failure of growth plate. Further slipping can occur at any time – urgent treatment needed
Fractures – common ones seen in children include fractures of: neck or shaft of humerus supracondylar fracture of humerus distal third of radius and ulna distal radial physis femoral shaft, tibia or fibula	Break in the continuity of a bone or cartilage usually caused by direct or indirect violence (Miller and Miller, 1985), by repeated stress and strain or by pathological processes (Pagdin, 1996). Children's bones are softer than adults and can withstand a greater degree of deformity before breaking. Greenstick fractures are unique to children; bone breaks at one cortex and bends at the other – there is no complete loss of bony continuity. Injuries of the epiphyseal plate unique to children. Fractures heal more quickly than in adults
Bone tumours osteosarcoma	Occur mainly in adolescents; in the metaphysis of long bones (particularly around the knee). Highly malignant, destroying the cortex, extending into soft tissue and metastasising early via bloodstream to the lungs
Ewing's sarcoma	Highly malignant occurring mainly in diaphysis of long bones and flat bones of children and adolescents. Metastasises early to lungs and bone marrow

Table 2.2

Acquired problems of bones, joints and muscles

- *Loss of function* – due to pain and instability of the fracture.
- *Swelling* – caused by oedema and effusion of blood. Takes time to appear, increases over the first 12–24 hours after surgery.
- *Deformity* – limb is bent or has a step in its alignment. There may be angular deformity, shortening of the limb, rotational deformity.

It will be important that the child is systematically assessed for any other injury on admission to the ward.

Mobility

In assessing a child's mobility you should consider the following:

Cross reference

Motor development – page 69

- Has the child reached the normal milestones in motor development? Delayed walking is sometimes evident in children with congenital dislocated hip (CDH).

- Watch the child walking. Is there a limp (Perthes' disease, CDH, bone tumour)? Is there an abnormal gait? A waddling gait is evident in CDH as is the Trendelenburg sign; note movement of the feet, legs, knees.

Trendelenburg's sign

The pelvis drops on the normal side when the child stands on the abnormal leg

- Look at the child's posture. Is there any abnormality which might indicate scoliosis – poor posture, one shoulder higher than the other, one hip which seems more prominent, crooked neck, lump on the back?

- Is there any evidence of joint swelling which may be indicative of arthritis? General swelling may accompany bone tumours.

- Is the child complaining of pain? Back pain is likely in scoliosis; pain in the hip referred to the knee, inner thigh and groin may accompany Perthes' disease; a reluctance to move a limb may be indicative of osteomyelitis. Pain can be a feature of bone tumours.

- Is the child generally unwell showing signs of infection (reluctance to eat and drink, fever) – linked to osteomyelitis.

- Examine the child – limited abduction and internal rotation of the hip accompany Perthes' disease; asymmetry of the gluteal folds and leg length inequality are indicative of CDH.

Other diagnostic tests may be used to determine potential problems (Table 2.3).

Table 2.3

Diagnostic tests for bone, joint and muscle problems (Copyright is waived for the purpose of photocopying and enlarging this table.)

Investigation	When and what for?	Role of the nurse
Plain X-rays		
Bone scan		
Blood cultures		
ESR		
Leucocyte count		
Computed tomography		
Ultrasound (see LeMaistre, 1991)		

Further reading

LeMAISTRE, G. (1991) Ultrasound and dislocation of the hip. *Paediatric Nursing*, May, 13–16.

Activity

Explore each of the tests/investigations in Table 2.9 and make notes in the boxes.

You should also become familiar with two screening tests used to diagnose CDH – Barlow and Ortolani tests. Universal screening for CDH was first recommended in 1969, but since then debates about its role and effectiveness have been controversial (Leck, 1995). However, it is important to detect the condition early so that conservative treatment can be attempted thus avoiding the need for surgery. The screening tests may be carried out by midwives, health visitors, general practitioners or community medical officers.

Activity

Take an opportunity to observe one of the above professionals carrying out screening for CDH. Discuss the use of the test with them and the implications of detection of a problem.

NURSING INTERVENTIONS

You may be required to participate in implementing any one of a number of interventions for children with problems of bones, joints and muscles. This section will address a few of the more common interventions. You are advised to explore each one further as space precludes the inclusion of too much detail.

CARE OF THE IMMOBILISED CHILD

For many children, treatment of problems will entail immobility for varying lengths of time. You need to have a clear understanding of the effects of immobility so that appropriate care can be implemented to avoid complications. The main effects and complications of immobilisation and associated care are:

- Decreased muscle activity and atrophy – leads to weakness, loss of joint mobility – encourage both active and passive exercises – put joints through full range of movements where possible.
- Decreased metabolism – increase by encouraging activity within the child's limitations.
- Bone demineralisation which can lead to high serum calcium levels – ensure increased hydration and active remobilisation a soon as possible.
- Disruption of normal elimination processes – adequate hydration promotes bowel and renal function. Enable child to sit to use potty or bedpan wherever possible to encourage normal elimination – provide privacy.

1986 Expert Working Party recommendations
- All infants should have an examination within 24 hours of birth
- At the time of discharge or within 10 days of birth
- At 6 weeks
- At 6–9 months
- At 15–21 months
- The gait should be reviewed at 24–30 months and again at preschool examination

(Hall, 1996)

Cross reference
Care of the child confined to bed – pages 364

Processes involved in skin breakdown
Increased pressure on tissues leads to compression of small blood vessels; this in turn leads to infarction of soft tissues with a reduced supply of nutrients and removal of waste; this results in cellular necrosis which can cause open infected ulcers and the development of systemic infection

Cross reference
Prevention of pressure sores – pages 366–369

- Reduced integrity of the skin – change position frequently, keep skin clean and dry, pay particular attention to prominent bony areas. Make use of sheepskins, avoid pressure on skin from equipment, tubes, tape, ensure adequate hydration and nutrition.

Activity

Explore the devices available to contribute to the prevention of pressure sores.

- Loss of appetite – offer small attractive meals, with nutrition snacks in between. Give preferred foods where possible.
- Psychological effects – make use of therapeutic play, involve play therapists and teachers.

Activity

Plan a day's activities for a 2-year-old girl confined to bed on gallow's traction. Give reasons for your decisions.

PRINCIPLES OF CARING FOR CHILDREN IN PLASTER CASTS

A plaster cast is an immobilising device made up of layers of bandages impregnated with plaster of Paris (made from calcium sulphate dihydrate – gypsum) or synthetic lighter weight materials. Plaster casts are used to:

- immobilise and hold bone fragments in reduction;
- permit early weight bearing activities;
- correct deformities.

Nursing care is aimed at preventing complications and ensuring the child's comfort (Table 2.4). Specific care for certain types of cast may be needed (e.g. body cast or hip spica).

Types of plaster casts

- *Short arm casts* – from below elbow to proximal palmar crease
- *Gauntlet cast* – extends from below elbow to proximal palmar crease including the thumb
- *Long arm cast* – extends from upper level of axillary fold to proximal palmar crease (elbow usually immobilised at right angle)
- *Short leg cast* - extends from below the knee to base of toes
- *Long leg cast* – extends from junction of upper and middle third of thigh to base of toes
- *Spica or body cast* - incorporates trunk and an extremity
- *Hip spica* – extends from waist level to knees – holding the legs in the 'frog' position

Table 2.4

Nursing care for children in plaster casts

Potential complication	Nursing care
Plaster sores	Prevent irritation at edge of cast; avoid wetting the cast; do not place anything sharp down the side of the cast; monitor for signs – severe initial pain over bony prominence; increasing restlessness, fretful; (pain decreases when ulceration occurs): odour; drainage on cast. Report any of above
Circulatory disturbance – particularly after application of plaster	Elevate the body part to increase venous return; handle moist cast with palms of hands to avoid damage (dry POP sounds hollow when tapped; monitor for signs of inadequate tissue perfusion – swelling, blanching or discoloration of nail beds, tingling or numbness, inability to move fingers or toes, temperature change in skin – cold extremity may indicate ischaemia

Many children can be discharged with a plaster cast and parents must be given adequate information about the care of the cast. The main points for inclusion should be:

- the plaster will take 2–3 days to dry out – do not write on it until it is dry;
- keep the plaster dry;
- keep fingers and toes moving;
- do not cut or interfere with the plaster;
- do not let child put small toys down the plaster;
- avoid contact with direct heat;
- return to hospital immediately if any of the following occur: the plaster feels tight or there is swelling; fingers/toes go blue/pale, cannot be moved, tingle or go numb; there is severe pain, there is an odd smell from the plaster; the plaster becomes wet or damaged.

Activity

Design a handout to give to children using the points above. Give reasons for your choice of design. If you get an opportunity try it out and reflect on its effectiveness.

MANAGING TRACTION

> *When forces having both direction and magnitude act on an object at the same point simultaneously from opposite directions, the object either changes its state of rest or motion or remains in equilibrium.*
>
> **(Campbell and Glasper, 1995)**

Traction uses the direct application of these forces to produce equilibrium at a given site. The two essential components of traction are the forward traction (produced by attaching weight to the distal bone) and the counter-traction (backward force of the muscle pull). There are two main types of traction:

- *Skeletal traction* – the pull is applied directly to the skeletal structure

Indications for traction

- To relieve pain or muscle spasm
- To ensure rest of a limb during the healing period
- To maintain correct alignment
- To restore length where shortening after a fracture has occurred
- To reduce dislocation of joints
- To maintain the position of unstable fractures
- Pre-operatively prior to external fixation
- To maintain good positioning after surgery

(Pritchard and David, 1990)

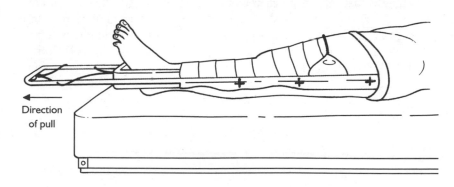

Direction of pull

Figure 2.2

Thomas' splint: the traction works against the force of the child's body.

Figure 2.3

Gallow's traction: the child's weight serves as counter-traction to the vertical pull of the weights

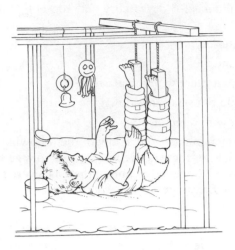

Points to remember when applying skin traction

- Careful explanations should be given – may be painful
- Maintain privacy
- Wash and dry the limb and check for any signs of injury or soreness prior to applying strapping; the use of solutions to enhance adhesiveness may be advocated (e.g. tincture of benzoin)
- Keep the ankle free
- Avoid folds and creases in the strapping
- Check temperature and colour of skin after application to ensure that tension is correct

by a pin inserted into or through the diameter of the bone (e.g. Steinemann's pin, halo traction).

- *Skin traction* – the pull is applied directly to the skin surface and indirectly to the skeletal structure. Adhesive strapping is applied to the skin with cords that can be attached to weights and pulleys (e.g. Thomas' splint – Figure 2.2, gallow's traction – Figure 2.3).

Traction imposes degrees of immobilisation and therefore care aimed at preventing the complications of immobilisation should be considered. In addition you should implement care to:

- Maintain effective traction – check apparatus at regular intervals to ensure that ropes/pulleys/weights are in the right position and freely movable; maintain the child in the appropriate position, e.g. in gallow's traction the infant's buttocks should be elevated and clear of the bed.
- Maintain skin integrity – keep skin clean and dry, examine skin regularly. Remove covering bandages from skin traction and reapply daily; monitor skin for signs of soreness.
- Avoid infection at pin sites – a review of the literature by Rowe (1997) suggests that there is no clear consensus regarding the cleaning of pin sites. Very often surgeons' preferences are the determining factor. Care varies from non-treatment to pin site care every 2 hours; the use of various cleansing agents including hydrogen peroxide (Jones-Walton, 1991), 70% alcohol, povidine iodine (Collins, 1984) and normal saline (Rowe, 1997; Gill, 1994); whether to cover or not – some surgeons prefer the pin sites to be left uncovered, others advocate the use of woven gauze (Henry, 1995, cited by Rowe, 1997).

Activity

Critically explore how pin site care is managed in your area and compare with the ideas given here.

Traction is a very effective form of conservative treatment but generally has to be carried out in hospital because of the problems of accommodating traction equipment at home. Clayton (1997) describes the successful implementation of a 'traction at home' scheme. Care was shared between hospital and community staff. Although caring for children on traction at home is not appropriate for everyone, the scheme evaluated positively and this service is now offered to families.

CARING FOR CHILDREN WITH JUVENILE CHRONIC ARTHRITIS (JCA)

Children with JCA require support from their families and health professionals as the disease can affect almost every aspect of their lives. Nursing care is based on the goals of treatment and is aimed at:

- Relieving pain – using drugs (NSAIDs – including ibuprofen, naproxen, mefenamic acid; SAARDs – gold, hydroxychloroquine); using moist heat, particularly by warm baths, hot packs, immersion of hands or feet in hot water.

- Promoting general health – well balanced diet; weight control may be needed to avoid excessive strain on inflamed joints; regular rest periods.

- Maintenance of good posture and body mechanics – firm mattress to maintain good alignment of spine, hips and knees; no pillow or at least a very thin one; the use of splints or supports to maintain positioning for children confined to bed.

- Physiotherapy – focused on strengthening muscles, mobilising restricted joint movements, preventing or correcting deformities.

- Psychological care – helping the child to cope with the demands of the disease whilst attempting to reach their potential. May need counselling.

SUPPORT AND ADVICE

Children with problems of bones joints and muscles require support from a variety of sources.

Activity

Some of the support agencies are listed below. Contact some of these to find out what information and support is available. Make up a resource pack for your ward/department.
- STEPS, 15 Statham Close, Lymm, Cheshire WA13 9NN. Hotline: 0925 757525.
- Children's Chronic Arthritis Association, c/o Caroline Cox, 47 Battenhall Avenue, Worcester WR5 2HN.
- Osteogenesis Imperfecta Support Group, Brittle Bone Society, 112 City Road, Dundee DD2 2PW.
- Perthes' Association, 42 Woodlands Road, Guildford, Surrey GU1 1RW.
- Scoliosis Association (UK), 2 Ivebruy Court, 323–327 Latimer Road, London W10 6RA.

Suggested process for planning and implementing home traction
- Involve community team
- Inform all parents of possibility of home care for traction
- Family must be committed to 24 hour care
- Family must have been observed caring for the traction
- Home circumstances should be assessed
- All equipment is available before discharge
- Transport home is arranged
- GP informed of discharge
- Open access to ward should be allowed

Adapted from Clayton (1997)

Goals of treatment for JCA
- To preserve joint function
- To prevent physical deformity
- To relieve symptoms without iatrogenic harm

(Campbell and Glasper, 1995)

JCA medication

NSAIDs – non-steroidal anti-inflammatory drugs

SAARDs - slower-acting anti-rheumatic drugs

3   PRINCIPLES OF CARE – CHILDREN WITH A CIRCULATORY DISTURBANCE

INTRODUCTION

The common disorders affecting the heart can be categorised into congenital cardiac anomalies (Table 3.1) and acquired cardiac disease (Table 3.2). Congenital heart defects are anatomical defects which are present at birth and impair normal cardiac function. The incidence of congenital heart disease is 0.8:1000 live births (Holmes, 1996). Acquired cardiac disorders are those which develop after birth in response to infection, autoimmune disease, environmental and familial factors.

COMMON CARDIOVASCULAR DISORDERS

To understand the consequences of congenital and acquired heart disease it is important to have a knowledge of the anatomy and physiology of the heart before and after birth.

Activity

Draw two large diagrams of the heart showing normal blood flow in the fetus and postnatally and use these to identify the position and consequences of the anomalies described in Table 3.1.

Causes of cardiac anomalies

Chromosomal anomalies
- trisomy 21
- Turner's syndrome
- Marfan's syndrome
- Rubella syndrome

Environmental factors
- teratogens, e.g. thalidomide

Maternal health
- insulin-dependent diabetes
- alcoholism
- cytomegalovirus
- parental congenital heart disease

Maternal age
- >40 years

The primary feature of impaired circulation is cyanosis and congenital anomalies are usually classified into cyanotis and acyanotic defects (Figure 3.1). Many of these congenital defects eventually lead to cardiac failure. Cardiac failure occurs when the heart is no longer able to maintain an adequate circulation of oxygenated blood to meet the body's metabolic demands. Cardiac failure can also result from myocardial failure. Cardiomyopathy, certain drugs and electrolyte imbalance can all weaken the contractability of the myocardium and cause cardiac failure. Failure of other body systems, especially the respiratory system, also causes heart failure. Initially the body tries to compensate for a failing heart by using several compensatory mechanisms. This cardiac reserve includes hypertrophy and dilation of the cardiac muscle and stimulation of the sympathetic system. Hypertrophy of the cardiac muscle increases the pressure within the ventricle and dilation enables the muscle to increase the force of each contraction thus increasing cardiac output. However, these compensatory mechanisms can only benefit the situation temporarily. Eventually, compliance is lost from the hypertrophied ventricle and the increased muscle mass prevents adequate myocardial oxygenation. Additionally,

Anomaly	Description
Acyanotic defects	
ventricular septal defect (VSD)	An opening in the ventricular septum. A small defect will allow blood to shunt from the left to right ventricle and into the pulmonary circulation. The increased pulmonary blood flow may cause pulmonary vascular disease
atrial septal defect (ASD)	A hole in the atrium which causes left-to-right shunting of blood because the right ventricle is more compliant than the left. The consequent volume overload of the right ventricle may not result in hypertrophy and heart failure until adulthood
patent ductus arteriosus (PDA)	Continued patency of the fetal ductus arteriosus which should constrict within hours postnatally. Blood shunts from the aorta into the pulmonary artery. A large shunt increases pulmonary blood flow, pulmonary venous return and a volume overload of the left ventricle. Left ventricular hypertrophy and heart failure results
pulmonary stenosis	The pulmonary valve is thickened and fused reducing the lumen of the valve. The increased resistance to blood causes an increase in the pressure generated by the right ventricle. Right ventricular hypertrophy and fibrosis ensues
aortic stenosis	Obstruction to the outflow of the left ventricle causes the left ventricle to generate greater pressure to maintain its flow. Consequently, left ventricular hypertension and hypertrophy occurs. Left coronary artery blood flow may be limited to diastole, causing tachycardia or angina on exercise
coarctation of the aorta	Aortic narrowing increases the resistance from the ascending to the descending aorta. The renal arteries which are served by the descending aorta receive a hypotensive flow and stimulate the release of renin which increases the aortic pressure above the coarctation. Collateral arteries may develop to allow the continuation of normal perfusion
Cyanotic defects	
tetralogy of Fallot	The association of four cardiac anomalies: VSD, pulmonary stenosis, right ventricular hypertrophy and dextroposition of the aorta. With mild forms of these defects resistance to pulmonary blood flow is usually equal to the resistance in the systemic circulation and minimal features are present. Right ventricular hypertrophy develops with larger defects to maintain a normal pulmonary blood flow. When this fails to prevent chronic arterial oxygen desaturation, a pulmonary collateral circulation and polycythaemia develops
tricuspid atresia	Absence of the tricuspid valve causes blood to leave the right atrium through some interatrial communication, usually a patent foramen ovale. If this is too small, right atrial hypertension and systemic venous congestion occur
transposition of the great arteries	Inappropriate septation and migration of the trunctus arteriosus during fetal development causes the aorta to arise from the right ventricle and the pulmonary artery to arise from the left ventricle. Thus, the right side of the heart receives systemic venous blood and is returned to the systemic circulation via the aorta. Similarly, oxygenated blood circulates back and forth through the lungs and the left side of the heart. Signs of arterial oxygen desaturation are immediately present at birth unless some other defect allows shunting of blood to occur
truncus arteriosus	Inadequate division of the truncus arteriosus during fetal cardiac development. Instead of dividing to form the pulmonary artery and the aorta a single great vessel arises from the ventricles. This single vessel receives the output from both ventricles and mixed venous blood is circulated, resulting in cyanosis

Table 3.1

Congenital cardiac anomalies

Common palliative operations for congenital heart defects

- *Pulmonary artery banding.* Performed for defects with a high pulmonary blood flow (e.g. VSD). A silk suture is tied around the pulmonary artery to reduce blood flow and reduce the risk of pulmonary vascular disease. Can be difficult to remove at the time of corrective surgery

- *Blalock–Taussig shunt.* End-to-side anastomosis of the subclavian artery to the pulmonary artery to increase pulmonary blood flow. Can occlude due to clotting

- *Modified Blalock–Taussig shunt.* A gortex tube is inserted between the subclavian and pulmonary arteries to increase pulmonary blood flow. Smaller shunts are likely to clot and prophylactic dipyrimadole is usually administered

- *Waterson's shunt.* A direct side-to-side anastamosis between the ascending aorta and the pulmonary artery to increase pulmonary blood flow. Although less likely to clot it may cause distortion of the pulmonary artery making later repair difficult

- *Glenn procedure.* The azygos vein is ligated and the superior vena cava is resected and anastamosed to the transected right pulmonary artery to increase blood flow selectively to the right lung. It reduces the work of the heart but eventually causes damage to the pulmonary vessels within the right lung. It also makes it almost impossible to restore normal anatomy at the time of the correct repair

- *Bi-directional Glenn procedure.* The azygos vein is ligated and the superior vena cava is transected and an end-to-end anastamosis is performed with the pulmonary artery to increase blood supply to both lungs. This procedure allows more chance of appropriate reconstruction at the time of corrective surgery

Table 3.2

Acquired cardiovascular disorders

Primary cardiomyopathy	Idiopathic disease of the myocardium which becomes progressively more thickened around the ventricles. As a result the ventricles are significantly reduced in size and there is associated impairment of their dilatation and contraction. Cardiac failure will eventually result. Reduced pressure in the left ventricle may cause mitral valve regurgitation. Sudden death may also occur as a result of ventricular arrythmia or complete obstruction of the ventricles
Primary hypertension	High arterial blood pressure forces the heart to pump harder to release blood against this resistance. As a result the heart muscle becomes enlarged and thickened. The increased demand for more oxygen may result in ischaemic changes. Increased pressure in the arterioles also causes thickening and narrowing of the lumen. Reduced renal perfusion stimulates the production of renin which exacerbates the high pressure
Subacute bacterial endocarditis	Microorganisms from any localised infection grow on a part of the endocardium which has been subject to some abnormal blood flow or turbulence. Areas of vegetation, fibrin deposits and thrombi develop which can break off and travel in the circulation to form renal, cerebral, splenic, pulmonary or skin emboli
Rheumatic fever	Inflammatory lesions develop in the heart, brain, pleura and joints from an autoimmune response to a group A, beta-haemolytic streptococcal sore throat. Lesions in cardiac tissue cause valvitis, myocarditis, pericarditis and endocarditis. Progressive valvular disease may eventually result in heart failure (rheumatic heart disease) and require surgery
Kawasaki disease	A microvascular inflammatory disease which progresses into myocarditis, pericarditis and sometimes valvitis. The myocardium is infiltrated with white cells, and the conduction system is impaired by oedema. Coronary artery dilatation may develop into aneurysms which may lead to coronary insufficiency, myocardial ischaemia and cardiac failure or infarction
Henoch–Schönlein purpura	Inflammation of small blood vessels causes widespread vasculitis of dermal capillaries, extravasation of red blood cells and a characteristic petechial rash. This inflammation and haemorrhage may also occur in the renal, gastro-intestinal or central nervous system

there is a limit to the amount of possible dilation and beyond this limit the contractability force decreases.

Stimulation of the sympathetic nervous system occurs in response to a reduced cardiac output. This stimulation is initiated by stretch receptors and baroreceptors in the blood vessels and catecholamines are released. Catecholamines increase cardiac contractions and also cause peripheral vaso-constriction which results in increased peripheral resistance and venous return, and reduced blood flow to the limbs, kidneys and abdominal organs. Whilst this increases blood flow to the vital organs, prolonged sympathetic stimulation reduces diastole which impairs coronary artery circulation. Continued increases in peripheral resistance requires the myocardium to work harder and reduced renal perfusion activates the production of renin, angiotensin and aldosterone. Renin and angiotensin cause further vaso-constriction which stimulates the production of aldosterone to cause retention of sodium and water. Sodium and water retention initially helps heart failure by increasing blood volume but this soon becomes excessive resulting in oedema and putting a further strain on the failing heart.

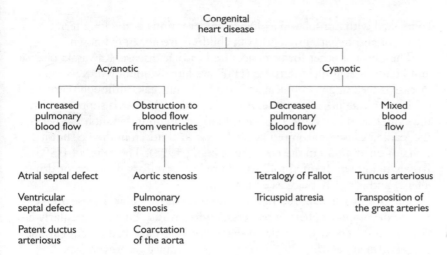

Figure 3.1

Classification of congenital heart disease.

The commonest cause of sudden death in previously healthy children is cardiac disease, especially cardiomyopathy. Very fit athletes often demonstrate an enlarged heart, but this is the result of fitness training rather than a pathological condition. Cardiopathy can be primary and idiopathic or secondary to other problems. Hohn and Stanton (1987) suggest that primary cardiomyopathy is linked to familial or genetic causes. Approximately 1:500 children are affected and in 1997 the first mass screening of children was introduced (Fletcher, 1997). Duchenne muscular dystrophy, Kawasaki disease, thyroid dysfunction and collagen diseases are all known causes of secondary cardiomyopathy (Purcell, 1989).

Hypertension can also be categorised as primary (essential) or secondary. Primary hypertension is more common in adolescents and appears to be related to genetic and environmental factors. Obesity, high salt intake, smoking and stress, which are often related to poor health behaviour in children, have all been identified as possible risks (Gillman *et al.*, 1993). Primary hypertension was traditionally thought to be a disease of adulthood, but now there is evidence of this disorder in children more emphasis has been made on routine screening of blood pressure. Secondary hypertension is more common in younger children. The most common cause is renal disease (90%), but cardiovascular, neurological, metabolic and endocrine disorders and some drugs may also be responsible. The American Academy of Pediatrics (1987) suggests that children whose blood pressure measurements fall consistently between the 95th and 99th percentiles should be considered to have significant hypertension. They define severe hypertension as blood pressure which is consistently above the 99th percentile. Measurements recorded in a doctor's surgery may bear little relationship to the child's blood pressure during a normal day's activities and Portman and Yetman (1994) recommend the use of the ambulatory blood pressure monitor to provide an overall profile of blood pressure patterns. Mild hypertension is usually

Cross references

BP norms – page 285
Recording children's BP – page 284

controlled with non-pharmacological interventions as the long-term effects of anti-hypertensive drugs in children are not fully known.

The cause of other forms of acquired cardiac disease, Kawasaki disease and Henoch–Schönlein Purpura (HSP) are largely unknown. Kawasaki disease is seen in geographical and seasonal outbreaks although there is no evidence for an infective cause. An environmental cause is supported by the evidence of its occurrence – it is most common in Japan, it has become the leading cause of acquired heart disease in children in the US, but it remains uncommon in the UK (Leung *et al.*, 1993). The cause of HSP is largely unknown. It often follows an upper respiratory infection or drug allergy and is nearly twice as common in boys.

Children with acquired or congenital cardiovascular disease are at risk of developing subacute bacterial endocarditis. Those particularly at risk are children with valvular disease and who have had recent cardiac surgery. Dajani *et al.* (1990) stress the importance of prevention, recommending individual prophylactic antibiotic therapy before and after any dental procedures or invasive procedures of the throat and respiratory, genito-urinary and gastro-intestinal tracts which are known to increase the risk of bacterial contamination.

This prophylactic treatment is also recommended for children with rheumatic fever who are subsequently susceptible to recurrent rheumatic fever for the rest of their lives. Rheumatic fever was a devastating problem and the leading cause of childhood deaths in the 1920s (Bland, 1987). Its decline from 1920 to 1990 was explained by the development of antibacterial drugs but it now seem to be re-emerging in parts of America and the UK (Veasey *et al.*, 1994).

ASSESSMENT

Any critically ill child requires cardiovascular assessment. Severe illness in children tends to result in shock and hypoxia as well as being likely to induce heart failure and cardiopulmonary arrest. Shock is commonly associated with haemorrhage, infection, drug toxicity, fluid and electrolyte imbalances, hypoxia or trauma. Hypoxia may be a primary problem for children with respiratory problems or cyanotic congenital heart defects. Cardiac failure is also a problem for children with congenital cardiac problems as well as being secondary to myocarditis and cardiomyopathy.

Hazinski (1992) succinctly describes the child with severe circulatory failure as 'looks bad'. However, Figure 3.2 describes the features more objectively.

Activity

Look at the features demonstrated by the child with cardiac failure listed in Figure 3.2 and determine the rationale for each feature.

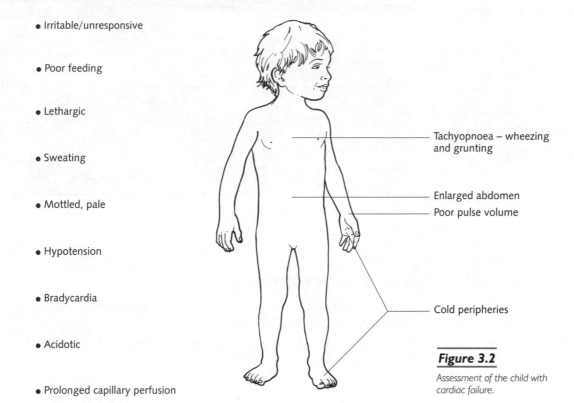

- Irritable/unresponsive
- Poor feeding
- Lethargic
- Sweating
- Mottled, pale
- Hypotension
- Bradycardia
- Acidotic
- Prolonged capillary perfusion

Tachyopnoea – wheezing and grunting

Enlarged abdomen
Poor pulse volume

Cold peripheries

Figure 3.2

Assessment of the child with cardiac failure.

In addition to these general features of cardiac disease there are some features which are characteristic of specific disorders. Clubbing of the fingers is thought to be the result of chronic tissue hypoxia and polycythaemia which occur in cyanotic heart disease. Small children with unrepaired Fallot's tetralogy try to overcome this chronic hypoxia by squatting. This position reduces their desaturated venous return and diverts more blood into the pulmonary artery by increasing systemic resistance. Hypercyanotic spells occur in children with large ventricular septal defects or pulmonary stenosis whenever there is an unmet need for increased oxygen. They commonly occur in infancy during feeding, crying or defaecation.

As well as making a nursing assessment of the child with a cardiac problem the nurse will be involved in caring for the child before, during and after any medical investigations.

Activity

Look at the common cardiac investigations listed in Table 3.3 and discover when and why these are performed. Make notes of the role of the nurse in each investigation.

Table 3.3

Common investigaitons of the cardiovascular system (Copyright is waived for the purpose of photocopying and enlarging this table.)

Investigation	When and what for?	Role of the nurse
Chest X-ray		
Electrocardiography		
Echocardiography		
Cardiac catheterisation		
Exercise stress test		

NURSING INTERVENTIONS

Specific nursing interventions which may be implemented for the child with cardiovascular disorder are:

- providing care to help decrease cardiac demands in the child with cardiac failure;
- administering medication to improve cardiovascular function;
- providing specific post-operative care following cardiac surgery.

The child in cardiac failure needs to rest and save energy to decrease the demands made on the failing heart. Nursing activities should be organised carefully to enable the child to rest between interventions. Feeding the child in cardiac failure is a particular challenge. Increased heart and respiratory rates increase the metabolic rate which needs to be met by a greater calorie intake. However, the breathless and exhausted child in cardiac failure has insufficient energy to suck.

Activity

Taking the above comments into consideration, plan care for the child detailed in Table 3.4.

One of the commonest medications given for cardiac disease is digoxin but this is highly toxic and the nurse must be alert for signs of toxicity when administering it. As soon as toxic effects are noted the next dose should be omitted. Once the therapeutic blood levels of digoxin (0.8–2.0 mg/l) are exceeded Opie (1991) suggests that it may be several days before they return to normal. Before administration of digoxin the apical pulse should be measured for a full minute to gain an accurate rate

Alan is a 10-week-old infant who has been admitted to the ward in heart failure following a diagnosis of ventricular septal defect. On admission he is sweating, lethargic and irritable. His vital signs are: T 36: P 160: R 80. His mother reports that he is feeding poorly and that his hands and feet are always cold.

Problem	Aim	Nursing actions
Alan is having difficulty in breathing		
Alan has cold peripheries		
Alan is only able to suck for short periods		
Alan is at risk of skin breakdown due to poor perfusion		
Alan is at risk of renal failure due to poor renal perfusion		
Alan is irritable and tires easily		
Alan's parents are very concerned		

Table 3.4

The child in cardiac failure: nursing care
(Copyright is waived for the purpose of photocopying and enlarging this table.)

and rhythm and the nurse should be aware of the prescribed pulse range within which the administration is considered therapeutic.

Activity

Identify the uses, dosage/kg and side effects of common medications used in cardiovascular disease (Table 3.5).

Cardiac surgery may be corrective or palliative. It may not be possible to undertake immediate corrective surgery due to the child's size or the severity of the condition. In such cases palliative surgery may be undertaken to stabilise the child until the corrective procedure can be performed. Immediate post-operative care following any cardiac surgery is undertaken in specialist intensive care units. The technology required to provide continuous observation of the child, including arterial pressure and central venous pressure (CVP) monitoring usually requires critical care facilities. This section will concentrate on the specific care of the child in this immediate period. Rehabilitation and ambulation

Post-operative care

Maintaining the airway
- ventilation for 24 hours
- continuous monitoring of respirations and O_2 saturations
- change of position and chest physio-therapy to promote lung re-expansion

Maintaining the circulation
- continuous ECG monitoring to observe for arrhythmias
- intra-arterial monitoring provides continuous BP measurements
- intracardiac monitoring gives constant readings of CVP
- measure chest drainage (Hazinski, 1992, indicates that drainage >3 ml/kg/hour for more than 3 hours is indicative of haemorrhage)
- observe for complications of intra-arterial monitoring (aerial thrombosis, infection, air emboli or blood loss)
- observe for complications of CVP monitoring (dysrhythmias, haemothorax, pneumothorax)
- care of IV infusions (heparinised saline to keep vein open for intra-arterial line, IV fluids via CVP line)

Maintaining body temperature
- keep child warm for first 24 hours to allow gradual return of heat after hypothermia procedures
- pyrexia after 48 hours usually indicates infection

Provide rest and comfort
- continuous IV opioid infusion (Maguire and Maloney, 1988)
- plan care to allow adequate rest between procedures
- observe child for features of depression due to pain and stress

Maintain fluid balance
- measure all intake and output
- hourly urine measurements (<1 ml/kg/hour is a sign of renal failure)
- daily weight
- nil by mouth for initial 24 hours or until extubation

Recognise complications of heart surgery
- mechanical trauma to red cells can cause haemolysis and anaemia
- haemorrhage may occur if clotting mechanisms are impaired by heparini-sation
- impure blood entering the circulation can cause fat emboli, infection or thromboemboli
- neurological observations to identify cerebral oedema and/or neurological damage which can result from cerebral ischaemia or emboli
- pericardial and pleural effusions can occur 1–3 weeks after surgery

Table 3.5

Common medications used in cardiovascular disease (Copyright is waived for the purpose of photocopying and enlarging this table.)

Medication	Uses	Dose/kg	Side effects
Digoxin			
Anti-arrhythmics propanalol			
Angiotensin converting enzyme (ACE) inhibitors catopril			
Vasodilators hydrallazine			

Diuretics
  frusemide
  spironolactone			

Cardiac surgery – advice on discharge

- Education about medication (e.g. anticoagulant therapy, digoxin)
- Restrictions to mobility
- Diet and nutrition
- Prevention of bacterial endocarditis
- Features of post-operative complications – recognition and reaction
- Follow-up appointments
- Wound care
- Medic-Alert identification (or similar) for children with a pacemaker, anticoagulation therapy
- Return to nursery or school
- Prognosis
- Effects on growth and development

usually commence 48 hours after surgery when ventilation, monitoring and drainage tubes can be removed and the child returned to the ward. Pain from thoracotomy incisions can limit lung expansion and remobilisation so it is important that regular assessment of pain and appropriate intervention is continued.

EDUCATION FOR DISCHARGE

Discharge planning after cardiac surgery needs careful preparation. Parents need much reassurance and advice. Some cardiac surgery procedures can only be palliative and others may need repeating. Continued medical and emotional support is vital to help parents of children with such an uncertain prognosis. Holmes (1996) argues that this is the role of a cardiac liaison nurse.

Acquired cardiac disease such as hypertension may be preventable and advice in childhood about the prevention of cardiovascular disease may prevent later problems in adulthood.

Activity

You are asked to talk to a group of primary school children about heart disease. Consider the best way to teach them about prevention of heart problems.

PRINCIPLES OF CARE – CHILDREN WITH A 4
METABOLIC OR ENDOCRINE DISORDER

INTRODUCTION

Inborn errors of metabolism are relatively rare but they include a large number of different disorders. They are all caused by the absense or deficiency of a substance essential to cellular metabolism. It is becoming more possible to screen and detect these inherited disorders and such processes enable early diagnosis and treatment. Prompt recognition and management of metabolic problems are essential if physical and mental retardation is to be avoided.

The most common endocrine disorder of childhood is diabetes mellitus (McEvilly, 1997). The British Diabetic Association (1996) reports that it occurs in:

- 1:50 000 infants
- 1:1500–2000 preschoolers
- 1:500 schoolchildren.

This section will therefore concentrate on the care and management of children with diabetes and only briefly discuss the principles of caring for children with metabolic disorders and other problems related to the endocrine system.

Activity

Complete Tables 4.1 and 4.2 to ensure that you can recall the principles of metabolism and the functions of the endocrine system.

COMMON DISORDERS OF METABOLISM AND THE ENDOCRINE SYSTEM

Phenylketonuria and galactosaemia are probably the two most commonly known errors of metabolism (Figures 4.1 and 4.2 – page 448). Phenylketonuria is an autosomal-recessive inherited absence of phenylalanine hydroxylase, an enzyme necessary for the metabolisation of phenylalanine, an essential amino acid. The accumulation of phenylalanine in the blood stream disturbs normal nervous system maturation by degeneration of grey and white matter and abnormal development of myelin and cortical lamination.

Galactosaemia is also an autosomal-recessive disorder and occurs in about 1:50 000 births. It affects normal carbohydrate metabolism by interfering with the normal conversion of galactose to glucose. The affected child is usually normal at birth but develops symptoms within a

Gland	Hormone	Function	Effect of hyposecretion	Effect of hypersecretion
Anterior pituitary	1 2 3 4 5 6 7 8			
Posterior pituitary	1 2			
Thyroid	1 2			
Parathyroid	1			
Pancreas	1 2 3			
Adrenals	1 2 3			
Ovaries	1 2			
Testes	1			

few days of commencing milk feeds. Vomiting, diarrhoea and weight loss are early signs which quickly progress to drowsiness, lethargy coma and sometimes death due to the accumulation of galactose in the blood stream.

Activity

Identify the prenatal and neonatal screening processes for inborn errors of metabolism.

The incidence of insulin-dependent diabetes in infancy and childhood is increasing (Metcalf and Baum, 1991). It is thought to be an autoimmune disorder which is triggered by a viral, dietetic or environmental factor in children who have a genetic susceptibility to the

Hormone	Effect upon the regulation of metabolism
Insulin	
Glucagon	
Epinephrine	
Human growth hormone	
Thyroxine	
Cortisol	
Testosterone	

Table 4.2

Principles of metabolism (Copyright is waived for the purpose of photocopying and enlarging this table.)

Absorbed nutrients may be oxidised for energy, stored to provide heat and energy or converted into other molecules. The control of these different pathways is largely regulated by hormones.

Disorder	Pathophysiology
Hypopituitarism	Growth retardation, absent or delayed puberty, hypothyroidism and adrenal hypofunction occur due to an impaired secretion of pituitary hormones. Usually due to pituitary or hypothalamic tumours
Congenital hypothyroidism (cretinism)	A deficiency of thyroid hormones which can be due to maldevelopment of the thyroid gland, pituitary dysfunction or abnormal thyroxine synthesis. Features of a decreased metabolic rate, which usually appear at 6 weeks of age when the maternal hormonal supply has ceased to have an effect, include bradycardia, hypothermia, lethargy and dry skin. If untreated normal nervous system maturation is impaired and mental retardation results
Lymphatic thyroiditis	The commonest cause of hypothyroidism in children aged 6–16 years. An autoimmune disorder in which lymphocytes infiltrate the thyroid gland and replace thyroid tissue with fibrous tissue, causing hyperplasia and enlargement of the gland
Hyperthyroidism	An autoimmune response of the thyroid stimulating hormone receptors causing an over-secretion of thyroxine. Irritability, hyperactivity, tremors, insomnia, tachycardia, heat intolerance, diarrhoea and vomiting can all result. Exopthalamus and visual disturbances are common although the exact rationale for these is unknown
Congenital adrenogenital hyperplasia	The commonest cause of adrenal hypofunction in children. An inborn deficiency of the enzymes necessary for the biosynthesis of cortisol causes an increased secretion of adrenocorticotrophic hormone. This causes hyperplasia of the adrenal cortex, reduced secretion of cortisol and aldosterone with the secretion of a large amount of immature steroids. These incompletely formed steroids have a masculising effect on the developing fetus

Table 4.3

Common endocrine disorders

disorder (Figures 4.3 and 4.4 – page 449). The mumps virus has been implicated as there appears to be a seasonal variation in the onset of diabetes in school-aged children. Karjalainen *et al*. (1992) identified cows' milk as a likely trigger factor. Environmental factors appear to be

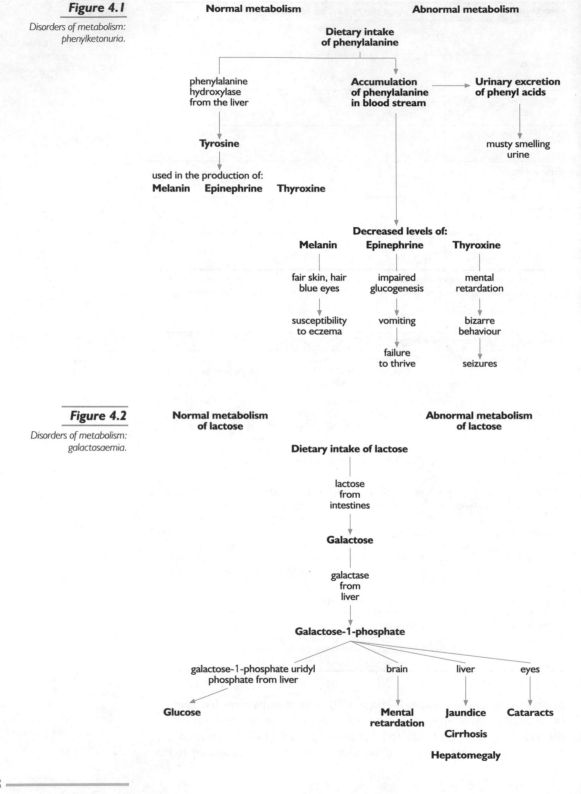

Figure 4.1

Disorders of metabolism: phenylketonuria.

Figure 4.2

Disorders of metabolism: galactosaemia.

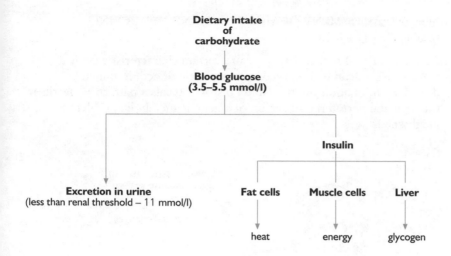

Figure 4.3

Normal carbohydrate metabolism.

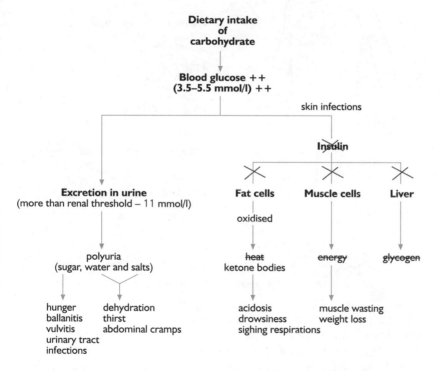

Figure 4.4

Carbohydrate metabolism in diabetes.

significant as the geographic distribution of the disorder is so variable. The incidence of diabetes in Sweden and Finland is 3–4 times the incidence in the UK and diabetes is almost unknown in Japan.

The trigger factor initiates an autoimmune process in the beta cells of the islets of Langerhans in the pancreas. As a result, the beta cells are destroyed and no insulin is available to support carbohydrate metabolism.

SPECIFIC ASSESSMENT OF METABOLIC AND ENDOCRINE DISORDERS (FIGURE 4.5)

Arn *et al.* (1988) report that there are certain characteristic clinical features which can be observed in any genetic or acquired metabolic disorders. If, in addition, the family history reveals a pattern of deaths in the neonatal period the suspicion of a genetic metabolic problem is heightened.

Specific assessment of metabolism

- Seizures
- Abnormal skin or hair
- Dysmorphic features
- Persistent vomiting
- Hepatomegaly
- Intractable diarrhoea
- Hypothermia
- Lethargy
- Abnormal eating patterns (aversion to certain foods, vomiting and/or diarrhoea after eating certain foods)

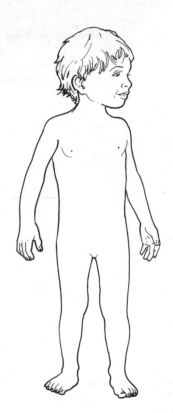

Specific assessment of the endocrine system

- Behavioural changes
- Excessive thirst
- Repeated skin infections
- Polyuria
- Signs of early puberty
- Weight loss *and* increased appetite
- Intolerance to changes of temperature

Figure 4.5

Specific assessment of the child with a metabolic or endocrine disorder.

It may be a family history of diabetes which first alerts parents to the possibility of this condition. The first features are often insidious and some children are not diagnosed until they present with ketoacidosis. The presence of excess glucose in the urine produces an osmotic diuresis and children who were previously dry at night may start bed wetting. This polyuria causes an extreme thirst and children may start to wake at night for a drink. Glycosuria may also cause a white sugary deposit around the toilet or urinary or genital infections. Repeated skin infections may also be apparent as the high blood glucose prevents the phagocytic action of white blood cells. Mature onset diabetes in adults is often diagnosed by a glucose tolerance test but this has not been found to be a reliable diagnostic test for children. Instead, the diagnosis is confirmed by the presence of characteristic features:

- fasting blood sugar >6.7 mmol/l;
- random blood sugar >10 mmol/l (Higgins, 1995).

Activity

Find out how to use the blood glucose meter and measure your own blood glucose. Reflect on how you felt about this procedure and how you might react if you needed to repeat it every day.

Other specific investigations are commonly used to diagnose metabolic or endocrine problems. Use Table 4.4 to make notes about these tests and their uses. Check your role in the preparation for these and the care needed by the child during and after the tests.

NURSING INTERVENTIONS

The main role of the nurse in the care of children with metabolic disorders is the education of the family about dietary restrictions. Dietary management in phenylketonuria aims to meet the child's nutritional needs for normal growth and development whilst maintaining phenylalanine levels within a non-toxic range (2–8 mg/dl). Brain damage occurs when levels exceed 10 mg/dl and protein stores are utilised for heat and energy, resulting in growth retardation if levels fall below 2 mg/dl. Therefore the low phenylalanine diet should contain 20–30 mg phenylalanine/kg body weight/day and be commenced as

Assessment of diabetic control

Blood glucose
- spot check for hypoglycaemia
- spot check for hyperglycaemia
- 24 hour profile
- at least once a day, increase at times of illness

Urine testing
- for ketones when blood glucose >17 mmol/l
- does not accurately reflect current blood glucose

Haemoglobin A
- glycosylated haemoglobin reflects control over previous 6–8 weeks

Monitor
- weight
- blood pressure
- eyesight

Investigation	When and what for?	Role of the nurse
Bone scan		
Chromosome analysis		
Fasting/random blood glucose		
Guthrie test		
Thyroid function tests		
Thyroid scan and uptake		
Urinary catecholamines		

Table 4.4

Metabolic and endocrine investigations (Copyright is waived for the purpose of photocopying and enlarging this table.)

soon as possible unless the mother is breastfeeding. Normal breast-feeding may be possible as breastmilk contains little phenylalanine (Lawrence, 1994). As the child grows older most high protein foods must be avoided or restricted. Aspartame, the artificial sweetener, must also be restricted as it converts to phenylalanine once ingested.

Treatment of galactosaemia is a lactose-free diet. This includes the elimination of breastfeeding. Although this diet is easier to manage than the low phenylalanine diet, care must be taken to avoid medicines such as penicillin which may contain lactose. Unfortunately, the outcome for children with metabolic problems even with dietary control is not good. The Medical Research Council (1993) reports that a high percentage of affected children demonstrate a degree of mental retardation.

Activity

Assess the contents of your food cupboard for catering for a child with phenylketonuria and galactosaemia. When you next do your food shopping assess how easy it is to shop for these children.

Activity

Study the list of drugs commonly used in endocrine disorders (Table 4.5) and find out their usual doses, uses, actions and side effects.

Table 4.5

Drugs commonly used in endocrine disorders (Copyright is waived for the purpose of photocopying and enlarging this table.)

Drug	Dose (mg/kg)	Action/use	Side effects
Aldosterone			
Cortisone			
Glucose			
Glycogen			
Growth hormone			
Hydrocortisone			
Sex hormones			
Thyroxine			

McEvilly (1997) states that the aims of care for the child with diabetes are initially to:

- correct dehydration and electrolyte imbalance;
- stabilise the blood sugar;
- educate and support the child and family in coming to terms with the diagnosis.

Once these initial aims have been met the long-term objectives of care are to:

- achieve good control of carbohydrate metabolism;
- reduce the risk of the acute and chronic complications of diabetes;
- maintain near-to-normal blood glucose levels;
- provide sufficient education and support to enable the transfer care from the multidisciplinary diabetic team to the child and family.

Swift *et al.* (1993) suggest that children with newly diagnosed diabetes are best managed at home rather than in hospital because it is so much easier to adjust their treatment around their usual routine and, as a result, subsequent hospital admissions are reduced. However, home management requires the support of a community diabetic team which should include the paediatric diabetic nurse (British Diabetic Association, 1995).

The majority of children with diabetes are treated with insulin which should be administered 20–30 minutes before a main meal. Initially they will probably be given a mixture of short and intermediate acting insulin morning and evening. The child, if old enough, and the family need to be taught how to:

- obtain and store insulin and injection device;
- time their injections;
- use an aseptic technique;
- mix insulins;
- choose injection sites;
- inject insulin;
- dispose of sharps.

Activity

Find out what to tell the child and family about the above.

Activity

Reflect upon a child you have known with diabetes and how they coped with their injections.

Complications of diabetes

Acute
- hypoglycaemia (insulin coma)
- ketoacidosis (diabetic coma)

Chronic
- diabetic retinopathy
- diabetic neuropathy
  - sensorimotor
  - autonomic
- diabetic foot
  - neuropathy
  - infection
  - ischaemia
- cardiovascular disease
  - coronary artery disease
  - cerebrovascular disease
  - peripheral vascular disease

Table 4.6

Types of insulin (Copyright is waived for the purpose of photocopying and enlarging this table.)

Insulin	Short action	Intermediate action	Long action
Human actrapid			
Humulin S			
Humulin insulatard			
Humulin I			
Human monotard			
Human ultratard			
Human mixtard 10			
Human mixtard 20			
Human mixtard 30			
Human mixtard 40			
Human mixtard 50			
Humulin M1			
Humulin M2			
Humulin M3			
Humulin M4			
Humulin M5			

Dietary control of diabetes

Guidelines

- Total daily calories = 1000 calories + 100 calories/year of age until 10 years
- Carbohydrate = 45–50% of daily intake (20–25% for main meals, 10–15% for snacks)
- Other content = high fibre/low animal fats

Principles

The diabetic child's dietary intake:

- of carbohydrate must balance with the dose of insulin
- should maintain normal body weight for the child's sex, age, height and level of activity
- of carbohydrate must be sufficient to prevent ketoacidosis
- must satisfy appetite, prevent hunger and meet individual tastes and routines
- should provide for a regular intake of carbohydrate

Activity

Find out the duration of action and the time of peak action for short, intermediate and long acting insulins. Then, using the list of insulins in Table 4.6, identify the length of action for different types of insulin.

Insulin treatment must be balanced with diet to promote a normal blood sugar and maintain normal growth and development. There is a clear association between this control and the onset of chronic complications of diabetes in later life (Diabetes Control and Complications Trial Research Group, 1993). Ansell (1995) suggests that the dietician visits the child and family on the day of diagnosis to begin teaching the basic principles of dietary control. This should be followed by a series of short teaching sessions to expand and consolidate the information they will need.

However well controlled a child's diabetes is, it is likely that at least occasional hypoglycaemic attacks may occur (Ansell, 1995). At one time, hypoglycaemic attacks were induced as part of diabetic education. This is no longer thought to be good practice but the child and family should be taught how to recognise and manage an attack (Figure 4.6). Hyperglycaemia can occur as result of illness when stress hormones, produced to fight infection, cause a rise in blood sugar. The child and family should be aware that insulin should not be stopped during illness, even if the child is unable to eat normally. Instead carbohydrate should be given in the form of a snack or drink and if this is not possible medical advice should be sought. Blood glucose should be tested more frequently and the urine tested for ketones.

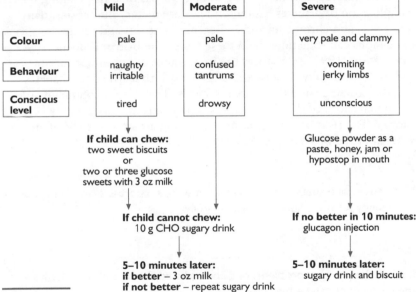

Figure 4.6

Management of hypoglycaemia.

Activity

Consider what carbohydrate snacks or drinks you could offer a diabetic child who was feeling unwell and nauseous.

There are many situations which predispose to poor control of diabetes. The varying growth of children as well as their changeable levels of activity and emotions do not help diabetic control.

Management of hyperglycaemia

Correct hypoperfusion and shock

- IV infusion normal saline 20 ml/kg for first 2 hours
- IV infusion saline 0.45% + 4% dextrose 20 ml/kg for next 2 hours
- IV infusion saline 0.18% + 4% dextrose thereafter
- monitor pulse, respirations, fluid balance and oxygen saturations

Correct hyperglycaemia

- IV insulin (1 unit insulin : 1 ml saline)
- 0.1 unit/kg/hour initially
- 0.05 unit/kg/hour when blood sugar <15 mmol/l
- discontinue 1 hour after first subcutaneous injection of insulin
- monitor blood glucose hourly for the first 4 hours

Correct electrolyte imbalance

- add potassium chloride (KCl) to infusion after 1 hour if serum K <5 mmol/l
- if serum K 3.5–5 mmol/l add KCl 20 mEq/l
- if serum K <3.5 mmol/l add KCl 40 mEq/l
- monitor urea and electrolytes hourly for first 4 hours

Recognise and treat possible cause

- IV antibiotics
- urine and blood specimens for culture
- chest X-ray
- swabs/specimens from any obvious sites of infection

Recent advances in the management of insulin-dependent diabetes

- Pancreatic transplantation
- Islet transplantation
- Insulin delivery systems
  - subcutaneous insulin infusions
  - implantable peritoneal pumps
  - implantable glucose sensors
  - intranasal insulin
  - insulin pens
- 'Designer' insulins

Problem solving in diabetes

1 David's mother has brought him to the clinic for a checkup. She is concerned that David has been having consistently high blood glucose levels although he is eating as usual and has not changed his insulin dose or level of activity. The diabetic nurse checks David's injection sites. Why?

2 Amanda, who is 15, is denying her diabetes and hiding it from her friends. When you ask her the reason for this she replies, 'They don't want to hang around with someone who is always ill'. How could you help Amanda to overcome these feelings about her condition?

3 Neil, aged 12, controls his diabetes fairly well with insulin and three meals and three snacks each day. He tells you that he has been chosen for his school football team and that he now needs to train with the team twice a week after school. What adjustments would you suggest he makes to maintain his control on these days?

4 Several months ago, Marie, aged 2 years, was diagnosed as a diabetic following convulsive hypoglycaemic reactions. Since then, her mother has been terrified of low blood sugars. At clinic, it is obvious that she is trying to keep Marie on a strict regimen to keep the diabetes under complete control 24 hours per day. How can you help Marie and her mother?

5 Michael, aged 15, is brought into the Accident and Emergency department by a friend. He has a fruity smell on his breath, flushed face, strong but slow pulse, and dilated pupils. He is sweating profusely and is confused about where he is. You discover a Medic-Alert bracelet stating that he is an insulin-dependent diabetic. What would you expect his diagnosis to be?

Useful address

British Diabetic Association, 10 Queen Anne Street, London W1M 0BD

Activity

Consider the particular problems of controlling diabetes in the:

- infant
- toddler
- schoolchild
- adolescent

Activity

Consider how to solve the problems of controlling diabetes outlined in the case histories: 'Problem solving in diabetes'.

DISCHARGE ADVICE

The impact of being given the diagnosis of diabetes may be very stressful for some parents, especially if a grandparent has died from a long-term complication of diabetes. Common fears are dietary limitations, daily injections, and chronic invalidity. Teaching sessions and group discussions can sometimes help these fears. The British Diabetic Association (1997) emphasises the importance of consistent support for the child and family because there is so much to learn about diabetes and the growing child has changing needs. They also recommend at least an annual check of the child's development and the onset of any complications. The risks of complications occurring are known to be greater 5 years after the onset of puberty (McEvilly, 1997).

Activity

Visit your local diabetic clinic and find out what support is available in your community for the diabetic child and family.

Activity

Look at the practical problems of diabetes listed below and consider how these situations can be managed.

Practical problems for children with diabetes

- Schooling/employment
- Travel/holidays (sickness, change of diet, time changes, storage of equipment, etc.)
- Dental treatment
- Surgery
- Minor illness
- Pregnancy

PRINCIPLES OF CARE – CHILDREN WITH EYE, EAR, NOSE AND THROAT DISORDERS **5**

INTRODUCTION

After the first year of life upper respiratory tract infections are more common than infections involving the lower respiratory tract and preschool children have about six upper respiratory tract infections per year (Valman, 1993). The pharynx and middle ear are so close together in these small children that infection in either area readily spreads to the adjacent organ. The most common disorder related to the nose is allergic rhinitis, affecting mostly older children.

Congenital problems affecting the upper respiratory tract are usually considered to be relatively minor defects which can be corrected by surgery. They include cleft lip and palate and abnormalities of the larynx, trachea and the subglottal area. Although mostly not life-threatening conditions, these problems are often just as devastating for parents who may be disappointed, angry and rejecting of their 'abnormal' baby, especially when the defects are very obvious.

Visual impairment is a another common problem during childhood which can cause emotional problems for parents and the child.

Activity

Test your knowledge of the structure and function of the eyes, ears, nose and throat by answering the questions in the margin. Check your answers with your anatomy and physiology textbook.

COMMON DISORDERS OF THE EYES (TABLE 5.1)

Visual impairment is the term used to describe children who are blind and partially sighted. There are many pre- and postnatal causes of visual impairment but the cause of most problems is unknown. Visual impairment can impair motor function and learning and prevention and early detection of problems is vital.

COMMON DISORDERS OF THE EARS (TABLE 5.2)

Flood (1989) suggests that few children escape childhood without some symptoms of secretory otitis media or 'glue ear'. Surgery to the middle ear is the commonest cause of surgical admissions of children to hospital in the UK, at a cost of approximately £30m per year, although there is increasing controversy about the benefits of such surgery (Audit

---

Test your knowledge of the structure and function of the eyes, ears, nose and throat

What is the normal process of vision?

What is the function of the:

- ciliary body?
- retina?
- lens?
- anterior cavity?
- vitreous chamber?

What structures lie close to the middle ear and are at risk from the spread of infection from otitis media?

What are the functions of the nose and the sinuses?

Why does the nose bleed readily?

Identify the position of the following:

- maxillary sinuses
- frontal sinuses
- ethmoid sinuses
- pharyngeal tonsils (adenoids)
- palatine tonsils

Where is a tracheostomy formed?

Disorder	Pathophysiology
Refractive disorders	
myopia	The eyeball is too long causing the image to fall in front of the retina. The individual only sees clearly when objects are close by (short-sightedness)
hyperopia	The eyeball is too short, causing the image to fall beyond the retina. The individual only sees clearly when objects are at a distance (long-sightedness)
astigmatism	Unequal curvatures in the cornea or lens cause light rays to bend in different directions resulting in blurred or distorted vision
anisometropia	Each eye has a different refractive strength causing the individual to avoid the use of the weaker eye
Amblyopia	Reduced visual acuity in one eye caused by a lack of stimulation and resulting in each retina receiving different images (double vision). Lack of use of visual cortex eventually results in loss of response and loss of vision in the affected eye
Cataract	Opacity of the lens prevents light rays from entering the eye
Conjunctivitis	Inflammation of the conjunctiva – usually bacterial in children – causing inflammation (pinkness) of the eyeball and the lining of the eyelids, pain and discomfort
Glaucoma	Increased intraocular pressure caused in children by a congenital defect in the flow of aqueous humor. The increased pressure eventually leads to atrophy of the optic nerve and blindness
Strabismus	A congenital defect, poor vision or muscle imbalance or paralysis results in unparallel visual axes causing the brain to receive two images

Table 5.2

Common disorders of the ears, nose and throat

Disorder	Pathophysiology
Otitis media	Obstruction of the eustachian tube from the inflammation and oedema of upper respiratory tract infections, allergic rhinitis or hypertrophic adenoids, causes the accumulation of secretions in the middle ear (acute otitis media). If this fluid is not released, it thickens to develop a glue-like consistency which reduces the movements of the tympanic membrane and impairs hearing (secretory otitis media, 'glue ear')
Allergic rhinitis (hayfever)	Inhaled water soluble allergens diffuse into the respiratory epithelium and react with antigen-specific immunoglobulin E on the susceptible child's nasal mast cells. As a result histamine is secreted causing vasodilation and swelling. Hypersecretion of nasal mucus and sneezing results
Tonsillitis	Infection of the palatine tonsils leads to inflammation and oedema. Obstruction of the passage of air and food results in difficulty in mouth breathing and swallowing
Infectious mononucleosis (glandular fever)	Infection by the Epstein–Barr (EB) virus causes mononuclear infiltration of lymph glands causing generalised lymphadenopathy and splenomegaly

Commission, 1993). Because of the prevalence of otitis media much attention has been paid to possible causes. Strachan *et al.* (1989) indicate that passive smoking is a significant factor. They suggest that the inhalation of smoke impairs mucocilliary function and this causes congestion of the nasopharyngeal tissues, predisposing the child to upper respiratory infection and blockage of the eustachian tube. Duncan *et al.* (1993) have found that breastfeeding appears to protect children from developing otitis media. They propose that breastfed babies are likely to be protected against respiratory allergies and viruses by maternal immunity and that the semi-prone position used for breastfeeding is less likely to cause reflux of milk into the eustachian tube. The commonest approach to the treatment of glue ear is surgical myringotomy and insertion of a grommet (incision into the tympanic membrane and the insertion of a small drainage tube). However, Black *et al.* (1990) found that 34% of ears had improved spontaneously by the time of surgery. In addition, some children gain no or little improvement from surgical intervention and sometimes the grommet falls out too soon necessitating repeat surgery (Audit Commission, 1993). These findings have led to a more 'watch and wait' policy towards treatment but recent evidence shows that this may also have disadvantages. Hogan *et al.* (1997) found that susceptible children develop frequent episodes of otitis media which can result in hearing losses which can be as great as 50 decibels. In the young child hearing loss prevents normal development of speech and language and the older child may fall behind in school and may be unfairly labelled as slow, backward, difficult or disobedient.

Adenoidectomy may also be performed to relieve glue ear. The adenoids tend to hypertrophy in response to repeated upper respiratory tract infections and cause obstruction of the eustachian tube, predisposing to glue ear. However, Widemar *et al.* (1985) express doubt that adenoidectomy prevents or treats glue ear and Flood warns that the longer hospital stay and risk of haemorrhage for such surgery may not outweigh the possible benefits.

Otitis media causes conductive deafness which is the most common type of hearing loss which results from an impairment of the transmission of sound to the middle ear. Sensorineural hearing loss or perceptive deafness is caused by inner ear and auditory nerve defects which distort sound and prevent its differentiation. Hearing impairment is one of the commonest disabilities of childhood and can vary from a slight deafness (below 30 decibels) to extreme deafness (above 90 decibels).

COMMON DISORDERS OF THE NOSE (TABLE 5.2)

Hayfever or allergic rhinitis affects about 20% of the UK population and usually begins in childhood before the age of 10 (Rees, 1994). Dewers (1990) found that it is two to three times more common in first born or only children and suggested that these children experienced less exposure to viral infections which prevent the development of allergies. Although not a serious disorder, hayfever causes extreme discomfort and affects sleeping and concentration. Both of these can have serious consequences for schoolwork. The major cause of hayfever is pollen and pollen counts are now often given during weather forecasts to help hayfever sufferers determine the risk. These counts are measured in units of pollen per cubic metre. Symptoms usually occur at a count of 50

Causes of sensory loss

Deafness
- family history of hearing problems
- anatomical craniofacial malformations
- low birth weight (< 1500 g)
- significant deprivation of oxygen at birth
- maternal infection (cytomegalovirus, rubella, herpes, syphilis, toxoplasmosis)
- postnatal infection (meningitis, measles, mumps)
- chronic ear infection
- ototoxic drugs (e.g. gentamycin, streptomycin, tobramycin)
- syndromes known to include sensorineural hearing loss

Blindness
- maternal infection (herpes, chlamydia, gonorrhoea, syphilis, rubella, toxoplasmosis)
- retinopathy of prematurity
- congenital defects causing glaucoma or cataracts
- meningitis
- trauma
- tumours (retinoblastoma)

Indications for surgery

- pus on the tonsils confirming bacterial infection more than three times in two consecutive years
- causative organism is found to be group A haemolytic streptococci more than three times in two consecutive years
- gross enlargement of the tonsils between infections, causing stridor or apnoea during sleep
- recurrent febrile convulsions related to repeated bouts of tonsillitis
- peritonsillar abscess (quinsy)

Contra-indications for surgery

- acute infections at the time of surgery; inflamed tissues are more likely to bleed
- bleeding disorders
- uncontrolled systemic disorders (e.g. asthma)
- cleft palate; tonsils help the escape of air during speech

(Newman-Turner, 1992). Antihistamines are the preferred medication as they counteract the histamine secretion but their undesirable side effects make them unpopular with all patients and may be the reason why most sufferers do not start treatment before symptoms appear. Rees (1994) stresses the importance of prevention and recommends the use of prophylactic nasal sprays. Topical sodium cromoglycate inhibits cell degranulation and can be used regularly. A corticosteroid spray reduces the responsiveness of the nose to allergens but is safest when used regularly on a short-term basis.

Clefts of the lip and palate are congenital malformations which occur to some degree in 1:700 births in the UK, affecting more females than males (Martin, 1995). These malformations are often associated with other chromosomal abnormalities but environmental factors and tetragens may also interrupt normal embryonic development of the palate. Clefts of the lips may be unilateral or bilateral and may range from a notch in the upper lip to complete separation of the lip extending to the base of the nose. They may or may not be associated with a cleft palate. Cleft palates are less obvious deformities but may have more serious consequences such as inadequate nasal airways and malposition or missing teeth.

COMMON DISORDERS OF THE THROAT (TABLE 5.2)

Children have much larger tonsils than adults and this is thought to be a protective mechanism against respiratory tract infections. Tonsillitis is common in childhood and may be caused by a viral or bacterial infection. Putto (1987) found that viral tonsillitis, which should be treated symptomatically, was more common in children under 3 years of age. Bacterial tonsillitis usually responds to penicillin so tonsillectomy for chronic tonsillitis is controversial. Because of their protective function and the potential complications of this type of surgery it is sometimes argued that they should not be removed unless they are hugely enlarged or causing other severe problems. In preschool children the tubal and lingual tonsils can enlarge to compensate for removal of the palatine tonsillar lymphatic tissue and pharyngeal and eustachian tube obstruction continues. Alternatively, because repeated bouts of tonsillitis may mean the child is consistently generally unwell and repeatedly missing school, surgery may sometimes provide significant improvement in health and social life.

More severe obstruction of the upper airways, sometimes necessitating formation of a tracheostomy to bypass the obstruction and maintain a clear airway, may result from a number of congenital or acquired causes.

ASSESSMENT

Hearing and visual impairment can severely affect the normal social, physical and psychological development of children and early detection and management of any problems can minimise these problems. Routine hearing and vision tests are carried out during developmental checks, but it is not always easy to test small children; sometimes their apparent inability to see or hear may be due to tiredness or boredom. Other testing may be necessary if developmental checks are abnormal or inconclusive.

Activity

Find out in what circumstances and why the hearing and visual tests listed in Tables 5.3 and 5.4 are performed. Identify the role of the nurse in each test.

The nursing assessment of the ears, nose and throat can be largely gained by simply looking and listening to the child (Figure 5.1). However, the nurse should be aware of strategies to restrain the child if more detailed medical examination of these structures is required (Figure 5.2). The child should be unable to suddenly move away as this could result in tissue damage. During otoscopic examination the ear lobe of the infant should be pulled down and back to straighten the upward curving ear canal and visualise the tympanic membrane. In children over 3 years the canal curves downward and forward and the earlobe is pulled up and back.

Test	When and what for?	Role of the nurse
Developmental hearing tests		
Conduction test		
Audiometry		
Brainstem – auditory evoked response (BSAER)		

Table 5.3

Hearing tests (Copyright is waived for the purpose of photocopying and enlarging this table.)

Test	What for and why?	Role of the nurse
Developmental sight tests		
Snellen chart		
Peripheral vision test		
Colour vision test		

Table 5.4

Visual assessment (Copyright is waived for the purpose of photocopying and enlarging this table.)

Figure 5.1

Assessment of the ears, nose and throat.

Ears
Discharge
Complaints of earache (younger children may rub ear)
Poor hearing and/or speech

Nose
Discharge – thin and watery
              – thick and purulent
Cough – expectorant
           – dry
Mouth breathing

Throat
Sounds – stridor
            – hoarseness
Difficulty in swallowing
Refusing to eat and drink
Enlarged cervical lymph glands
Bad breath caused by dry mouth from mouth breathing

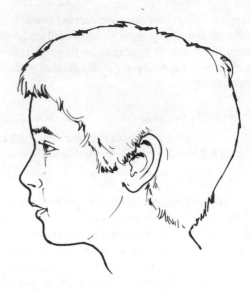

As with respiratory problems, listening can provide useful information. Enlarged adenoids obstruct the passage of air from the nose to the throat and this affects the resonance of the voice, causing the child to talk nasally. Stridor is noisy breathing caused by obstruction in the pharynx, larynx or trachea. Most cases are due to acute laryngitis and are self-limiting (Valman, 1993) but stridor can also result from more severe infections, trauma and congenital defects. Valman (1993)

Figure 5.2

Holding children for ear examination.

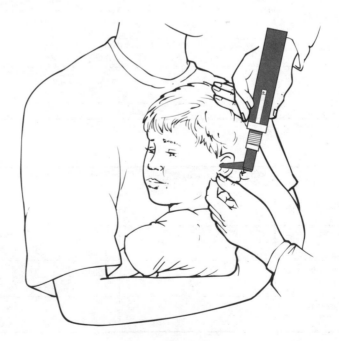

warns that stridor is one of the most ominous sounds in childhood and recommends that, unless urgent treatment is required, all unpleasant procedures which may agitate the child and cause further hypoxia are avoided. In non-emergency situations a detailed history of the development of the stridor should reveal the likely cause as the type of sound is determined by the type of obstruction. Gilbert *et al.* (1993) suggest that the three most important questions are:

- Has the stridor been present since birth?
- Does the child cry, speak and cough normally?
- Is there any chance the child may have inhaled a foreign body?

NURSING INTERVENTIONS

Nursing care of the visually or hearing impaired child aims to support the child and family and enables the child to achieve optimum independence. This will include teaching the child self-help skills, alternative methods of communication and helping them to come to terms with their disability. Children can become depressed by teasing about abnormalities such as squints, or the wearing of glasses and hearing aids (Swanwick, 1986).

Activity

- Find out what alternative methods of communication are available for deaf or blind children.
- Susan, aged 10, who is blind, is anxious to go on the school holiday to France. How can you help her to identify colour coordinating clothes?
- Consider how you would explain pre-operative care to a deaf child.

Other nursing interventions for children with eye, ear, nose or throat problems in this section are related to specific pre- and post-operative care of:

- eye surgery;
- ear surgery;
- nasal surgery;
- cleft lip and palate repair;
- tonsillectomy;
- tracheostomy.

The commonest type of eye surgery is squint repair which may be performed if corrective lenses or patching the non-diverging eye are unsuccessful. This repair involves lengthening or shortening the appropriate muscles of the eye. This is usually performed as a day case and has no specific complications. The operated eye may be swollen and

Causes of stridor
Infection
- acute laryngitis
- epiglottitis
- croup
- bacterial tracheitis

Traumatic obstruction
- foreign body
- steam/smoke inhalation burns

Congenital abnormalities
- laryngocoele
- vocal cord paralysis
- subglottic stenosis
- subglottic haemangioma
- laryngocoeles
- laryngeal webs, cysts
- tracheomalacia
- tracheal stenosis
- compression of the trachea by vascular anomalies

Stridor – types of sounds
- *Foreign bodies* – tend to change position with the airflow during respiration. Consequently, they create changing sounds according to their position
- *Fixed airway lesions* – produce nearly the same sound regardless of the phase of respiration
- *Supraglottic airway abnormalities* – create noise in the initial phase of inspiration because the loose tissue in this area collapses inwards with inspiratory pressure. This, together with the abnormality, causes obstruction on inspiration which is relieved on expiration as the loose tissue returns to its normal position. These abnormalities also prevent normal air movement over the vocal cords and alter the sound of crying, speaking or coughing
- *Glottic and subglottic obstructions* – cause stridor on inspiration and expiration because the lumen of these areas is of fixed size

uncomfortable. Parents are advised to bathe the eye with cooled boiled water to remove any discharge or crusts. Intraocular surgery usually requires intervention to avoid:

- raised intraocular pressure, strain on the sutures and bleeding;
- the child interfering with the dressing and causing injury or infection;
- frightening the child whose eye(s) are bandaged;
- causing discomfort or infection during dressing changes or instillation of medication.

Activity

Consider what care you would give to avoid the potential problems listed above.

As discussed previously the commonest type of ear surgery is myringotomy and insertion of grommets. This is also a day surgery procedure with no specific complications. Advice on discharge is a controversial issue. Some surgeons believe that water in the affected ear during hair washing and swimming poses an infection risk. Flood (1989) indicates that there is no evidence for this precaution and that the incidence of otorrhoea is the same for swimmers and non-swimmers. However, she warns against the entry of irritant soapy water and water entry under pressure when diving and swimming under water. Isaacson and Rosenfeld (1994) recommend that parents are shown a grommet so they can recognise it if it falls out and know that this is normal. Grommets usually become blocked 6–9 months after insertion and are then gradually extruded from the ear. Other more complicated ear surgery is associated with the potential problems of giddiness and nausea due to interference with the inner ear.

Nasal surgery in children is usually relatively minor. Children may need reduction of a nasal fracture, removal of a foreign body or drainage of infected sinuses which are mostly day cases. Post-operative care may involve the care and removal of a nasal pack. Nasal packs are very uncomfortable as they prevent nasal breathing, and interfere with normal speech, and eating and drinking.

Activity

Consider how you could minimise the discomfort for a child with a nasal pack *in situ*.

Cleft lip and palate repair are performed at different times. The cleft lip is usually repaired during the first weeks of life. The palate repair is performed when the child is between 12 and 18 months old to make some allowance for the palate changes which occur during childhood but also to correct the deformity before the development of speech is too impaired. Cleft palate often require long-term treatment. Depending on the extent of the deformity extensive orthodontic treatment may be needed for some time after the initial repairs and most children require some speech therapy. The only further treatment for cleft lip repair may be revision of the scar although specialist centres usually have successful results (Martin, 1995). The immediate problems before the surgical repair are the support of the parents and the development of a feeding regime. Cleft lip and palate both impair the ability to suck, and feed taken into the mouth may escape through the cleft palate into the nose. Martin (1995) recommends assessment of the individual child to determine the most appropriate feeding technique. Breastfeeding is possible with the baby in an upright position, and a variety of teats and feeding devices are available to assist bottle-feeding. These methods help the baby to develop the sucking muscles as well as meeting sucking needs but cup feeding or naso-gastric tube feeding may be necessary if these do not ensure good weight gain.

Tonsillectomy – advice on discharge

- Analgesia 30 minutes before meals
- Encourage rough foods to deslough wound and promote healing
- Seek GP advice if child seems feverish
- Some associated earache on swallowing is normal
- Avoid crowded places and contact with those who have coughs and colds for 10 days after discharge
- Stay away from school or nursery for 10 days post-operatively
- Call 999 for an ambulance if fresh bleeding from the throat occurs

Activity

Identify the nursing actions to overcome the potential problems before and after cleft lip and palate repair (Table 5.5).

Problem	Aim	Nursing actions
Pre-operative care Risk of inadequate nutritional intake, choking and excessive wind	Feed/fluid chart shows adequate intake (ml/kg); no choking or excessive wind	
Risk of loss of parent–child attachment due to deformity	Parents demonstrate acceptance of child	
Post-operative care Risk of aspiration	Secretions and feed not aspirated	
Risk of trauma to site of repair	Site of repair remains undamaged	
Risk of inadequate nutrition due to feeding difficulties	Fluid/feed chart shows sufficient intake (ml/kg)	

Table 5.5

Cleft lip and palate repair: specific pre- and post-operative care
(Copyright is waived for the purpose of photocopying and enlarging this table.)

Tonsillectomy is beginning to be performed as a day case but is associated with asphyxia and haemorrhage because of the vascularity and position of the tonsils.

Indications for tracheostomy

Allergy
- angioneurotic oedema
- anaphylaxis

Prophylactic
- prolonged endotracheal intubation
- head and neck surgery

Degenerative
- vocal cord paralysis

Congenital
- choanal atresia
- microglossia
- Pierre Robin syndrome
- laryngomalacia
- laryngeal webs, cysts, stenosis

Trauma
- facial or oral injury/fractures
- facial burns/burn inhalation
- foreign body inhalation
- pharyngeal oedema

Toxic
- ingestion of corrosives

Infection
- epiglottitis
- croup
- diphtheria
- tetanus
- rabies
- retro-pharyngeal abscess

Neoplastic
- papillomatosis
- haemangioma
- lymphangioma

Activity

Identify the time of occurrence, causes and features of asphyxia, primary, reactionary and secondary haemorrhage.

Tracheostomy is often performed as a temporary measure to bypass an acute upper airway obstruction or provide access for long-term ventilation. Occasionally it is a more permanent treatment for a congenital obstruction of the airway. Children with a tracheostomy require frequent suctioning during the initial post-operative period to maintain their airway. After this time they may still need periodic clearance of secretions. Suctioning is a potentially hazardous procedure with well documented risks and some associated procedures such as the installation of saline prior to suctioning are debatable practices (Table 5.6). Although saline may loosen secretions and facilitate their removal Prasad and Hussey (1995) do not recommend its regular use and suggest that good hydration and humidification is a better way of ensuring loose secretions. The child with a tracheostomy requires highly skilled care to maintain the airway and promote a normal lifestyle.

Activity

Find out the following:
- what is needed at the bedside of a child with a tracheostomy?
- procedures for changing tracheostomy tapes and tube
- the nursing care required to overcome the problems listed in Table 5.7

If the tracheostomy is a temporary measure there is a gradual return to normal airway breathing. A smaller tube is inserted and if this does not cause respiratory problems the tube is occluded for 24 hours under close observation. If no problems occur the tube is removed and the stoma occluded.

Table 5.6

Tracheal suctioning – potential risks

Risk	Prevention
Damage to the tracheo-bronchial mucosa (Sumner, 1990)	Perform suction when required – not at pre-determined intervals Insert and withdraw the suction catheter gently Occlude suction pressure during catheter insertion
Hypoxia (Kerem *et al.*, 1990)	The external size of the catheter should not exceed half the internal diameter of the tracheostomy tube (Imle and Klemic, 1991). Duration of suctioning is ideally 15 seconds (Sumner, 1990). Limit suction pressure to 70–100 mmHg (Kusenski, 1978). Hyperoxygenate and hypoventilate with 100% O_2 before, during and after suction (Kerem *et al.*, 1990)
Cardiac arrythmias	Only suction when necessary Do not suction for more than 30 seconds
Bacterial infection	Use clean or sterile procedure Change suction tubing and bottles at least daily Rinse suction tubing with sterile water between suctions

Problem	Aim	Nursing actions
Tracheostomy may become blocked or dislodged	Clear airway maintained	
Irritation of tube in stoma and nursing interventions may cause infection	Site remains free from infection	
Loss of function of upper respiratory tract	Air is filtered, warmed and moistened	
Air flow diverted from vocal cords	Child develops effective method of communication	
Bibs, dribbling may occlude airway	Child able to eat and drink without endangering airway	
Fluff from toys or small toys may be inhaled and obstruct airway	Child has no potentially dangerous toys	
Water and talcum, fluff from clothing may occlude airway	Washing and dressing avoids inhalants	
Small children reluctant to lie prone to learn to crawl	Child develops normal mobility	
Inability to call/cry for help at night	Strategies in place to monitor child at night	

Table 5.7

Care of the child with a tracheostomy (Copyright is waived for the purpose of photocopying and enlarging this table.)

EDUCATION FOR DISCHARGE

Discharge advice following insertion of grommets and tonsillectomy have already been explored. Your answers to the previous activity should give you an idea of the tremendous responsibility the parents of a child with a tracheostomy at home have.

Activity

Consider all the teaching needs of the parents taking home a child with a tracheostomy. Decide how you could sequence and organise this teaching to ensure they had the optimum preparation before discharge.

6 PRINCIPLES OF CARE – CHILDREN WITH ALTERED GASTRO-INTESTINAL FUNCTION

INTRODUCTION

Processes related to gastro-intestinal function (eating, drinking and elimination) fill all aspects of our daily lives, and are important physically, socially and psychologically. Indeed much of the talk of young mothers centres around infant feeding and nappies. When a child has problems with elimination, the issues can cause psychological upset and can lead to a preoccupation with toileting. Problems of the gastro-intestinal tract are common in childhood. The nurse needs to understand the implications of such problems in order to help the child and his family cope with treatment and care.

Activity

Before reading any further you should refresh your memory on anatomy and physiology of the gastro-intestinal tract. You should look at structure, the functions of digestion, absorption and elimination, and acid–base balance.

Some of the problems which children face (and related pathophysiology) are given in Tables 6.1–6.4.

ASSESSMENT

When assessing gastro-intestinal function the nurse needs to take into account more than just the physical signs. She must look at the whole child and his/her family and lifestyle. Familial problems may be identified or there may be psychological problems which might affect management and care of the child. As part of the assessment process (on

Table 6.1 *Problems of motility*	Gastro-oesophageal reflux	Incompetent/malfunctioning lower oesophageal sphincter; on inspiration stomach contents move into oesophagus which in turn leads to vomiting; oesophagitis; scarring; stricture. Can also result in aspiration pneumonia
	Hirschsprung's disease	Absence of parasympathetic ganglion cells in intestinal muscle wall (usually sigmoid colon and rectum); no peristalsis as bowel is spastic and contracted; no faecal material can pass through; proximal bowel becomes distended and filled with faecal material and gas; internal sphincter fails to relax; no elimination; abdominal distension and constipation
	Chronic constipation with soiling	Constipation caused by a variety of factors becomes so severe that the bowel becomes distended and eventually insensitive and unable to prevent soft faeces passing round the hard impacted masses and oozing out

Coeliac disease	Changes in mucosal lining of small intestine caused by gluten; irregularity of epithelial cells; a reduction in normal villi which become flattened; disaccharide deficiency and depression of peptidase activity; malabsorption of fats, fat soluble vitamins, minerals, some protein and carbohydrates
Short bowel syndrome	Diminished ability of the intestine to function normally following resection for bowel anomalies, inflammatory problems. Loss of more than 75% results in malabsorption (Campbell and Glasper, 1995)
Cystic fibrosis	Defective CFTR gene; disruption of normal electrolyte and water secretion by cells; increased loss of sodium and chloride in sweat; reduced hydration of secretions from exocrine glands (Cree, 1997); viscid secretions from pancreas and gastro-intestinal tract (and respiratory system); malabsorption

Table 6.2

Problems of absorption

Cross reference

Cystic fibrosis – pages 515–516

Pyloric stenosis	Pyloric muscle is increased in length and diameter; there is marked increase in thickness in the circular muscle and attenuation of the longitudinal muscle (Cree, 1997); pyloric lumen is narrowed; stomach emptying is delayed causing distension; vomitting (often projectile) after feeds; dehydration and weight loss
Intussusception	'Invagination of a length of bowel into the succeeding bowel segment' (Cree, 1997, page 261); mesentery pulled into intestine as invagination occurs; intestine becomes curved; blood supply cut off; bowel begins to swell; complete obstruction may occur; necrosis

Table 6.3

Obstructive problems

Appendicitis	Acute inflammation of the mucosa; inflammatory changes throughout wall of appendix; oedema compromises blood flow; ischaemia and ulceration of epithelial lining; necrosis and perforation; peritonitis
Meckel's diverticulum	Failure of obliteration of the omphalomesenteric duct; out-pounching of bowel wall close to ileo-caecal valve; lined by small intestine mucosa; presence of acid-secreting gastric mucosa can lead to ulceration; inflammation
Gastro-enteritis	Loss of water and electrolytes leads to dehydration, electrolyte imbalance and metabolic acidosis
Crohn's disease and ulcerative colitis	See Figure 6.1

Table 6.4

Inflammatory problems

admission and subsequently) the nurse should use her skills to ascertain information about a wide variety of aspects (Figure 6.2).

Activity

One of the most dangerous consequences of gastro-intestinal problems can be dehydration. Giving rationale, describe the possible effects of severe dehydration on a small child. Use information given in this book and other references to help you.

Cross references

Maturation – page 65

Fluid balance – page 339

Figure 6.1

Cross section of small intestine to show comparison of pathology: (a) Crohn's disease and (b) ulcerative colitis. (Adapted from Cree, 1997.)

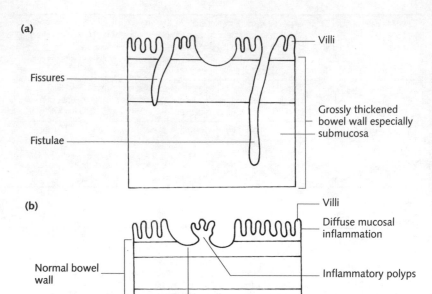

(a)
- Villi
- Fissures
- Grossly thickened bowel wall especially submucosa
- Fistulae

(b)
- Villi
- Diffuse mucosal inflammation
- Normal bowel wall
- Inflammatory polyps
- Shallow ulcers

Figure 6.2

Specific assessment of the child with gastro-intestinal problems.

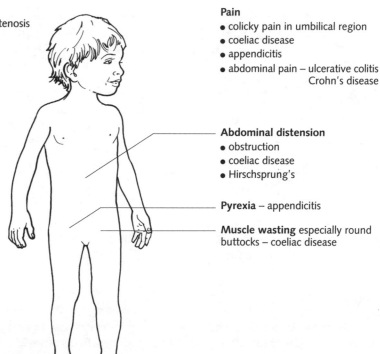

Dehydration → electrolyte/fluid imbalance, e.g. gastroenteritis, pyloric stenosis
- skin tone
- colour
- behaviour
- urine output
- fontanelle

Vomiting
- projectile (pyloric stenosis)
- bile stained – obstruction
- faecal – low obstruction
- regurgitation
- haematemesis

Abnormal bowel pattern
- diarrhoea – infection
  – inflammatory problems
- pale bulky offensive stools – coeliac disease
- constipation with or without overflow – Hirschsprung's
  – encopresis

Pain
- colicky pain in umbilical region
- coeliac disease
- appendicitis
- abdominal pain – ulcerative colitis Crohn's disease

Abdominal distension
- obstruction
- coeliac disease
- Hirschsprung's

Pyrexia – appendicitis

Muscle wasting especially round buttocks – coeliac disease

These observations together with the results of medical investigations will enable an accurate decision to be made about treatment and care. Table 6.5 shows the various investigations which may be done to diagnose problems of the gastro-intestinal tract.

Activity

Find out in what circumstances each one might be used, what it might show and what the role of the nurse would be. Make notes in the boxes for future reference

Test	When and what for?	Role of the nurse
Blood Hb haematocrit sodium potassium pH CO_2 WCC		
Biopsies jejunal rectal		
Manometry oesophageal rectal		
pH studies oesophageal stool		
X-rays plain barium		
Endoscopy		
Rectal examination		
Xylose absorption test		
Faecal fat excretion		

Table 6.5

Medical investigations (Copyright is waived for the purpose of photocopying and enlarging this table.)

INTERVENTIONS

This section concentrates on discussing care related to four of the specific interventions which may be implemented for children with gastro-intestinal problems. These are:

- specific pre- and post-operative care;
- bowel retraining;
- colostomy care;
- rehydration therapy.

Specific pre- and post-operative care

Intervention	Rationale	Notes
Pre-operative care: IV therapy	To restore fluid, electrolyte and acid–base balance; in conditions where there is metabolic alkalosis, super-imposition of this on the respiratory alkalosis which follows mechanical ventilation can cause major problems in re-establishing spontaneous respirations (MacMahon, 1991)	
Naso-gastric tube – aspirated with possible gastric washout	To empty stomach contents to prevent vomiting and possible aspiration	
Bowel clearance using either rectal washouts with saline or via naso-gastric tube using a bowel cleansing preparation (e.g. Kleanprep)	To clear the bowel	
Low residue diet progressing to fluids only	To keep stools soft and complement bowel clearance	
Preparation for formation of colostomy	To identify most appropriate site; to prepare child/family psychologically	
Post-operative care: Naso-gastric tube on free drainage – aspirated as directed	To prevent abdominal distension	
Nil by mouth until bowel sounds return	To ensure that peristalsis has returned before re-introducing feeding	
Gradual re-introduction of oral feeding	Rate at which this is done will depend on operative procedure	

Care of colostomy
  observe drainage
 	
  observe colour
	
	to ensure adequate bowel function
	to detect reduction in blood supply	

Activity

Find out in what circumstances each of the above interventions may be implemented. Make notes in column 3 of Table 6.6.

Bowel retraining

The first step in managing encopresis, when there is found to be a severe degree of retention, is to empty the bowel. This may be done by the short-term administration of a laxative such as Senokot. This is often accompanied by longer term administration of lactulose. This treatment can usually be given at home reducing the necessity for hospital admission. Where this conservative treatment does not work alternative therapies may be tried including suppositories and/or enemas. These will often necessitate hospital admission. It is extremely important if this is the case, to establish trusting relationships with the child before administering the treatment. When there is no faecal retention management can move directly on to step two which is a period of re-training using behaviour modification principles. Behaviour therapy is based on the principles of learning theory and on the belief that problem behaviours can be eliminated by the introduction of new learning experiences (Barker, 1995). It is important that a detailed assessment is carried out prior to developing an individual therapy plan for each child. In each case realistic goals need to be drawn up in discussion with the child and family. The context in which the family is operating must be taken into consideration and recognised as important in planning any treatment.

According to Herbert (1987) there are two basic learning tasks:

- The acquisition of a desired behaviour in which the child is deficient – in this case bowel control.
- The extinction of an undesired response – in this case soiling.

Achieving these can be done using reinforcement, either positive or negative. Positive reinforcement is anything which will increase the likelihood of a previous behaviour being repeated. It stands therefore that any desired behaviours (which should be agreed in the planning stage), e.g. clean pants, should be positively reinforced. Negative reinforcement is an alternative and occurs when attention-seeking behaviour is not reinforced. In this case, for example, soiled pants would be ignored. Dealing with the problem of bowel re-training requires patience and perseverance on behalf of the child and family. Family therapy may be required to help families cope with stresses and tensions which may be an underlying factor. The nurse's role is to support and encourage adherence to the programme and to be aware of the distress this problem can cause.

Colostomy/ileostomy care

A colostomy/ileostomy may be temporary or permanent. In either case the child and family will need considerable support and education to

- **Senokot** – a stimulant laxative – encourages bowel movement by acting on nerve endings in the wall of the intestine that trigger contraction of intestinal muscles. This speeds up the passage of faecal matter through the intestine therefore allowing less time for water to be absorbed. The faeces become more liquid and more frequent. Used as a short-term treatment
- **Lactulose** – increases the amount of water in the large intestine and softens the stools. Used for long-term management

Cross references

Family therapy – pages 537–538
Behaviour modification – pages 538–539

Examples of positive reinforcers (rewards)

- *Tangible* – stars (on a star chart), points, money, food, sweets, treats such as trips out, small toys, privileges such as watching television
- *Intangible* – praise, attention, hugs, time with parent, smiles, words of thanks

Reinforcement must be immediate for young children. Delaying tactics will not act as a reinforcer manage at home. Time will be needed to adjust to the colostomy and to learn the principles of colostomy care. A study by Johnson in 1996 found that the support and advice given to children and families was often inadequate. Some of the concerns raised by parents/carers are highlighted. The principles of managing a colostomy are as follows:

- *Hygiene and skin care.* Bathing can take place as normal either with the appliance on or off. The skin around the stoma should be examined for signs of inflammation or excoriation whenever the appliance is changed. The skin around an ileostomy is particularly liable to become sore. Distal loop washouts may be required if the child has a colostomy. The purpose of these is to evacuate faeces and mucus from the distal bowel in order to minimise infection. They also assist in preparing the bowel for possible later surgery (Adams and Selekof, 1986).

- *Using appliances.* The stoma therapist should be involved in choosing the most appropriate appliance and giving advice on changing the bags. Bags should be removed carefully and slowly. The skin around the stoma is washed and dried carefully and a barrier cream/gum applied. The bag should fit snugly round the stoma to prevent leakage.

- *Observation of the stoma and its function.* The stoma should be bright red; signs of complications include a change in colour, ribbon-like stool, diarrhoea, bleeding, failure of evacuation of stool, prolapse, retraction and stenosis.

- *Diet.* There are no real restrictions to normal diet unless medically indicated. However, low residue diet may be advocated to decrease the stool bulk. As the risk of fluid loss is increased due to reduced colon absorption (particularly in hot weather) parents should be advised to ensure an adequate fluid intake. It is wise to avoid carbonated drinks as this increases flatus.

- *Psychological aspects of care.* The nurse must be aware of the effects of a change in body image and give support accordingly. Privacy and dignity must be maintained when dealing with the colostomy. Time must be set aside to discuss problems and concerns. Children and parents can be encouraged to contact support agencies as talking to families with similar difficulties can act as a powerful coping strategy:

British Colostomy Association, 15 Station Road, Reading, Berkshire RG1 1LG. Tel: 01734 391537.

National Advisory Service for Parents of Children with a Stoma, 32 Sules Drive, Norwich, Norfolk NR8 6UU.

Rehydration therapy

This type of therapy is normally implemented for infants and young children who present with dehydration as a result of diarrhoea (with or without vomiting):

- Mild dehydration (5% or less) – clear fluids for at least 24–48 hours. A range of formulas are available which are based on the principle that oral rehydration works best when glucose or sucrose is added to an electrolyte solution (Hull and Johnston, 1987). It is important that the solution is made up according to instructions on the packet. Young children often find the solution unpalatable; Moulai and Huband (1996) advocate the use of very weak fruit juice in this instance. Recent experience has shown that 'flat' fizzy drinks also work well. Milk should be avoided as it tends to prolong the diarrhoea and vomiting. After the initial period of 24 hours, intake can gradually be re-introduced according to local policy.

- Moderate to severe dehydration (more than 5%) – IV therapy with or without fasting. The type of fluid infused will depend on electrolyte results. The child's condition is monitored daily and when appropriate a regrading programme is introduced.

Activity

Find out the policy for rehydration therapy in your local children's ward or department. Make a note in the margin for future reference.

EDUCATION FOR DISCHARGE

Many children with problems of the gastro-intestinal tract can be managed at home. Others will need admission to hospital for surgical treatment which may be followed up by many months of additional treatment. The community children's nurse plays a vital role in helping to plan for discharge, ensuring that support and advice is available in the community. Children may go home with:

- total parenteral nutrition;
- gastrostomy, jejunal, naso-gastric feeding systems;
- stoma;
- dietary restrictions;
- drug therapy;
- surgical wounds.

In each case the nurse must ensure that an individual teaching plan is drawn up as soon after admission a possible to teach aspects of home care to the child and/or family.

Activity

A 10-year-old girl has been diagnosed as having colitis. Draw up a teaching plan to ensure that she can manage her diet and drug therapy correctly following discharge.

Rehydration formulas
- Dioralyte
- Dextrolyte
- Pedilyte
- Rehydrat

Cross reference

Calculation of IV fluid rates – page 341

Research suggestion

Explore the use of 'flat' fizzy drinks in the treatment of dehydration for young children with diarrhoea and vomiting

---

7 PRINCIPLES OF CARE – CHILDREN WITH GENITO-URINARY PROBLEMS

INTRODUCTION

Problems of the genito-urinary system are relatively common in childhood. One reason for this could be that the system has a high percentage of congenital and genetic abnormalities compared with other organ systems (Taylor, 1996). Some problems can improve with surgery or conservative treatment, others develop chronic disease and progress towards renal failure. Chronic disease invades all aspects of the child's life with dietary and activity restrictions and altered elimination and growth patterns. To appreciate the impact renal disease can have on a child and family, the nurse needs a clear understanding of the development and function of the genito-urinary system.

Activity

Draw a labelled diagram of a nephron. Critically examine the functions of each part.

Problems of the genito-urinary system can be divided into:
- inherited and congenital anomalies (Table 7.1);
- acquired disorders (Table 7.2).

    When the function of the kidney is compromised as a result of renal disease, renal failure may occur.

Activity

Consider the physiological explanations for the following manifestations of chronic renal failure:
- sustained metabolic acidosis
- significant bone demineralisation and impaired growth
- anaemia
- intractable itching
- loss of energy and increased fatigue on exertion

Then do the same for the manifestations of acute renal failure.

ASSESSMENT

Skilled assessment of the child with potential renal problems is vital for prompt diagnosis. Problems may be difficult to identify as presenting

---

Causes of acute renal failure

Pre-renal – reduction of renal perfusion in a normal kidney:
- dehydration secondary to diarrhoea/vomiting
- surgical shock
- trauma

Renal – diseases which damage the glomeruli, tubules or renal vasculature
- glomerular disease
- ischaemia
- nephrotoxins

Post-renal
- obstructive lesions

Causes of chronic renal failure – end stage renal disease which occurs following progressive deterioration over months or years as a result of
- chronic glomerulitis
- recurrent pyelonephritis
- renal hypoplasia
- Alport syndrome

symptoms are sometimes rather obscure, for example in the case of urinary tract infections. Many of the clinical manifestations of renal disease are common to a variety of other childhood disorders and therefore careful follow-up may be necessary. Figure 7.1 (page 479) gives an indication of the specific aspects which should be addressed when assessing the child. Table 7.3 (page 480) gives an indication of the signs of urinary tract infections in different age groups.

In assessing the child you will be required to carry out a routine urinalysis. It is important that you are familiar with the various ways of

Problem	Pathophysiology
Renal agenesis – unilateral or bilateral	In unilateral agenesis the remaining kidney becomes hypertrophied. Bilateral agenesis or Potter's syndrome, usually stillborn. May be associated with pulmonary hypoplasia.
Renal hypoplasia – unilateral or bilateral	Kidneys are normally formed but small. Bilateral hypoplasia results in renal failure
Polycystic disease	Autosomal recessive disorder with gradual severity. The kidneys are grossly enlarged and renal function is impaired. There are cystic changes in the liver and other organs
Obstructive malformations ureteropelvic junction obstruction ureteric duplication posterior urethral valves	Obstruction to the flow of urine from the kidney or bladder results in backflow of urine into the kidney leading to hydronephrosis and impaired kidney function
Primary vesicoureteric reflux (VUR)	An inherited disorder where there is failure of the mechanisms which prevent reflux of urine; prevention of reflux is mainly due to the following process – when the pressure in the bladder is increased during micturition, the detrusor muscle contracts and the submucosal ureter is passively compressed increasing the resistance to reflux (Dunne and Gibbons, 1992). Failure of this process is usually due to an inadequate length of the submucosal ureter. VUR predisposes to infection
Bladder extrophy	Failure of development of the anterior bladder wall and the overlying abdominal wall. The ureters open onto the exposed anterior wall mucosa which is prone to infection and metaplastic change. In boys the penis is up-turned, the pubic bone unfused and the lower limbs apparently rotated. In girls the genital tract is normal but with possible vaginal stenosis
Wilm's tumour – nephroblastoma	Originates from embryonal kidney – peak incidence age 3 years, more common in boys than girls, more often affecting the left kidney
Undescended testes incomplete descent ectopic or maldescended	Testes follow normal descent route but fail to reach scrotum. May be impalpable. Testes often grossly abnormal with poor spermatogenesis. Testes follow abnormal route. Easily palpable and normal in appearance, normal spermatogenesis
Hypospadias	The urethra opens on the ventral aspect of the penis instead of at the end. Site of opening may be anywhere along the length of the penis. May be accompanied by ventral curvature or chordee of the penis distal to the abnormal urethra. Failure of fusion of the ventral part of the foreskin results in a redundant dorsal hood
Inguinal hernia and hydrocele	Caused by persistency of the processus vaginalis, the pouch of peritoneum which accompanies the descent of the testis

Table 7.1

Inherited and congenital anomalies

Manifestations of acute renal failure

- Oliguria (volume less than 0.5–1.0 ml/kg/hour)
- Scant bloody urine
- Lethargy
- Nausea and vomiting
- Diarrhoea
- Dry skin and mucous membranes
- Drowsiness, headache, muscle twitching, convulsions

Table 7.2

Acquired disorders

Problem	Pathophysiology
Urinary infections	Caused by a variety of organisms – *Escherichia coli* most prevalent. May involve the urethra, bladder, ureters, renal pelvis, calyces or parenchyma. Ascension of organisms from perineal area is the most common scenario. Inflammation of the urethra can occur within 30 minutes of bacterial invasion (Wong, cited by Miller, 1996). Organisms then ascend into the bladder causing cystitis. A transient vesicoureteral reflux allows urine to ascend up to the kidneys causing pyelonephritis. Inflammatory changes can result in incompetence of the vesicoureteral valve leading to continuing reflux and renal scarring. Recurrent renal infections may lead to chronic renal failure
Acute post-streptococcal glomerulonephritis	Primarily affects early school-age children (6–7 years); more common in boys than girls. An immune compex disease with an onset 10–14 days after a beta-haemolytic streptococcal throat infection
Minimal change nephrotic syndrome (MCNS)	Idiopathic disease occurring mainly in preschool children. Cause is uncertain but the glomerular membrane becomes abnormally permeable allowing proteins (especially albumin) to pass through into the urine. This leads to a reduced serum albumin level which in turn decreases colloidal osmotic pressure in the capilliaries; fluid leaks out from the circulation into interstitial compartments (tissues and body cavities) leading to oedema; shift of fluid reduces vascular fluid volume (hypovolaemia)
Renal tubular acidosis proximal (type II) distal (type I)	Defect in bicarbonate absorption; hyperchloraemic metabolic acidosis; growth failure, tachypnoea; possible severe acidosis. Inability of the kidney to establish a normal pH gradient between tubular cells and tubular contents. Inability to secrete hydrogen ions causes accumulation producing a sustained acidosis; retards growth, demineralisation of bone occurs, increased levels of calcium and phosphorus predisopose to formation of stones
Renal disease associated with systemic disease	Diabetes mellitus, systemic lupus erythematosus, Henoch–Schönlein purpura, amyloidosis
Enuresis	Common problem in childhood – involuntary voiding of the bladder when there is no organic cause. It may occur by day (diuresis) or by night (nocturnal enuresis)
Phimosis	Stenosis of the preputial orifice mostly caused by recurrent balanitis or traumatic retraction of the foreskin. Leads to ballooning and a poor stream during micturition and further attacks of balanitis

Observations of urine – the implications

- Smell – strong amoniacal smell – urinary infection
- Appearance
  - red urine – frank blood usually due to renal trauma; dyes present in food, e.g. beetroot, and some drugs, e.g. rifampicin
  - pale urine – dilute
  - dark yellow – concentrated
  - deep orange – obstructive jaundice
- Urinalysis – in many cases there is no cause of urinary tract infection
  - proteinuria – small amount is normal; if present in large amounts may indicate renal disease, e.g. infection or glomerulonephritis
  - glucose – possible implications include diabetes mellitus, renal tubular disease (e.g. Fanconi's syndrome); can also occur as a result of total parenteral nutrition and steroid therapy
  - ketones – found in children who are fasting or on a weight reducing diet, children who are pyrexial or those who have a metabolic disorder (e.g. diabetes mellitus)
  - pH – normal urine should have a pH greater than 5.5; a low pH means that the urine is very dilute. The pH is constant in renal failure

collecting urine for this purpose and of the implications of your findings. The methods for collection include:

- *Clean catch* – this method is suitable for babies and young children who have not yet gained bladder control. It can be rather time consuming but is often an approach preferred by parents as it causes least distress. The vulval area or penis should be cleaned with saline and the child left without a nappy. When the child micturates the urine is caught in a sterile pot.
- *Supra-pubic aspiration (SPA)* – this is a reliable method of collecting an uncontaminated specimen from a child who is not toilet trained. However, it is traumatic and needs to be carried out when the bladder is full. A needle is inserted through the skin into the bladder and urine aspirated through a syringe. The first few cubic centimetres should be discarded.

Oedema
- pre-orbital ⎤ glomerulonephritis
- generalised ⎦ nephrotic syndrome

Urine
- proteinuria – nephrotic syndrome
- haematuria – UTI trauma
- dark, opalescent frothy
  – nephrotic syndrome
- cloudy/smoky brown
  – glomerulonephritis
- reduced volume
  – glomerulonephritis
  – acute renal failure
- dysuria/urgency – UTI
- strong smelling – UTI
- eneuresis – UTI

Blood pressure
- mild to moderate elevation
  – glomerulonephritis
- normal or slightly low – nephrotic
  syndrome
- raised – renal damage

Fever
- high fever with rigors – pyelonephritis
- fever – UTI

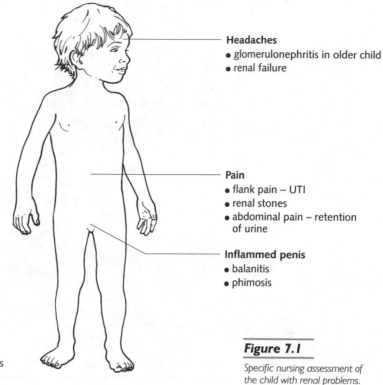

Headaches
- glomerulonephritis in older child
- renal failure

Pain
- flank pain – UTI
- renal stones
- abdominal pain – retention
  of urine

Inflammed penis
- balanitis
- phimosis

Figure 7.1

Specific nursing assessment of the child with renal problems.

Activity

You are asked to assist in an SPA on a 12-year-old girl who has severe spina bifida. The urine is wanted for a routine urinalysis – there is no specific reason to suggest the young girl has any renal disease. Consider your role as advocate in this instance.

- *Midstream urine (MSU)* – a useful means of collecting urine from a cooperative child who has bladder control. The vulval area or penis should be cleaned as before and the child instructed to either retract the foreskin or hold the labia apart during micturition. Allow the child to pass some urine before collecting your sample. A young child will need assistance.

- *Bag urine* – least reliable method of collecting an uncontaminated specimen especially in females (Miller, 1996). Waddington and Watson compared three commonly used urine collection bags and concluded that the Urinicole bag (Cliniflex, High Wycombe, Buckinghamshire) was the most favourable.

- *Catheter specimen* – used when a catheter is already *in situ* or if a child uses intermittent catheterisation for incontinence. This can also be used to collect urine from a stoma.

An alternative method for urine collection from infants

Vernon (1995) discusses the development of the 'Urine Collection Pad' (available nationally). This technique uses a pad to collect the urine from babies and infants who are in nappies. The method has been found to be cheap, reliable and simple. For further information about the pads contact: Sue Vernon 0191 232 5131.

Table 7.3

Age-related signs of UTI

Neonates	Infants	Preschooler	School age	Adolescent
Unstable temperature				
Jaundice				
Apnoeic episodes				
Pallor	Pallor			
Sepsis	Sepsis			
Abdominal distension	Abdominal tenderness			
Nappy rash	Nappy rash			
Poor feeding	Failure to thrive	Anorexia		
Irritability	Irritability			
Lethargy	Lethargy			
Vomiting	Vomiting	Vomiting	Vomiting	Vomiting
Hypothermia	Fever	Fever	Fever	Fever
Diarrhoea	Diarrhoea	Diarrhoea	Diarrhoea	
		Strong urine	Strong urine	Strong urine
		Haematuria	Haematuria	Haematuria
		Frequency	Frequency	Frequency
		Urgency	Urgency	Urgency
		Dysuria	Dysuria	Dysuria
			Enuresis	
			Mood swings	
				Chills

Further reading

TOMSETT, A. and WATSON, A. (1996) Renal biopsy as a day case procedure. *Paediatric Nursing*, **8** (5), 14–15.

Laboratory studies will help to identify renal problems which can be further evaluated using radiological studies and renal biopsy (Thomsett and Watson, 1996). Table 7.4 shows the various investigations which may be done.

Interventions for children with genito-urinary problems

- Blood pressure monitoring
- Daily weight
- Catheterisation and catheter care
- Pre- and post-operative care
- Care of an ileal conduit
- Fluid restriction
- Administration of a salt free diet
- Dialysis – peritoneal/ haemodialysis
- Bladder training
- Management of oedema
- Administration of drugs

Activity

Find out in what circumstances each of the investigations in Table 7.4 might be used, what it might show and what the role of the nurse would be. Make notes in the boxes for future reference.

In caring for children with genito-urinary problems you may be involved with implementing a variety of interventions. The following interventions will be discussed in more detail here:

- catheter care;
- the management of oedema;
- the administration of specific drugs;
- peritoneal dialysis.

Investigation	When and what for?	Role of the nurse
Glomerular filtration rate and creatinine clearance		
Laboratory urinalysis		
Urine culture		

Blood
    urea, creatinine,
    sodium, potassium,
    phosphate,
    haemoglobin,
    serum albumin		

ASO titre		

Radiologic studies:
    – micturating
      cysto-urethrogram
    – IV pyelogram
    – ultrasound
    – dimercaptosuccinic
      acid scan		

Renal arteriogram		
Radionuclide imaging		
Urodynamics		

Table 7.4

Medical investigations (Copyright is waived for the purpose of photocopying and enlarging this table.)

Further reading

JADRESIC, L. (1993) Investigation of urinary tract infection in childhood. *British Medical Journal*, **307**, 761–764.

TAYLOR, C. M. and CHAPMAN, S. (1989) *Handbook of Renal Investigations in Children*. Sevenoaks: Wright.

Reasons for use of indwelling catheter

Short-term
- severely ill child requiring intensive care
- surgery to the renal tract
- surgery to the genital area
- reconstructive surgery

Long-term
- unconscious child
- child with deteriorating/disabling condition
- to overcome obstruction to outflow of urine

CATHETER CARE

Urinary catheters are usually passed via the urethra into the bladder to allow drainage of urine. Some children will require an indwelling catheter which is inserted on a short-term or long-term basis. An aseptic technique must be used when inserting the catheter and the following points noted:

- cleanse the area around the urethral meatus using an antiseptic solution;
- avoid contamination of the surface of the catheter;
- ensure the catheter is well lubricated (use packet of sterile lubricant);
- ensure that the catheter is the correct size – use the smallest size capable of providing adequate drainage.

Children who have indwelling catheters are prone to urinary tract infection and particular care should avoid this by:

- Keeping the area around the urethral meatus clean – normal bathing should be sufficient. Too much cleansing around the meatus in boys can cause irritation and infection (de Sousa, 1996).

- Ensure that there is patency of the catheter with no kinking of tubes. If the child is ambulatory ensure that the catheter and bag are strapped to the leg securely.
- Ensure a high fluid intake to promote free flow of urine and prevent blockage of the catheter – monitor output.
- Observe urine regularly – check for colour and smell.

Some children will require intermittent catheterisation which is often carried out by the child (self-catheterisation). The use of this type of catheterisation is indicated in children who have a neurogenic bladder (e.g. those with spina bifida). The catheters used are self-lubricating and can be washed and re-used. The advantage of using this intervention is that children can learn to empty the bladder efficiently and therefore become dry by day and by night. This can promote self-confidence and allow the child to take a more active part in everyday life.

SPECIFIC DRUGS

Table 7.5 shows some of the more common drugs which would be used for children with genito-urinary problems. You should ensure that you are aware of the potential side effects of each drug and of any particular role you should play in their administration.

Activity

Consider the drugs listed in Table 7.5. Explore when each may be used, note normal dosage and any further important points to note regarding administration. Make notes in the margin and in the table for future reference.

THE MANAGEMENT OF OEDEMA

Some children with renal problems may exhibit varying degrees of oedema. You need to take great care of the child's skin as oedematous skin is extremely susceptible to infection and breakdown. Keep the following points in mind when delivering care:

- keep skin clean and dry;
- avoid friction between oedematous parts of the body by applying non-perfumed talcum powder or by using rolls of cotton, pillows;
- support the scrotum with cotton pads held in place by T-bandage;
- avoid using tape on the skin as this can cause tearing when removed;
- keep child on bed rest only in the acute phase – encourage to move position frequently;
- follow instructions regarding fluid restriction and salt restriction.

Fluid restriction

Fluid restriction is contra-indicated in children with nephrotic syndrome. The oedema leads to hypovolaemia – restricting fluids would therefore deplete circulating volume further causing hypercoagulability and possible arterial/venous thrombosis Maughan (1994)

Drug	Potential side effects	Role of the nurse
Antibiotics (for UTI)		
sulphonamides	Nausea, vomiting, drug fever, rashes, photosensitivity	Keep child well hydrated – avoids crystallisation of drug in urine
gentamycin	renal and auditory toxicity	Minimise toxic effects by using slow IV infusion
		Assist with taking blood for levels
cephalexin	Diarrhoea nausea and vomiting	Must be taken with food
Immunosuppressives		
cyclophosphamide	Nausea, vomiting, hair loss, irregular menstruation, mouth ulcers	Encourage high fluid intake and frequent bladder emptying to prevent bladder irritation
Steroids		
prednisolone	Increased appetite, obesity, decreased resistance to infection, growth retardation, mood changes, adrenal suppression	
Antihypertensives		
hydralazine	Headache, dizziness, rapid heart beat; lupus erythematosus may occur with prolonged use	
nifedipine	Dizziness on rising, headache, flushing	
Diuretics		
frusemide	Dizziness; rare side effects include noises in ears, cramps, rash	Ensure potassium rich diet to combat reduction by the drug
metolazone		

Table 7.5

Specific drugs used for children with renal problems

PERITONEAL DIALYSIS (PD)

This intervention uses the peritoneum as a semi-permeable membrane to filter and remove toxins and fluid. Sterile dialysis solution is instilled through a permanent silastic catheter into the peritoneal cavity. The solution is left to dwell (time will depend on method and reason for dialysis and can range from 30 minutes to 4–5 hours) and then drained off. PD may be implemented for children who are in acute renal failure where oliguria continues after 24–48 hours. In this case dialysis will be for a short period of time. Longer term PD may be used for children with acute renal failure where it gives more freedom than haemodialysis and can be done at home more easily. In the latter circumstances there are two main methods of implementing the process:

- *Continuous ambulatory peritoneal dialysis (CAPD)* – this method allows for continuous dialysis but does not necessitate bed rest or hospitalisation. Dialysis solution is left to dwell for about 4–6 hours allowing for four to five exchanges daily. During the dwell time, the bag is clamped and strapped to the child's abdomen leaving him to be relatively active. The dwell time can be lengthened overnight to allow for uninterrupted sleep.

- *Continuous cycling peritoneal dialysis (CCPD)* – a machine is used to deliver the desired exchanges automatically at night while the child sleeps.

Principles of dialysis

PD removes water and electrolytes from the blood by virtue of the osmotic gradient that exists between the dialysate and the blood across the peritoneal membrane. By manipulating the concentration of the dialysis solution the quantity and speed of fluid movement can be altered

(Hazinski, 1992)

Although this form of treatment has its advantages, it should be acknowledged that it is not necessarily that easy to cope with at home. In a small study, MacDonald (1995) explored mothers' experiences of living with chronic renal disease. Although the mothers were delighted to be able to take their children home from hospital they quickly realised how their expectations of home life with dialysis were unrealistic. They found the technical procedures and monitoring stressful, they had to forfeit their own needs and they indicated a fear of losing control of themselves.

When providing nursing care for a child receiving PD you should be aware of the complications of the procedure and take appropriate steps to prevent them (Table 7.6).

Table 7.6

Nursing care for a child receiving peritoneal dialysis

Complication	Nursing care
Peritonitis – mild to severe and ultimately resulting in loss of membrane integrity prohibiting further use of the peritoneum as a filter	Keep catheter exit site clean and covered with dry dressing; use aseptic technique throughout procedures; take care not to raise dialysate bottle above level of the bed as this allows reflux of drained solution; meticulous daily hygiene – showers not baths; monitor for signs of infection – cloudy dialysate, abdominal pain and tenderness, fever
Catheter problems obstruction leakage round catheter	Ensure that the tubing hangs freely straight down from the bed to the collection bottle Check for overflowing of abdomen – abdomen should not feel rigid; check insertion site; pack weighed, sterile dressings round site – weigh when changed to measure volume and notify doctor
Pulmonary complications – infusion of fluid into abdomen can cause abdominal fullness which can compromise movement of the diaphragm leading to hyperventilation and atelectasis	Assess breath sounds frequently, check effectiveness of ventilation. Encourage child to cough and take deep breaths; elevate head of the bed
Fluid and electrolyte imbalance	Maintain accurate records of all fluid in and out; implement fluid and sodium restrictions as prescribed. Monitor for signs of fluid and electrolyte imbalance – dehydration, peripheral oedema, blood sugar levels

Activity

Explore the use of the other interventions listed in the margin on page 480. When might they be implemented and what would be your role?

HEALTH EDUCATION FOR DISCHARGE

Secondary education – preventing the reoccurrence of urinary tract infections

It is important to educate parents and children so that they understand the rationale for steps which can be taken to reduce the risk of urine infections. Begin by ensuring an understanding of the anatomy of the renal tract using pictures and diagrams and non-jargon terminology.

Activity

Draw a labelled diagram of the renal tract which you could use to teach children and parents basic anatomy and physiology. Try it out and then critically evaluate.

Preventive measures are related to the factors which predispose to infection:

- In girls the urethra is very short (about 2 cm in young girls, 4 cm in mature women). This means that there is an increased chance of contamination from a close proximity to the anus. Males are less susceptible due to the longer urethra and antibacterial properties of prostatic secretions. However, the presence of a foreskin is associated with an increase in periurethral bacteria that can easily ascend (Wiswell *et al.*, 1988) particularly in the first year of life. It is important therefore to teach about basic hygiene and the need for frequent baths; clean from front to back when cleaning the vulval or anal area during nappy changing or toileting.

- Urinary stasis is perhaps the single most important predisposing factor for urinary tract infections (Miller, 1996). Normally regular emptying of the bladder flushes away any organisms before they can multiply. Incomplete emptying leaves urine in the bladder providing an ideal culture medium for bacterial growth. Teach to avoid 'holding on' and delaying micturition; encourage frequent voiding and complete emptying. Children are sometimes in a hurry to get back to play and may finish before the bladder is empty. Double voiding is useful and involves returning to micturate after a short time. Increased fluid intake encourages flushing of the bladder.

Causes of incomplete emptying of the bladder

- Neurogenic bladder
- Obstructive lesions
- Anomalies in the urinary tract
- Constipation
- Infrequent voiding

- Normal urine is slightly acidic with a pH of 5. This helps to hamper the multiplication of bacteria. However, alkaline urine predisposes to bacterial growth. Urine can be made more acidic by offering apple juice, cranberry juice or a diet high in animal protein.

- Essential oils in some bubble baths and soaps can irritate the urethra thereby predisposing to bacterial growth – use of these should be avoided.

Tertiary education – managing infections at home to reduce the risk of renal damage

Include the following points in a teaching plan:

- instructions regarding the administration of antibiotics;
- specific guidelines on fluid intake – it is not sufficient to say 'encourage fluids' – offer a suggested amount, e.g. based on weight

Further reading

BERRY, A. C. and CHANTLER, C. (1986) Urogenital malformations and disease. *British Medical Bulletin*, **42** (2), 181–186.

GARTLAND, C. (1993) Partners in care. How families are taught to care for their child on peritoneal dialysis. *Nursing Times*, **89** (30), 34–36.

POSTLETHWAITE, R. J. (ed.) (1994) *Clinical Paediatric Nephrology*, 2nd edn. Oxford: Butterworth Heinemann.

Helpful addresses

British Kidney Patient Association, Bordon, Hants.
Tel: 01420 472021/2

Enuresis Resource and Information Centre (ERIC), 65 St Michael's Hill, Bristol, BS2 8DZ.
Tel: 01272 264920

(100 ml/kg/day). Give ideas on how to encourage oral intake in reluctant children (use of bendy straws, frozen lollies, reward systems, e.g. stars). Give ideas on types of fluid to offer (should avoid caffeine and carbonated drinks as these may irritate bladder mucosa; Miller, 1996).

Activity

Design a teaching plan for a 4-year-old girl and her carers to prepare them for discharge following hospitalisation for a severe urinary tract infection.

PRINCIPLES OF CARE – CHILDREN WITH PROBLEMS RELATED TO THE IMMUNE SYSTEM

8

INTRODUCTION

The body is protected from harmful agents by a complex system. The effects of dysfunction in this complex system can involve any or all of the body systems and as such can present the child with many varied problems. It is likely that you will meet the challenges presented by children with problems of the immune system and therefore it is essential that you have a working knowledge of the system's normal function and the mechanisms of dysfunction. Some aspects of anatomy and physiology are reviewed here for you but you will need to revise your knowledge more fully.

The organs which contribute to protection of the body:

- Non-immunological host defences – skin, cilia, mucous membranes, tears and saliva.
- Inflammatory response – vascular and cellular changes that eliminate dead tissue, microorganisms, toxins, and inert foreign matter.
- Mononuclear phagocytic system (reticuloendothelial system) – removes pathogens from blood and tissue by phagocytosis – mainly by macrophages.
- Immune system – includes organs, tissue and cells circulating in the blood. Primary organs – bone marrow and thymus. Secondary organs – lymph nodes, spleen, tonsils, Peyer's patches and appendix. The main cells of the immune system are lymphocytes – T and B cells. There are two mechanisms by which the immune system responds to antigens – humoral and cell mediated (Figure 8.1). These usually work together to produce a combined response.

Activity

Having read so far you should explore some aspects of anatomy and physiology further (Nurse's Clinical Library, 1985):
- the role of the complement system and cascade
- the role of macrophages
- the process of phagocytosis.

The problems associated with the immune system are numerous and are categorised here as:
- immunodeficiency disorders (Table 8.1);

Definitions

The key to understanding the complex immune system is to have an understanding of the interactions of antigen and antibody:

- *antigen* – any substance capable of eliciting an immune response
- *antibody (immunoglobulin)* – serum proteins that bind to specific antigens and begin the processes that start lysis or phagocytosis of the antigen; produced by plasma cells

---

The immunoglobulins (Ig)

- **IgG** – major Ig (75%). Smallest. Only one that crosses the placenta; second Ig to respond to antigen in primary response BUT major one to respond on subsequent exposure. Activates the complement system
- **IgM** – found mainly in the blood. Largest Ig, first Ig to respond to an antigen. Binds with viral and bacterial agents in blood to activate complement cascade
- **IgA** – concentrates in exocrine secretions (colostrum, milk, tears, sweat, saliva) respiratory, gastro-intestinal and urogenital secretions. Provides specific protection
- **IgD** – found on surface of B cells; may be involved in differentiation
- **IgE** – present in trace amounts normally. Elevated in allergic disorders

Figure 8.1

Humoral and cell-mediated response to antigens.

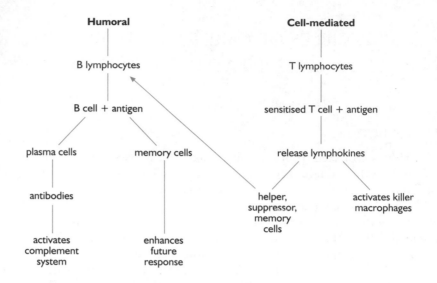

Lymphocytes

- *B cells* – precursors of antibody producing plasma cells. Recognition of an antigen activates B cells to proliferate (to increase response) and differentiate into antibody secreting cells (which synthesise immunoglobulin and memory cells able to respond more rapidly in subsequent attack)
- *T cells* – either promote (helper cells) or suppress (suppresser cells) the immune response, kill antigens directly or participate in other immune responses. Helper cells assist B cell proliferation

- allergic disorders (Table 8.2);
- autoimmune disorders (Table 8.2);
- infectious diseases (Table 8.3).

Table 8.1

Immunodeficiency disorders

Further reading

GROER, M. E. and SHEKLETON, M. E. (1979) *Basic Pathophysiology: A Conceptual Approach*. St Louis: Mosby

Complement system

The complement system is 'composed of an interacting series of glycoproteins that, when triggered, are activated in an orderly sequence to produce biologically active substances that enhance the inflammatory reaction, promote removal of particular matter from the bloodstream, or possibly cause lysis of cells or micro-organisms'.

(Shyur and Hill, 1996)

Problem	Pathophysiology
Congenital stem cell deficiency – severe combined immunodeficiency (SCIDS)	Early lack of stem cell which would normally give rise to lymphocytes resulting in striking lymphopenia. Absence of cellular immunity and antibody synthesis. Invariably leads to fatal infection.
B cell deficiency – infantile X-linked agammaglobulinaemia	Humoral immunity is impaired; symptoms become evident at about 9 months of age when maternal immunity decreases. Leads to a susceptibility to severe infections caued by pyogenic organisms
T cell abnormality – DiGeorge's syndrome T and B cell deficiency – Wiskott–Aldrich syndrome	Partial or total absence of the parathyroid and thymus glands. Normal B cell humoral immunity but no cellular immunity. Immune system unable to initiate a response to antigens
Acquired Iatrogenic: steroids, chemotherapy, antibodies infections: transient (via infections); permanent (human immunodeficiency virus HIV) antibody loss; nephrotic syndrome, protein losing enteropathy	HIV virus targets helper T cells, enters them and uses them to produce. The virus then destroys the host cell, replicates and attacks other lymphocytes
Immunoproliferative disorders: leukaemia	Proliferation of abnormal white cells which accumulate in blood, bone marrow and body tissues
lymphoma – Hodgkin's disease and non-Hodgkin's disease	Abnormal proliferation of lymphoid stem cells

Problem	Pathophysiology

Allergenic problems
  asthma
  hay fever
  eczema
  anaphylactic shock
	Atopic individual combines certain antigens (allergens) with IgE. This complex then attaches itself to the surface membranes of basophils and mast cells. These cells respond by degranulation – the granules contain histamine which when freed causes weal formation, itching, bronchoconstriction and hypotension. Exact mechanisms are different for each type of reaction

Autoimmune disorders (immune complex disease)
  glomerulonephritis
  systemic lupus erythematosus (SLE)
	Self-tolerance (i.e. tolerance of own cells and tissues) is thought to develop early in embryonic life. When this system fails autoantibodies are produced which become complexed with self-antigens resulting in a variety of reactions depending on which tissues are involved

Table 8.2

Allergic and autoimmune disorders

Infectious disease	Causative organism	Incubation period: infectious period
Chicken pox (varicella)	*Varicella zoster*	14–21 days after exposure: onset of fever until last vesicle has dried (5–7 days)
Diphtheria	*Corynebacterium diphtheriae*	2–6 days: 2–4 weeks untreated, 1–2 days with antibiotics. Child clear after two consecutive clear cultures
Roseola	Human herpes virus type 6	5–15 days: not known – probably not highly contagious
Measles (rubeola)	Measles virus, RNA-containing paramyxovirus	10–12 days: day 5 until 5–7 days after rash appears
Mumps	Mumps virus, paramyxovirus	14–28 days (average 18): until all swelling has disappeared, not less than 14 days from start of illness
Pertussis (whooping cough)	*Bordetella pertussis*	5–21 days: 7 days after exposure to 3 weeks after onset of paroxysms
Poliomyelitis	Enteroviruses, type 1, 2 + 3	7–14 days: not exactly known, virus is present in throat and faeces shortly after infection and persists for about 1 week in the throat and 4–6 weeks in faeces
Rubella (German measles)	Rubella virus	14–21 days: 7 days before rash – 5 days after rash
Scarlet fever	Group A beta-haemolytic streptococci	2–4 days (range 1–7 days): during incubation period and clinical illness, approximately 10 days

Table 8.3

Infectious diseases

Incubation period

The time between exposure to a pathogenic organism and the onset of symptoms of a disease

Infectious period

The time during which the infective agent may be transmitted (directly or indirectly) from the infected person to an uninfected person

ASSESSMENT

Assessing children with potential immune problems can be confusing and requires you to keep many different aspects in your mind at once. Immune problems often produce multi-system effects and you need to take a thorough history and a general physical assessment. You need the ability to recognise immune related signs and symptoms keeping in mind the different types of immune dysfunction identified above. The first step in assessing the child is to talk to him and his carers. Ask questions about the following (try to get the child to answer wherever possible):

- Bleeding/bruising tendencies – this helps to identify platelet/clotting dysfunction which can occur in some deficiencies and immune disorders.
- Any swellings which might have been noticed in the neck, armpits or groin. If so find out their nature (painful, tender red). Swollen lymph nodes may be indicative of infection, inflammation, certain leukemias or lymphatic tumours.
- Energy levels. Find out if the child has shown fatigue or weakness. Ask questions about normal energy levels and any noticeable changes. Relate to child's normal daily activities.
- Temperature. Has the child had a fever? If so has it been constant or intermittent in nature? Frequently recurring fevers may indicate impaired immune system or increased cell proliferation.
- Joint pain – if so where and what has been the nature of the pain?
- Take a full immunisation history.
- Ask questions about general health.
- Does the child have any allergies?
- Is the child taking any medications? – steroids, some chemotherapy agents and some antibiotics can compromise the immune system.
- Take a family history – this may highlight any potential hereditary problems.

Activity

You are taking a history from a 9-year-old boy who has been admitted with a possible immune problem. His mother is present and every time you ask him a question, she answers for him. Think critically about this situation and explore ways in which you might encourage the mother to allow her child to answer. Why is it important that the child answers?

Your physical assessment of the child should begin as soon as you meet him. You may pick up cues by just 'looking' before actually examining him or taking any vital signs. Figure 8.2 shows the specific signs which might alert you to an immune disorder.

During the assessment phase you may be required to assist in a variety of medical investigations. Many of the investigations are too complex to explain in detail here and some are listed in the margin for you to explore more fully at a future date. One of the initial tests that will be done will be a full blood count and differential which provides quantitative values for haemoglobin, haematocrit, platelets, red blood cells and white blood cells. Table 8.4 shows the implications of an altered white cell count.

Tests specifically related to the lymphocytes may be done:

- T and B cell proliferation tests – evaluate the mitotic response of T

Examples of investigations for immune disorders

- Immunohaematologic test
- Schick test
- Complement function
- Rosette test
- Delayed hypersensitivity skin test
- Immunoelectrophoresis
- Tests for antinuclear antibodies and anti-DNA antibodies
- Skin tests, food challenges, elimination diets
- Bone marrow aspirate and biopsy
- Lymph node biopsy
- Lymphangiography
- CT scan
- MRI scan

Cross reference

Normal blood values – page 420

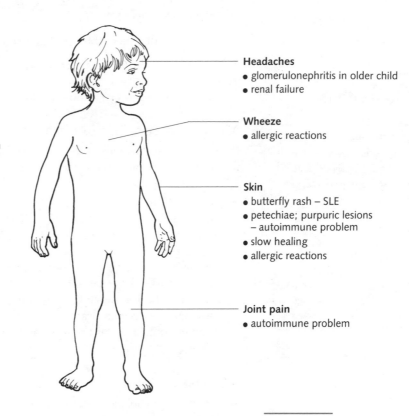

Signals of autoimmune problem
- nausea
- vomiting
- loss of appetite
- bowel changes

Lymphadenopathy
- infection
- inflammation
- increased lymphocyte production

Unusual bleeding
- immunodeficiencies

Fever
- frequently recurring – impaired immune system?

Infection (repeated)
- signs of infection in any system?
- immunodeficiency

Headaches
- glomerulonephritis in older child
- renal failure

Wheeze
- allergic reactions

Skin
- butterfly rash – SLE
- petechiae; purpuric lesions – autoimmune problem
- slow healing
- allergic reactions

Joint pain
- autoimmune problem

Figure 8.2

Specific assessment for immune disorders.

and B cells to foreign antigens. A lowered response implies decreased available cells or functional defect.

- T and B cell counts – this can help to diagnose deficiencies, evaluate immuno competence in autoimmune disease and monitor response to therapy. An abnormal count suggests specific disease. However, a normal count does not necessarily rule it out.

Cell type	Increased by	Decreased by
Neutrophils	Infection, cancer, poisoning, stress, haemorrhage, myelocytic leukaemia	Chemotherapy, radiotherapy, deficiency of vitamin B12 or folic acid
Lymphocytes	Hepatitis, herpes simplex and zoster, mononucleosis, lymphocytic leukaemia	Wiskott–Aldrich syndrome; occasionally in SLE
Monocytes	Tuberculosis, cancer, anaemia, typhoid, myelocytic leukaemia	Rarely decreased
Eosinophils	Allergies, asthma, worm or parasitic invasion, inflammation plus many other conditions	SLE, stress, Cushing's syndrome
Basophils	Granulocytic leukaemia, basophilic leukaemia	Hyperthyroidism (occasionally) allergies

Table 8.4

Understanding the differential white cell count

NURSING INTERVENTIONS

This section will concentrate on exploring:

- Measures to prevent infection
- Care of children with HIV and AIDS
- The use of immunotherapeutic agents.

Measures to prevent infection

One of the main principles in the control and prevention of infection is to halt transmission and contamination. There are several measures which contribute to this:

- Handwashing – this has been identified as being the single most important method of preventing the spread of infection – if done properly (Lowberry, 1975; Taylor, 1978; Ayliffe *et al.*, 1992). Important aspects of handwashing include technique and frequency. The areas which are most frequently missed during handwashing are the tips of the fingers, the thumbs, the wrist, the palms and the backs of the hands. Too much handwashing can cause sore skin which in turn can lead to colonisation by pathogens. It is important therefore to wash your hands at the most appropriate times and avoid overwashing.

Activity

Test your own technique! Before reading any further wash your hands as if preparing to enter the cubicle of a child who is immuno-suppressed. Critically reflect on your technique – could it be improved upon?

Activity

Test your colleagues' handwashing techniques. How long do they wash for, watch how well they wash, do they use soap? Discuss the techniques together.

- The use of gloves, masks and gowns (protective clothing) – gloves should always be worn when handling or having contact with blood or body fluids (e.g. changing nappies, changing suction tubing). Gloves must be discarded after use, never washed and reused. The use of gloves should not preclude handwashing. The use of gowns has been a controversial issue for some time and their use has not been established as an effective way of preventing infection (Carter, 1993). Donowitz (1986) questioned the use of gowns in paediatric intensive care units. The use of plastic aprons is common but these only serve to protect the wearer's clothes. The use of masks is usually indicated to prevent the spread of droplet infection. However, the effectiveness of this protection has been questioned. Filter masks may be used but should be changed if they become moist or if the wearer coughs or sneezes (Ayliffe *et al.*, 1992).

• Correct disposal of waste guidelines for the disposal of waste and linen are laid down by the Department of Social Services (DSS).

Activity

Investigate your hospital's policies for the disposal of waste and linen. Make notes in the margin for future reference.

There are also a number of isolation techniques:

• Source isolation (barrier nursing) – for children who are infectious and need to be nursed away from other children. The principle is not to take infection out of the cubicle.

• Protective isolation (sometimes called reverse barrier nursing) – for children who need protecting from infection. The principle is to keep infection out of the cubicle.

• Laminar air flow rooms – provides a germ free room for children at high risk. The room contains a high efficiency air filter – filtered air flows across the room providing several hundred air exchanges per hour.

Activity

Find out if your hospital has laminar air flow rooms – make arrangements to visit and talk to staff about caring for a child.

Activity

Make arrangements to spend time with members of the control of infection team. Discuss topical issues and find out about any new policies and research which might affect nursing care.

Categorising waste

Linen
• used (domestically dirty)
• foul or infested
• infected (used by child with infectious disease)
• high-risk (contaminated by blood, body fluids from child in high-risk category)

Waste
• household waste
• other clinical waste (includes dressings, nappies, stoma and urine bags)
• sharps
• glass

Caring for children with HIV disease

The number of children with HIV disease is on the increase. In 1992, 403 children under 15 had been diagnosed as HIV-positive (47 of whom had died) (Woodroffe *et al.*, 1993). By October 1996 this had increased to 450 reported cases (PHLS, 1996). It is considered highly likely that there may be more children who are HIV-positive but who remain well and undiagnosed.

Activity

Find out the current figures and compare with those given here. What is the trend? Analyse the reasons for the trend.

The majority of children (200 babies in 1993, 380 in 1996) are infected by vertical transmission of the virus – from the mother before or during birth (PHLS, 1994, 1996). Babies of mothers who are HIV-positive before birth will test positive. However, maternal antibodies can persist until about 18 months when many will test negative having seroconverted. Other sources of infection include :

- blood and blood products – this is rare now as a result of screening, heat treatment and the use of monoclonal antibodies;
- unprotected sexual activity – abuse or sexually active young people;
- sharing of injections by drug users;
- social contact (rare).

AIDS – acquired immune deficiency syndrome

The final phase of the chronic disease HIV infection. Characterised by a progressive decline in cell-mediated immunity and the consequent development of opportunistic infections, tumours and death

(Cree, 1997)

HIV disease can now be considered a chronic illness in childhood with a range of complex problems which can affect the whole family (MacKenzie, 1994) especially as in the majority of cases the mother is also HIV-positive. Progression from HIV infection to AIDS occurs over an undefined time which is different for every child (Figure 8.3). It may be that an infected parent will witness the deterioration and eventual death which could forecast their own fate (Brown and Powell-Cope, 1991). Thus a family approach to care is vital. Reidy *et al.* (1991)

Figure 8.3

Course of HIV disease. (Adapted from Cree, 1997.)

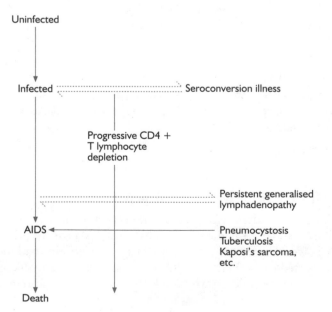

suggests that the role of the nurse in caring for a child with HIV disease can be based upon five needs – the need to:

- *Maintain physical integrity* – one of the most important aspects of care is infection control (a) to prevent the spread of the virus and (b) to protect the child from infection (particularly important when the child is admitted to hospital). Each hospital will have its own infection control policies but you need to be aware of the principles of universal precautions.

- *Communicate* – many difficult issues arise when considering this aspect of care. Firstly it is imperative that the family are given room and opportunity to communicate with health care staff. You should be aware of when to involve others who are perhaps more skilled at discussing feelings or concerns. The channels for communicating should be obvious and available to the child and family. One of the main concerns may be 'who to tell'. There is no legal requirement to divulge information about the child's HIV status and any decision to tell (school, nursery or playgroup) must rest with the family and support for their decision given by all members of staff.

- *Learn* – you must ensure that families and children receive up-to-date information. The family need a sound understanding of the nature of HIV disease and its modes of transmission. In order to do this you need to keep up to date and know where to send them for additional help and support. Sources of support include:

  - Paediatric Aids Resource Centre (PARC), Edingburgh.
  - Black HIV/AIDS Network (BHAN), 111 Devonport Road, London W12 8PB. Tel: 0181 749 2828.
  - Mildmay Mission Hospital, Hackney Road, London E2 7NA. Tel: 0171 729 5361.
  - Terence Higgins Trust, 52–54 Gray's Inn Road, London WC1X 8JU. Tel: 0171 831 0330. Helpline 0171 242 1010 (12 noon –10 p.m. daily).

- *Feel worthwhile and useful* – MacKenzie (1994) highlights the importance of developing a close relationship with the family based on trust and mutual respect. Acknowledgement of the caring skills of the family is vital so that you avoid making them feel inadequate.

- *Act according to a set of beliefs and values* – according to Friedemann (1989) it is important that the nurse and the family share the same goals. This may be difficult if the values and goals of the family are different from those held by the nurse. However, to maintain an effective relationship the nurse must be able to set aside her own beliefs and respect those of the family. Facing personal prejudices was highlighted as being a factor when caring for children with HIV disease in a study by Nettleship (1994/5).

Universal precautions

The main principle of universal precautions is to acknowledge that it is impossible to identify all those children who are seropositive to HIV (or Hepatitis B). It is therefore good practice to assume that any individual could carry the virus and to *routinely* use appropriate barrier methods to prevent contamination by body fluids/blood. Additionally you should:

- avoid injury with potentially contaminated sharp objects (do not resheathe needles before disposal)
- use gloves, aprons and eye protection as per hospital policy
- dispose of contaminated waste in yellow sacks and leave for incineration as per hospital policy

(DoH, 1990; Duggan, 1996)

The Department of Education and Science (1991) stated that children with HIV should be allowed to attend school freely and that there was no obligation for parents to disclose the child's HIV status. (DES, 1991)

Further reading

CLAXTON, R. and HARRISON, T. (eds) *Caring for Children with HIV and AIDS*. London: Edward Arnold

GIBB, D. and WALTERS, S. (1993) *Guidelines for the Management of Children with HIV*, 2nd edn. West Sussex: Avert

ORR, N. (ed.) (1995) *Children's Rights and HIV: A Framework for Action*. London: National Children's Bureau

Firstly consider your views towards HIV disease. Then draw up a short questionnaire asking about attitudes to caring for children with HIV disease. Give out to your colleagues and then analyse the results. Perhaps you might hold a meeting afterwards to discuss the points raised.

The use of immunotherapeutic agents:

Table 8.5 shows some of the immunotherapeutic agents that may be used for children. Table 8.6 gives an immunisation schedule.

Activity

Explore the use of these agents as and when you come across them making your own notes with particular reference to dosages for children.

MANAGING INFECTIOUS DISEASES AT HOME

The majority of children with infectious diseases can be cared for at home. However, carers need adequate support and information to enable them to carry out appropriate care. Rickard and Finn (1997) surveyed 120 parents accompanying children to an Accident and Emergency department to explore parental knowledge of infectious diseases. The results indicated that lack of knowledge could lead to inappropriate use of medical time and resources. The research also found that some parents were unaware of potentially dangerous interventions (e.g. that aspirin should not be given to a febrile child). Finally lack of knowledge about when to seek medical intervention could put the child at risk. Information about caring for children at home should therefore be made available from a variety of sources. Leaflets and booklets could be made available in chemists, GP surgeries, wards and Accident and Emergency departments. The principle goals of care include:

- preventing the spread of infection to others;
- prevention of complications;
- maintaining comfort – including managing a fever and skin symptoms.

Activity

Using information given in this section and elsewhere in the book, draw up a leaflet or handout which will give appropriate guidelines for parents to enable them to care for a child with (a) chicken pox and (b) measles. Pilot the information and then critically evaluate its effectiveness.

Immunotherapeutic agent	Notes	Your notes/dosages

Anti-inflammatory drugs
  non-steroidal anti-inflammatory drugs (NSAIDs)
  corticosteroids
	Care must be taken in the administration of aspirin
	Oral preparations should be given with or shortly after meals to reduce gastro-intestinal side effects. Warn not to discontinue without medical approval – can cause life-threatening adrenal insufficiency	

Immunosuppressive agents	Suppress immune responses to control disease activity. Major side effect is bone marrow suppression and an increased susceptibility to infection (mouth sores and ulcers, fever, chills). Teach about side effects and need to monitor for infection	

Antiallergic agents
  antihistamines
 	
  decongestants
	Block histamine receptors. Generally well tolerated but may produce drowsiness and dry mouth. Administer with food to avoid gastro-intestinal side effects
	Stimulate alpha-adrenergic receptors of vascular smooth muscle to constrict dilated blood vessels in nasal mucosa. May elevate blood pressure	

Immunoenhancing agents inteferon	Inhibit viral replication and tumour cell growth, enhance natural lymphocyte activity and phagocytosis. Side effects include fever, pain at injection site, shivering and fatigue	

Immunisation
  active immunisation
 	
  passive immunisation
	Natural exposure to an infecting organism or use of vaccines and toxoids. May produce fever, malaise, soreness at injection site. Serious complications are rare. Caution with children allergic to eggs; live vaccines should not be given to children who are immuno-suppressed; advise caution with live oral polio – inadequately immunised people can contract polio when exposed to viral excretions in stools
	Administration of preformed antibodies to a non-immunised child. Animal serum can cause allergic reactions and life-threatening anaphylaxis; serum sickness reactions. Adverse reactions to human serum are rare, usually confined to injection site	

Other immunotherapies
  bone marrow transplant
  apheresis
  radiotherapy
  biological therapies
	Space precludes giving details about these therapies. Investigate them if you come across them	

Table 8.5

Immunotherapeutic agents (Copyright is waived for the purpose of photocopying and enlarging this table.)

Cross reference

Aspirin – safety of the drug – page 314

Table 8.6

Immunisation schedule (DoH, 1996)

Cross references

Immunisations – pages 126 and 186

When is the immunisation due?	Which immunisation?	Route
2 months	Polio	Oral
	HIB, diphtheria, tetanus, whooping cough	Injection
3 months	Polio	Oral
	HIB, diphtheria, tetanus, whooping cough	Injection
4 months	Polio	Oral
	HIB, diphtheria, tetanus, whooping cough	Injection
12–15 months	Measles, mumps, rubella	Injection
3–5 years (usually before child starts school).	Measles, mumps, rubella	Injection
	Diphtheria, tetanus	Injection
	Polio	Oral
10–13 years (sometimes shortly after birth)	Tuberculosis	Skin test plus injection (BCG) if needed
14–19 years (school-leavers)	Diphtheria, tetanus	Injection
	Polio	Oral

PRINCIPLES OF CARE – CHILDREN WITH A NEUROLOGICAL PROBLEM 9

INTRODUCTION

Cerebral blood flow and oxygen consumption in children under 6 years of age is almost double that of adults to meet the younger child's needs for rapid growth and development. The brain grows rapidly during the first 6 years of life especially during infancy when half of its postnatal growth occurs. Consequently any problems occurring at birth or during early childhood which impair the cerebral circulation or oxygen consumption can have far-reaching effects on normal growth and development. The degree and type of impairment which result from such disturbances depends upon the function of the part of the brain involved. Therefore, the nurse needs an understanding of the structure and function of the central nervous system to be able to appreciate, recognise and implement appropriate care for the disorders which may occur.

Activity

Answer the questions in the quiz (right) about the structure and function of the nervous system. Check your answers with an anatomy and physiology text.

Neurology quiz

Identify the areas of the brain which control:
- temperature
- respiration, pulse and blood pressure
- posture and balance

Which cranial nerve is responsible for controlling pupil size?

Identify the sites of a:
- sub-dural haemorrhage
- sub-arachnoid haemorrhage

Where are the fontanelles and at what age do they close?

What is the position and function of the following:
- frontal lobes
- parietal lobes
- occipital lobes
- temporal lobes

COMMON NEUROLOGICAL PROBLEMS IN CHILDREN (TABLE 9.1)

Febrile convulsions are one of the most common neurological disorders of childhood affecting about 3% of children aged 6 months to 3 years. The cause of these seizures is not proven. Berg (1993) notes that the height of the temperature rather than the speed of the increase appears to be the significant factor. The pyrexia is usually over 38.8°C and the convulsion usually occurs during the rise rather than after it. Bethune *et al.* (1993) identify children at particular risk from febrile convulsions as those who meet all the following criteria:

- have a family history of febrile convulsions;
- are in full-time day care;
- demonstrate delayed developmental milestones;
- were nursed in special care units for at least 28 days.

It may be that these criteria link with an increased risk and susceptibility to infection rather than any predisposition to seizures in relation to fever. Febrile convulsions are not associated with epilepsy, 95–98% of children recover with no lasting neurological damage.

Table 9.1

Common neurological problems of childhood

Problem	Pathophysiology
Cerebral palsy	A group of disorders caused by prenatal or postnatal anoxia. The consequences depend upon the area of brain deprived of oxygen but it usually involves impaired movement and posture due to disordered muscle tone and coordination. Sensory and mental impairment may also be present
Epilepsy	Spontaneous electrical discharges are initiated in the brain by hyper excitable cells (epileptogenic focus) in response to a variety of physiological stimuli. These stimuli overcome the normal inhibitory mechanisms and the increased electrical activity is able to spread to normal cells via synaptical pathways. When the activity reaches the midbrain and reticular formation a generalised seizure occurs
Febrile convulsion	A pyrexia stimulates peripheral and central thermoreceptors in the skin and mucous membranes and impulses are sent to the pre-optic area of the hypothalamus. In children over 5 years this stimulates the heat-losing centre resulting in vasodilation, perspiration and decreased metabolism. In younger children this centre is too immature and its stimulation causes a convulsion
Head injury	Intracranial contents are damaged if the force of the injury is too great to be absorbed by the skull and diffuse swelling occurs. Cerebral oedema and increased intercranial pressure can result in hypoxia, hypercapnia and inadequate perfusion
Hydrocephalus	Impaired absorption or obstruction to the outflow of cerebrospinal fluid causes an accumulation of fluid in the ventricles which dilate, putting pressure on to cerebral tissue
Meningitis	Acute inflammation of the meninges caused by a variety of bacterial and viral agents. Organisms enter the cerebral spinal fluid via the blood stream from infections or trauma of neighbouring sites and spread throughout the sub-arachnoid space. Inflammation, exudation and tissue damage to the brain result causing pyrexia and raised ICP. Septic shock and rashes may occur in severe infections

Epilepsy (Table 9.2) affects about one in 200 people but its incidence varies greatly with age and the highest proportion of those affected are children (Shorvon, 1990). Valman (1993) estimates that six in 1000 schoolchildren are epileptic. Epilepsy can be idiopathic (primary) or symptomatic (secondary) and can present as generalised or partial seizures. Until recently epilepsy in childhood was considered to be a progressive disorder which required early treatment. This concept began to be questioned in 1997 with research findings which suggested that children may grow out of epilepsy, or that their convulsions decrease in frequency without treatment (Van Donselaar *et al.*, 1997). Epilepsy can be found with some types of acquired spastic cerebral palsy.

Cerebral palsy (Table 9.3) is the most common permanent disability of childhood although the degree of severity may vary from mild, when the child has impairment of only fine precision movements, to severe, when the child is unable to perform most of the daily activities of living independently. The incidence of cerebral palsy has risen by 20% since the 1960s and Bhushan *et al.* (1993) suggest that this increase is due to increased technology which now enables the survival of very pre-term babies. Pre-term delivery is associated with a higher risk of cerebral palsy and Murphy *et al.* (1997) believe that an integrated approach to antenatal, intrapartum and neonatal care is the only way to decrease the incidence in these babies. They found that neonatal sepsis,

Type of seizure	Description
Generalised	Seizures which occur simultaneously in both cerebral hemispheres and cause a brief loss of consciousness at onset
Absence	Brief losses of consciousness lasting only seconds; onset and completion are sudden and the affected child may only appear to be briefly distracted
Myoclonic	Sudden, brief muscle contractions which result in sudden jerking movements of the limbs
Atonic	'Drop' attacks where the child suddenly loses muscle tone and falls to the ground
Tonic	Widespread muscle contraction which causes the child to fall to the ground due to muscle rigidity which prevents a coordinated posture
Clonic	Intense jerking movements of the limbs, trunk and facial muscles
Infantile spasms	Sudden repetitive limb flexion which causes the affected infant to fall backwards (Salaam attacks). Occurs in babies between the age of 3 and 12 months
Partial seizures	Seizures which arise in a specific area of the brain and therefore affect only one part of the body; *simple partial (focal) seizures* arise in the cerebral cortex and cause disturbances in sensation or movement without loss of consciousness; *complex partial seizures* cause impairment of conscious level, behaviour and memory
Secondary generalised	Partial seizures which develop into a generalised fit as the abnormal cerebral discharges spread from a localised area of the cortex to the sub-cortical areas of the brain

Table 9.2

Types of epilepsy

pneumothorax, and blood transfusion were all significantly associated with cerebral palsy regardless of adverse factors antenatally and at delivery. It can also be acquired in association with meningitis or severe head injury.

Pre-term babies are also at risk from hydrocephalus as the result of intraventricular haemorrhage, but in most cases hydrocephalus results from congenital developmental defects which cause obstruction to the flow of cerebral spinal fluid. Postnatal causes include cerebral tumours and infections or trauma.

Trauma in children often results in a head injury. The three major causes of head injuries in children are falls, road traffic accidents and bicycle accidents. Younger children are more prone to head injuries from falls and car accidents as their heads, which are relatively large and heavy compared with the rest of their bodies, tend to lead the fall. Valman (1993) reports that 40% of injuries at home to children under 5 years are due to falls. Great efforts have been made to promote the use of cycle helmets to prevent the number of head injuries in older children caused by bicycle accidents.

One of the complications of an open head injury is bacterial meningitis. Bacterial meningitis is considered to be a problem of childhood with over 66% of cases occurring in children under 15 years of age and the peak incidence being between 3 and 12 months (Davies, 1996). The causative bacteria are also age related. Viral meningitis is less severe and the affected child usually recovers in 3–10 days without

Bacterial meningitis – causative organisms

Neonates
- *Escherichia coli* and B streptococcus (acquired from maternal infection during birth or via umbilical cord or respiratory infection)
- *Listeria monocytogenes* – maternal listeria

>2 months
- *Haemophilus influenzae*, *Neisseria meningitidis* (meningococcus) and *Streptococcus pneumoniae* (pneumococcus) (droplet infection)

Rarer causes
- *Staphylococcus* – secondary to head wounds, upper respiratory tract infections
- *Myobacterium tuberculosis* – primary TB or secondary to pulmonary TB

Table 9.3	Spastic (50–60%)	Defect in the motor cortex of the pyramidal tract causes hypertonicity of certain muscle groups
Types of cerebral palsy		Hemiparesis is the most common form (30–40%), but quadriparesis is seen in 15–20% of children
		Hypertonicity causes poor posture, balance and coordination
		Unbalanced muscle tone predisposes to orthopaedic complications (scoliosis, contractures)
		Abnormal postures in movement and at rest
		Likely to include mental retardation
	Dyskinetic (20–25%)	Defect of the extra pyramidal tract and basal ganglia causes uncontrollable movements of the affected muscle groups
		Athetosis (slow, writhing involuntary movements of the extremities)
		Stress may cause movements to become jerky or disordered
		Drooling and difficulty in speech can result from involvement of the pharyngeal, laryngeal and oral muscles
		Drooling may cause an increase in dental caries
	Ataxic (1–10%)	Defect of the cerebellum impairs balance
		Wide-based gait
		Intention tremor
		Incoordination of gross and fine motor skills
	Mixed type (15–40%)	Combination of spastic and athetosis

treatment. Certain pre-disposing factors appear to increase susceptibility to meningitis:

- maternal factors (premature rupture of membranes, maternal infection);
- immune deficiencies of the newborn;
- pre-existing central nervous system anomalies;
- open head injuries/neurosurgery;
- upper respiratory tract infections before the development of acquired immunity.

SPECIFIC ASSESSMENT OF THE CHILD WITH A NEUROLOGICAL DISORDER (FIGURE 9.1)

Specific neurological observations are important for almost any child with a neurological impairment. These observations include:

- level of consciousness;
- pupil size and reaction to light;
- vital signs;
- motor function;
- posture.

A decreasing level of consciousness is well known as an important initial sign of serious neurological damage. However, this is not always so in infants under 18 months of age. When the fontanelle is still open any swelling of the brain, which would normally create raised

Cross reference

Assessment of consciousness level – page 300

Vital signs
- pulse
- blood pressure
- temperature
- respirations

Movement
- symmetrical
- twitching

Level of development

Temperature
- irritability
- high-pitched cry?

Motor function

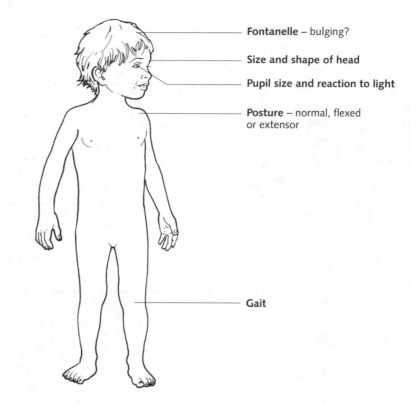

Fontanelle – bulging?

Size and shape of head

Pupil size and reaction to light

Posture – normal, flexed or extensor

Gait

intracranial pressure (ICP) and unconsciousness, can be accommodated by these open sutures causing bulging of the fontanelle.

Assessing level of consciousness in a child of any age is complicated by a child's lack of understanding and ability to respond appropriately to the common questions used to determine orientation to time and space. In addition, children commonly react to stressful situations by sleeping or non-communication (Reeves, 1989). The Glasgow Coma scale (GCS) was introduced in 1974 by Teasdale and Jennet to meet clinical nurses' needs for a set of objective criteria to assess conscious level. The original scale was designed for use with adult patients and the need for an adapted version for children, which took account of the difficulties outlined above, was quickly recognised. In 1982, Simpson and Reilly produced a modification of the GCS for children. This recognised that young children may only verbalise by crying or making sounds other than recognisable speech. The type of cry is important to note as raised ICP causes the young child to have a characteristic highpitched cry. The modified GCS also accepted that fear may prevent a child from being able to demonstrate orientation. See Figures 9.2 and 9.3.

The assessment of level of consciousness does not just involve verbal response but also eye opening and motor response but these are also difficult to assess in young children. Assessment of children's pupil size

Figure 9.1

Specific assessment of the child with a neurological disorder.

Cross reference

Neurological assessment – pages 300–302

OBSERVATION CHART

| | | DATE |
| | | TIME |

COMA SCALE

Eyes Open Score	4. Spontaneous 3. To shout 2. To pain 1. No response	Eyes closed by swelling = C
Verbal Score	5. Smiles & appropriately cries 4. Cries 3. Inappropriate crying 2. Grunting 1. No response	Endotracheal tube or tracheostomy = T
Motor Score	4. Localises to pain 3. Flexion to pain 2. Extension to pain 1. No response	Usually record the best arm responses

B.P. BLACK

PULSE RED

TEMP GREEN

Pupil scale (mm)

1
2
3
4
5

TOTAL

Blood pressure and pulse rate

230
220
210
200
190
180
170
160
150
140
130
120
110
100
90
80
70
60
50
40
30
20
10

Respiration

Temperature °C

40
39
38
37
36
35
34
33
32
31
30

| PUPILS | right | Size
Reaction | | + reacts
− no reaction
C eye closed |
| | left | Size
Reaction | | |

LIMB MOVEMENT

| ARMS | Normal Power
Mild weakness
Severe weakness
Spastic flexion
Extension
No response | Record right (r) and left (L) separately if there is a difference between the two sides. |
| LEGS | Normal Power
Mild weakness
Severe weakness
Extension
No response | |

Figure 9.2

Luton and Dunstable Hospital NHS trust paediatric neurological chart. Children below 1 year.

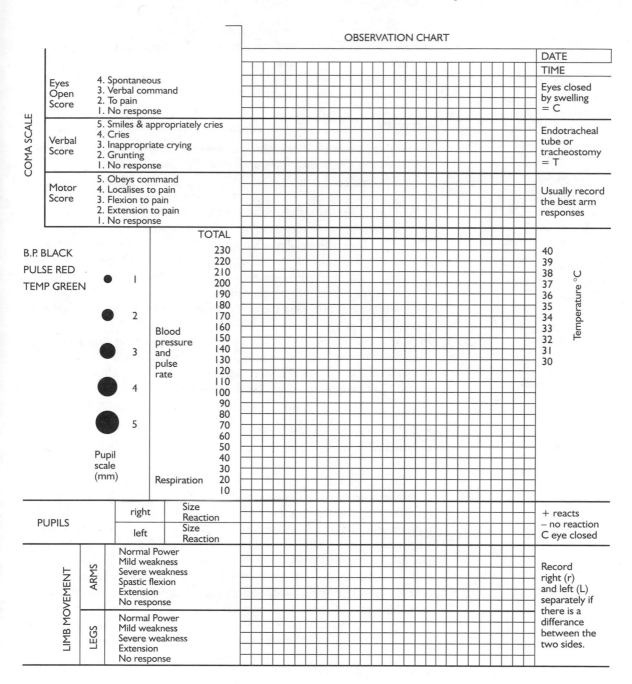

Figure 9.3

Luton and Dunstable Hospital NHS trust paediatric neurological chart. Children 1–2 years.

and reaction to light is also complicated. Young children cannot always understand or obey the necessary instructions. Reeves (1989) suggests that nurses turn off the main lights and hand the child a pen torch. The natural response for most children is to turn the torch on and look at the light enabling the assessment to take place.

Activity

Try out pupil assessment of healthy children and make a note of the normal pupil sizes and reactions in different lighting.

Motor responses are also impaired by immaturity. A 6-month-old baby has a best motor response of flexion whilst older children may obey commands and localise pain although the ability to localise pain in preschool children is questionable. Frightened children may be unwilling and uncooperative to respond rather than unable to do so. Providing the child with appropriate toys and watching them play may prove a more successful way of assessing motor response than trying to push and prod the child.

Many authors recognise the importance of involving parents in the assessment of the level of consciousness. As Williams (1992) notes, parents' views are vital if an accurate assessment of the child is to be made. They should be asked about their child's:

- milestones in development;
- language, hearing and visual abilities;
- usual response to pain.

The GCS is a useful predictor of outcome and a score of 8 or less is generally accepted as a definition of coma and a sign of the severity of the neurological damage (Grewal and Sutcliffe, 1991). However, it should be remembered that it is not able to accurately determine the responses of all children. For example, a child with cerebral palsy may achieve a very low GCS because of physical inability rather than raised ICP. Together with the GCS score other neurological measurements are necessary to provide useful information about the site of involvement and the probable cause of the neurological damage. Changes in pulse and blood pressure are important indicators of disturbed autonomic activity which occurs in deep coma and brain stem lesions. The bradycardia and hypertension seen in adults in response to the inability of the cerebral arterial vessels to dilate further when the ICP is raised and maintain cerebral perfusion pressure, is rarely seen in children. When it occurs it is a very late sign. Respirations are slow and deep after seizures or in cerebral infections. Rapid, deep breathing may be the result of metabolic acidosis or poisoning. Damage to the brain stem usually produces irregular respirations. Hyperpyrexia which is unresponsive to treatment usually suggests a dysfunction of the hypothalamus.

Widely dilated and fixed pupils are indicative of paralysis of the oculomotor nerve due to pressure from herniation of the brain through the tentorium (coning). When this occurs in one eye only the cerebral lesion is likely to be on the same side. When both eyes are affected brain stem damage is likely. However, such things as mydriatic drops, poisons and hypothermia also cause dilated unresponsive pupils and a pre-existing strabismus also complicates accurate assessment.

Asymmetric or absence of movement suggests paralysis and dysfunction of the motor cortex or nerve pathway, muscle tone may be flaccid or rigid and muscle tremors or twitching may occur. This hyperactivity is more likely to occur in acute febrile and toxic states than in association with raised ICP. When dysfunction of the motor cortex occurs or nerve pathways are lost primitive postural reflexes occur. These reflexes demonstrate an imbalance between the central stimulating and inhibiting influences upon motor function enabling stronger muscles to overcome weaker ones. When the lesion affects the motor cortex in the cerebrum, decorticate posturing is seen (Figure 9.4). Bilateral decerebrate posturing may be caused by tentorial herniation. Care should be taken to ensure that true postural reflexes are seen and not merely a flexion or extension of one limb in response to pain.

Posturing is not always evident until the administration of painful stimuli. Nurses need to ensure that they explain the purpose of this activity to parents and that they do not use methods which can cause tissue damage or bruising. Allan and Culne-Seymour (1989) advocate the use of nail-bed pressure by pressing the side of a pencil or similar object onto the proximal nail-bed.

As with adults, children can often suffer from headache with raised ICP but they are less skilled at vocalising their distress. Reeves (1989) suggests that restless irritability, immobility or rubbing of the head may

(a)

(b)

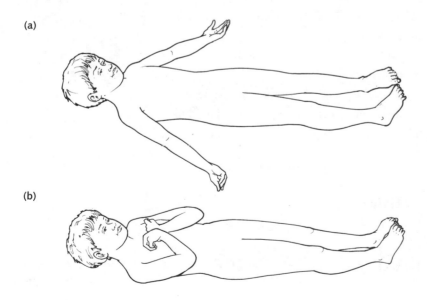

Figure 9.4

Primitive postural reflexes:
(a) decerebrate posturing;
(b) decorticate posturing.

Case history – neurological observations

Liam O'Donnell, aged 6, had been playing on a swing in the playground and fell. He sustained a scalp wound which bled profusely. His mother reported that he had been unrousable 'for a couple of minutes' and she had rung for an ambulance

On admission to A&E

Liam is conscious and able to give his name, age and address to the triage nurse. His mother gives the details of the accident as above also adding that 'the ground was covered with blood'. The ambulance paramedic reports no change in conscious level during the journey to hospital

On examination

Liam says he has a headache which is worse over the site of the injury. He has a 4 inch laceration over the right parietal area and, on examination, a small artery can be seen spurting blood. The Casualty officer immediately ligates the vessel and Liam is admitted to the paediatric ward

On admission to the ward

Liam appears quite lucid and rational although he is uncertain of events in A&E. He appears in pain but is trying to be brave. Both parents are now present. The admitting nurse notes that Liam:

- is of average weight for his age
- appears rather pale
- has rather large pupils which respond briskly to light
- has cool, moist peripheries
- demonstrates a strong grip with both hands and motor power in both legs appears normal
- has a regular pulse 100/min, BP 100/70, respirations 22/min

Cross reference

Care of the child confined to bed – page 364

be indicators of headache in small children. Vomiting due to raised ICP, especially as a result of a head injury, tends to occur more frequently in children than in adults (Reeves, 1989).

Activity

Read the case history 'neurological observations' and analyse the information you are given. Consider the significance of this information and the implications for the nurse.

Activity

Find out what chart is used for neurological observations in your area of work and critically evaluate its (a) appropriateness for children and (b) ease of use.

It is essential that whichever neurological chart is used that all practitioners are aware of the significance of the observations taken and that each assessment is documented in a simple, objective and easily interpreted manner. This enables an easy comparison of previous and current findings which is especially important when nurses are changing over shifts.

Activity

Complete Table 9.4 to ensure you know the common neurological investigations performed and the nurse's role in these.

NURSING INTERVENTIONS

Nursing interventions for children with neurological problems often include:

- care of the unconscious child;
- management of seizures;
- care of the child with meningitis;
- management of an intraventricular shunt;
- administration of drugs used in neurology.

Care of the unconscious child

Activity

Using Roper's activities of daily living, plan care for an unconscious child.

Particular problems in the care of the unconscious child may include ICP monitoring, management of pain and fluid balance. ICP monitoring is an

Investigation	What for and why?	Role of the nurse
Computerised axial tomography (CAT) scan		
Electroencephalogram (EEG)		
Fundoscopic examination		
Lumbar puncture		
Magnetic resonance imaging (MRI) scan		
Skull X-ray		
Subdural tap		
Ventricular tap		

Table 9.4

Specific neurological investigation (Copyright is waived for the purpose of photocopying and enlarging this table.)

Intracranial pressure monitoring

Types of monitors:

- intraventricular catheters
- sub-arachnoid bolt
- epidural sensor
- anterior fontanelle pressure monitor

Specific nursing care

Care

Elevate head of bed 30° and maintain head position in the midline

Rationale

Compression of the neck veins impairs venous return and increase ICP

Care

Avoid causing the child pain and administer appropriate pain relief

Rationale

Crying raises ICP

Care

Minimise environmental stimuli

Rationale

Stress increases ICP

Care

Plan care to avoid over stimulation of child

Rationale

Stress increases ICP

Care

Use pressure relieving/decreasing devices

Rationale

Turning side to side may compress the neck veins

Care

Prevention of constipation with regular use of laxatives

Rationale

Straining at stools raises ICP

intensive care procedure which was introduced in the 1960s but its value is now beginning to be questioned. Reynolds (1992) suggests that such monitoring does not reflect the degree of the initial cerebral damage which is the most important factor in determining outcome. ICP may be measured in different ways and the nurse caring for the child needs to be able to understand the type of monitoring used and be able to analyse the monitor readings. Nursing interventions may need adaptation to avoid increasing ICP further.

ICP may be increased by pain but the use of analgesia or sedation can complicate the assessment of level of consciousness. Codeine phosphate (0.5–1 mg/kg/dose 4–6 hourly) can be useful in such situations. The assessment of pain in the unconscious child is in itself a skill.

Activity

Consider how you could assess pain in an unconscious child.

Fluid and electrolyte balance is particularly crucial in the child with raised ICP. Osmotic diuretics such as mannitol 20% 1–2 g/kg may be used but should be administered slowly unless herniation is occurring. An indwelling urinary catheter is necessary to monitor the urine output and assess the diuretic response. Intravenous fluids are indicated initially for any unconscious child but the volume should be carefully calculated to two-thirds normal maintenance intake to avoid aggravating any cerebral oedema. Other means of providing fluid and nutrition will be necessary if there has been no improvement in conscious level in 48 hours.

Management of seizures

Seizures are associated with recovery from head injury in about 5% of children (Ghajar and Hariri, 1992). They may also be due to pyrexia in young children or occur as a post-operative complication of brain surgery. Treatment of a febrile convulsion is usually related to the treatment of the underlying cause. Rectal diazepam may be administered if the seizure continues until medical intervention. Environmental measures to reduce the temperature (opening windows, use of a fan) should be used with care as they often induce shivering. Shivering maintains the pyrexia as it increases the metabolic rate and thus produces heat. Tepid sponging is no longer recommended because it tends to cause shivering and also does not significantly reduce the temperature (Camfield and Camfield, 1993). Probably the most effective treatment is the use of an antipyretic (paracetamol or ibuprofen). Epileptic seizures are a feature rather than a disease and children with epilepsy should be encouraged to lead as normal a life as possible. One of the roles of the nurse caring for the child with epilepsy is to teach the child and family to manage the seizure so that the child's safety is maintained.

Activity

Find out how to care for the epileptic child:
- who complains of an aura
- during the clonic–tonic phase of a seizure
- after the seizure.

Treatment of status epilepticus
- Maintain airway
- Monitor oxygen saturation
- IV diazapam 0.3 mg/kg over 1–5 minutes*
- IV phenytoin 10 – 20 mg/kg over 5–20 minutes
- Phenobarbitone 5 – 20 mg/kg*
- Rectal paraldehyde 0.1–0.3 ml/kg diluted 1:1 in olive oil
- Consider intubation, ventilation and transfer to ICU

*Diazepam can cause respiratory arrest if given too rapidly or when followed by phenobarbitone

Generally a seizure is self-limiting and the child will recover spontaneously. The British Epilepsy Association (1995) suggests that in a first aid situation an ambulance need only be called if:
- the child is not a known epileptic;
- the seizure follows a head injury;
- the child is injured during a seizure;
- the seizure is continuous and shows no sign of stopping after 4 minutes.

Status epilepticus is a seizure in which the tonic–clonic phase is continuous for 30 minutes or more, or in which the child does not regain consciousness between bouts of tonic–clonic activity for this length of time. Dieckmann (1994) recommends the use of rectal diazepam 0.3–0.5 mg/kg for pre-hospital treatment. In hospital treatment is directed at the maintenance of vital functions, sedation and anti-epileptic drugs.

In most recent cases epilepsy can be controlled by medication but compliance and awareness of side effects is crucial. Surgery is a relatively recent option for children who suffer repetitive uncontrollable seizures. Partial or full temporal lobectomy may benefit children whose lesions initiate in the temporal lobe and partial colostomy may prevent generalised seizures. Careful assessment is necessary to identify the children whose epilepsy is most likely to benefit from surgery and the benefits of brain surgery must be weighed against the potential risks.

Activity

Find out and make a list of the actual and potential problems after brain surgery.

Care of the child with meningitis

Meningitis is one complication of brain surgery but is more likely to be encountered as a childhood infection. As soon as it is suspected the child should be hospitalised and a lumber puncture performed unless the child shows features of raised ICP. If the child is shocked or has a petechial rash or if there is any suspicion of bacterial meningitis the GP should start antibiotic treatment immediately with IV or IM benzyl penicillin (Markovitch, 1990). Cefotaxime is the treatment of choice once the diagnosis has been confirmed. IV dexomethasone 0.15 mg/kg 6 hourly for the first 4 days has been shown to hasten the reduction of meningeal inflammation (Schaad *et al.*, 1993) and lessen the risk of permanent hearing impairment (Bhatt *et al.*, 1993).

Activity

Identify the specific nursing actions required to care for a child with bacterial meningitis (Table 9.5).

Bacterial meningitis may be the cause or effect of hydrocephalus. Hydrocephalus, or the accumulation of cerebral spinal fluid in the ventricles, can be the result of a congenital or acquired problem. Maldevelopment of the central nervous system or maternal infection are the commonest causes of congenital hydrocephalus. Causes of acquired hydrocephalus are infection, neoplasm or cerebral haemorrhage. When the accumulation of fluid occurs before closure of the fontanelles the head enlarges as a result. If the accumulation is allowed to progress the increasing ICP will eventually prevent brain stem functioning. The usual treatment is surgical removal of the ventricular obstruction or the insertion of a shunt to drain the excess fluid from the ventricles. A ventriculoperitoneal (VP) shunt is the preferred procedure for most children. The proximal end of the shunt is inserted into the lateral ventricle and the distal end is inserted into the peritoneal cavity. Although the insertion of a shunt significantly improves the survival rate

m
Neo
3 week
- cefo
  100 m
  12 hourly
- benzyl peni
  100 mg/kg/2
  12 hourly
- gentamycin
  2.5 mg/kg/24 hour
  12–18 hourly

Infants and children
7–10 day course of:
- cefotaxime
  200 mg/kg/24 hourly

Prophylaxis for the immediate family
2–4 day course of:
- rifampicin
  5–10 mg/kg/12 hourly

Prophylaxis for other close contacts
- <6 years
  rifampicin 5–10 mg/kg × 1 dose
- 6–12 years
  ciprofloxacin 250 mg × 1 dose
- >12 years
  ciprofloxacin 500 mg × 1 dose

Complications of intraventricular shunts

Malfunction
- kinking of catheter
- plugging of catheter by tissue or exudate
- migration of tubing
- obstruction of the distal end of the catheter by thrombosis
- displacement of the distal end of the catheter due to growth

Infection
- septicaemia
- wound infection
- meningitis
- ventriculitis
- cerebral abscess
- peritonitis

Abdominal complications
- paralytic ileus
- perforation of abdominal organs at insertion of the shunt
- peritoneal fistulas

Table 9.5

Specific care of the child with bacterial meningitis (Copyright is waived for the purpose of photocopying and enlarging this table.)

Problem	Nursing action
Potential spread of infection to others in hospital and at home	
Altered conscious level due to raised ICP	
Pyrexial with cold, cyanosed peripheries due to septicaemic shock	

Potential development of:
 	
   cerebral abscess
 	
   ventriculitis
 	
   hydrocephalus
 	
   inappropriate anti-diuretic hormone secretion
 	
   hearing loss
 	
   motor or learning disability	

Unable to feed as usual due to alterations in conscious levels	

of children with hydrocephalus, it is not without complications and may not prevent mental retardation.

Management of an intraventricular shunt

Activity

Look at the complications (p. 511) associated with shunts and consider how you would recognise these.

Administration of drugs used in neurology

Activity

Identify the uses, usual dosages and side effects of the drugs used in neurology (Table 9.6).

DISCHARGE ADVICE

Neurological problems such as head injury and meningitis can be prevented by good health care advice.

Drug	Dose/kg	Use	Side effects
Carbamazepine			
Clonazepam			
Diazepam			
Lamontrigine			
Paraldehyde			
Phenobarbitone			
Phenytoin			
Sodium valproate			
Vigabactrin			

Table 9.6

Medication used in neurology (Copyright is waived for the purpose of photocopying and enlarging this table.)

Activity

Design two posters for your area of work to give parents advice about the prevention of:
- head injuries
- meningitis caused by listeria or haemophilus influenza type 'B'.

Febrile convulsions cannot always be prevented, but Miller (1996) suggests that parents need more information about the prevention and treatment of these seizures before they experience this traumatic and frightening event.

Activity

Find out what information about febrile convulsions is available to parents in your area of work.

Families of children with epilepsy need information about the prevention of trigger factors and the management of the condition as well as psychological support to help them overcome the prejudice others may have about this condition.

Activity

Consider which day-to-day activities could pose risks for the child with epilepsy and the advise to be given in relation to them.

Useful address

British Epilepsy Association Crowthorne House, New Wokingham Road, Wokingham, Berks RG11 3AY

10 PRINCIPLES OF CARE – CHILDREN WITH ALTERED BREATHING

INTRODUCTION

Acute problems affecting the respiratory tract are the commonest cause of illness in infancy and childhood. Fifty per cent of illnesses in children under 5 years, and 30% of illnesses for children aged 5–12 years are due to respiratory problems. Respiratory problems can present as very mild illnesses, the onset of chronic problems or be life threatening. They can be the primary cause of the illness or they may occur as secondary complications to other problems. Because an adequate circulation relies upon an adequate oxygen intake they commonly affect the cardio-vascular system.

Children are particularly prone to respiratory problems because of a number of differences between their respiratory tract and that of adults.

Activity

Test your knowledge of the structure and function of the respiratory system by answering the quiz in the margin. Check your answers with an anatomy and physiology textbook.

COMMON DISORDERS OF THE RESPIRATORY TRACT

Infection is the cause of most childhood respiratory disorders. The cause and the effect of the infection depends upon the individual child's age, medical history and environment. Most childhood respiratory infections (Table 10.1) are caused by viruses and tend to cause only a mild illness in older children but severe problems in the younger age group. The reason for this varied severity is partly due to the anatomical differences in the respiratory tract of the younger child but also to the older child's greater resistance to infection. Resistance to infection is influenced by the amount of lymphoid tissue, passive immunity developed by exposure to infective organisms, pre-existing chronic respiratory or cardiac problems and the environment. Exposure to cigarette smoking by a child's main carer increases the likelihood of infection (Holberg *et al.*, 1993).

The commonest of the chronic respiratory problems (Table 10.2) affecting children is asthma. Speight (1996) suggests that 20–25% of children will experience a significant degree of clinical asthma during childhood and that 5% of these will have frequent and severe problems which will continue into adulthood. The cause of this increased incidence is debatable, but it seems likely that environmental factors are

The respiratory tract in children

Compared with the adult, the airway of the small child has:

- narrow nasal passages
- more anteriorly and cephalad positioned glottis
- longer epiglottis
- a 4 mm diameter larynx
- its narrowest portion at the level of the cricoid cartilage
- an upper airway which is funnel-shaped, pliable and may narrow with inspiration
- a very compliant chest wall
- increased resistance to airflow (16-fold) in the presence of 1 mm circumferential oedema
- a greater reduction (50%) in laryngeal radius in the presence of 1 mm oedema

Respiratory quiz

Draw a diagram of the lower respiratory tract to identify the trachea, segmental bronchi, bronchioles and alveolar ducts

At what age do the lungs complete their development?

Identify three conditions which can affect lung development

Explain the mechanism of inhalation and exhalation

How is respiration regulated?

Identify the function of the following structures:

- respiratory cilia
- epiglottis
- respiratory mucous membranes

Infection	Usual age range	Pathophysiology
Bronchiolitis	Infancy	Viral colonisation of the bronchiolar mucosa – spreads to bronchiolar epithelium causing necrosis of ciliated cells and proliferation of non-ciliated cells. Impaired clearance of secretions, increased mucus production and desquamation of cells leads to bronchiolar obstruction and lung collapse
Croup	6–36 months	Inflammation of the laryngeal and tracheal mucosa narrow the airways. The effort involved to inhale air past the obstruction causes an inspiratory stridor and sternal retractions. If air entry is insufficient, hypoxia will occur. Impaired exhalation of carbon dioxide will lead to respiratory acidosis and respiratory failure
Epiglottitis	2–5 years	Acute bacterial infection of the epiglottis and surrounding areas causing inflammation and swelling of the mucous membranes in this area which can completely obstruct the airway. Complete obstruction can be precipitated by stimulating the gag reflex by examination, manipulation or suctioning of the airway
Pneumonia	All ages	Inflammation of the pulmonary parenchyma, caused by viruses, bacteria, mycoplasmas and aspiration, involving: • lobar pneumonia – one or more lobes • bronchopneumonia – terminal bronchioles • interstitial pneumonia – within alveolar walls Inflammation impairs gaseous exchange and can lead to pulmonary effusion
Whooping cough	<4 years	The presence of *Bordetella pertussis* causes an inflammatory reaction in the mucosal lining of the upper airways. The bacteria adhere to the ciliated epithelial tissue in these areas inhibiting its function. As a result, cellular debris, mucus and pus collect and can cause plugging of the bronchial tree and necrosis of the bronchial epithelium. Stasis of secretions can lead to secondary infection. Paroxysms of severe coughing to expel secretions can increase ICP causing rupture of cerebral vessels, bradycardia, hypoxia and apnoea. If prolonged deprivation of oxygen occurs, permanent cerebral damage may result

Table 10.1

Respiratory infections in children

implicated. Atmospheric pollution and home furnishings which are favourable to the house dust mite may be significant triggers. Hunt (1997) suggests that bronchodilator drugs used to treat asthma could be responsible for the rising incidence and severity of this condition.

Cystic fibrosis is the commonest recessively inherited disease in the Caucasian population affecting approximately 1:2500 (Davies *et al.*, 1996). Although other organs are affected the effects on the respiratory system are more likely to be the presenting feature and the cause of death. Ninety-five per cent of cystic fibrosis patients die from respiratory failure. Cystic fibrosis is due to various different mutations in the cystic fibrosis transmembrane regulator (CFTR) gene situated on chromosome 7. CFTR appears to function as a chloride channel and mutations affect chloride and sodium movement across epithelial cells but it is still not clear how this affects the respiratory system (Koch and Hoiby, 1993).

Bronchopulmonary dysplasia (BPD) is a chronic iatrogenic respiratory disease which mainly affects babies who were born prematurely with lungs which were too immature to function independently. To support their inadequate respiratory function they are

Table 10.2

Chronic respiratory problems

Disorder	Pathophysiology
Bronchopulmonary dysplasia	Interstitial oedema and epithelial inflammation of the small airways results in fibrosis of the alveolar walls, reduced lung compliance, increased airway resistance and a severe reduction in expiration. This causes over-inflation and alveolar collapse leading to hypercapnia, and hypoxaemia. Chronic disease results in pulmonary hypertension and right sided heart failure
Cystic fibrosis	Thick viscous secretions pre-dispose the individual to recurrent infections which cause chronic inflammation and oedema of the small airways. Excessive pooling of secretions leads to mucus plugging, increases the susceptibility to bacterial infections (*Staphylococcus aureus*, *Haemophilus influenzae* and *Pseudomonas aeruginosa*), and distorts the airways causing bronchospasm and airway collapse. Abnormal secretions in other exocrine organs cause intestinal and bile duct obstruction, pancreatic enzyme deficiency, agenesis of the vas deferens. The primary defect causes elevated sodium and chloride levels
Asthma	Increased bronchoconstriction, oedema and hypersecretion of mucus occur in response to an allergen and result in narrowed resistant airways. Obstruction of exhalation causes wheezing, hyperinflation of the chest, air hunger and anxiety. Decreased ventilation causes insufficient oxygenation of blood

treated with high concentrations of oxygen and positive pressure ventilation. However, prolonged use of these treatments causes long-term pulmonary damage and many infants who survive are oxygen dependent, require repeated periods of hospitalisation and have increased susceptibility to respiratory infection (Northway *et al.*, 1990).

ASSESSMENT

Much information can be gained about a child's respiratory status by merely looking and listening (Figure 10.1). If the child is very distressed by the hospital environment this is a useful method of assessment, allowing the nurse to make an immediate assessment of the severity of the child's condition and the child time to acclimatise to the situation. No observation is meaningful unless the nurse is aware of the normal parameters in children and the significance of any abnormalities.

Older children may complain of chest pain related to respiratory disease. This pain may sometimes be referred to the abdomen and abdominal pain can be the primary complaint of younger children with a respiratory problem. Infants often grunt to indicate chest pain which is usually caused by inflammation of the pleura. Grunting can also be an indication of respiratory distress as it increases end-expiratory pressure prolonging the time available for alveolar exchange of oxygen and carbon dioxide.

Accurate observations of children with respiratory problems enable the nurse to determine the most appropriate nursing interventions. The information provided by nursing observations may be enhanced by

Cross references

Normal respiratory rates – page 299

Significance of respirations – page 281

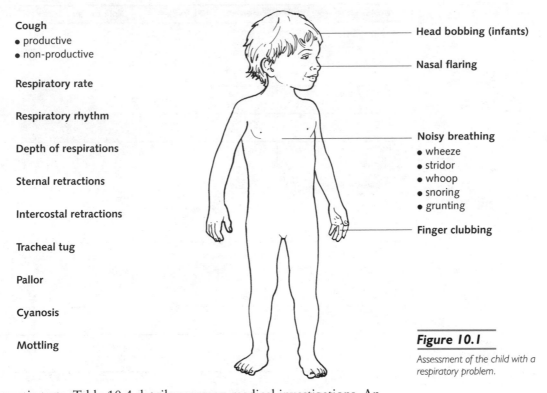

Cough
- productive
- non-productive

Respiratory rate

Respiratory rhythm

Depth of respirations

Sternal retractions

Intercostal retractions

Tracheal tug

Pallor

Cyanosis

Mottling

Head bobbing (infants)

Nasal flaring

Noisy breathing
- wheeze
- stridor
- whoop
- snoring
- grunting

Finger clubbing

Figure 10.1

Assessment of the child with a respiratory problem.

diagnostic tests. Table 10.4 details common medical investigations. An understanding of common diagnostic tests enables the nurse to appreciate their findings and also to help prepare and care for the child before, during and after the investigation. Some of these investigations (Table 10.5) are commonly performed by nurses. Pulse oximetry can be monitored at the bedside to give information about the need for or the efficacy of oxygen therapy. Although it can be measured intermittently, continuous monitoring will provide more information about the effect of activity upon oxygen consumption. Sensors should be covered to avoid ambient light interfering with the accuracy of the reading. The

Test	Normal value	Acidosis	Alkalosis
pH	7.35–7.45	<7.35	>7.45
pCO_2 (mmHg)	35–45	>45	<35
pO_2 (mmHg)	80–100	<80	>100
HCO_3 (mmHg)	22–26	<22	>26
Base	±2	More negative	More positive

Respiratory acidosis
Increased pCO_2, decreased pO_2 – caused by obstructive lung disease or hypoventilation

Respiratory alkalosis
Decreased pCO_2, increased pO_2 – caused by hypoxia or hyperventilation

Table 10.3

Blood gas analysis: normal values

Table 10.4

Medical investigations of the respiratory system (Copyright is waived for the purpose of photocopying and enlarging this table.)

Investigation	When and what for?	Role of the nurse
Pulmonary function tests spirometry peak flow		
Blood gas analysis		
Exercise tests		
Radiography CXR Ba swallow CT scan MRI scan		
Operative procedures bronchoscopy lung biopsy		
Sweat test		

Table 10.5

Nursing investigations

Capillary refill	Capillary refill is a quick and easy method for determining efficacy of respiratory function. A raised digit is pressed for 5 seconds and the time taken for blood to return to the area is estimated in seconds. A capillary refill time of over 2 seconds in a child (3 seconds in a neonate) is a sign of poor oxygenation
Oximetry	Determination of oxygen saturation (SaO_2) which can be a continuous or intermittent measurement. A light-emitting sensor and a photodetector are placed in an opposing position around a digit, hand, foot or earlobe. The diode emits red and infrared lights which pass through the skin to the photodetector. Oxyhaemoglobin absorbs more infrared light than deoxyhaemoglobin and a microprocessor measures the difference between the amount of absorption of red and infrared light and displays the percentage of oxyhaemoglobin
Peak expiratory flow rate (PEFR)	Peak flow measurement can be easily measured using a Wright's peak flow meter or a mini peak flow meter. Children can usually learn to use these from about 4 years. They need to be able to a take a deep breath and a fast and forced expiration. Peak flow rates are useful to monitor asthma and the efficacy of inhaled or nebulised medication. PEFRs vary with sex, age, height and race but a variation of up to 8% of normal values is acceptable
Naso-pharyngeal aspiration	Aspiration of the naso-pharynx is performed to identify the presence of respiratory syncytial virus (RSV) in infants with bronchiolitis

probe site should be changed every 4 hours to prevent pressure necrosis or burns from incompatible sensors and oximeters (Murphy *et al.*, 1990). Nurses should also be aware that using an extremity which is already being utilised for blood pressure monitoring or as the site for an arterial catheter will prevent the sensor from identifying pulsation and produce inaccurate readings. Movement of the child has the same effect.

Activity

Find out the rationale for using the investigations listed in Table 10.4 and determine the role of the nurse before, during and after each investigation.

NURSING INTERVENTIONS

Specific nursing interventions which may be implemented for a child with a respiratory problem are:

- easing respiratory effort;
- oxygen therapy;
- chest physiotherapy;
- administration of respiratory drugs;
- care of chest drains.

Easing respiratory effort is mainly achieved by ensuring maximum lung expansion. This is aided by positioning – usually breathless children will determine whichever position best enables them to breathe and the nurse can then use pillows to help them maintain this optimum position. Clothing and bedclothes should not constrict the neck or chest. Not only does this increase the child's comfort but it also makes observation of respiratory effort easier. Dyspnoea is a frightening symptom for both the child and the parents. For the child, the sympathetic nervous system reaction to fear leads to bronchodilation and an increased respiratory rate. This results in an increase in pCO_2 which produces bronchocon-striction and further breathlessness and panic. It is therefore important that the breathless child feels reassured by being treated in a calm and competent manner.

Oxygen therapy may be necessary to maximise respiratory efficiency (Table 10.6). Oxygen is a drug which should be prescribed by dose. Prolonged exposure to high percentages of oxygen causes complications and Higgins (1990) suggests that long periods of oxygen therapy above 50% should be avoided. Toxic effects include retrolental fibroplasia in premature neonates, lung collapse, increased destruction of red blood cells and carbon dioxide narcosis. Children with chronic respiratory disease are at risk from carbon dioxide narcosis which occurs when they are given high percentages of oxygen. The principle respiratory stimulus for these children is a falling pO_2 (the hypoxic drive) because their diseased lungs and poor ventilation cause them to always retain carbon dioxide and to always be hypercapnic. High percentages of oxygen depresses their respirations leading eventually to unconsciousness and death. Oxygen may be given by a variety of methods, which all have their advantages and disadvantages (Table 10.6), but should ideally be accompanied by humidification. In health, the mucus-secreting cells of the naso-pharynx humidify the inhaled air and this process compensates

Method	Advantages	Disadvantages
Headbox	Delivery of high O_2% possible	High humidity – condensation can obscure child
	Enables observation of chest and control of O_2 concentration	Needs removal to give most care
		Can rub infant's chin or shoulder
Nasal cannula	Enables care to continue Facilitates observation Ideal for low flow oxygen	Not always well tolerated Cannot attach to humidity Cannot give high flows of oxygen Difficult to control O_2 concentration
Oxygen masks	Different sizes available Known O_2 concentration	Not well tolerated by children Discomfort Interferes with talking and eating

Table 10.6

The administration of oxygen

for the loss of water which occurs on expiration (Foss, 1990). This normal humidification process is often impaired in respiratory disease and added gas will exacerbate the dehydration of mucous membranes and pulmonary secretions. The method used for oxygen therapy should also suit the child. A method which distresses the child and causes crying will only cause further respiratory distress and it may be more effective to nurse the child sitting on a parent's lap with the oxygen administered through a funnel held as close to the child's nose and mouth as possible.

Chest physiotherapy aims to remove retained bronchopulmonary secretions, and reduces the airway obstruction and re-inflates the areas of lung collapse caused by the excess secretions. It therefore improves ventilation and reduces the effort of breathing. The techniques of chest physiotherapy include:

- positioning;
- postural drainage;
- chest percussion;
- chest vibrations;
- manual hyperinflation;
- breathing exercises.

Activity

Arrange to join a physiotherapist performing chest physiotherapy. Identify each of the techniques listed above giving the rationale for each.

In certain conditions chest physiotherapy may be inappropriate. Infants with acute bronchiolitis usually only have increased secretions in their upper airways which is best managed by humidified oxygen and naso-pharyngeal suction (Prasad and Hussey, 1995). Chest physiotherapy may further impair respiratory embarrassment due to severe bronchospasm and is best avoided unless mucus plugging is evident. Inhaled foreign bodies are best removed by bronchoscopy; chest physiotherapy may only cause the object to move into a central airway or into the larynx with disastrous results (Phelan *et al.*, 1990).

Medications for respiratory problems are often given by inhalation via inhalers or nebulisers. Common medications include bronchodilators, anticholinergics and anti-inflammatory agents including corticosteroids (Table 10.7). Whilst bronchodilators are useful for a range of respiratory problems, it is only children over 2 years who respond to such treatment. Only 50% of wheezy infants react to bronchodilators. Anticholinergics such as ipratropium bromide, which cause less hypoxaemia in young children, are recommended for children under 2 years (Wilson, 1996).

The British Thoracic Society (1993) recommends the use of a 4–6 week course of cromoglycate as the primary anti-inflammatory treatment for asthma, and that steroids should only be given if this has no effect. Speight (1996) reports that 80% of GPs do not follow these recommendations and prescribe steroids straight away. There are concerns about children using inhaled steroids on a long-term basis, with fears about adrenal suppression, stunted growth and inhibition of normal lung development in preschool children. Speight (1996) indicates that the efficacy of inhaled steroids outweighs these potential and unproven complications. He suggests that asthmatic children are given steroids in doses which are high enough to control their asthma and administered via a spacer device to enhance lung deposition and to reduce the risk of systemic absorption. He also promotes a 'crash course' of oral steroids (prednisolone 1–2 mg/kg for 3–5 days) for acute episodes for children over 18 months. There is no evidence that such treatment is effective for children under this age (Wright, 1996). Prophylactic prednisolone 10 mg daily may also be useful to cover short

Medication	Use	Route	Dose/kg	Side effects
Bronchodilators salbutamol terbutaline salmeterol				
Anticholinergics ipratropium bromide				
Methylxanthines aminophylline				
Anti-inflammatory agents sodium cromoglyconate prednisolone hydrocortisone				
Mucolytics rhDNase				
Virostatic Ribavirin				

Table 10.7

Common respiratory medications
(Copyright is waived for the purpose of photocopying and enlarging this table.)

periods such as holidays or examination times when an acute attack would be a major inconvenience (Speight, 1996).

Nebulised steroids in the form of budesonide have recently been found to improve the symptoms of children with severe croup, improving their symptoms in 2 hours and reducing their length of stay in hospital by one third (Godden *et al.*, 1997).

Recent evidence shows that ibuprofen, a non-steroidal anti-inflammatory drug, given orally twice daily, provides a significant reduction in deterioration of lung function for children with cystic fibrosis (Konstan *et al.*, 1995). (Ibuprofen cannot be given to asthmatic children.) Another relatively new treatment for cystic fibrosis, human recombinant DNase alpha (rhDNase) was introduced in 1994. RhDNase, administered via a nebuliser, breaks down the DNA strands in the respiratory secretions, thus reducing their viscosity, and has been shown to improve lung function and general health as well as reducing bacterial colonisation of the lungs (Scott, 1994).

Another relatively new medication is Ribavirin which is recommended by the American Academy of Pediatrics (AAP) for certain infants with respiratory syncytial virus bronchiolitis (AAP, 1993). Although it is used in some parts of the UK, not all British paediatricians are convinced that this is a beneficial treatment and Rakshi and Couriel (1994) suggests that the cost and uncertain efficacy of Ribavirin do not recommend it as the treatment of choice. However, they also recognise that there is no current evidence that any treatment reduces the severity or duration of viral bronchiolitis.

Activity

Find out the uses, dosages/kg, routes of administration and side effects of the common respiratory medications listed in Table 10.7.

Care of chest drains is a very specific intervention for children with respiratory disorders. Chest drains are inserted into the pleural or mediastinal space to drain air and/or fluid from a:

- pneumothorax;
- haemothorax;
- chylothorax;
- empyema;
- pleural effusion.

Since interpleural pressure is normally subatmospheric, drainage of this space requires a special collecting system which uses an underwater seal. For drainage to occur the pressure in the collecting chamber must always be lower than the pressure in the interpleural or mediastinal space. This is achieved by the creation of a water seal in the collection chamber and the distal end of the chest tube is submerged in at least

2 cm of water. Increased amounts of water increase the resistance to drainage from the chest. Disposable chest drainage units are now common which incorporate the collection chamber, water seal chamber and a suction control chamber in a closed system. Suction will facilitate drainage of viscous fluid. To ensure the drainage system is properly functioning the nurse should observe the:

- child for respiratory distress;
- chest drain for bubbling and fluctuation of water during respiration;
- quantity and appearance of drainage.

Activity

Study the box 'Management of chest drains' and answer the questions about the care related to chest drainage.

Two chest drain clamps should be kept at the child's bedside at all times in case of need. Hospital policies vary about their routine use. Some units advise clamping whenever the child is moved whilst others believe that this routine clamping delays healing. However, if staff are unused to caring for chest drains this may be the safer policy.

When the level of the water in the drain stops fluctuating the lung has probably re-expanded. A chest X-ray is taken to confirm this and the drain is then removed. The chest drain is stitched in place with a 'purse-string' suture. Following administration of analgesia it is removed by two nurses as one person is required to pull the suture tight while the other removes the tube to avoid air entry and tension pneumothorax from occurring. Older children can be asked to breathe in and hold their breath at the point of removal of the drain. This minimises the risk of air entry.

Management of chest drains

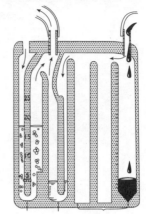

In the diagram above, identify the:
- water seal
- attachment to the child
- attachment for suction
- collection chamber

What fluid is put into chest drainage systems in your hospital?

Why is this fluid chosen?

How much fluid is put in?

Why does the nurse need to know how much fluid is in the system?

Which is more important and why? To have:
- a standard amount of fluid in the system?
- enough fluid to cover the end of the drainage tube?

What should you do if the chest drain:
- slips out of the child?
- becomes disconnected?

What is your hospital policy about clamping chest drains?

Problem	Significance	Action
Cessation of drainage	Pressure on chest drain tubing may impede drainage	Check, straighten and secure tubing
No fluctuation of water	Re-expansion of the lung Tubing obstructed Tubing kinked Failure of suction	Chest X-ray to confirm Ask child to cough Dislodge clots or fibrin by 'milking' tubing Check, straighten and secure tubing Check connections
Constant bubbling	Air leak	Clamp drain close to chest wall – if bubbling stops, air leak is below chest level. If it continues leak is in pleural space – unclamp and call doctor
Child in respiratory distress	Tension pneumothorax	Report to doctor

Table 10.8

Problem solving for the management of chest drains

EDUCATION FOR DISCHARGE

Active involvement of asthmatic children and their families in the management of asthma seems to not only improve parental knowledge, skills and confidence but also results in a significant reduction in the severity and frequency of acute attacks (Ramsay, 1994). Speight (1996) suggests that all families of asthmatic children should have a crisis pack of information and drugs to help them recognise and manage an acute attack. He found that 80% of childhood deaths (80–100 per year) could have been prevented by such a strategy.

It seems appropriate that children and families living with chronic disorders are empowered in this way. Module 4, chapter 4 (pages 225–231) discussed how coping skills are enhanced by improved understanding of the problem.

Activity

Find out what written information is available for children with asthma or cystic fibrosis and their families. Consider the helpfulness of this advice for managing acute problems.

Home oxygen therapy: parental teaching

- Changing nasal cannula
- Care of oxygen and cylinder
- Care of oxygen concentrator
- Setting up of low flow meter
- Discussion of anxieties
- Use of apnoea monitor[*]
- Recognition of hypoxia and appropriate action[*]
- Resuscitation[*]

[*] For parents of infants with bronchopulmonary dysplasia

Some children with chronic respiratory problems are oxygen dependent. Home oxygen therapy can promote family relationships and normal child development. It minimises health care costs and hospital acquired infection but it requires careful preparation and education. Usually certain criteria need to be met before discharge:

- child must tolerate nasal cannula;
- infants must be feeding well and gaining weight;
- O_2 requirements must be stable at 30% or below;
- absence of other medical problems requiring medical treatment;
- adequate community support, housing and telephone;
- willing and able parents.

Because oxygen supports combustion, it may be appropriate for parents to inform their insurance company and the fire brigade of the presence of oxygen in the home. An oxygen concentrator, which fits unobtrusively in the home, can manufacture oxygen from room air and eliminates the needs for the storage and delivery of bulky oxygen cylinders. It usually has two outlet points and ample tubing to maximise the child's mobility.

PRINCIPLES OF CARE – CHILDREN WITH SKIN DISORDERS

11

The structure and function of the skin

Give five functions of the skin

Explain how the skin helps to regulate body temperature. How does this differ in children?

Differentiate between the layers of the epidermis:

- stratum corneum (horny layer)
- stratum granulosum (granular layer)
- stratum spinosum (prickle cell layer)
- stratum basale (basal layer)
- stratum lucidum

What is the average life cycle for epidermal cells?

In which layer of skin do the hair follicles, sweat glands, nerves, lymph and blood vessels originate?

Where are the sebaceous glands found and what is their function?

INTRODUCTION

Skin rashes and problems are common during childhood. Although they are rarely life threatening, they cause much physical and psychological distress for the affected child. Many conditions cannot be cured and their treatment is sometimes as psychologically upsetting as the disorders themselves. Parents are often embarrassed at their child's appearance and may be wrongly accused of not maintaining good standards of hygiene. Children's nurses need to be able to offer support and advice to parents and children which will overcome this teasing and accusations by others. Lay people often shun children with obvious skin problems believing all skin problems to be infectious. Nurses need to counteract this behaviour by always showing a positive acceptance of the child's appearance whilst always remembering that some skin disorders are infectious or can be transmitted to other children and taking the necessary precautions against such transmission.

To recognise and care for skin disorders appropriately, nurses need to understand how the normal structure and function of the skin is impaired by various intrinsic and extrinsic factors.

Activity

Test your knowledge of the structure and function of the skin by answering the questions on the left. Check your answers with an anatomy and physiology textbook.

COMMON SKIN DISORDERS

Common skin disorders can be classified into problems in infancy, chronic disorders, infections and infestations of the skin (Tables 11.1–11.4). Chronic disorders include eczema which has many causes and can affect any age group. Eczema and dermatitis, which are interchangeable terms, may be caused by endogenous or exogenous factors or develop secondary to other disorders. One of the commonest forms in childhood is atopic eczema which affects about 5% of the population (Goolamali, 1993). This form of eczema is an immunologically determined genetic disorder often associated with asthma and hay fever. The first clinical signs of atopic eczema usually occur between 3 and 6 months of age and are found on the cheeks. Flexural lesions appear within the next year. Acute exacerbations may be precipitated by secondary bacterial or viral infections. Children with atopic eczema seem particularly susceptible to virus infections and staphylococci or streptococci infections are often caused by scratching. Childhood

Types of childhood eczema

Endogenous eczema

- atopic eczema – flexural eczema associated with a familial tendency to hay fever, asthma or eczema
- discoid eczema – chronic oval or round areas of erythematous, itchy, and vesicular or dry and scaly skin; more common in coloured children than those of Caucasian origin
- seborrhoeic eczema – occurs in sites of increased sebaceous activity; commonly found on infants scalps but can also affect any of the body folds in later life

Exogenous Eczema

- irritant contact dermatitis – inflammation of the skin in response to an external irritant (e.g. nappy rash)
- allergic contact dermatitis – eczema arising from sensitivity to nickel, chrome, chemicals and medicaments; uncommon in children
- photodermatitis – an interaction of light and chemicals absorbed by the skin (e.g. drugs such as sulphonamides, cosmetics, chemical substances)

Secondary eczema

- lichen simplex (neurodermatitis) – areas of eczema that seem to appear secondary to itching. Often preceded by an insect bite or minor trauma which causes irritation. Persistent scratching damages the skin to produce redness, scaling and thickening. Rare in children
- pompholox – intensely itchy vesicular lesions which occur on the palms and soles and between digits which occurs secondary to dysfunction of the eccrine sweat glands

eczema can be very distressing for the child and parents although its prognosis is usually good. Fifty per cent of children usually recover by the age of 6 years and 80% by the age of 10 years, but the years when the disorder is present are characterised by a miserable child who has severe itching and is constantly scratching causing skin damage and bleeding. These areas heal to form crusts which crack during movement

Table 11.1 *Skin problems of infancy*

Problem	Description
Milia	Distended sebaceous glands that appear as tiny white papules around the nose. They do not cause symptoms and disappear spontaneously
Mongolian spots	Irregular areas of deep blue pigmentation usually in the sacral and gluteal regions found in babies of African, or Asian origin. Can be mistaken for bruising
Congenital capillary malformations: port-wine stain	Flat, pink, red or purple 'stains' of the skin which often enlarge, thicken and darken as the child grows. The depth of colour varies according to whether superficial, middle or deep dermal vessels are involved. Goldman et al. (1993) recommend laser therapy to treat or minimise this deformity
Haemangiomas	Benign tumours consisting of closely packed small blood vessels which are sometimes apparent at birth or become noticeable within the first weeks of life ('strawberry mark'). They tend to enlarge during the first year of life and then resolve spontaneously
Cavernous haemangiomas	A less common type of birthmark. This benign capillary tumour has a soft spongy consistency and because of its fragility, which increases as it grows, it carries the risk of haemorrhage should injury occur. Early treatment by irradiation, surgery or injection of a sclerosing agent is recommended
Seborrhoeic eczema	Thick, adherent, yellowish, scaly and oily patches which usually appear within 2–8 weeks after birth. It mostly affects the scalp ('cradle cap'). Spowart (1995) indicates that the aetiology of this type of eczema is not well understood. Because the scalp has many sebaceous glands, it is thought to relate to a dysfunction of these glands. Although unsightly, this type of eczema does not disturb the baby and usually clears spontaneously within 3–4 weeks. Thick scaling can be relieved by the daily use of coconut or arachis oil massaged into the scalp followed by washing with a mild baby shampoo

Table 11.2 *Common skin disorders of childhood*

Disorder	Pathophysiology
Eczema	An inflammatory response of the epidermis which may be an innate response or a reaction to an external irritant. Erythema occurs and the burning sensations cause severe itching. Intercellular and intracellular oedema results in the formation of small vesicles and papules. The vesicles erupt and can become secondarily infected, especially if the skin is broken by scratching. Constant scratching produces dry, leathery and thickened skin which tends to exacerbate the irritation
Psoriasis	A familial loss of control of epidermal cells which causes epidermal hyperplasia and a rapid cell cycle of 37.5 hours as opposed to the normal 28 days. This results in thick scaly plaques of skin. The blood supply to the dermis is increased by the dilated capillaries causing marked erythema when the scales are shed
Acne	The formation of an excessive amount of sebum occurs as the result of increased androgen production in adolescence which stimulates the growth of the sebaceous glands and follicles. Alteration in the follicular lining prevents the excretion of sebum which accumulates and stagnates to form non-inflamed comedones or inflamed lesions which rupture to form papules, pustules, nodules and cysts

Disorder	Pathophysiology
Impetigo contagiosa	Bacterial infection caused by Gram-positive cocci causes an inflammatory epidermal reaction resulting in a papular erythema. This progresses into vesicles which weep seropurulent fluid and form yellow crusts
Herpes simplex	Type I herpes simplex virus causes inflammation of the epidermal cells which become inflamed and blistered
Verruca (warts)	Human papillomavirus causes epidermal inflammation and the epithelial cell react by proliferations
Tinea capitis	Fungal infection of the scalp. The fungus excretes an enzyme which digests the keratin of the hair. The dissolved hair breaks off to form the characteristic round areas of itchy, scaly skin or alopecia
Tinea corporis	Fungal infection which invades the stratum corneum layer of the skin of the body. The stratum corneum is dissolved by the action of the fungus and round or oval patches of erythematous scaly skin occur
Tinea pedis (athlete's foot)	Fungal infection of the feet involving the soles or between the toes. The dissolved stratum corneum in these areas causes itchy vesicles on the soles of the feet and maceration and cracking between the toes
Candidiasis (thrush)	The yeast-like fungus, Candida albicans, can affect the mouth or nappy area. In the mouth it causes white adherent patches on the tongue, palate and inner aspects of the cheeks. Infection of the warm, moist nappy area which encourages the infection, produces acute inflammation and redness. White patches may be visible in the genital area
Cellulitis	Inflammation of the skin and subcutaneous tissues from a staphylococcal or streptococcal infection often gained from a puncture wound which is no longer visible. Causes redness and swelling of the site, enlarged adjacent lymph nodes, pyrexia and malaise

Table 11.3

Common skin infections of childhood

Infestation	Pathophysiology
Scabies	The scabies mite burrows into the stratum corneum of the epidermis usually in intertriginous areas. The affected child becomes sensitised to the mite and this initiates an allergic inflammatory response. As a result itching, redness and a papular, vesicular rash occurs around the area of burrowing
Pediculosis capitis (head lice)	The female head louse lays her eggs at the junction of the hair shaft and the skin and feeds by sucking blood from the host. The crawling insect and its saliva causes itching and scratching may cause secondary infection. The eggs (nits) may be visible as white areas attached to the hair shaft

Table 11.4

Common skin infestations of childhood

causing further soreness and bleeding. The child cannot sleep because of itching and discomfort and the parents are unable to provide lasting relief. Often children with eczema fail to thrive because of protein loss from their inflamed skin, loss of sleep and poor appetite or restricted diet (Donald, 1995). Restricted diets are only recommended as the last line of treatment because results are disappointing and because of the risk of nutritional and growth problems. A strong family history of atopy, age of onset over 2 years and involvement of extensor skin surfaces are thought to be indicators of a prolonged disorder. Frank (1987) gives a harrowing account of the torture of incessant itching, the damage and disfigurement caused by constant scratching and the messy, repugnant treatments which plaqued her childhood and early adulthood.

Nappy rash or dermatitis is a type of exogenous eczema which is probably the most common skin disorder of childhood. The skin in this area can be in prolonged occlusive contact with urine and faeces. The warm, moist environment causes maceration of the skin and encourages bacterial conversion of the urine to ammonia. Ammonia is an alkaline irritant which then produces a contact dermatitis reaction. Secondary infection can easily occur.

Activity

How would you advise new parents about the prevention of nappy rash?

Psoriasis is thought to be due to hormonal and immunological factors as well as dermal factors (Buxton, 1993). It can appear at any age but usually presents during adolescence and affects about 2% of the population. It is very variable in its duration and course. In some individuals it may only affect knees and elbows whilst others have widespread lesions. It appears to be a genetic tendency which can be triggered by injury, throat infections, certain drugs, and both physical and mental stress. Stress is often cited as a possible cause for skin disorders but this has to be considered carefully as stress is also an effect of skin disorders. Severe psoriasis is unsightly and leaves a trail of scales wherever the affected person has been. Ann, aged 10 years, was very depressed because no-one would sit next to her at school in case her psoriatic scales fell on them. She never wore skirts or short sleeved shirts or dresses so she could keep the affected parts out of sight. (The one advantage of psoriasis is that it rarely affects the face.) Craig, aged 14, was confined to his bedroom when his psoriasis exacerbated and his parents burnt his clothes because they were full of scales. These examples show how difficult it is to separate cause from effect.

Acne is another skin problem where the cause is not fully understood. It can occur on the face of infants or be drug-induced (anabolic steroids, oral and topical corticosteroids) but these forms only last briefly and clear spontaneously. The usual age of onset is 12–14 years with a peak severity occurring at 16–18 years in girls and 18–19 years in boys (Buxton, 1993). Its severity appears to be related to the genetically determined sebum secretion rate (Rothman and Lucky, 1993). Its high occurrence in families and identical twins seem to confirm a hereditary predisposition. At one time the cause was thought to be abnormal sebaceous glands but this has now been disproved. The abnormality seems to be in the sebum, the secretion of which is stimulated by androgens. Androgens are a likely causative factor as acne improves during pregnancy, is rare during young childhood and has high occurrence in adolescent boys. It is also precipitated by androgen-producing tumours. However, some females experience an exacerbation of their acne pre-menstrually. Buxton (1993) suggests that this may be

Types of psoriasis

Guttate psoriasis
- widespread lesions are a few millimetres in diameter
- common in children
- often develops following an infection, especially a streptococcal sore throat

Plaque psoriasis
- commonest form of psoriasis
- coin-shaped and well-defined lesions all over the body
- scalp is also often affected

Flexural psoriasis
- confined to body folds
- erythematous inflammatory reaction which is often macerated and fissured at the centre
- no scaling

Pustular psoriasis
- lesions form pustules
- commonly affects palms and soles
- generalised type is very rare and causes an acute systemic illness

Psoriasis of the nails
- affects about 50% of individuals with psoriasis
- nails become thick and porous
- nail can detach from nail bed

Psoriatic arthritis
- seronegative arthropathy of the non-rheumatic type
- double normal incidence (2%) in individuals with psoriasis (Buxton, 1993)
- commonly involves distal interphalangeal joints
- familial psoriatic trait in 40% of those affected (Buxton, 1993)

due to fluid retention which increases the hydration of the skin to cause swelling and hypersecretion of the sebaceous ducts. Another historical cause was fatty or oily food, especially chocolate and pork. It now appears that these are not implicated other than for certain susceptible individuals but acne is known to be exacerbated by exposure to oily substances in the environment. Acne is of psychological concern for adolescents who are concerned about their appearance. Unfortunately, constant fingering of the lesions tends to perpetuate the problems and may cause scarring.

Two very rare skin conditions are known to be inherited disorders. Epidermolysis bullosa (EB) is a group of disorders in which the skin is extremely fragile and blisters at the slightest touch. The tissues which attach each epidermal cell to the next are absent or dysfunctional, causing the cells to separate and fluid to fill the gap. At a touch, the thin upper layer can peel away to leave raw areas of sore and painful skin. Internal organs can also be affected. Congenital lamellar icthyosis is almost always fatal due to loss of fluid, protein and electrolytes from the thick, inelastic and very permeable skin.

ASSESSMENT OF SKIN DISORDERS

The specific assessment of the child with a skin disorder involves:

- *Listening to the history of the problem.* A family history of a skin disorder or an onset related to another illness, medication or contact with plants, insects, or animals may be very significant.
- *Listening to symptoms.* Alterations in feeling or sensation help to determine nursing interventions as well as helping in the diagnosis.
- *Looking at the lesions.* The distribution, size and appearance of the lesions can help to identify allergic or irritant rashes, and differentiate between infections and other problems. It is useful to record your findings on a body outline. This helps to monitor progression or improvement.

In addition to this assessment, it may be necessary to carry out more detailed dermatological investigations.

Activity

Find out when and why the dermatological investigations listed in Table 11.5 are performed. What is the role of the nurse in each investigation?

NURSING INTERVENTIONS

Caring for children with a skin disorder involves relief of their physical and psychological distress. This distress is common to nearly all skin disorders so there are certain principles of care which can be applied regardless of the diagnosis.

Skin disorders – terminology
- *Bullae* – large fluid-filled lesion
- *Burrow* – linear lesion caused by the scabies mite
- *Crusts* – dried areas of exudate (serum, pus, dead skin and debris) from lesions
- *Erythema* – reddened skin
- *Excoriation* – superficial loss of skin often caused by scratching
- *Fissure* – deep linear split through the epidermis into the dermis
- *Macule* – flat, round area of colour change less than 1 mm in diameter (e.g. freckle)
- *Nodule* – solid, round or ellipsoid raised area which originates in or below the dermis
- *Papule* – small, round, solid raised area less than 1 mm in diameter which lies mainly above the skin surface
- *Plaque* – large flattened disc-shaped raised area
- *Pustule* – pus-filled lesion
- *Vesicle* – small fluid-filled lesion
- *Scales* – flakes of dead tissue on the skin surface
- *Scar* – permanent dermal change formed by excess collagen in response to damage to the dermis

---

Specific assessment of the child with a skin disorder

Where?
- where are the lesions distributed?

When?
- when was the onset, did it relate to:
- medication?
- other illness?
- changes in occupation?
- changes in the home environment?
- when were there any previous episodes?

What?
- what symptoms are the lesions causing – itching, burning, scaling, blistering?
- what type and size of lesions are they?

Who?
- who else is affected?

How?
- how long have the lesions been present?
- how are the lesions now, compared with previous problems or since onset? (better or worse?)

Investigation	When and why?	Role of the nurse
Skin scrapings		
Skin biopsy		
Patch testing		
Woods light		

Activity

The common problems of children with skin disorders are identified in Table 11.6. Consider the aims of care and nursing actions for each of these problems.

As discussed above, the cause of many skin disorders is not clear. As a result much of the treatment is symptomatic rather than curative. For this reason much work has been done to look at the efficacy of complementary therapies in the management of skin disorders. Traditional Chinese herbal treatments have been shown to be beneficial for the treatment of eczema but the long-term effects of this treatment are unclear and one study has shown that liver damage may ensue (Harper, 1994). Skin treatments usually involve some kind of local application which is determined by the type of lesion involved and its site on the body. It is important for nurses to wash their hands before and after the

Problem	Aim	Nursing action
Itching and irritation		
Potential risk of secondary infection due to scratching or rubbing		
Feelings of isolation and rejection due to altered body image		
Parental anxiety due to child's appearance		
Potential exacerbation of condition due to stress		

application of these topical treatments, not only to prevent cross infection, but to minimise the risk of absorption for themselves. The use of gloves for applications is debatable. Alderman (1988) argues that gloves may increase the child's feelings of being socially unacceptable. Topical treatments are usually drugs which have been suspended in a base. The choice of drug and base are both important and depend upon the disorder and state of the skin. Table 11.7 gives indications for uses of bases with their advantages and disadvantages. Most of these applications have to be covered by some kind of gauze body suit to help their adherence and absorption by the lesions. Other more specific interventions are bathing, wet dressings and occlusive therapy.

Bathing helps to remove scales, crusts and topical medications and provides hydration for dry skin. Donald (1995) recommends a lukewarm bath to avoid dilation of blood vessels and exacerbation of itching. Cleansing of old applications should be performed after the child has soaked in the bath for about 10 minutes and may be helped by soap, oils or colloidal oatmeal. The benefit of hydration is increased dramatically if topical applications are renewed immediately after the bath (Clark *et al.*, 1990). The benefit of hydration is also found with wet wraps which are used to soothe weeping, crusting and purulent lesions. They cool the skin by relieving the inflammation and enhancing the absorption of the topical treatment. They are often used in acute eczema in conjunction with emollients.

Occlusive therapy is sometimes used to encourage penetration of topical steroids but concern has been expressed about the use of such treatment in children because of the risk of systemic absorption (Hunter *et al.*, 1989). Steroids should therefore be used with care as under-use will not overcome the disorder and over-use may cause steroidal side effects. Hunter *et al.* (1989) recommend that nothing stronger than hydrocortisone 1% should be used on the face or for infants. Donald (1995) suggests that a blob of cream on the finger tip is about 0.5 g and that no more than 6 g should be used for a single application to the whole body for a small child.

Use of wet wraps
- Bathe and cleanse the skin
- Apply emollient liberally, so that it no longer sinks into the skin
- Soak tubifast bandages in warm water and then squeeze so they are not dripping wet
- Apply wet bandages to limbs and trunk
- Apply dry tubifast bandages to cover wet bandages, tying wraps together at the shoulders and tops of the legs

Base	Uses	Action	Advantages/disadvantages
Powder	Between flexures	Lessens friction	Can clump and irritate
Watery/shake lotions	Acutely inflammed wet and oozing lesions	Dries, soothes and cools	Tedious to apply; frequent changes needed
Creams	Moist and dry skin	Cools, moisturizes and softens	Short shelf-life; fungal and bacterial growth possible
Ointments	Dry and scaly skin	Occludes and softens	Messy to apply; stains clothes
Pastes	Dry, scaly and lichenified skin	Protects and softens	Messy and tedious to apply; most protective
Sprays	Weeping, acutely inflammed skin	Drying, non-occlusive	Evaporate quickly; no need to touch inflamed sore skin

Table 11.7

Types of topical treatments and their uses

Treatment	Uses	Dose/kg	Instructions for use/side effects
Topical benzyl benzoate dithranol malathion			
Systemic acyclovir cyproterone acetate trimeprazine griseofulvin nystatin tetracycline			
Physical cryotherapy cautery phototherapy			

Specific treatments are available for the treatment of infections and infestations of the skin (Table 11.8). Compliance with instructions for these is important if the problem is to be completely eradicated and nurses should be aware of the instructions and advice to give parents using such treatments. Recent evidence appears to indicate that head lice are more prevalent because they have become resistant to popular treatments. Harper (1994) estimates that 10–20% of urban schoolchildren are affected by head lice. For this reason most health districts have a policy of rotating recommended treatments. There is also some concern that some preparations may be carcinogenic.

Activity

Your local infant school asks you to give a talk to parents about the recognition and treatment of head lice. Prepare the content of your talk.

ADVICE ON DISCHARGE

Activity

Consider all you have learnt about the problems and treatment of chronic skin disorders such as eczema and psoriasis. How would these disorders affect your normal lifestyle?

You will probably realise that such problems can affect every aspect of a usual lifestyle. Apart from a possible avoidance of mixing with others because of embarrassment, scaly skin disorders are not acceptable for some occupations, of which nursing is one example. Nurses with eczema of the hands often find that their skin cannot tolerate constant washing and contact with antibacterial lotions. The weather also affects the skin. Hot weather and sweating tends to increase the itching of eczema and psoriasis tends to flare up in the winter due to the constriction of extra clothes. Work environments may therefore not be conducive to certain skin disorders. Environmental factors, including the dust mite, are thought to be as important as genetic factors in atopic asthma and controlling such factors may help to reduce itching. An allergic reaction to dust mite excreta may trigger eczema (Donald, 1995). Parents can be given advice about reducing dust mites in the home.

Useful support agencies for parents are:

- National Eczema Society, 164 Eversholt Street, London NW1 1BU. Tel: 0171 388 4097.

- The Psoriasis Association, 7 Milton Street, Northampton NN2 7JG. Tel: 01604 711129.

Avoidance of the dust mite: advice to parents

- Keep the child's bedroom cool
- Avoid the use of central heating and carpets in the bedroom
- Cover the mattress with an impermeable cover
- Vacuum the base of the bed and the room at least weekly
- Damp dust the room daily
- Wash all bed linen with a non-biological washing powder at 55°C
- Avoid soft toys or wash regularly

12 MENTAL HEALTH IN CHILDHOOD

INTRODUCTION

According to the DoH (1991, page 86) mental health problems account for 23% of NHS in-patient costs and 25% of pharmaceutical costs with 'the total direct and indirect costs of depression and anxiety estimated at up to £4.6 billion a year'. The recognition, treatment and resolution of young people's mental health problems is vital in the fight to reduce these costs and to promote mental well-being in adulthood. The very nature of childhood exposes children to a wide variety of factors which can influence their development and it is clear that emotional and behavioural problems are increasing as a result (Kurtz, 1992). The role of children's nurses in promoting mental health is to be able to communicate with the child and family and be able to assess problems and needs, referring to the specialist team where necessary. The purpose of this section is to introduce you to the nature and management of mental health problems in children and young people so that you will be able to take the appropriate steps to support and help them.

THE NATURE AND EXTENT OF MENTAL HEALTH PROBLEMS IN CHILDHOOD

Defining mental health

Activity

Before reading on jot down your own definition of 'mental health'. Do you consider yourself to be mentally healthy? Why?

For many, mental health is linked to mental illness and therefore extreme states of incapacity. However, this is a very narrow view to take and one which fails to recognise the diverse nature of mental health problems especially in childhood. Wilson (1995, page 90) suggests that mental health is essentially about emotional development and refers to 'the robustness, soundness and healthy functioning of the mind, consisting as it does of an individual's cognitive, emotional and volitional capacities'. Three further definitions are offered here for you to consider:

- 'The components of mental health include the following capacities: the ability to develop psychologically, emotionally, intellectually and spiritually; the ability to initiate, develop and sustain mutually satisfying personal relationships; the ability to become aware of others and to empathise with them; the ability to use psychological distress as a developmental process, so that it does not hinder or impair further development' (Health Advisory Service, 1995).

- 'Mental health problems in children and young people may be defined as abnormalities of emotions, behaviour or social relationships sufficiently marked or prolonged to cause suffering or risk to optimal development in the child or distress or disturbance in the family or community' (Kurtz, 1992, page 6).

- Mental health in young people is indicated by:
  - an ability to form and sustain mutually satisfying relationships;
  - a continuing progression of psychological development;
  - an ability to play and learn, achieving appropriately for age and intellectual level;
  - developing a moral sense of right and wrong;
  - a degree of psychological distress and maladapted behaviour within normal limits for the child's age and context (Wilson, 1995).

The extent of mental health problems in young people has been estimated by a variety of sources. Although the figures vary, there can be no doubt that many children and young people have behavioural and emotional problems which need help and as result are failing to make the most of their potential:

- Graham (1986) – estimated that 20% of the child population had mental health problems with 7–10% of those being moderate to severe.

- Bone and Meltzer (1989) – carried out a survey in 1988 and suggested that disabling emotional or behavioural problems were evident in 2.1% of all children in Great Britain.

- Mental Health Foundation (1993) – approximately 2 million children under the age of 16 in England and Wales.

- HAS (1995) – between 10 and 20% of children may require help because of mental health problems at any one time.

- Various studies have attempted to estimate the prevalence of problems in different age groups (see Table 12.1): (a) preschool – 22% of children in the UK (7% severe, 15% mild) suffer common behavioural and emotional problems (Richman *et al.*, 1982), (b) middle childhood – Rutter *et al.* (1975) found that up to 25% of children living in inner cities had mental health problems compared with 12% in rural areas and (c) adolescence – all studies seem to indicate that a higher proportion of this age group (between 10 and 20%) suffers from mental health problems. Worrying statistics show that teenage suicide is on the increase. According to the Samaritans (1997) 19% of deaths among 15–24 year olds were attributed to suicide in 1995.

Common behavioural problems of preschool children
- Bed wetting
- Soiling
- Waking at night
- Over-activity
- Poor appetite

Problem	Child	Adolescent
Nocturnal enuresis	8%	
Sleep problems	13% difficulty settling	
	14% wake persistently	
Feeding difficulties	12–14%	
Abdominal pain (with no organic cause)	10% (5%)	
Severe tantrums	4–20%	
Major depression	0.5–2.5%	2–8%
Encopresis	0.7–2.3%	0.3–1.3%
Anorexia		0.5–1%
Bullaemia		1%
Attempted suicide		2.4%
Suicide		7.6:100 000
Alcohol misuse		29%
Solvents and illegal drugs		16%

The classification of childhood mental health problems is complex and you are referred to more specialist texts (see Barker, 1995, chapter 3). Graham (1986) identified the most common disorders as being:

- emotional disorders – depression, anxiety states, phobias and psychosomatic disorders;
- conduct disorders – stealing, truancy, aggression, fire setting and persistent delinquency;
- attention deficit disorder, with or without hyperactivity;
- depressive disorder leading to suicide;
- developmental disorders, e.g. language delay and autism;
- severe eating disorders, e.g. anorexia nervosa;
- elimination disorders, e.g. enuresis and encopresis.

THE CAUSES OF MENTAL HEALTH PROBLEMS IN CHILDHOOD

There are various factors which interact to cause mental health problems in childhood. The result is that no two children react in the same way to the tasks associated with development. Some cope well with the demands placed upon them. Others do not cope so well with the same demands. Even children within the same family, with similar upbringings, can differ in their emotional development. The factors which seem to contribute to the development of mental health problems are grouped into four categories according to Barker (1995):

- Constitutional including genetic factors, the effects of chromosomal abnormalities, the consequences of intrauterine injury and the results of birth injury.

- Physical disease and injury including brain damage caused by injury, infection and tumours; chronic illness which can impose restrictions on children's lives leading to emotional problems.

- Temperamental factors. A study by Chess and Thomas (1984) identified three types of temperament – easy children, difficult children and those who were 'slow-to-warm-up'. However, there is no optimal temperamental type, rather it is the fit between the temperaments of the child and that of the parents.

- Environmental factors. These include the influence of the family, school and the wider social environment.

Kurtz (1992) identifies several situations in which there appears to be greater risk of mental health problems:

- in families where there is socioeconomic disadvantage or family disharmony;

- in families where there is a history of parental psychiatric illness particularly maternal depression;

- following child abuse;

- in association with physical illness especially chronic illness, very severe conditions and sensory deficit.

MANAGING MENTAL HEALTH PROBLEMS IN CHILDHOOD

A range of interventions may be used for the treatment of mental health problems in childhood. Some may need the involvement of a specialised team on an in-patient or out-patient basis. The team may include a variety of professionals working within a multidisciplinary framework:

- psychiatrists;

- social workers;

- community psychiatric nurses;

- child psychotherapist;

- music therapists;

- art therapists;

- occupational therapists;

- other medical staff.

Other interventions may be implemented within the general paediatric area. For this reason you should become familiar with some of the variety of treatments available. Two examples of interventions will be considered here.

Family therapy

Module 1 examines the nature of the family and highlights its diverse nature and important role in the development of children. The family is

Easy children
- Quickly fall into regular sleep and feeding patterns
- Take readily to new foods, strangers, new schools
- Accept frustration without much fuss

Difficult children
- Have irregular biological functions
- Have negative withdrawal responses to new situations
- Show slow adaptability to change
- Have intense mood expressions which are often negative
- Often have temper tantrums

Slow-to-warm-up children
- Show negative responses of mild intensity to new experiences
- Generally have reactions which are of a mild intensity
- Less irregular biological functioning than difficult child

Groups of children likely to have greater incidence of mental health problems
- Young offenders
- Children with a criminal background
- Children in the care of the local authority
- Children with learning disabilities
- Children with emotional and behavioural difficulties
- Abused children
- Children with a physical disability
- Children with sensory impairment
- Children who have parents with mental health problems
- Children with a chronic illness
- Children who experience/witness sudden extreme trauma
- Refugees

(DoH, 1996)

Interventions for mental health problems
- Family therapy
- Behaviour therapy
- Psychotherapy
- Group therapy
- Pharmacotherapy
- Hypnosis and hypnotherapy
- Speech therapy

Further reading

ANDERSON, T. (1990) *The Reflecting Team*. Broadstairs: Bergman

BARKER, P. (1992) *Basic Family Therapy*, 3rd edn. Oxford: Blackwell Scientific

Cross reference

Bowel retraining – page 473

a complex, ever changing entity and factors which affect its function can affect family members in various ways. Family therapy aims to change the dynamics of the family system which inevitably leads to individual change (McMahon, 1995). The family group is the focus of treatment, not just the individual child. The therapist looks at the family as a whole and the dynamics within it, with the aim of establishing healthy family functioning. Assessing the way the family functions is important in identifying areas in which the family may be experiencing difficulties. Steinhauer *et al.* (1984) give an example of a scheme for understanding families and how they function along six dimensions:

- task accomplishment (problem solving) – basic tasks, those which provide the essentials of life; developmental tasks, those which ensure the healthy development of family members; crisis tasks, those which must be dealt with in the face of unexpected or unusual events;
- role performance;
- communication;
- affective involvement – the degree and quality of the family members' interest and concern for each other;
- control – the influence family members have over each other – rigid, flexible, *laissez-faire* or chaotic;
- values and norms.

Activity

Consider a child you have cared for/are caring for with behavioural or emotional problems. Using the six dimensions outlined above explore the possible difficult areas that the family may be experiencing.

Activity

Arrange to talk to a family therapist about the different schools of thought and the use of family therapy for children with behavioural or emotional problems.

Behaviour therapy

This type of therapy is based upon work from the field of social-learning theory and draws ideas from theorists such as Pavlov and Skinner. It focuses on the factors which maintain certain behaviours and how they can be altered. Assessment of the nature of the child's behaviour is paramount and includes ascertaining the:

- frequency of occurrence of the behaviour;
- the developmental appropriateness of the behaviour, e.g. temper

tantrums are to be expected in the 2 year old but would warrant more concern in an 11 year old;

- the social relevance of the behaviour;
- the intensity and focus of the behaviour;
- the costs and gains to the child (Varma, 1990).

Behaviour can then be categorised into that which is lacking or that which is in excess. Behaviourists are not concerned with exploring the nature and meaning of problem behaviour. Rather they believe that problem behaviours are learned and can be replaced by new learning experiences. Three main types of intervention are (Barker, 1995):

- *operant and respondent conditioning* – concerned with altering the conditions following (operant) or preceding (respondent) a problem behaviour;
- *cognitive behaviour therapy* – attempts to teach the child to think differently about things so that their behaviour changes;
- *modelling* – behaviour learned by observing and imitating another person; parents often do not realise how powerfully they can influence their child's behaviour in this way.

Activity

Reflect critically on the management of a child you have cared for where this behaviour approach has been used. Consider the factors involved in influencing its outcome.

SUICIDE IN YOUNG PEOPLE

The suicide rate among young people has risen alarmingly, especially among males, since 1980. Suicide is now the second most common cause of death among young people aged 15–24 (Whitefield *et al*. (1995). Parasuicide (attempted suicide) is also prevalent but is more common in young females than males. According to Leenars (1988) there may be as many as 100 attempts for every successful suicide and many more young people contemplate killing themselves. Thus the prevention of suicide in young people is an important issue and one which should concern all who work with young people in whatever setting.

The cause of suicide is complex and arises from multiple factors acting together. Factors which have been shown to contribute to suicide and parasuicide in young people include:

- extreme and traumatic events (e.g. physical and sexual abuse);
- alcohol and substance abuse – drugs and alcohol can 'affect thinking capacities and may act as a catalyst for suicidal thoughts by reducing inhibitions' (Borton, 1997);

Further reading

MURDOCH, D. and BARKER, P. (1991) *Basic Behaviour Therapy*. Oxford: Blackwell Scientific

SCHAFFER, D., et al. (1995) *The Clinical Guide to Child Psychiatry*. London: The Free Press, Collier and Macmillan.

Between 1980 and 1990 the rate of suicides and deaths due to undetermined cause have increased by 85% in males aged 15–24 (Hawton, 1994)

Definitions of suicide

' ... suicide is a conscious act of self-induced annihilation, best understood as a multidimensional malaise in a needful individual who defines an issue for which suicide is perceived as the best solution'. (Shneidman, 1985)

' ... suicidal behaviour in children can be defined as self-destructive behaviour that has the intent to seriously damage oneself or cause death'. (Pfeffer, 1986)

- psychiatric illness, e.g. depression, excessive fears and anxieties, conduct and emotional disorders (Shaffer, 1974); a family history of mental illness is also more common in young people who kill themselves (Barton, 1995);
- family dysfunction, e.g. broken homes (through death or divorce), parental unemployment, poor support mechanisms.

Although suicide can never be totally eradicated the aim of prevention should be to reduce the number of suicides to the lowest possible level. The DoH (1992) set a target for reducing overall suicides by 15% by the year 2000. A multi-agency, multi-faceted approach to the three levels of prevention is essential in order to develop focused strategies.

Primary prevention – to prevent the contemplation of suicide:

- detecting and treating mental disorders in young people;
- restricting access to alcohol and drug abuse;
- reducing access to lethal means of suicide, e.g. firearms;
- reducing media influences;
- educating young people about the importance of talking through feelings and promoting mental health.

Secondary prevention – providing help for those who are already suicidal:

- hotlines (e.g. the Samaritans and Childline);
- identifying those at risk – children's nurses (particularly those working in A&E) play a vital role here in picking up cues from young people in their care. Borton (1997) suggests signs of suicide to which we should be alert:

  – withdrawn behaviour;

  – having definite ideas about how to kill themselves;

  – talking about feeling isolated;

  – losing self-esteem and expressing feelings of failure and uselessness;

  – constantly dwelling on problems for which there seems to be no solution.

The risk is increased if there are any of the contributory factors mentioned above.

Tertiary prevention – providing support for those who have attempted suicide. All young people who self-harm or attempt suicide should be referred. Diekstra (cited by Barton, 1995) suggests that only 1:4 cases lead to contact with medical or other professionals. According to Barton (1995) ideally all young people should be assessed by a child and adolescent psychiatrist following a parasuicide attempt.

The Samaritans are available on: 0345 90 90 90

e-mail at jo@samaritans.org

web site http://www.samaritans.org

and at: 10 The Grove, Slough, SL1 1QP

Childline for children in trouble or danger

0800 1111

Further reading

JENKINS, R., et al. (eds) (1994) *The Prevention of Suicide*. London: HMSO.

ANOREXIA NERVOSA

The most important eating disorder which occurs mainly in adolescent girls is anorexia nervosa – a profound aversion to food. Particularly high prevalence figures have been noted among students of fashion (3.55%) and professional ballet students (8.6%) (Garner and Garfinkel, 1980). The individual loses weight and has a distorted body image, seeing herself as grotesquely fat even when thin and emaciated. The anorexic young woman sees starvation as a positive thing helping her to achieve the aim of being thin. The effects of starvation eventually lead to clinical signs. The young woman becomes weak and lethargic, with a slow pulse and blood pressure, menstruation ceases and in severe cases heart failure can occur. Factors associated with the condition are depression, dissatisfaction with life and a poor self-image, perfectionism. According to Wright (1991) the death rate from complications arising from anorexia is about 4%. Important aspects of management include:

- The establishment of rapport with all concerned.
- A firm, accepting, non-punitive approach. Adults involved in care must be supportive towards each other and united. Non-eating is not negotiable, and privileges may have to be dependent on eating or preferably gaining weight.
- It must not be possible for food to be disposed of, e.g. down the toilet.
- The possible use of family therapy once a target weight has been achieved.

PROMOTING MENTAL HEALTH IN CHILDREN AND YOUNG PEOPLE

A variety of measures have been identified which can contribute to the promotion of mental health and the prevention of problems.

Primary level

Offord (1987) suggests dividing primary measures into:

- *Milestone programmes* – these concentrate on children at particular ages of stages of development.
- *High-risk programmes* – aimed at children believed to be at above average risk for a disorder. These may include children admitted to hospital, children with chronic illness, bereaved children, abused children and those in the care of welfare agencies. Caplan (1980) encourages the use of positive steps to help children cope with crises such as admission to hospital involving anticipatory guidance (preparation) and preventive intervention (dealing with the here and now, understanding what is happening and developing coping skills).
- *Community-wide measures* – many factors associated with the community in which the child lives can influence the development of

---

Bulaemia

- An eating disorder similar to, and often associated with, anorexia nervosa
- Word is derived from Greek and means 'ox hunger'
- Characterised by repeated episodes of binge eating followed by a variety of weight controlling activities:
  - self-induced vomiting
  - diuretics
  - laxatives
  - rigorous exercise
- Eating episodes are followed by periods of depression and self-deprecation

---

Cross reference

Levels of health promotion – page 136

Other high-risk programmes may include

- Self-help groups for children with chronic illness
- Bereavement counselling
- Child guidance clinics
- Counselling clinics

---

a healthy emotional state and the development of mental health problems.

Measures to promote mental health include:

- Good obstetric and neonatal care to minimise the mental health problems associated with birth injury.
- Genetic counselling and screening.
- Parent craft sessions.
- Development screening.
- Life skills sessions for children to help them communicate effectively.
- School counselling services – schools play a very important role in the promotion of mental health. Faulconbridge and Spanswick (1995) give an account of how school nurses were helped to provide counselling to adolescents. The scheme enhanced the school nurses' ability to deal with problems and recognise the need for early referral.

Activity

Consider the potential role of the children's nurse in this level of mental health promotion. Design a programme to help your colleagues understand the need for mental health promotion.

Secondary level

This involves the early detection and treatment of mental health problems:

- Screening – screening for behavioural and emotional problems is considered part of the 1996 programme for child health (Hall, 1996). Whilst the difficulties associated with it are acknowledged, the important role of all those who work with children (particularly at preschool level) is recognised. In order to recognise behavioural and emotional problems in children primary care staff need to be aware of normal development and the variations that can be expected.
- Treatment of problems will be dependent on the type of problem as discussed earlier. Some interventions, for example managing minor problems, can often be dealt with successfully by health visitors. Others can be managed through counselling and guidance services. Others will need referral to specialist services.

In preventing mental health problems and promoting mental health it is important to recognise the role of healthy public policy. Many of the factors which influence the development of mental health problems are outside the control of the individual. Consideration needs to be given to such issues as:

Services for mental illness in children and young people

According to Kurtz (1992) the essential elements of service provision are:

- a multidisciplinary child and adolescent psychiatric service with a management team which coordinates the service and encourages liaison with other children's services
- an NHS base with appropriate secretarial and administrative support with access to database
- clearly identifiable budget within the control of the service manager
- a multidisciplinary team consisting of psychiatrists, psychologists, therapy staff, child psychiatry nurses and a specialist social worker
- a confidential service where information is only extended on a 'need to know basis'
- provided in a variety of settings other than health services – within social services, education and voluntary services

- poverty;
- the environment;
- child abuse;
- the family and dysfunction within it;
- unemployment;
- homelessness;
- education.

Activity

Explore any policies which exist to deal with any of the issues cited above. How well do they reflect the needs of the population?

In conclusion we must recognise the vital role of health promotion in the development of healthy minds as well as bodies. Children need to be encouraged to develop to their full potential and those who work with children and young people must be aware of the potential factors which can contribute to mental health problems in this age group.

13 CARE OF THE SICK NEONATE

INTRODUCTION

The advancement of medical technology, a deeper knowledge of neonatal physiology and the development of a research based body of nursing knowledge has led to vast improvements in the care of the sick neonate. This is evidenced by a dramatic fall in perinatal and neonatal mortality rates over recent years. However, the first 4 weeks after birth remains a vulnerable time for many babies. Indeed mortality rates are generally at their highest immediately after birth with 1:5 deaths under the age of 15 occurring in the first 24 hours of life (Kelmar *et al.*, 1995). One important risk factor is weight at birth. Infants weighing less than 1500 g are 100 times more likely to be stillborn or die within the first month of life than babies weighing 3000 g or more (Platt and Pharoah, 1996). Problems related to immaturity are identified as being the main cause of death in 50% of babies who die in the first 4 weeks of life. The other main cause of neonatal deaths is congenital abnormalities.

Table 13.1 gives an overview of some of the more common problems faced by the sick neonate. As there are too many to cover in detail, this section will concentrate on the main principles of managing care for the sick neonate.

GENERAL PRINCIPLES OF CARE FOR THE SICK NEONATE

Assessing the neonate

Assessment is perhaps one of the most important aspects of caring for the sick neonate. Skilled observation and monitoring with minimal disturbance are essential if the nurse is to detect any deterioration in a baby's condition. Figure 13.1 (page 545) shows the types of observations which may be made and some of the possible associated problems.

Vital signs are normally monitored using sophisticated cardio-respiratory monitors which allow continuous measurement of temperature, pulse, blood pressure and oxygen saturation. Arterial lines allow for regular blood sampling/monitoring without the need for traumatic venepuncture.

Activity

Make arrangements to visit a special care baby unit. Take time to find out about the different types of monitors available and what they can monitor.

Definitions

- *Neonate* – term given to describe a baby from day 1 to 27
- *Pre-term* – a baby born before the 37th completed week of gestation
- *Post-term* – a baby born during or after the 42nd completed weeks (294 days)
- *LFD/SFD* – light- or small-for-dates – a baby who weighs below the 10th percentile at birth (at any gestational age)
- *LBW* – low birth weight – a baby weighing less than 2.5 kg at birth
- *VLBW* – very low birth weight – a baby weighing less than 1.5 kg at birth
- *ELBW* – extremely low birth weight – a baby weighing less than 1.0 kg at birth

Further reading

Texts on care of neonates needing maximal intensive care:

CRAWFORD, D. and MORRIS, M. (1994) *Neonatal Nursing*. London: Chapman & Hall

NIXON, H. and O'DONNELL, B. (1992) *Essentials of Paediatric Surgery*. London: Butterworth Heinemann

ROBERTSON, N. R. C. (1993) *A Manual of Neonatal Intensive Care*. London: Hodder & Stoughton

Respiratory	Transient tachypnoea of the newborn Respiratory distress syndrome Congenital diaphragmatic hernia Choanal atresia Tracheo-oesophageal atresia Meconium inhalation Drug-induced respiratory depression
Gastro-intestinal	Jaundice Oesophageal atresia Imperforate anus Meconium ileus Gastroschisis Exompalous
Renal	Acute renal failure Chronic renal failure Congenital abnormalities, e.g. ectopic vesicae
Cardiac	Cardiac failure Tetralogy of Fallot Tricuspid atresia Coarctation of the aorta Transposition of the great vessels Ventricular septal defect Patent ductus arteriosus
Blood	ABO incompatibility Rhesus incompatibility
Nervous	Seizures Birth asphyxia and trauma Structural deformities, e.g. spina bifida, hydrocephalus Intracranial haemorrhage Meningitis Neonatal hypotonia
Infection	Neonatal septicaemia Thrush Conjunctivitis Omphalitis Necrotising enterocolitis HIV

Table 13.1

Common problems of the sick neonate

Temperature control

Under normal circumstances a neonate can maintain his body temperature within a small range. However, any significant environmental changes can compromise his condition considerably. Poor vaso-motor control of surface blood vessels means that vaso-constriction is less effective. This and a large surface area in relation to body weight make the conservation of heat more difficult for the neonate. Heat loss through radiation, convection, evaporation and conduction is therefore increased. The neonate's main method of heat production is non-shivering thermogenesis. This involves the metabolism of brown fat, found in the neck and abdomen. This fat has a high enzyme content and is capable of rapid conversion to energy and heat. This process is unique to infants and relies on the consumption of oxygen. Hypothermia will therefore increase a baby's oxygen consumption as he attempts to raise

Figure 13.1

Observing the sick neonate.

Cry
- excessive crying/abnormally quiet – infection
- high pitched cry – meningitis

Breathing patterns
- increased costal recession and grunt – RDS
- backward movement of head on inspiration; asymmetrical chest – pneumothorax
- dyspnoea
  - acidosis
  - obstructive problems
- dyspnoea during feeding
  - heart failure

Behaviour
- unusual lethargy or irritability – subtle signs of cardiac/respiratory distress
- lethargy and sleepiness – infection

Urine
- renal problems

Meconium – delayed passage
  - Hirschsprung
  - meconium ileus
  - obstruction

Colour
- pallor
- jaundice
- cyanosis

Posture
- hypotonia
  - common in ill babies
  - cerebral depression
  - Down's syndrome
  - neuromuscular disorder
- hypertonia
  - cerebral palsy
  - birth injury
  - drug addict mother

Convulsions
- repetitive jerky movements
- jitters
  - meningitis
  - hypoglycaemia
  - hypocalcaemia
  - birth injury

Vomiting
- bile stained – obstruction
- frothy mucoid – TOF
- blood stained – volvulus

Thermo-neutral environment

The environmental temperature at which an infant can maintain his rectal temperature at 37°C with minimal oxygen consumption

his temperature. This will in turn accentuate any existing hypoxaemia.

To avoid this a neonate must be nursed in a thermo-neutral environment. There is an ideal range of environmental temperature for each individual baby which will depend on his size (Table 13.2), whether he is nursed naked or clothed, in an incubator or in a cot.

Loss of heat through the four different methods can be reduced by:

- the use of Perspex shields or bubble sheeting in incubators, clothes such as hats – minimises heat loss through radiation;

- drying the baby immediately and thoroughly after birth and after washes – minimises heat loss through evaporation;

- never laying the baby on a cold surface (e.g. theatre table) as this increases heat loss through conduction – make use of warm blankets, sheepskins;

- minimising the number of times the portholes of the incubator are opened as this creates cool draughts increasing heat loss via convection.

Weight (g)	Age (hours)	Temperature range (°C)
<1200	0–24	34.0–35.4
	24–96	34.0–35.0
>2500	0–6	32–33.8
	6–24	31.4–33.8
	24–48	30.7–33.5
	48–96	29.8–32.8

Table 13.2

Suggested thermo-neutral environmental temperatures for infants in incubators. (Adapted from Klaus and Fanaroff, 1979.)

Particular care must be taken with pre-term and light-for-dates babies as they have small deposits of brown fat, little subcutaneous fat and a relatively larger surface area.

At the same time as preventing hypothermia it is important not to overheat the neonate. He will then attempt to lower his temperature by increasing respiratory rate and fluid losses by evaporation. This in turn can increase weight loss, dehydration and jaundice (Morris, 1994).

Activity

Investigate the various means of maintaining a neonate's temperature. What are the advantages and disadvantages of each one?

Infection control

The neonate is more prone to infection than older children and adults due to an immature immune system. The neonate has reduced immunoglobulin stores and lacks previous antigen exposure to infections (Hazinski, 1992). Premature infants may be deficient in immunoglobulin G (IgG) as passive immunity is normally passed across the placenta during the last trimester. Adult levels of IgG are not reached until about 4 years of age; adult levels of IgM are reached by about 2 years. Neonates have a reduced ability to make new antibodies and polymorphonuclear leukocyte function and stores are deficient during the first weeks of life (Wilson, 1986).

The most effective way of reducing cross infection in neonatal units is the use of strict and rigid handwashing routines. Parents must be taught the importance of thorough handwashing. Strict adherence to other infection control procedures must also be observed. Other aspects of care to prevent infection include (Kelmar *et al.*, 1995):

- isolating infected or potentially infected babies;
- floors, incubators and lockers must be regularly cleaned;
- breastfeeding should be encouraged with strict procedures for human milk banks;
- babies should not be crowded together;

Cross reference

Children with problems related to the immune system – page 487

- babies admitted from home should be regarded as potentially infected until proved otherwise;
- babies must be examined daily for signs of infection;
- visitors with active infections should keep away.

Activity

Critically examine the infection control procedures in your nearest special care baby unit. How do they compare with those on the ward?

It is important to note that neonatal infection is difficult to assess – there is not always accompanying fever and the baby may in fact become hypothermic. Other features are non-specific and include poor weight gain, reluctance to feed, jaundice, lethargy, irritability and tachypnoea.

Skin care and handling

The main principle of nursing sick neonates is minimal handling. Excessive handing can cause exhaustion – the skin is delicate and easily damaged. The smaller and more premature the infant the more the skin is prone to damage. Attention should be paid to minimising skin damage by careful cleansing and drying, the use of sheepskins, regular change of position, and careful positioning of tubes and wires. Small-for-dates babies tend to have very dry and cracked skin which is particularly prone to infection. Sunflower oil or baby lotion can be used to gently massage intact skin to prevent cracking (Morris, 1994).

Nappy changing need not be carried out frequently unless the nappy area is reddened, sore or excoriated. The use of tapes to secure tubes, drains and vascular lines cannot be avoided and some damage is almost inevitable. Consideration should therefore be given to the type of tape used and its application and removal. Care of the umbilicus varies between units. Some advocate the use of alcohol wipes and Sterzac (Bain, 1993), others advocate leaving the cord alone to heal. Whichever method is used, the umbilicus should be examined daily for signs of infection as it is a prime site for colonisation in the neonate, particularly when the infant is pre-term or has an umbilical catheter *in situ*.

Careful consideration should be given to positioning the pre-term infant. Pre-term infants demonstrate physiological muscle hypotonia which can lead to a flattened posture – the infant assumes a frog like position – due to the effects of gravity. According to Updike *et al.* (cited by Hallsworth, 1995) this can lead to pronounced extension leading to the development of 'toe walking'. Other effects of this flattened posture include rotation of the hips and problems with sitting and crawling due to shoulder girdle retraction (Georgioff and Bernbaum, 1986). The skull of the pre-term infant is usually thin, soft and rather pliable, and therefore liable to postural deformity. Prolonged immobility can therefore result in a narrow, elongated head which can be quite distressing for parents. The pre-term infant should be nursed in supported positions with hip support recommended in all positions (Hallsworth, 1995). Babies may be nursed prone, supine or on their side but no one position should be used for long periods of time. Support can be achieved through the use of rolls, sheepskins, water pillows and soft toys.

Managing nutrition

Meeting the infant's nutritional requirements is an important part of care. As each baby must be treated according to his individual requirements only the principles will be considered here. Points to consider when planning and implementing feeding regimes include:

- infants under 34 weeks' gestation have poorly coordinated sucking and swallowing reflexes – this makes them prone to reflux;
- neonates have a small stomach capacity (reduced even more in pre-term infants) with slow gastric emptying;
- small babies have poor energy reserves;
- an infant has a high metabolic rate requiring more calories per kilogram of body weight than an adult;
- gastric motility is reduced but gastric emptying is more rapid in neonates.

The method of feeding chosen will depend on the age, size and condition of the infant:

- *Parenteral feeding* – clinical indications for this method include the need for surgery, gut pathology such as necrotising enterocolitis (NEC) and an inability to tolerate enteral feeding due to gut immobility or immaturity (Dear, 1992). Babies weighing less than 2000 g are likely to require this type of nutrition initially.
- *Enteral feeding* – clinical indications for this method include any baby who has considerable difficulty in sucking or is unable to suck (Kelmar *et al.*, 1995). Feeds can be passed through a tube into the stomach, jejunum or duodenum. The tube may be passed through the nose or through the mouth. Although nasal tubes are easier to secure in place, Sporik (1994) suggests that the presence of such a tube increases mucosal oedema and secretions which compromises an already narrow nasal airway. Research by Greenspan *et al.* (1990) and van Someren *et al.* (1984) shows that infants weighing less than 2000 g with nasal tubes have more periodic breathing, central apnoea and lower transcutaneous oxygen tension values when compared with those fed by oral tubes. Enteral feeding may be given by continuous infusion or by intermittent gavage. When using gastric feeding the stomach should be aspirated every 3–4 hours to ensure that milk is not collecting in the stomach, as the risk of aspiration into the lungs is high.

Aims of good positioning

The aims of good positioning are to:
- stimulate active flexion of the trunk and limbs
- achieve more rounded heads
- encourage a balance between extension and flexion
- allow for more symmetrical postures
- enhance midline orientation (contributes to hand–eye co-ordination)
- facilitate smooth anti-gravity limb movement

(Updike *et al.*, cited by Hallsworth 1995)

Prone position

It is acknowledged that the use of the prone position in the term infant nursed at home is to be discouraged due to its association with Sudden Infant Death Syndrome (SID). However, its use in the special care baby unit is permissible where a baby is closely monitored. The prone position has been shown to improve oxygenation, lung mechanics and volume, reduce energy expenditure, gastric reflux and the risk of aspiration

(Merenstein and Gardner, 1979)

Cross references

Enteral feeding – page 329
Parenteral feeding – page 332

Necrotising enterocolitis

The most commonly acquired gastrointestinal problem among sick neonates (Hylton Rushton, 1990). The cause is unclear but it is thought that there is reduced blood flow to the gut due to hypoxaemia, hypogly-caemia or hypothermia. This in turn leads to mucosal oedema and ulceration allowing colonisation by Gram-negative organisms (e.g. *Escherichia coli, Klebsiella*)

- *Oral feeding* – breastfeeding or bottle-feeding can be introduced whenever the baby demonstrates an ability to suck and when his condition allows (e.g. after surgery). Patience and support will be needed for the mother who wishes to breastfeed particularly when this has been delayed for some time. Encouraging mothers to express breastmilk for their pre-term and sick infants will help with the establishment of breastfeeding when the baby is ready. The use of breastmilk for sick and pre-term infants should be actively encouraged as its benefits (both long and short term) have been clearly documented (Lucas *et al.*, 1989, 1990; Lucas and Cole, 1990). It may be feasible for some babies to alternate oral and enteral feeding to give an opportunity for the baby to rest, particularly if feeds are frequent.

Activity

Arrange to visit a dietician to talk about the nutritional needs of pre-term and light-for-dates babies.

Managing pain and discomfort

Cross reference

Care of children in pain – page 348

Although much attention has been focused on pain in infancy and childhood there are still concerns about the management of pain in neonates. According to Sparshott (1994) those who suggest that neonates do not feel pain do so perhaps to assuage their own guilt at having to inflict pain on tiny infants. There is increasing evidence to show that neonates do respond to pain, be it acute, extreme or chronic (Figure 13.2).

Pain in neonates should be assessed using an appropriate tool. Horgan *et al.* (1996) looked particularly at post-operative distress in neonates and devised a tool to assess the effectiveness of various

Figure 13.2

Neonate response to pain and discomfort.

Facial expression	**Crying**
• furrowed brow • flared nostrils • unnaturally open mouth • eyes tightly shut • pallor	• sudden long and strong initial cry – then long period of silence (apnoea) short gasping inhalations
Temperaure • deficit between core and peripheral temperature – stress	**Palmar sweating** • during painful procedure from 37 weeks
Body movements • violent thrashing/extension of all extremes, sometimes withdrawal of affected limb from site of injury	**Respirations** • hyperventilation • decreased rate • apnoea

Figure 13.3

Minimising pain and discomfort for neonates.

Attendance to light and sound levels
- dimmer switches
- day and night light
- noise reduction
- gentle voice
- careful use of radio

Infusions/blood taking
- good techniques
- mechanical lancets
- careful siting of IVs

Clothing
- swaddling
- barriers against which to rest – gives security
- warmth

Analgesia
- morphine
- paracetamol

Minimal handling
- allowing periods of rest

Equipment
- careful siting of electrodes, tubes, etc., and use of strappings

analgesic protocols. They suggest that it is possible to score an infant's behavioural responses to an operation over a period of 24 hours. Sparshott (1995) describes a framework against which to assess the behaviour of the pre-term infant. She suggests that through behaviour the infant can show when he wants to be left to rest and when he is ready for stimulation.

Figure 13.3 gives some ideas on how to minimise pain and discomfort for neonates.

Activity

Find out if your local special care baby unit uses specific assessment tools for assessing pain in neonates. If they do, critically compare them with those used for older infants and children.

Managing unstable blood sugars

Infants have high glucose needs and low glycogen stores so often develop hypoglycaemia during periods of stress. In fact hypoglycaemia is quite common during the first 48 hours of life (Johnston, 1994). What exactly constitutes hypoglycaemia seems to be controversial ranging from 1.6 to 2.6 mmol/l in term babies and from 1.1 to 1.4 mmol/l in low birth weight babies. Balfour-Lynn and Valman (1993) suggest that it is sensible to opt for the higher safety margin.

Activity

What does your unit/ward classify as hypoglycaemia in a term neonate? Note your findings in the margin for future reference.

Causes of hypoglycaemia

- Small-for-dates babies
- Infants of diabetic mothers
- Poor feeding/delayed feeding
- Severe birth asphyxia
- Sick babies where the illness is severe
- Haemolytic disease of the newborn
- Polycythaemia
- Inborn errors of metabolism

Prolonged low blood glucose levels can cause brain damage – leading to developmental abnormalities including cerebral palsy and severe mental retardation. The aim of management should be to prevent hypoglycaemia in all babies. This can be achieved by commencing feeding within 4 hours of birth. Falling blood glucose levels in sick neonates can be counteracted by smaller more frequent enteral feeding or intravenous infusion. Clinical signs of jitteriness, apnoea, cyanosis or fits may or may not be obvious. If a baby demonstrates any of these signs a bolus of glucose needs to be given urgently and followed by a dextrose infusion. Certain groups of babies are more prone to develop hypoglycaemia and their capillary blood glucose should be monitored 4 hourly initially.

Managing jaundice

Jaundice occurs in 80% of pre-term babies and up to 50% of term babies (Crawford, 1994). It is a symptom of underlying pathology and is a yellow discoloration of the skin and mucous membranes which occurs when serum bilirubin is raised.

Activity

Before reading on please take time to refresh your knowledge of the metabolism of bile pigments. Figure 13.4 might help you.

There are many varied causes of jaundice in the neonatal period which can be classified as:

- *Jaundice occurring at birth or within 24 hours*. This type of jaundice is often associated with haemolysis of red cells as a result of

Figure 13.4

Metabolism of bile pigments.

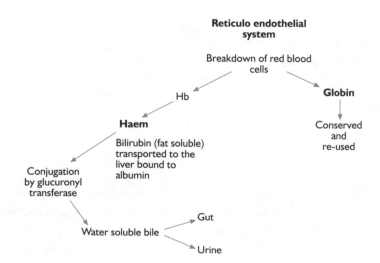

incompatibility. The level of unconjugated bilirubin rises and the cause should be investigated immediately.

- *Jaundice occurring from days 2 to 5.* Physiological jaundice is accepted as 'normal'. It occurs as a result of a temporary deficiency in the levels of glucuronyl transferase in the newborn. At the same time there is a rapid breakdown of fetal red cells after birth. There is a consequent rise in unconjugated bilirubin levels. Serum levels usually peak by about day 3/4 and are normal by day 10/11.
- *Prolonged jaundice.* In these cases there may be a rise in either conjugated or unconjugated bilirubin or both.

It is important to assess serum bilirubin levels particularly if there is a rise in *unconjugated* bilirubin. High levels of fat soluble unconjugated bilirubin can pass across the blood–brain barrier and cause kernicterus – damage to the basal ganglia and brain stem (deSa, 1995). Clinical signs include opisthotonous, limb rigidity, tremors or convulsions and fever. Infants who survive kernicterus can present with mental retardation, deafness and other neurological problems (deSa, 1995). According to Balfour-Lynn and Valman (1993) neurological problems are unlikely to occur when the serum bilirubin is less than 170 mmol/l even in babies under 1250 g. However, Johnston (1994) suggests that any jaundice which results in serum levels of over 200 mmol/l should be investigated while Kelmar *et al.* (1995) advocates investigating serum levels over 150 mmol/l at 2 weeks of age.

Activity

At what level would your local special care baby unit investigate jaundice? Note your findings in the margin for future reference.

Treatment for jaundice includes:

- *Exchange transfusion* – an effective rapid means of removing bilirubin from the blood particularly if serum levels are near danger point. This procedure may now be done *in utero*.
- *Phototherapy* – this treatment can often prevent unconjugated bilirubin from rising to danger levels. The infant is placed under fluorescent light tubes which emit blue light which converts bilirubin in the skin to harmless water soluble metabolites. These are then excreted in the urine and bowel.

Nursing management of babies having phototherapy must take account of the following:

- The baby must be nursed naked to maximise the area of skin exposed to the light – maintenance of temperature is important.
- The use of phototherapy often provokes anxiety in parents. Full explanations must be given.

Causes of jaundice occurring at birth or within the first 24 hours
- ABO incompatibility
- Rhesus incompatibility
- Congenital infection
- Haemolytic anaemia, e.g. sickle cell anaemia

Causes of jaundice occurring between day 2 and 5
- Physiological jaundice
- Drugs
- Infection
- Metabolic diseases
- Excessive bruising

Causes of prolonged jaundice
- Breastmilk jaundice
- Neonatal hepatitis
- Bilary atresia
- Endocrine disorders

– Radiation from blue light has been shown to cause retinal damage in animal experiments. The baby's eyes must therefore be protected by the use of eye shields or a tinted screen. The protection must be checked regularly as small babies can often wriggle out from under the screen or push off eye shields.

– There is often increased fluid loss from the skin during phototherapy. The treatment can also decrease bowel transit time leading to diarrhoea. Jaundiced infants are often drowsy and do not always wake for feeds. Consideration must therefore be given to increasing fluid intake.

Activity

Investigate the types of phototherapy equipment used in your special care baby unit. Examine the advantages and disadvantages of each.

PLANNING FOR DISCHARGE

Planning for discharge should ideally begin as soon as a neonate is admitted to the unit. Going home with a small baby or one that has been very ill can be a daunting prospect for any parent. Some hospitals have transitional care wards where the babies are cared for by their parents under supervision from the nurses. This can help to build confidence and allow the parents time to adjust to their baby. Each family is unique and will have unique needs so a careful teaching plan should be drawn up to ensure that all aspects of the baby's care are covered. Some babies will go home with continuing care needs such as oxygen therapy, gastrostomy feeding, colostomies, wound dressings. In these cases parents will need support from community children's nurses. Some areas have special community nurses whose role is mainly to visit and support parents with special care babies in the first few days and weeks at home. Whichever type of support is available the nurse must take time to develop a trusting relationship with the family. Voluntary support agencies such as Blisslink/Nippers (17–21 Emerald Street, London WC1N 3QL, Tel: 0171 831 9393) give valuable written information and are able to put parents in touch with other families with similar problems. Other voluntary organisations exist for some of the special problems such as tracheo-oesophageal fistula (TOF).

Cross reference

Home oxygen therapy – page 524

Activity

Visit a special care baby unit and find out what resources are available to support parents and their babies on discharge from the unit.

LONG-TERM PROBLEMS FOR SICK NEONATES

The vast majority of pre-term babies who survive do so with no medical, physiological or psychological problems. However, other evidence shows that the younger the gestation, the higher incidence of long-term problems (Cooke, 1994; Morell, 1994). Potential problems faced by these babies include:

- *Neurological problems.* Cerebral palsy, developmental delay, severe learning difficulties, sensory, visual motor and attentional problems, hydrocephalus, microcephaly, blindness, deafness and epilepsy. Some children display more subtle problems such as lower than average IQ, clumsiness, poor hand–eye coordination and poor speech articulation, behavioural problems.

- *Respiratory problems.* Bronchopulmonary dysplasia – a chronic inflammatory lung disease characterised by an increased oxygen demand. It occurs in pre-term infants who have been mechanically ventilated.

- *Sensory problems.* Retinopathy of prematurity – this normally occurs in babies who are less than 30/32 weeks' gestation as a result of raised partial pressure of oxygen in arterial blood. This damages the retinal blood vessel network causing blindness.

- *Nutritional problems.* Weak and uncoordinated suck, prolonged tube feeding, delayed weaning, poor weight gain, aneamia of prematurity, gastro-oesophageal reflux.

All infants who have spent time in the special care baby unit need close follow-up to:

- assess growth and development;
- detect complications;
- detect emergence of problems related to new treatments;
- provide reassurance to parents and give continuing advice and support.

Further reading

LUDHAM, L. (1992) Emotional development after major neonatal surgery. *Paediatric Nursing*, May, 20–22.

14 PRINCIPLES OF CARE – CHILDREN UNDERGOING CYTOTOXIC TREATMENT AND RADIOTHERAPY

INTRODUCTION

Childhood malignancies are rare, affecting only 1:600 children under 16 years (Hollis, 1997) and in 1996 Hawkins estimated that 60–65% of children in Britain who were diagnosed with cancer would survive. Over the last 20 years there has been a huge improvement in the survival rates of children with cancer largely due to cytotoxic therapy. Chemotherapy for the treatment of childhood cancers really began in the 1970s and since then new, complex and multidrug regimes have evolved and contributed to the steady rise in cure rates. The most promising results have been demonstrated in children with acute lymphoblastic leukaemia (ALL) but solid tumours of childhood have also responded well to cytotoxic drugs when used in conjunction with radiotherapy and surgery (Hollis, 1997). Leukaemia is the most common cancer of children of all ages, accounting for one-third of all childhood cancers.

The acute leukaemias comprise over half of the leukaemias seen in clinical practice. Eighty per cent of leukaemias in children are of the acute lymphoblastic type. The incidence of ALL is highest at 3–4 years, falling off by 10 years. There is a low frequency after 10 years with a secondary rise after 40 years of age. Acute myeloid leukaemias (AML) occur in all age groups but are more common in adults and form only a fraction of childhood leukaemias.

The prognosis of acute leukaemia in children has been greatly improved by the use of chemotherapy, radiotherapy, better supportive therapy and the development of specialist leukaemia units.

* 30–50% of children with ALL are now alive and have been off treatment 5 years from presentation;
* relapsed disease is more difficult to treat, and has a worse prognosis;
* AML progress in treatment has not been as good as ALL.

As drug therapy plays the main role in the treatment of many cancers it is important to understand what action each drug has in order that nursing care can be given accordingly. The drugs fall into five main areas (Tables 14.1–14.4):

* Cytotoxic therapy – the curative part of the treatment.
* Prophylactic drugs – to prevent or minimise the effects of cytotoxic therapy.
* IV antibiotics – to treat isolated or suspected infections.
* Pre- and bone marrow transplant drugs – to prevent 'graft versus

Table 14.1

Drugs used to treat childhood cancers

Drug	Mechanism of action	Specific side effects	Nursing care
Cyclophosphamide	Alkylating agent	Severe haemorrhagic cystitis, cardiomyopathy, alopecia	MESNA infusion runs concurrently (this inactivates the toxin acrotion) Give dose early morning to enable high fluid intake later Test all urine for blood, pH and sugar Ensure a high urine output is maintained
Methotrexate	Antimetabolite – inhibits the formation of folic acid, essential for metabolism pneumonitis, and DNA synthesis	Severe gut toxicity, liver and renal damage, CNS toxicity, pneumonitis, mouth ulcers	Gut toxicity is reduced by the administration of 'folinic acid' (calcium leucovorin rescue); if this is not given after a high dose of methotrexate the toxicity may be fatal Observe for signs of neurotoxicity Avoid the use of folic acid-containing vitamins
Cytosine arabinoside (cytarabine)	Antimetabolite – a powerful depressant of bone marrow function	Hyperuricaemia, liver damage, gut toxicity, haemolytic anaemia, conjunctivitis	Observe for sore eyes, jaundice
6-mercaptopurine	Antimetabolite – has a valuable suppressive action in acute leukaemia and can produce a remission of the disease; however, response to a repeated course may be less dramatic and repeated treatment leads eventually to a refractory state unresponsive to further treatment	Unusual – hyperuricaemia, liver damage	None specific
6-thioguanine	Antimetabolite – similar to 6-mercaptopurine, but mainly used in AML; a powerful myelo-suppressive drug	As for 6-mercaptopurine	None specific
Doxorubicin (adriamycin)	Cytotoxic antibiotic – binds with DNA to interfere with mitosis	Cardiac toxicity, causing tachycardia and arrythmias, alopecia, colours urine red (but this is not significant)	ECG monitoring, warn child and parents of red urine up to 12 days after administration
Daunorubicin	Cytotoxic antibiotic -similar to doxorubicin	As for doxorubicin	As for doxorubicin
Vincristine	Vinka alkaloid	Neuropathy (peripheral, bladder or gut), abdominal colic, constipation and alopecia	Observe for signs of neurotoxicity, monitor bowel movements, administer stool softeners (e.g. lactolose)
Etanoside (VP16-231)	Miscellaneous – similar to the vinka alkaloids as it is a mitotic inhibitor	Alopecia, oral ulceration, hypotension, bradycardia, allergic reaction (rare)	Give slowly as IV infusion with emergency drugs available to treat anaphylaxis and/or shock
L-asparaginase	Miscellaneous – an enzyme which derives the cells of asparaginase	Allergic reactions (urticaria, hypotension, anaphylaxis), fever, anorexia and weight loss, low albumin, pancreatitis, renal and liver dysfunction	Daily weight, emergency drugs available to treat anaphylaxis

Mucositis

All patients are commenced on the following drugs on diagnosis and continue them throughout periods of chemotherapy:

- amphoteracin suspension – anti-fungal prophylaxis of mouth
- betadine/chlorhexidine mouthwash – for prevention of mucosal sepsis
- ciprofloxacillin – used instead of neomycin in patients over 14 years old
- colistin – useful to prevent Gram-negative infection of the intestine
- flucanazole – an oral triazole anti-fungal used as prophylaxis against local and systemic candidiasis and cryptococcal infections
- neomycin – an aminoglycoside antibiotic used to prevent intestinal infection

Herpes

Acyclovir is given to all bone marrow transplant patients with pre-transplant IgC antibodies to the herpes simplex virus. It is given for 100 days from transplant. It is also used for patients who have had contact with chickenpox. It is an antiviral drug which is inactive until it enters a virus infected site. It is then activated by a viral enzyme to form acyclovir phosphate, which blocks the replication of viral DNA

Tuberculosis (TB)

Prophylaxis with isoniazid is required for 6 months post BMT if there is a previous history of TB or an abnormal chest X-ray. Isonazid is a highly selective antibacterial drug which has virtually no action against organisms other than *Myobacterium tuberculosis*. It is rapidly absorbed and penetrates easily into the tissues and fluids, including the cerebrospinal fluid. As it is thought to interfere with normal pyridotine metabolism, pyroxodine is also given

P. neumocistis carinii

Prophylactic treatment with Septrin is required for all BMT patients for 1 week prior to transplant and 6 months post transplant (or until counts increase). Septrin acts as an antibacterial agent by a combination of blocking the formation of folic acid and preventing its conversion to folinic acid

Other infections

Other than the specific treatments listed above, the following are the most commonly used prophylactic drugs:

- **amikacin** – a semi-synthetic aminoglycoside, effective against Gram-negative organisms and some staphylococcal infections
- **amphoteracin B** – is the most effective drug for the treatment of deep fungal infections such as cryptococcosis, histoplasmosis and systemic candidiasis
- **azlocillin** – a broad spectrum antibiotic with significant anti-pseudomonal activity
- **ceftazidime** – a bacterial cephalosporin antibiotic, active against a wide range of Gram-positive and gram-negative bacteria
- **erythromycin** – effective against Gram-positive and a few Gram-negative organisms. Active against many respiratory infections, including *Mycoplasma pneumoniae*. Useful against penicillin-resistant organisms
- **metronidazole** – effective against anaerobic infections, e.g. peritonitis
- **vancomycin** – effective against many Gram-positive organisms and severe staphylococcal or streptococcal infections which do not respond to other antibiotics

host' disease and to stimulate the action of the new bone marrow.

- Miscellaneous drugs – to correct or prevent the complications of the treatment or illness or given as part of the non-cytotoxic curative treatment.

CYTOTOXIC TREATMENT

The aim of cytotoxic treatment is initially to induce a remission (absence of any clinical or laboratory evidence of the disease) and then to continue to reduce the hidden malignant cell population by repeated courses of therapy. Cyclical combinations of two, three or four drugs are

MODULE 6 Specific care of sick children

Anti-human granulocyte colony (ALG) stimulating factor
Used in haematology to treat severe aplastic anaemia or to treat 'graft versus host' disease post BMT. It is a purified solution of horse anti-human lymphocyte immunoglobulin. It is obtained by hyper-immunisation of horses with human lymphocytes. Thus, its acts by attacking lymphocytes and causes immunosuppression. It requires monitoring during infusion for signs of fever, hypotension, respiratory distress and urticaria. (ATG, which is a rabbit serum derivative may be used where there is intolerance to horse proteins)

Campath
This is an unlicensed investigational drug. It is used prior to bone marrow transplantation in order to prevent graft rejection or 'graft versus host'. It contains an antibody to human lymphocytes and monocytes which is produced in rats, and hence is an immunosuppressive. As it is a rat protein it may provoke hyper-sensitive reactions when the test dose is given, and monitoring is required during the infusion of further doses. Side effects include fever, chills, rigors, nausea, urticaria, bronchospasm and hypotension

Cyclosporin 'A'
An immunosuppressive agent which will reduce the risk of 'graft versus host' disease. It has a selective action on the T lymphocytes (which react with foreign proteins), but unlike other immunosuppressive drugs it does not depress the general bone marrow activity

Human granulocyte colony stimulating factor (G-CSF)
Is a glycoprotein which regulates the production and release of function neutrophils from the bone marrow. It is used post BMT or following a period of prolonged neutropenia post-chemotherapy. Marked increases in peripheral blood neutrophil counts can occur within 24 hours. G-CSF is usually restricted to non-myeloid leukaemia because of the possibility of its action causing an increase of malignant cells. However, this has not been established. Specific side effects include mild or moderate musculoskeletal pain and dysuria

Table 14.3

Pre- and post-bone marrow transplant drugs

given with treatment-free intervals to allow the bone marrow to recover. This recovery depends upon the differential re-growth pattern of normal haemoietic and malignant cells.

There are five types of cytotoxic drugs:

- *Alkylating agents* – act on the nucleus of the cell and cause DNA strands to break or cross-link abnormally, preventing normal DNA replication and cell growth.
- *Antimetabolites* – replace cell metabolites or inhibit their activity so that the normal cell growth is interrupted.
- *Cytotoxic antibiotic* – (similar to alkylating agents), as they break down the system of DNA/RNA replication and interfere with protein synthesis. Appear to increase sensitivity to radiation therapy.
- *Vinca alkaloids* – inhibit cell division at the metaphase stage of chromosome separation and so have a growth-inhibiting action.
- *Miscellaneous drugs* – a group of ill-defined, unrelated substances that have a cytotoxic action.

Prednisolone, vincristine and asparaginase are the drugs usually used in ALL to achieve remission in over 90% of children in 4–6 weeks. Daunorubicin or doxorubicin (adriamycin) is added to the regimen either in the induction phase or in the consolidation once remission has been achieved. The following carry a less favourable prognosis:

- males compared to females;

559

Table 14.4

Miscellaneous drugs used in oncology

Allopurinol
Given post-chemotherapy to reduce uric acid formation which is produced by the breakdown of neoplastic cells. As there is mass cell destruction after a course of chemotherapy, increased uric acid may cause gout to develop. Allopurinol prevents this by inhibiting the action of an enzyme concerned with purine metabolism and so indirectly reduces uric acid formation

Amiloride
A potassium sparing mild diuretic which is usually given to reduce potassium loss during a course of amphoteracin

Analgesics
A variety are used according to the severity of the pain

Anti-emetics
Should be given regularly during courses of chemotherapy. Metoclopramide is used in children only for the severe nausea associated with cytotoxic therapy due to potential acute dystonic reactions. Ondansetron is a more effective, longer lasting anti-emetic, the action of which may be enhanced by dexamethasone

Azothiaprine
Has a marked depressant effect on the bone marrow and hence slows the disease process

Piriton and hydrocortisone
May be used prophylactically prior to the administration of blood derivatives whan previous reactions have occurred. They may also be used to minimise reactions to ALG/ATG and campath

Prednisolone
A glucocorticosteroid which increases the resistance of the body to stress and shock and has the power of suppressing the inflammatory processes generally. It inhibits the development of lymphocytes and in leukaemia a high degree of remission of symptoms may result. Although it cannot prevent an ultimate relapse, as well as initiating a remission it may restore a sensitivity to other forms of treatment. Side effects include delayed tissue repair, increased gastric acidity causing or exacerbating peptic ulcers, electrolyte imbalance, muscle wasting, loss of calcium, hypertension, Cushing's syndrome and diabetes

Ranitidine
May be used for either active or prophylactic treatment of peptic ulcers/mucositis. Unlike antacids which neutralise the gastric acid, ranitidine acts by inhibiting gastric acid secretion and pepsin output. This is done by blocking the histamine H_2 receptors which are chiefly found in the gastric parietal cells and are concerned with acid and pepsin secretion. Conventional antihistamines only block the H_1 receptors, hence cannot inhibit the acid secretion response to histamine

Vitamin and mineral supplements
Required to overcome the poor nutritional intake associated with the toxic effects of chemotherapy as well as the deficiencies caused by the intensive drug therapy. The commonly used supplements include pyridoxine (B_6), vitamin K, Parentrovite, folic acid, Sando K, Sando Cal and Sando-phosphate

- those with an initial high leukocyte count;
- meningeal involvement at presentation;
- very young (under 2 years) or older (adolescent or adult) patients.

In all these cases, more intensive induction regimens improve chances of long-term survival. Maintenance chemotherapy usually follows for 2–3 years with daily mercaptopurine and weekly methotrexate (vincristine, steroids and other drugs are added in some cases).

Cytoxic therapy for AML is similar to that of ALL, but with worst results. The most commonly used regimen for AML is cytosine, daunorubicin and 6-thioguanine. Compared with ALL the:

- remission rate is lower (60–80%);
- remission often takes longer to achieve;
- myelotoxic drugs are of major value, with less selectivity between leukaemic and normal marrow cells;
- marrow failure is severe and prolonged;
- remissions are shorter, maintenance therapy is less effective.

Central nervous system prophylaxis is not routinely given in AML, although intrathecal methotrexate may be used as a prophylactic.

Drugs used for their cytotoxic action are not selective and therefore their effect on rapidly dividing malignant cells is duplicated on healthy cells which have a high rate of proliferation. These include the cells of the bone marrow, hair, skin and the epithelial cells of the gastro-intestinal tract. Problems caused by the destruction of these healthy cells are often more debilitating and traumatic to the child than the disease itself.

The actual administration of cytotoxic drugs is potentially dangerous. Many of these drugs are sclerosing agents which can cause severe cellular damage if extravasation occurs. The resulting inflammation and ulceration can progress slowly over several weeks. They should only be administered by specialist nurses using a patent vein which has been initially tested with isotonic saline. The injection site should be constantly observed for signs of infiltration and irrigated with saline after the administration to avoid leakage of the drug as the needle is removed. Suspected extravasation can be treated by:

Cross reference

IV fluid therapy – page 341

- cessation of administration;
- changing the syringe but leaving the needle in place and withdrawing as much of the drug as possible;
- 100 mg hydrocortisone infiltrated into the surrounding tissue;
- immediate application of warm compresses to the site to increase circulation and absorption of the drug into the bloodstream;
- cold compresses after one hour to relieve pain and swelling;
- referral to a plastic surgery team.

In addition, many cytotoxic drugs may cause an anaphylactic reaction. After administration, the child should be observed for at least 20 minutes and emergency equipment must be close at hand. If a reaction is suspected the administration should be discontinued and the line flushed with isotonic saline.

Many children have a surgically inserted indwelling intravenous access line to overcome the problems of repeated venous access required for intensive courses of cytotoxic therapy, blood analysis and the frequent administration of blood products. However, blood required to monitor antibiotic levels must be taken peripherally to ensure accuracy (Pinkerton *et al.*, 1996).

Skin care during radiotherapy

Do:

- use soft loose clothing
- keep the area clean, using only water to wash
- dress moist areas with non-adherent dressings, tubular bandages and non-allergic tape
- apply prescribed cream to area at least twice daily until the skin has returned to normal
- use sunscreen with a protection factor of 15 or more

Don't:

- rub or massage the area
- alter or wash off the indelible marks which delineate the area for treatment
- expose the area to the sun during treatment and for up to a year after treatment
- use perfumes, deodorants or perfumed toiletries on the area

RADIOTHERAPY

Radiotherapy is usually used to treat or relieve childhood cancer in conjunction with chemotherapy and/or surgery. It may be beneficial in palliative care because its action shrinks tumours and thus reduces symptoms. It is the palliative treatment of choice for isolated bone secondaries as it relieves pain and prevents pathological fractures. Radiotherapy has a cytotoxic effect by:

- damaging the pyrosine bases essential for nucleic acid synthesis;
- causing breaks in DNA or RNA molecules.

Side effects of radiotherapy are mostly due to the cytotoxic effects of radiation but the specific problem is skin damage. The affected area of skin and mucous membranes can initially become blanched or erythematous, later reactions include dryness, itching, peeling, blistering and loss of tissue. The area targeted for radiation should be monitored daily to enable early recognition and treatment of problems.

SIDE EFFECTS OF CYTOTOXIC TREATMENT AND RADIOTHERAPY

Cytotoxic treatment and radiotherapy have many side effects but the most life threatening is bone marrow depression (Table 14.5). Overwhelming infection may occur secondary to neutropenia and thrombocytopenia may cause haemorrhage. The child is most at risk from infection:

- at the time of diagnosis when the leukocytes have been largely replaced by malignant cells;
- during immunosuppressive treatment;
- after prolonged antibiotic treatment when resistant organisms may develop.

The child undergoing cytotoxic treatment will often not show the usual overt features of infection and the first sign may be pyrexia. The care of neutropenic children is usually outlined in strict local protocols which usually include protective isolation. However, research shows that such isolation neither decreases the infection risk nor improves survival (Frenck *et al.*, 1991). Reasonable precautions should be continued at home to protect the child from infection but this has to be moderated by the need for the child to resume a normal lifestyle which includes returning to school. Haematopoietic growth factors have recently been produced in the laboratory to stimulate the bone marrow and reduce the duration of high dose cytotoxic therapy induced neutropenia. Haemorrhage associated with thrombocytopenia can be prevented by the administration of platelets whenever the platelet count falls below 20. Packed red cells are usually transfused when the haemoglobin falls below 8 g.

Problem	Effect	Intervention
Due to bone marrow failure		
anaemia	Pallor, lethargy, dyspnoea	Blood transfusions
leucopenia	Fever, malaise, infections of mouth, throat, skin, lungs and risk of septicaemia	Isolation or clean care, antibiotics for specific infections, clean food
thrombocytopenia	Spontaneous bruising, purpura, bleeding gums and major haemorrhage risk	Platelet infusions, mouth care and mouth washes
Due to organ infiltration of		
bones	Joint pain, lytic bone lesions	Analgesia
lymph glands	Superficial lymphadenopathy	Analgesia
spleen	Moderate splenomegaly	Analgesia
liver	Hepatomegaly	Analgesia
gums	Gum hypertrophy	Action to minimise localised infection
bowel	Rectal ulceration	
skin	Skin involvement	
central nervous system	Headaches, nausea and vomiting, blurred vision diplopia, papilloedema, and haemorrhage	Intrathecal chemotherapy
testes	Swelling	Localised radiotherapy
Due to combined effect of above		
anorexia, nausea and vomiting	Loss of weight and muscle wasting	Anti-emetics, high calorie drinks and diet
long-term hospitalisation and effects of treatment (e.g. alopecia)	Delayed development, psychological problems of patient and parents	Involvement of psychosocial team, teaching staff and play leaders
long-term prognosis	Anxiety for family	Support of whole family

Table 14.5

Nursing care of children with cancer undergoing cytotoxic treatment or radiotherapy

Care of the pyrexial neutropenic child

Identify any potential sources of infection:
- central line site
- mucosal ulceration
- skin tears, abrasions
- blood, stool, urine and naso-pharyngeal cultures
- chest X-ray

Treat the infection:
- IV administration of a combination of broad spectrum antibiotics for a minimum of 10 days

Prevent further infection:
- protective isolation
- restriction of visitors with infection or history of contact
- varicella immunoglobin (ZIG) within 48 hours for children who have been exposed to chickenpox

Cross reference

Dental hygiene – page 184

Nausea and vomiting are probably the most distressing side effects of chemotherapy (Knapman, 1993) and the most difficult to control. A small study by Cook and Gallagher in 1996 revealed that chemotherapy induced nausea and vomiting is poorly controlled and remains a challenge to children's nursing. However, for the children themselves, it appears that alopecia is the most traumatic side effect of cytotoxic treatment (Reid, 1997). Wigs are available but most children prefer to wear hats, caps or scarves. Some kind of head protection is important to prevent hypothermia or over-heating and sunburn. Children can be reassured that regrowth usually occurs in 3–6 months but should be warned that the new hair is often darker, thicker and curlier than before.

Porter (1994) suggests that 90% of children undergoing chemotherapy experience oral complications. The cause of this is not only the direct cytotoxic effect on the rapidly dividing cells of the oral mucosa but also the child's susceptibility to oral infections due to neutropenia, thrombocytopenia, anorexia and malnutrition. It may be also due to poor recognition of the problem. Campbell (1987) indicated that nurses did not have the knowledge to assess oral complications of cytotoxic therapy. Since then various assessment tools have been developed to assess and score the condition of the mouth (Table 14.6) and the importance of prophylactic mouth care has been recognised. Pinkerton *et al.* (1996)

Table 14.6

Oral assessment scoring scale

Assessment	Scoring		
	1	2	3
Listening to child talking or crying	Normal	Deep or hoarse	Difficulty/pain when talking or crying
Observation of swallowing	Normal	Some pain	Inability to swallow
Looking and feeling the lips and corners of the mouth	Smooth, pink and moist	Dry and/or cracked	Ulcerated or bleeding
Looking at the tongue	Pink, moist with obvious papilla	Coated or smooth and shiny	Blistered or cracked

recommend 6 hourly teeth cleaning with a soft toothbrush and toothpaste (and sterile water if neutropenic), Corsodyl mouthwash held in the mouth for 30–60 seconds and Fluconazole.

Anorexia is often a side effect of cytotoxic therapy which may be related to a sore mouth, nausea and vomiting, constipation or anxiety and depression. It appears to distress parents more than the child (Brady, 1994). Steroids will sometimes alleviate anorexia but their side effects often outweigh their benefits especially if the anorexia is not concerning the child. An altered sense of taste may change the child's usual likes and dislikes and it may need some experimentation to re-stimulate the appetite. Small, frequent and varied snacks may help the child to eat. Poor nutrition not only affects the child's general well-being but also exacerbates the child's susceptibility to infection and decreases their tolerance to cytotoxic therapy. Pinkerton *et al.* (1996) suggest that the vicious cycle of poor intake, poor appetite and weight loss is overcome by naso-gastric feeding until the child can return to normal eating. Total parenteral nutrition is usually only required by children on intensive chemotherapeutic regimes such as those required in AML, prior to bone marrow transplantation and for stage IV neuroblastomas.

BONE MARROW TRANSPLANTATION (BMT)

Children who have malignancies which cannot be treated by other means may be given a bone marrow transplant. BMT involves the administration of lethal doses of chemotherapy, often in conjunction with radiation, to eradicate all the malignant cells and suppress the immune system to prevent rejection of the transplanted marrow. A transfusion of donor marrow cells can then be given to produce normal blood cells.

Three types of BMT are possible:

- *Allogenic* – a match with a histocompatible donor (sibling or unrelated donor);
- *Autologous* – uses the patient's own peripheral blood stem cells or marrow;
- *Synogenic* – uses donated marrow from an identical twin.

Activity

Find out the procedure to become a bone marrow donor. Discuss this with friends and relatives to assess how many people outside the health service are aware of the bone marrow donor register. Consider how children's nurses could raise this awareness.

Allogeneic BMT is now used during the first remission with AML and in ALL patients who relapse and achieve a successful second remission after re-induction chemotherapy. It is also considered in poor prognosis ALL patients after the first remission.

Prior to BMT, intensive chemotherapy and total body irradiation (TBI) is given to kill all remaining leukaemic cells. Preliminary results of trials show 50% long-term survivors but the first month after transplant is potentially the most risky as the child is completely neutropenic and thrombocytopenic. In addition to the risk of overwhelming infection and life-threatening haemorrhage the child is also at risk of graft versus host disease (GVHD). GVHD is caused by the donor T lymphocytes which perceive the host as a foreign protein and begin to attack the cells of the skin, gastro-intestinal tract, liver, heart, lungs lymphoid tissue or bone marrow. Treatment is by immune-suppressant drugs.

LONG-TERM COMPLICATIONS

Pinkerton *et al.* (1996) estimate that over 9000 young adults in the UK have survived childhood malignancy. Improved survival rates have made the late effects of successful treatment more apparent. As a result long-term survivors are monitored yearly both to monitor their long-term survival and also to identify and treat late effects of treatment. See Table 14.7 and Figure 14.1.

Site of radiotherapy	Potential problems
Central nervous system	Hypothalamic/pituitary dysfunction, psychological dysfunction, skeletal mass
Spine	Breast hypoplasia/malignancy, lung or gonadal dysfunction, adverse pregnancy outcome, bladder fibrosis, skeletal mass
Head	Cataracts, caries, hypoplasia of gums, dysfunction of salivary glands
Neck	Thyroid dysfunction/malignancy
Thorax	Breast hypoplasia/malignancy, lung dysfunction, cardiovascular disease
Liver	Dysfunction, fibrosis, malignancy
Gastro-intestinal tract	Dysfunction, fibrosis, malignancy
Kidneys	Renal dysfunction, hypertension, adverse pregnancy outcome
Bladder	Bladder fibrosis, adverse pregnancy outcome
Gonads	Infertility, hormone deficiency, adverse pregnancy outcome
Bone	Hypoplasia, pathological fractures, malignancy
Skin and soft tissue	Malignancy, pigmented naevi

Table 14.7

Potential long-term problems of radiotherapy

Figure 14.1

Five-year survival rates for childhood malignancy.

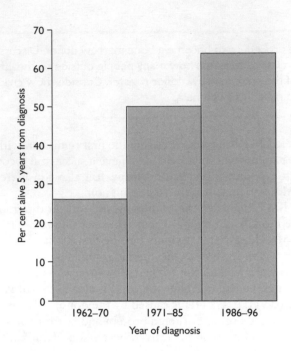

References

ADAMS, D. A. and SELEKOF, J. L. (1986) Children with ostomies: comprehensive care planning. *Pediatric Nursing*, **12** (6), 429–433.

ALDERMAN, C. (1988) Starting from scratch. *Nursing Standard*, 28 August, 36–37.

ALLAN, D. and CULNE-SEYMOUR, C. (1989) Paediatric Coma Scale. *Nursing Times*, **85** (20), 26–28.

AMERICAN ACADEMY of PEDIATRICS (1987) Report of the second task force on blood pressure control in children. *Pediatrics*, **79** (1), 1–25.

AMERICAN ACADEMY OF PEDIATRICS (1993) Committee of Infectious Diseases: Use of Ribavirin in the Treatment of RSV. *Pediatrics*, **92** (3), 501–504.

ANSELL, K. (1995) Let us show the way – dietary advice for children with diabetes. *Child Health*, **3** (2), 54–56.

ARN, P., VALLE, D. and BRUSILOW, S. (1988) Inborn errors of metabolism: not rare, not hopeless. *Contemporary Pediatrics*, **5** (12), 47–63.

AUDIT COMMISSION (1993) *Children First*. London: HMSO.

AYLIFFE, G. A. J., LOWBERRY, E. J. L., GEDDES, A. M. and WILLIAMS, J. D. (1992) *Control of Hospital Infection. A Practical Handbook*, 3rd edn. London: Chapman & Hall.

BAIN, J. (1993) Umbilical cord care. *The Neonatal Nurse's Year Book 1993*. London: Neonatal Nurses Association.

BALFOUR-LYNN, I. M. and VALMAN, H. B. (1993) *Practical Management of the Newborn*. London: Blackwell Scientific Publications.

BARKER, P. (1995) *Basic Child Psychiatry*, 6th edn. Oxford: Blackwell Scientific Publications.

BARTON, J. (1995) A cause for public concern – suicide in children and young people. *Child Health*, **3** (3), 106–109.

BERG, A. (1993) Are febrile convulsions provoked by a rapid rise in temperature? *American Journal of Diseases of Childhood*, **147**, 1101–1127.

BETHUNE, P., *et al.* (1993) Which child will have a febrile convulsion? *American Journal of Diseases of Childhood*, **147**, 35–39.

BHATT, S., *et al.* (1993) Progression of hearing loss in experimental pneumococcal meningitis. *Journal of Infectious Diseases*, **167**, 675–683.

BHUSHAN, V., PANETH, N. and KIELY, J. (1993) Impact of improved survival of very low birth weight infants on recent secular trends in the prevalence of cerebral palsy. *Pediatrics*, **91** (6) 1094–1105.

BLACK, N., SANDERSON, C., FREELAND, A. and VESSEY, M. (1990) A randomised controlled trial of surgery for glue ear. *British Medical Journal*, **300**, 1551–1556.

BLAND, E. (1987) The way it was. *Circulation*, **76**, 1190–1195.

BONE, M. and MELTZER, H. (1989) *The Prevalence of Disability among Children*. OPCS Surveys of Disability in Great Britain. Report. London: HMSO.

BORTON, E. (1997) Young people at breaking point. *Nursing Times*, **93** (21), 32–33.

BRADY, M. (1994) Symptom control in dying children. In HILL, L. (ed.), *Caring for Dying Children and their Families*. London: Chapman & Hall.

BRITISH DIABETIC ASSOCIATION (1995) *The Principles of Good Practice for the Care of Young People with Diabetes*. London: BDA.

BRITISH DIABETIC ASSOCIATION (1996) *Babies and Children with Diabetes*. London: BDA.

BRITISH DIABETIC ASSOCIATION (1997) *What Care to Expect when Your Child has Diabetes*. London: BDA.

BRITISH EPILEPSY ASSOCIATION (1995) *Living with Epilepsy*. London: BEA.

BRITISH THORACIC SOCIETY (1993) BTS guidelines. *Thorax*, **48**, S1–S24.

BROWN, M. A. and POWELL-COPE, G. M. (1991) AIDS family caregiving: transition through uncertainty. *Nursing Research*, **40** (6), 338–345.

BUXTON, P. (1993) *ABC of Dermatology*, 2nd edn. London: BMJ.

CAMFIELD, C. and CAMFIELD, P. (1993) Febrile seizures: an Rx for parent fears and anxiety. *Contemporary Pediatrics*, **10** (4), 26–44.

CAMPBELL, S. (1987) Mouthcare in malignancy patients. *Nursing Times*, **87** (29), 59–60.

CAMPBELL, S. and GLASPER, A. (eds) (1995) *Whaley and Wong's Children's Nursing*. St Louis: Mosby.

CAPLAN, G. (1980) An approach to preventive intervention in child psychiatry. *Canadian Journal of Psychiatry*, **25**, 623–630.

CARTER, B. (1993) *Manual of Paediatric Intensive Care Nursing*. London: Chapman & Hall.

CARTER, B. (1994) *Child and Infant Pain. Principles of Nursing Care and Management*. London: Chapman & Hall.

CHESS, S. and THOMAS, A. (1984) *Origins and Evolution of Behaviour Disorders from Infancy to Early Adult Life*. New York: Bruner/Mazel.

CLARK, R., *et al.* (1990) *Principles and Practice of Dermatology*. London: Churchill Livingstone.

CLAYTON, M. (1997) Traction at home: the Doncaster approach. *Paediatric Nursing*, **9** (2), 21–23.

COLLINS, B. (1984) Prevention of infection in orthopaedic wards. *British Association of Orthopaedic Nursing*, 4/5, part 2, March.

COOK, J. and GALLAGHER, A. (1996) Evaluation of an anti-emetic protocol. *Paediatric Nursing*, **8** (7), 21–23.

COOKE, R. W. (1994) Factors affecting survival and outcome at three years in extremely pre-term infants. *Archives of Disease in Childhood*, **71**, 28–31.

CRAIG, C. (1995) Congenital talipes Equinovarus. *Professional Nurse*, **11** (1), 30–32.

CRAWFORD, D. (1994) Nursing care of a baby with jaundice. In CRAWFORD, D. and MORRIS, M. (eds), *Neonatal Nursing*. London: Chapman & Hall.

CREE, I. A. (ed.) (1997) *Pathology*. London: Chapman & Hall.

DAJANI, A., *et al.* (1990) Prevention of bacterial endocarditis: recommendations by the American Heart Association. *Journal of the American Medical Association*, **264** (22), 2919–2922.

DAVIES, D. (1996) The causes of meningitis and meningococcal disease. *Nursing Times*, **92** (6) 25–27.

DEAR, P. (1992) Total parental nutrition of the newborn. *Care of the Critically Ill*, **8** (6), 252–257.

DES (1991) *HIV and AIDS: A Guide for the Education Service*. London: HMSO.

deSA, D. J. (1995) *Pathology of Neonatal Intensive Care: An Illustrated Reference*. London: Chapman & Hall.

DEWERS, R. (1990) Rhinitis and intranasal fluticasone propionate. *Royal Society of Medicine Symposium*, 10 July 1990.

DoH (1990) *Guidance for Clinical Health Care Workers: Protection against Infection with HIV and Hepatitis Viruses*. London: HMSO.

DoH (1991) *The Health of the Nation*. London: HMSO.

DoH (1992) *The Health of the Nation: a Strategy for Health in England*. London: HMSO.

DoH (1994) *Weaning and the Weaning Diet*. London: HMSO.

DoH (1996) *A Handbook on Child and Adolescent Mental Health*. London: HMSO.

DIABETES CONTROL AND COMPLICATIONS TRIAL RESEARCH GROUP (1993) The effect of intensive treatment of diabetes on the development and progression of long-term complications in insulin-dependent diabetes. *New England Journal of Medicine*, **329**, 977–986.

DIECKMANN, R. (1994) Rectal diazepam for pre-hospital pediatric status epilepticus. *Annals of Emergency Medicine*, **23**, 216–224.

DONALD, S. (1995) Atopic eczema: management and control. *Paediatric Nursing*, **7** (2), 30–34

DONOWITZ, L. G. (1986) Failure of the overgrown to prevent nosocomial infection in paediatric intensive care unit. *Paediatrics*, **77** (1), 35–38.

DUGGAN, C. (1996) HIV infection in children. *Paediatric Nursing*, **8** (10), 32–34.

DUNCAN, B., *et al.* (1993) Exclusive breast-feeding for at least 4 months protects against otitis media. *Pediatrics*, **91** (5), 867–872.

DUNNE, E. and GIBBONS, D. (1992) In FOWLER, J. (ed.), *Urologic Surgery*. London: Little Brown.

FAULCONBRIDGE, J. P. and SPANSWICK, S. M. L. (1995) Back up when you need it. Teaching and support for school nurses involved in counselling. *Child Health*, **3** (3), 111–114.

FLETCHER, D. (1997) Sports day screening to curb heart risks. *Daily Telegraph*, 44,158,9.

FLOOD, J. (1989) Glue ear. *Nursing Times*, **85** (36), 38–41.

FOSS, M. (1990) Oxygen therapy. *Professional Nurse*, **6** (4), 180–190.

FRANK, G. (1987) Scratching the surface. *Nursing Times*, 83 (39).

FRENCK, R., KOHL, S. and PICKERING, L. (1991) Principles of total care: infections in children with cancer. In FERNBACH, D. and VIETTI, T. (eds), *Clinical Pediatric Oncology*, 4th edn. St Louis: Mosby.

FRIEDEMANN, M. L. (1989) The concept of family nursing. *Journal of Advanced Nursing*, 14, 211–216.

GARNER, D. M. and GARFINKEL, P. E. (1980) Sociocultural factors in the development of anorexia nervosa. *Psychological Medicine*, 10, 647–656.

GEORGIOFF, M. and BERNBAUM, J. (1986) Abnormal shoulder girdle muscle tone in premature infants during their first 18 months of life. *Paediatrics*, 77, 664–669.

GHAJAR, J. and HARIRI, R. (1992) Management of paediatric head injury. *Paediatric Clinics of North America*, 39 (5), 1093–1123.

GILBERT, E., RUSSELL, K. and DESKIN, R. (1993) Stridor in the infant and child. *American Operating Room Journal*, 58 (1), 23–41.

GILL, K. (1994) External fixation: the erector sets of orthopaedic nursing. *Canadian Nurse*, 80 (5), 29–31.

GILLMAN, M., *et al.* (1993) Identifying children at high risk for the development of essential hypertension. *Journal of Pediatrics*, 122, 837–846.

GODDEN, C., CAMBELL, M., HUSSEY, M. and COGSWELL, J. (1997) Double blind placebo controlled trial of nebulised butesonide for croup. *Archives of Disease in Childhood*, 76, 155–158.

GOLDMAN, M., FITZPATRICK, R. and RUIZ-ESPARZA, J. (1993) Treatment of port-wine stains with the flash-lamp-pumped pulse dye laser. *Journal of Pediatrics*, 122 (1), 71–77.

GOOLAMALI, S. (1993) Paediatric dermatology. In VALMAN, H. (ed.), *ABC of One to Seven*, 3rd edn. London: BMJ.

GRAHAM, P. J. (1986) Behavioural and intellectual development in childhood epidemiology. *British Medical Bulletin*, 42 (2), 155–162.

GREENSPAN, J. S., WOLFSON, M. R., HOLT, W. J. and SHAFFER, P. G. (1990) Neonatal gastric intubation: differential respiratory effects between nasogastric and orogastric tubes. *Pediatric Pulmonology*, 8, 254–258.

GREGORY, J. R., COLLINS, D., DAVIES, P. S. W., CLARKE, P. C. and HUGHES, J. M. (1997) *National Diet and Nutrition Survey of Children Aged 1½ to 4½*. London: HMSO.

GREWAL, M. and SUTCLIFFE, A. (1991) Early prediction and outcome following head injury: an assessment of GCS score trends. *Journal of Paediatric Surgery*, 26, 1161.

GROER, M. E. and SHEKLETON, M. E. (1979) *Basic Pathophysiology – A Conceptual Approach*. St Louis: Mosby.

HALL, D. (1996) *Health for All Children*. Oxford: Oxford University Press.

HALLSWORTH, M. (1995) Positioning the pre-term infant. *Paediatric Nursing*, 7 (1), 18–20.

HARPER, J. (1994) Traditional Chinese medicine for eczema. *British Medical Journal*, 308, 409.

HAS (1995) The commissioning role and management of child and adolescent mental health services: together we stand. *The NHS Health Advisory Thematic Review*. London: HMSO.

HAWKINS, M. (1996) The long-term survivors. *British Medical Bulletin*, 52 (4), 898–923.

HAWTON, K. (1994) Causes and opportunities for prevention. In JENKINS, R.,

WYLIE, I., HAWTON, K., MORGAN, G. and TYLEE, A. (eds), *The Prevention of Suicide*. London: HMSO.

HAZINSKI, M. (1992) *Nursing Care of the Critically Ill Child*, 2nd edn. St Louis: Mosby.

HERBERT, M. (1987) *Conduct Disorders of Childhood and Adolescence: A Social Learning Perspective*, 2nd edn. Chichester: John Wiley.

HIGGINS, C. (1995) Pathology testing and blood glucose levels. *Nursing Times*, **91** (3), 42–44.

HIGGINS, J. (1990) Pulmonary oxygen toxicity. *Physiotherapy,* **76** (10), 588–592.

HOGAN, S., STRATFORD, K. and MOORE, D. (1997) Duration and recurrence of otitis media with effusion in children from birth to 3 years. *British Medical Journal*, **314**, 350–353.

HOHN, A. and STANTON, R. (1987) Myocarditis in children. *Pediatric Review*, **9** (3), 83–88.

HOLBERG, C., WRIGHT, A. and MARTINEZ, F. (1993) Child day care, smoking by care givers, and lower respiratory tract infections in the first 3 years of life. *Pediatrics*, **91**, 885–892.

HOLLIS, R. (1997) Childhood malignancy into the 21st century. *Paediatric Nursing*, **9** (3), 12–15.

HOLMES, A. (1996) The role of the cardiac liaison nurse. *Paediatric Nursing*, **8** (1), 25–27.

HORGAN, M., CHOONARA, I., AL-WAIDH, M., SAMBROOKS, J. and ASHBY, D. (1996) Measuring pain in neonates: an objective score. *Paediatric Nursing*, **8** (10), 24–27.

HULL, D. and JOHNSTON, D. I. (1987) *Essential Paediatrics*, 2nd edn. Edinburgh: Churchill Livingstone.

HUNT, E. (1997) The big wheeze. *Nursing Times*, **93** (7), 32–33.

HUNTER, J., SAVIN, J. and DAHL, M. (1989) *Clinical Dermatology*, vol. 3. Oxford: Glaxo/Blackwell Scientific Publications.

HYLTON RUSHTON, C. (1990) Necrotising entero-colitis. Part I. Pathogenesis and diagnosis. Part II. Treatment and nursing care. *American Journal of Maternal/Child Nursing*, **15**, 296–313.

IMLE, P. and KLEMIC, N. (1991) Methods of airway clearance: coughing and suctioning. In MacKENZIE, C., IMLE, P. and CIESLA, N. (eds), *Chest Physiotherapy in the Intensive Care Unit*. Baltimore: Williams & Wilkins.

ISAACSON, G. and ROSENFELD, R. (1994) Care of the child with typanoplasty tubes: a visual guide for the pediatrician. *Pediatrics*, **93** (6), 924–929.

JOHNSON, H. (1996) Stoma care for infants, children and young people. *Paediatric Nursing*, May, 8–11.

JOHNSTON, P. G. B. (1994) *Vulliamy's the Newborn Child*, 7th edn. Edinburgh: Churchill Livingstone.

JONES-WALTON, P. (1991) Clinical standards in skeletal traction pin-site care. *Orthopaedic Nursing*, **10** (2), 12–16.

KARJALAINEN, J., *et al.* (1992) A bovine albumin peptide as a possible trigger of insulin dependent diabetes mellitis. *New England Journal of Medicine*, **327** (5), 302–307.

KELMAR, C. J. H., HARVEY, D. and SIMPSON, C. (1995) *The Sick Newborn Baby*, 3rd edn. London: Bailliere Tindall.

KEREM, E., YATSIV, I. and GOITEIN, K. (1990) Effect of endotracheal suctioning on arterial blood gases in children. *Intensive Care Medicine*, **16**, 95–99.

KLAUS, M. H. and FANAROFF, A. A. (1979) *Care of the High Risk Neonate*. Philadelphia: Saunders.

KNAPMAN, J. (1993) Controlling emesis after chemotherapy. *Nursing Standard*, 7 (1), 38–39.

KOCH, C. and HOIBY, N. (1993) Pathogenesis of cystic fibrosis. *Lancet*, 8852, 1065–1069.

KONSTAN, M., BYARD, P., HOPPEL, C. and DAVIS, P. (1995) Effect of high dose ibuprofen in patients with cystic fibrosis. *New England Journal of Medicine*, 332, 848–854.

KURTZ, Z. (1992) *With Health in Mind – Mental Health Care for Children and Young People*. London: Action for Sick Children.

KUZENSKI, B. (1978) Effect of negative pressure in tracheobronchial trauma. *Nursing Research*, 27, 260.

LAWRENCE, R. (1994) *Breastfeeding: A Guide for the Medical Profession*, 4th edn. St Louis: Mosby.

LECK, I. (1995) Congenital dislocation of the hip. In WALD, N. (ed.), *Antenatal and Neonatal Screening*. Oxford: Oxford University Press.

LEENAARS, A. A. (1988) Preventing youth suicide: education is the key. *Dimensions*, October, 22–24.

LEUNG, D., *et al.* (1993) Toxic shock syndrome toxin-secreting *Staphylococcus aureus* in Kawasaki syndrome. *Lancet*, 342, 1385–1388.

LeMAISTRE, G. (1991) Ultrasound and dislocation of the hip. *Paediatric Nursing*, May, 13–16.

LOWBERRY, E. J. (1975) *Control of Infection. A Practical Handbook*. London: Chapman & Hall.

LUCAS, A. and COLE, T. J. (1990) Breast milk and neonatal necrotising entero-colitis. *Lancet*, 336, 1519–1523.

LUCAS, A., BROOKE, O. G. and MORLEY, R. (1990) Early diet of preterm infants and development of allergic and atopic disease: randomised prospective study. *British Medical Journal*, 300, 837–840.

LUCAS, A., MORLEY, R. and COLE, T. J. (1989) Early diet in preterm babies and developmental status in infancy. *Archives of Disease in Childhood*, 64, 1570–1578.

MacDONALD, H. (1995) Chronic renal disease: the mother's experience. *Pediatric Nursing*, 21 (6), 503–507.

MacKENZIE, H. (1994) HIV and AIDS: a family approach to care. *Paediatric Nursing*, 6 (10), 18–21.

MacMAHON, R. A. (1991) *An Aid to Paediatric Surgery*, 2nd edn. Melbourne: Churchill Livingstone.

McEVILLY, A. (1997) Childhood diabetes. *Paediatric Nursing*, 9 (3), 29–33.

McMAHON, B. (1995) A family affair: understanding family therapy. *Child Health*, 3 (3), 100–104.

MAGUIRE, D. and MALONEY, P. (1988), A comparison of fentanyl and morphine in neonates. *Neonatal Network*, 7 (1), 27–35.

MARKOVITCH, H. (1990) Recognising meningitis. *The Practitioner*, 234, 539–541.

MARTIN, V. (1995) Helping parents cope. *Nursing Times*, 91 (31), 38–40.

MAUGHAN, N. (1994) Care of the child with nephrotic syndrome. *Paediatric Nursing*, 6 (3), 20–21.

MEDICAL RESEARCH COUNCIL WORKING PARTY ON PHENYLKETONURIA (1993) Phenylketonuria due to phenylalanine hydroxylase deficiency: an unfolding story. *British Medical Journal*, 306, 115–119.

MENTAL HEALTH FOUNDATION (1993) *Mental Illness – Fundamental Facts*. London: Mental Health Foundation.

MERENSTEIN, G. and GARDNER, S. L. (1979) *Handbook of Neonatal Intensive Care*, 2nd edn. St Louis: Mosby.

METCALF, M. and BAUM, J. (1991) Incidence of insulin dependent diabetes in children under 15 years in the British Isles in 1988. *British Medical Journal*, **302**, 443–447.

MILLER, K. L. (1996) Urinary infections: children are not little adults. *Pediatric Nursing*, **22** (6), 473–480, 544.

MILLER, M. and MILLER, J. H. (1985) *Orthopaedics and Accidents Illustrated*. London: Hodder & Stoughton.

MORELL, P. (1994) Low birth weight babies at school age. *Northern Neonatal Journal*, **2**, 44–48.

MORRIS, M. (1994) Nursing care of babies who arc born too soon or too small. In CRAWFORD, D. and MORRIS, M. (eds), *Neonatal Nursing*. London: Chapman & Hall.

MORRISON, R. A. and VEDRO, D. A. (1989) Pain management in the child with sickle cell disease. *Pediatric Nursing*, **15** (6), 595–599, 613.

MOULAI, S. and HUBAND, S. (1996) Nutrition and the digestive system. In McQUAID, L. M., HUBAND, S. and PARKER, E. (eds), *Children's Nursing*. Edinburgh: Churchill Livingstone.

MURPHY, D., HOPE, L. and JOHNSON, A. (1997) Neonatal risk factors for cerebral palsy in very pre-term babies: case-control study. *British Medical Journal*, **314**, 404–408.

MURPHY, K., *et al.* (1990) Severe burns from a pulse oximeter. *Anesthesiology*, **73**, 350–351.

NETTLESHIP, A. (1994/5) Do we have an attitude problem? *Child Health*, **2** (4), 150–153.

NEWMAN-TURNER, R. (1992) *The Hayfever Handbook*. London: Thorsons.

NORTHWAY, W., *et al.* (1990) Late pulmonary sequalae of bronchopulmonary dysplasia. *New England Journal of Medicine*, **323** (26), 1793–1799.

NURSE'S CLINICAL LIBRARY (1985) *Immune Disorders*. Pennsylvania: Springhouse.

OFFORD, D. R. (1987) Prevention of behavioural and emotional disorders in children. *Journal of Child Psychology and Psychiatry*, **28**, 9–19.

OPIE, L. (1991) *Drugs for the Heart*. Philedelphia: W. B. Saunders.

PAGDIN, J. (1996) The musculoskeletal system In McQUAID, L. M., HUBAND, S. and PARKER, E. (eds), *Children's Nursing*. Edinburgh: Churchill Livingstone.

PFEFFER, C. R. (1986) *The Suicidal Child*. New York: Guilford Press.

PHELAN, P., LANDAU, L. and OLINSKY, A. (1990) Pulmonary complications of inhalation. In PHELAN, P., LANDAU, L. and OLINSKY, A. (eds) *Respiratory Illness in Children*, 2nd edn. Oxford: Blackwell Scientific Publications.

PHLS (1994) *Communicable Diseases Report*. London: PHLS.

PHLS (1996) *Communicable Diseases Report*. London: PHLS.

PINKERTON, J., *et al.* (1996) *Supportive Care – Guidelines for Shared Care Centres*. London: Great Ormond Street Hospital NHS Trust.

PLATT, M. J. and PHAROAH, P. O. D. (1996) Child health statistical review, 1996. *Archives of Disease in Childhood*, **75**, 527–533.

PORTER, H. (1994) Mouthcare in malignancy. *Nursing Times*, **90** (14), 27–29.

PORTMAN, R. and YETMAN, R. (1994) Clinical uses of ambulatory blood pressure monitoring. *Paediatric Nephrology*, **8**, 367–376.

PRASAD, S. and HUSSEY, J. (1995) *Paediatric Respiratory Care*. London: Chapman & Hall.

PRITCHARD, A. P. and DAVID, J. A. (1990) *The Royal Marsden Hospital Manual of Clinical Nursing Procedures*, 2nd edn. London: Harper & Row.

PURCELL, J. (1989) Cardiomyopathy. *American Journal of Nursing*, **89** (1), 57–75.

PUTTO, A. (1987) Febrile exudative tonsillitis: viral or streptococcal? *Pediatrics*, **80** (6), 911–914.

QUINTERO, C. (1993) Blood administration in pediatric Jehovah's Witnesses. *Pediatric Nursing*, **19** (1), 46–48.

RAKSHI, K. and COURIEL, J. (1994) Management of acute bronchiolitis. *Archives of Disease in Childhood*, **71**, 463–469.

RAMSAY, J. (1994) The psychology of childhood asthma. *Paediatric Nursing*, **6** (8), 17–21.

REES, M. (1994) The season of discontent. *Child Health*, **2** (1), 22–26.

REEVES, K. (1989) Assessment of paediatric head injury: the basics. *Journal of Emergency Nursing*, **15** (4), 329–333.

REID, U. (1997) Stigma of hair loss after chemotherapy. *Paediatric Nursing*, **9** (3), 16–18.

REIDY, M., *et al*. (1991) Psychological needs expressed by the natural caregivers of HIV infected children. *AIDS Care*, **3** (3), 331–343.

REYNOLDS, E. (1992) Controversies in caring for the child with a head injury. *Maternal and Child Nursing*, **17**, 246–251.

RICHMAN, N., STEVENSON, J. and GRAHAM, P. (1982) *Pre-school to School: A Behavioural Study*. London: Academic Press.

RICKARD, S. and FINN, A. (1997) Parental knowledge of paediatric infectious diseases. *Ambulatory Child Health*, **3**, 13–19.

ROBERTS, I., DOKAL, I. and DALY, P. (1996) *Management Protocol for Patients with Beta Thalassaemia Major – Version 1.0*. London: Hammersmith Hospital.

ROTHMAN, K. and LUCKY, A. (1993) Acne vulgaris. *Advances in Dermatology*, **8**, 131.

ROWE, S. (1997) A review of the literature on the nursing care of skeletal pins in the paediatric and adolescent setting. *Journal of Orthopaedic Nursing*, **1**, 26–29.

RUTTER, M. (1975) *Helping Troubled Children*. Harmondsworth: Penguin.

SAMARITANS (1997) *Exploring the Taboo*. London: Samaritans.

SARTORI, P. C. E., GORDON, P. G. J. and DARBYSHIRE, P. J. (1990) Continuous papavertum infusion for the control of pain in painful sickling crisis. *Archives of Disease in Childhood*, March, 1151–1153.

SCHAAD, B., *et al*. (1993) Dexamethasone therapy for bacterial meningitis in children. *Lancet*, **324**, 457–461.

SCHECTER, N., BERRIAN, F. B. and KATZ, S. M. (1988) The use of patient controlled analgesia in adolescents with sickle cell pain crisis: a preliminary report. *Journal of Pain and Symptom Management*, **3**, 109–113.

SCOTT, M. (1994) A new treatment becomes reality. *CF News*, spring edition.

SHAFFER, D. (1974) Suicide in childhood and early adolescence. *Journal of Child Psychology and Psychiatry*, **15**, 275–291.

SHNEIDMAN, E. (1985) *Definition of Suicide*. New York: John Wiley.

SHORVON, S. (1990) *Epilepsy: A Lancet Review*. London: The Lancet.

SHYUR, S.-D. and HILL, H. R. (1996) Recent advances in the genetics of primary immunodeficiency syndromes. *Journal of Pediatrics*, **129** (1), 8–24.

SIMPSON, D. and REILLY, P. (1982) Paediatric coma scale. *Lancet*, ii, 450.

van SOMEREN, V., LINNETT, S. J., STOTHERS, J. K. and SULLIVAN, P. G. (1984)

An investigation into the benefits of resisting nasoenteric feeding tubes. *Pediatrics*, 74, 379–383.

de SOUSA, M. E. (1996) The renal system. In McQUAID, L., HUBAND, S. and PARKER, E. (eds), *Children's Nursing*. London: Churchill Livingstone.

SPARSHOTT, M. (1994) Nursing care of a baby in pain and discomfort. In CRAWFORD, D. and MORRIS, M. (eds), *Neonatal Nursing*. London: Chapman & Hall.

SPARSHOTT, M. (1995) Assessing the behaviour of the newborn infant. *Paediatric Nursing*, 7 (7), 14–16.

SPEIGHT, N. (1996) The changing face of childhood asthma management. *Paediatrics Today*, 4 (4), 78–80.

SPORIK, R. (1994) Why block a small hole? The adverse effects of nasogastric tubes. *Journal of the British Paediatric Association*, 71, 393–394.

SPOWART, K. (1995) Childhood skin disorders. *Paediatric Nursing*, 7 (3), 30–34.

STEINHAUER, P. D., SANTA-BARBARA, J. and SKINNER, H. (1984) The process model of family functioning. *Canadian Journal of Psychiatry*, 29, 77–88.

STRACHAN, D., JARVIS, M. and FEYERABEND, B. (1989) Passive smoking, salivary cotinine concentration and middle ear effusion in 7 year old children. *British Medical Journal*, 298, 1549–1552.

SUMNER, E. (1990) Artificial ventilation of children. In DINWIDDIE, R. (ed.), *The Diagnosis and Management of Paediatric Respiratory Disease*. London: Churchill Livingstone.

SWANWICK, M. (1986) The ugly duckling. *Nursing Times*, 3 December, 47–49.

SWIFT, P., *et al*. (1993) A decade of diabetes: keeping children out of hospital. *British Medical Journal*, 307, 96–98.

TAYLOR, J. H. (1996) End stage renal disease in children: diagnosis, management and interventions. *Pediatric Nursing*, 22 (6), 481–490.

TAYLOR, L. J. (1978) An evaluation of handwashing techniques. *Nursing Times*, part 1, 54–55.

TEASDALE, G. and JENNETT, W. (1994) Assessment of coma and impaired unconsciousness. Lancet, ii, 81–84.

VALMAN, H. (1993) *ABC of One to Seven*, 3rd edn. London: BMJ.

Van DONSELAAR, C., BROUWER, O. and GEERTS, A. (1997) Clinical course of untreated tonic-clonic seizures in childhood: prospective, hospital-based study. *British Medical Journal*, 314, 401–404.

VARMA, V. P. (ed.) (1990) *The Management of Children with Emotional and Behavioural Difficulties*. London: Routledge.

VEASEY, L., TANI, L. and HILL, H. (1994) Persistence of rheumatic fever in the intermountain area of the United States. *Journal of Pediatrics*, 124, 9–16.

VERNON, S. (1995) Urine collection from infants: a reliable method. *Paediatric Nursing*, 7 (6), 26–27.

WADDINGTON, P. and WATSON, A. (1997) Which urine collection bag? *Paediatric Nursing*, 9 (2), 19–20.

WATSON, J. (1990) Screening for congenital dislocation of the hip. *Maternal & Child Health*, October, 310–314.

WHALEY, L. F. and WONG, D. L. (1987) *Nursing Care of Infants and Children*, 3rd edn. St Louis: Mosby.

WHALEY, L. F. and WONG, D. L. (1995) *Nursing Care of Infants and Children*, 5th edn. St Louis: Mosby.

WHITEFIELD, W., LEEMIN, M. and PAPWORTH, P. (1995) Stemming the rising tide. *Paediatric Nursing*, 7 (4), 16–17.

WHO (1972) *Nutritional Anaemias*. WHO Technical Report Series 503. Geneva: WHO.

WIDEMAR, L., SVENSSON, C., RYNNEL-DAGOO, B. and SCHIROTZKI, H. (1985) The effect of adenoidectomy on secretory otitis media. *Clinical Otolaryngology*, **10** (6), 345–350.

WILLIAMS, J. (1992) Assessment of head injured children. *British Journal of Nursing*, **2**, 82–84.

WILSON, C. B. (1986) Immunological basis for increased susceptibility of the neonate to infection. *Journal of Pediatrics*, **112**, 104.

WILSON, N. (1996) Early childhood wheezing. *Paediatrics Today*, **4** (4), 91–93.

WILSON, P. (1995) Which way forward? Provision of child and adolescent mental health services. *Child Health*, **3** (3), 90–94.

WISWELL, T. E., *et al.* (1988) Effect of circumcisions status on periurethral bacterial flora during the first year of life. *Journal of Pediatrics*, **133**, 442.

WOODROFFE, C., GLICKMAN, M., BARKER, M. and POWER, C. (1993) *Children, Teenagers and Health*. Milton Keynes: Open University Press.

WRIGHT, S. (1991) Altered body image in anorexia nervosa. In GLASPER, A. (ed.), *Child Care: Some Nursing Perspectives*. London: Wolfe.

ZIPURSKY, J., *et al.* (1992) Oxygen therapy in sickle cell disease. *American Journal of Pediatric Hematology Oncology*, **14** (3), 222–228.

Genito-urinary problems

Further reading

BERRY, A. C. and CHANTLER, C. (1986) Urogenital malformations and disease. *British Medical Bulletin*, **42** (2), 181–186.

GARTLAND, C. (1993) Partners in care. How families are taught to care for their child on peritoneal dialysis. *Nursing Times*, **89** (30), 34–36.

JADRESIC, L. (1993) Investigation of urinary tract infection in childhood. *British Medical Journal*, **307**, 761–764.

POSTLETHWAITE, R. J. (ed.) (1994) *Clinical Paediatric Nephrology*, 2nd edn. Oxford: Butterworth Heinemann.

TAYLOR, C. M. and CHAPMAN, S. (1989) *Handbook of Renal Investigations in Children*. Sevenoaks: Wright.

Pathophysiology

CLAXTON, R. and HARRISON, T. (eds) *Caring for Children with HIV and AIDS*. London: Edward Arnold.

GIBB, D. and WALTERS, S. (1993) *Guidelines for the Management of Children with HIV Infection*, 2nd edn. West Sussex: Avert.

GROER, M. E. and SHEKLETON, M. E. (1979) *Basic Pathophysiology: A Conceptual Approach*. St Louis: Mosby.

HIV disease

ORR, N. (ed.) (1995) *Children's Rights and HIV: A Framework for Action*. London: National Children's Bureau.

Family therapy

ANDERSON, T. (1990) *The Reflecting Team*. Broadstairs: Bergman.

BARKER, P. (1992) *Basic Family Therapy*, 3rd edn. Oxford: Blackwell Scientific Publications.

Cognitive behaviour therapy
MURDOCH, D. and BARKER, P. (1991) *Basic Behaviour Therapy*. Oxford: Blackwell Scientific Publications.
SCHAFFER, D., *et al.* (1995) *The Clinical Guide to Child Psychiatry*. London: The Free Press, Collier and Macmillan.

Prevention of suicide
JENKINS, R., GRIFFITHS, S., WYLIE, I., HAWTON, K., MORGAM, G. and TYLEE, A. (eds) (1994) *The Prevention of Suicide*. London: HMSO.

Psychological problems of 'surgical' babies
LUDHAM, L. (1992) Emotional development after major neonatal surgery. *Paediatric Nursing*, May, 20–22.

Helpful addresses   British Kidney Patient Association, Bordon, Hants. Tel: 01420 472021/2.

Enuresis Resource and Information Centre (ERIC), 65 St Michael's Hill, Bristol BS2 8DZ. Tel: 01272 264920.

PART THREE

PROFESSIONAL ISSUES IN CHILD CARE

THE DEVELOPMENT AND PROCESS OF CHILDREN'S NURSING

Joan Ramsay

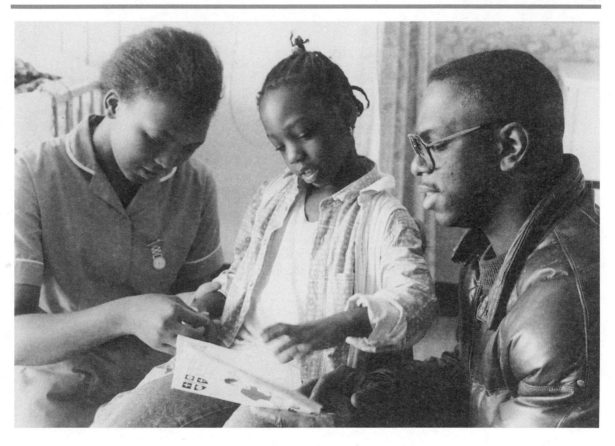

OBJECTIVES

The material contained within this module and the further reading/references should enable you to:

- Explore the history of children's nursing.
- Examine the different roles of the children's nurse.
- Discuss the value of models of nursing.
- Assess the appropriateness of different models of children's nursing.
- Explore the meaning and practice of family-centred care.
- Consider the future of children's nursing.

INTRODUCTION

This module is concerned with promoting children's nursing as a unique speciality which requires specific knowledge and understanding. It begins by looking at the history of children's nursing and considering how the speciality has developed since these early days. It discusses the different roles of the children's nurse in providing specific care for the sick child alongside caring, supporting and teaching the family. Children's nurses usually have a philosophy of family-centred care and this concept, and nurses' and families' understanding of it, is explored. Family-centred care is usually the basis of any model of nursing used in children's nursing but this module, whilst exploring how different models of nursing can be applied to children's nursing, also questions the usefulness of models. Finally the module discusses the future of children's nursing in the light of political changes to the health service.

THE HISTORY OF CHILDREN'S NURSING 1

INTRODUCTION

Children's nursing is a relatively new speciality which did not really commence until the mid-19th century. It began as a need to protect vulnerable children from disease and death, and, whilst that fundamental concept has never been lost, it has developed into a service for the whole family to enable the healthy growth and development of all children. In the beginning the nurses employed to care for the children were given no special training and were often less than satisfactory. Over the years children's nurse education has developed into a speciality with graduate and post-graduate programmes now available. There are also a number of recognised specialities within the field of paediatrics which nurses can study at degree level.

The first children's hospitals were very basic and could cater for only small numbers of children who were separated from their families during their stay in hospital. Nowadays, specialist children's hospitals have at least 300 beds, including facilities for intensive care, and cater for families as well as children. They employ not only a large number of medical and nursing staff, but also other professionals important to children's welfare, such as nursery nurses, play therapists and teachers. Families of sick children, who were once rejected as a disturbance to the children and the ward routine, are now welcome to participate in the care of their child.

In spite of these developments in the care of sick children, there is still room for further improvement. Children's nursing has been fortunate to have gained backing from various government reports over the last 50 years but the recommendations contained within these have still to be fully implemented. The number of registered children's nurses does not meet the growing demand for such specialist practitioners and their preparation needs review.

HOSPITALS FOR SICK CHILDREN

The origins of children's hospitals in the UK began in 1739 when Captain Thomas Coram retired from a life at sea and returned to London. He was horrified by the numbers of sick and dying children he encountered in the streets of the capital and set about gaining support to fund a place to care for these children. In 1739 he opened a foundling hospital to care for unwanted children. Yet he was still unable to stop the huge numbers of deaths amongst the children. During the next 20 years 15 000 children were admitted here, demonstrating the very great need at this time for a place of care for abandoned and unwanted children, but only 4400 of them managed to survive to adulthood (Besser, 1977). This high mortality rate of children in the 17th and early

---

Significant reports in the history of children's nursing

1959 *Welfare of Children in Hospital (Platt Report)*
A government report which recognised the adverse effects of hospitalisation for children and made recommendations to enable children to be nursed by specialist practitioners in a suitable environment

1976 *Fit for the Future: Child Health Services (Court Report)*
A government report which realised the disparity of health services for children and recommended a more coordinated integrated service which would shorten hospital admission and enable children to be nursed at home

1988 *Parents Staying Overnight with their Children*
A recommended standard for the provision of overnight accommodation for resident parents produced by the consortium Caring of Children in the Health Services (comprising ASC, RCN, British Paediatric Association and the National Association of Health Authorities and Trusts)

1988 *Hidden Children – An Analysis of Ward Attenders in Children's Wards*
A report from the Caring for Children in the Health Services group recommending good practice for the care of children who do not require a stay in hospital but still need to attend hospital

1989 *The Children Act: An Introductory Guide for the NHS*
Produced by the DoH to clarify the provisions of the Children Act and the duty of NHS Trusts in providing services for children in need and their families

1991 *Just for the Day*
A report by the consortium Caring for Children in the Health Services which suggested ways of improving the quality of health care for children and produced a comprehensive set of standards for day care

1991 *Welfare of Children and Young People in Hospital*
A government report re-iterating the principles of the Platt Report and making more specific recommendations about staffing levels in areas where children are nursed and stressing the involvement of parents in the care of their children in hospital

1993 *Children First – A Study of Hospital Services*
The findings of the Audit Commission's study into the hospital services for sick children, investigating why principles for good practice outlined in the Platt Report were not being met

1994 *The Allitt Inquiry (Clothier Report)*
The findings of the independent inquiry team into the deaths and injuries of the children cared for by Beverley Allitt which includes recommendations aimed to tighten procedures for safeguarding children in hospital and prevent a repetition of the tragedy

1995 *The Children's Charter*
A government produced charter to help children and their parents be aware of their rights in relation to health care

---

18th century was mostly due to ignorance about childhood infections, their cause and method of spread.

Coram also did not manage to change the attitudes of the time to children which were largely influenced by John Wesley. Wesley believed that children were evil and could only be saved by physical punishment. In light of such widely held views, it is not surprising that sick children were not catered for in hospitals and left to die. In 1843 the annual mortality rate was 50 000, yet children accounted for nearly half this figure. Of 2363 patients in the London hospitals, only 26 were children. At the London hospital children under 7 years were actually prohibited unless they required an amputation or 'cutting for stone'. In 1831 Guys hospital had 15 beds for children in a wooden building over some stables but this building was pulled down in 1850 and not replaced (De Mause, 1974).

However, as the industrial revolution progressed so did education and literacy and gradually, with the help of such authors as Charles Dickens and Charles Kingsley who highlighted some of the worst child care practices, attitudes towards children began to change. At the same time, Dr Charles West was taking an interest in childhood illnesses. He saw the children at local clinics or dispensaries where they were seen, treated and sent home. He put together his observations to form the first textbook on the diseases of childhood to be published in England. He also realised that the reason that most children did not recover from their illnesses was because they returned home to an overcrowded environment, poor sanitation and little or no healthy food. He resolved to open a children's hospital to overcome these problems.

Dr West had to battle to get his dream accepted. The arguments against a hospital for children were many. It would separate the children from their families and require one nurse for each child. The nurses would not agree with the mothers' care and the potential for the spread of infection would be great. However, Dr West did realise his dream in spite of these arguments and The Hospital for Sick Children, Great Ormond Street, was opened on 14th February 1852. Initially it had only 10 beds but these gradually increased so that by 1858 the hospital could cater for 75 children.

STANDARDS OF CARE

During the 1850s and for a long time afterwards it was believed that the child's parents should not be part of the child's care in hospital. This idea was partly due to the military philosophy of the Nightingale type of nurse training which commenced in 1860. Parents were seen as amateurs in the care of sick children who would distress themselves and the child if allowed to come into the hospital too often. Concern was also raised about the spread of infection and disruption to the hospital routine and consequently strict visiting hours for parents were imposed. Other members of the family were not allowed at all. Remember that at this time children were kept in hospital much longer than at present.

This state of affairs stayed unchanged for almost a century. For many years nurses used the fact that the children cried at the end of visiting time to support their beliefs that parental presence in hospital was upsetting and should not be encouraged. These beliefs began to be challenged in the post-war years. Concerned with the possible effects of the evacuation of children during the war and the consequence upon children of the changing role of women, psychologists began to study the effects of parental separation. Bowlby (1951) discovered that children formed an attachment with their parents from an early age and used this relationship as a source of comfort when distressed or stressed. The following year, evidence on film showed clearly the protest, despair and detachment which occurs in the child in hospital when parental separation occurs (Bowlby and Robertson, 1952). Later research by Robertson revealed that children in hospital who were separated from their mother took longer to recover from their illness and their development regressed (Robertson, 1958). As a result of this evidence, the government appointed Platt to report on the welfare of children in hospital. The report, published in 1959, revealed the restrictions imposed upon parents, the lack of proper facilities for children in hospital and the number of children being nursed in adult wards. It made several recommendations to change these bad practices. However, these recommendations involved a major change in current beliefs and practices as well as having financial and organisational implications. It is not surprising, therefore, that its implementation was slow and difficult. What is surprising is that nearly 40 years later some of the recommendations of the Platt Report are still to be met (Audit Commission, 1993).

Activity

Read the Platt Report recommendations and make a critical assessment of how your area of practice meets these.

Since the Platt Report other government reports have highlighted the importance of special resources for the care of children. In 1961 the National Association for the Welfare of Children in Hospital (NAWCH) was established to campaign for the rights of sick children and their families. Now known as Action for Sick Children (ASC), this pressure group has done much to improve the quality of care for children in hospital. In other countries progress has been even slower. Stenbak (1986) revealed that in many parts of Europe parental visiting is still prohibited or limited. In 1988 the European Association of Children in Hospital (EACH) was established with the aim of producing a charter for children in hospital across Europe. Now representing 18 countries, EACH has agreed to focus its efforts on emphasising the importance of children being nursed on children's wards. Even in the UK children are

Cross reference

Separation anxiety – page 210

The Platt Report recommendations

- Hospitalisation only when absolutely necessary and for the minimum length of time
- Mothers to be resident in hospital with their sick child
- Unrestricted visiting
- Appropriately qualified children's nurses on all wards where children are nursed
- Children's usual home routine to be maintained in hospital
- Children should be nursed in an appropriate child-friendly environment
- Provision of play and education for all children in hospital
- Children's wards should have a strategy for preparing children for elective admission

(MoH, 1959)

still admitted to adult ear, nose and throat, and ophthalmology wards (Audit Commission, 1993).

The 1990s saw a number of reports which highlighted the changes still to be met in order to comply with the Platt Report. These were particularly highlighted by the Beverley Allitt case in 1991. Allitt, a nurse working on a children's ward, murdered four children and attempted to kill at least eight others. The independent inquiry into the case recommended that there should always be a certain number of appropriately qualified children's nurses on a children's ward (DoH, 1994a). Whilst the rationale for such a recommendation may have been flawed, Allitt's mental state is surely unrelated to the absence or presence of a children's nursing qualification, the report's suggestions have not been acted upon. One year after the publication of the inquiry's report, 80% of children's wards were still lacking sufficient numbers of children's nurses.

Cross references

Allitt inquiry – page 258

Number of registered children's nurses – page 350

Activity

Study a month's duty roster in your own area and determine the numbers of appropriately qualified children's nurses on duty over a 24-hour period. Do these numbers meet with the DoH's guidelines of two registered children's nurses on duty at any time? Consider if two such nurses are enough.

Cross reference

Children's Charter – page 695

In 1995 the government followed their Patient's Charter with one for children. This was aimed to inform children and their parents of their rights in relation to health care. Surprisingly, it does not mention staffing issues other than to state that children can expect to have a named nurse in charge of their care.

Activity

Read the Children's Charter (page 695) and consider its implementation in your own area of work.

CHILDREN'S NURSE EDUCATION

At the time of Dr West's hospital for sick children there was of course no formal system of nurse education and most nurses resembled the notorious Sairey Gamp who lived close to Great Ormond Street. Reports from visitors to the hospital in these early years state that everything seems very satisfactory except for the nurses. Committee records make constant reference to nurses being found asleep, being 'dirty and disrespectful' and 'wholly incapable'. Consequently, Dr West decided to ensure his hospital nurses were properly trained.

From 1862 Dr West employed sisters and recommended that they and the other nurses and probationers should reach a certain standard.

He decreed that any nurse who hit a child should be dismissed immediately as this demonstrated an inability to keep children contented. He wrote a book entitled *How to Nurse Sick Children* and in 1878 he appointed Miss Catherine Wood as Lady Superintendent of Nurses to arrange the training of all probationer nurses at the hospital. During her first year in post, Miss Wood also published her own textbook for nurses, *Handbook of Nursing*. Ten years later she produced a second book, *The Training of Nurses for Sick Children*. It is interesting to read excerpts from her work as she writes clearly about her philosophy of nursing children, revealing ideas which are still fundamental to children's nursing. However, bearing in mind the social climate of the late 19th century, these ideas must have been seen as revolutionary in 1888.

Although Miss Wood developed the first training programme for children's nurses in 1878, it was not until the 1920s that children's nurses became registered. Initially nurses were trained specifically to care for children. Applicants who had to have their school certificate were taken on unpaid probation for the first 1–2 months and then, if deemed suitable, undertook 3 years' training. Their lectures were given by doctors with practical sessions taught by a sister tutor or ward sister.

The validity of nurses being trained only to nurse children then began to be considered rather narrow and it became accepted that a nurse should also have general nurse training to be able to manage a children's ward or hospital. Once parents became more involved in their children's care, this general qualification was also seen as necessary to appreciate and respond to parental needs. Obtaining two qualifications was difficult. The number of hospitals offering sufficient experience for children's nurse training was small and nurses who undertook their general training first were loathe to return to student status on qualifying. As the numbers of registered sick children's nurses (RSCNs) declined and the government pressure to provide appropriately qualified practitioners to care for sick children increased, a further change was required.

It is only relatively recently that this change has occurred. Children's nursing had always been considered to be less rigorous and significant than general training, and although Scotland retained and respected the single RSCN qualification, the rest of the UK was slow to accept that nurses wishing to care for children need only undertake a children's nursing course. In 1986, The United Kingdom Central Council (UKCC) for nursing, midwifery and health visiting proposed a new way of preparing nurses to practise (Project 2000) which included an 18 month branch programme in the care of children. This new nurse education programme at diploma level proposed a move away from the traditional apprentice style of nurse training and proposed that students of nursing were supernumerary and should be paid on a bursary. It also proposed that students undertook an 18 month common foundation programme (CFP) where they would gain experience in a supernumerary capacity in all the nursing specialities. At the end of this time the students would

Dr Charles West's standards of care for nurses and sisters

'The duty of attending on sick children calls not only for the ordinary amount of patience, gentleness and kindness necessary in the case of all sick persons, but also for the freedom from prejudice and a quickness of observation seldom found among the uneducated. No woman is to be admitted as a nurse who cannot read writing as well as printing, and who cannot repeat the Lord's prayer and the Ten Commandments and who is not acquainted with the principles of the Christian religion; and no-one is to be admitted as a Sister who is not able in addition to the above to write a legible hand. Further that it is to be the duty of every nurse not only to watch the children with care and to tend them with kindness, but also to try by all means to keep them cheerful and contented.'

The training of nurses for sick children

'I commence by stating two propositions, first that sick children require special nursing; and second, that sick children's nurses require special training.

The child can give no reliable help in detailing his symptoms or in giving a detailed account of his bodily functions … He must not be left alone, his attendant must always be on the watch for any change in his physical condition as such changes for good or ill occur most unexpectedly and run their course with startling rapidity.

The child will thrive best who is best mothered by his own nurse, for little sick ones are quick to discern those who love them and that nurse will have most success who makes an individual study of her patients …

It will not be found that the same regularity and order can be maintained amongst the children as among the adults. Order and discipline there must be, or the child will not be happy; but the ward that is tidied up to perfection, in which the little ones look like well drilled soldiers … is hardly suggestive of the happy heart of a child. Toys and games are as much part of the treatment as physic, and the ceaseless chatter and careless distribution of toys are surely consistent with a well-ordered children's ward.'

(Wood, 1988)

choose their speciality for the branch programme and their future qualification. This innovation should have helped to overcome the shortage of qualified children's nurses as it enabled more colleges of nursing to offer children's nurse training.

However, other changes in the health service prevented the new diploma programmes from making these reforms. In 1989, when the pilot schemes for the diploma programmes were being initiated, Trust status for health services was being discussed, and the movement of nurse education away from health service management and into the education sector was beginning. Whilst these changes may have improved the quality of patient service and given more academic credibility to nurse education, they may also have impaired the numbers of nurses entering the smaller branches of nursing, including children's nursing. Trust hospitals, responsible for their own budgets, had to consider carefully their need for trained nurses in the future to determine the number of students required for each speciality. The universities were then asked to meet these requirements. As a result, student nurses have to choose their speciality on entry and the ability to make an informed decision at the end of CFP is largely lost. The post-registration entry gate to children's nursing has also been largely lost. The placement experience has been given to diploma students and, because the original idea of PK2 was that the students chose their speciality, the need for a change of branch after qualification was not really considered and programmes were not developed. In addition, now that nurse education is managed by universities, most registered nurses wishing to change speciality have to return to a student bursary as well as finding funds to pay for the course.

At present, therefore, there is still a deficit of appropriately qualified children's nurses, especially in areas not specifically catering for children such as general intensive care units and A&E units. The Audit Commission (1993) discovered that most of the 31 children's wards studied were staffed with only one RSCN during the day and that 50% of the sample had no RSCNs on duty at night. Other areas, where children are the minority patient group, have no qualified children's nurses (DoH, 1991). Although the right of sick children to be cared for by appropriately qualified nurses who understand their special needs is not disputed and is supported by the government, the medical profession and pressure groups for the care of children (Colson, 1996), it appears that the argument is turning again, this time to consider the generic nurse. The important debate would appear to be is this merely a financial solution which ensures the provision of a cost-effective qualified work force rather than the best option for sick children?

Activity

Consider the advantages and disadvantages of the generic nurse for children and their families.

It must be remembered that many nurses still believe that a general nurse qualification is fundamental for any speciality and many students wanting to nurse children are given the wrong career advice from registered nurses. The professional bodies have also been slow to adapt to the single qualification. In 1997 (8 years after the first diploma programmes commenced), advertisements for senior posts in paediatrics were still requiring general and paediatric qualifications. In addition, child branch students have difficulty entering health visiting and midwifery without a general nurse qualification, and recognition of the child branch qualification for those wishing to work abroad is not always easy. Glasper (1995) suggests that a generic registration could precede a specialist advanced qualification relating to the UKCC's 1995 recommendations. Whilst this would have the advantage of enabling children's nursing to become an academic subject in its own right, would all nurses follow the specialist route? Would we be in danger of perpetuating a shortage of appropriately qualified children's nurses and re-creating the second level nurse?

In view of this generic versus specialist debate it is reassuring that the importance of specific children's nurses was recognised by the 1997 government reports, 'The Specific Health Needs of Children and Young People' and 'Health Services for Children and Young People in the Community: Home and School'. At the launch of these reports Mrs Marion Roe, chair of the Health Select Committee, said that: 'We recommend that all nurses for whom children comprise the focus of their work should be qualified children's nurses … '. Hopefully, the future of children's nursing as a separate speciality can be assured by such support, allowing it to flourish and add to its relatively short history.

➤ **Key points**

1. Services for sick children did not commence properly until the mid-19th century.
2. The first establishment to specifically care for sick children was established in the 18th century to look after unwanted children. Hospitals at this time had little or no facilities to care for children.
3. Hospital facilities for children arose initially in an effort to overcome their poor home environment and parents were seen as an infection risk and not made welcome.
4. Psychological research in the 1950s showed that sick children needed their parents and gradually families have been more involved in the care of their sick children.
5. There are still many recommendations about the special care needed by sick children which have yet to be implemented.
6. Specific training for children's nurses commenced in 1878 but discussion has been ongoing through the years about the appropriateness of specialist versus generic training for the children's nurse.

2 ROLES OF THE CHILDREN'S NURSE

INTRODUCTION

What is a children's nurse? What makes this type of nursing different from other branches of nursing? The next chapters about nursing models begin to explore the answers to these questions but the issue of the uniqueness of nursing children is so fundamental that it is worthy of further exploration. The history of children's nursing shows that government guidelines have always recommended that children are cared for by registered nurses who have a children's nursing qualification (MoH, 1959; DoH, 1991, 1996a, b). The Audit Commission (1993) stated categorically that:

> The special needs of children and their families cannot be met without staff who have the right skills to:
> * provide care and support for the whole family;
> * deal with the highly specific problems of childhood illnesses.

None of these reports really attempt to say what it is that children's nurses do that is so different from other nurses. Children's nurses care for every aspect of the growth and development of the child and their family. In developing a therapeutic relationship with the child and family their own individuality cannot be forgotten. In the present climate of relying more and more on unqualified health care assistants, who are less costly than registered nurses, to carry out nursing care, it is important for children's nurses to be able to define exactly what they do and protect their important role.

These roles have been identified in various ways by nurse educationalists attempting to develop schemes of assessing children's nursing practice. Using these and Peplau's (1952) ideas about the roles of the nurse it appears that children's nursing practice consists of nine roles, which link closely with each other:

* stranger;
* surrogate;
* technical expert;
* advisor;
* advocate;
* resource;
* teacher;
* leader;
* developing professional.

THE STRANGER

Peplau (1952) talks about the role of the stranger as being the role in which the nurse may first meet the patient; in children's nursing practice the patient would be the child *and* family. It is in this role that the nurse makes an initial assessment of the child and family, remembering that this is also the time in which the child and family are making an initial assessment of the nurse. It is in this role that the nurse builds up the therapeutic relationship which is so crucial to quality care (Price, 1993). Darbyshire (1994) records several parents who talked about a special relationship with the nurse who had been present at admission. Nurses also spoke of their particular closeness to children and families whom they had admitted. In this study nurses relied heavily upon their first impressions of children and families in forming a relationship with them. As one nurse noted, 'we can't help it, we're only human'.

Nichols (1993) believes that a therapeutic relationship cannot be formed until the patient knows the nurse as a person. Children and families will not be able to share their feelings with a nurse until they have had time to trust that nurse. This trust is often built at the time of admission when the nurse has spent some time with the child and family. Enabling children and parents to discover the person behind the nurse and for them to accept that nurse as a caring, open and honest person is not easy. For many years nurses were taught not to get involved with patients and to maintain a professional distance from them. Close involvement with patients was considered to be too stressful for nurses, whose consequent anxiety would impair the care that they could give. Now it is recognised that nurses need to relate to their patients meaningfully whilst recognising their own needs and emotions. In an effort to define the characteristics of the therapeutic relationship, Barnsteiner and Gillis-Donovan (1990) outlined those behaviours which both aided and inhibited such a relationship. To enable the development of a therapeutic relationship, the nurse should be self-aware and be able to recognise and express personal emotions in an appropriate way (Nichols, 1993).

THE SURROGATE

Surrogate is a difficult word to define. The dictionary definition includes such synonyms such as 'substitute', 'replacement' and 'stopgap'. Children's nurses are keen not to become replacement or substitute parents, and Darbyshire's (1994) research reveals clearly that one of the parents' anxieties is that they (the parents) are incompetent and the nurses would take over their parenting role. Yet, nurses do act as a stopgap when family is not present. As discussed in Module 5, (page 361), the role of surrogate is to follow the usual home care routine when family cannot be present. It is not an opportunity for the nurse to replace the family and change the normal home practices which, in the nurse's view, are not appropriate for that child.

Behaviour which enables a therapeutic relationship

The nurse is able to:

- explore families' strengths and needs
- teach parents rather than doing everything for them
- separate the families' needs from personal needs
- recognise personal emotions arising from contact with different children and families
- demonstrate interpersonal skills as well as technical skills
- maintain clear, open communication with parents
- explore families stressors and coping styles
- recognise own emotional overload and withdraw emotionally whilst remaining committed to the care of the child and family
- resolve conflicts and misunderstanding directly

(Barnsteiner and Gillis-Donovan, 1990)

Behaviour inhibiting a therapeutic relationship

The nurse:

- works overtime to care for an individual family
- spends off-duty time with families
- shows favouritism towards certain children
- competes with other staff or parents for the affection of certain children
- attempts to influence families' decisions
- is over-involved with children and under-involved with families
- is critical of families who cannot be resident with their child
- focuses on the technical aspect of care to the detriment of the emotional care

(Barnsteiner and Gillis-Donovan, 1990)

THE TECHNICAL EXPERT

Fundamental to all the roles of the nurse is the restoration of health. Although this includes meeting the psychological needs of the child and family, the nurse performs much of this activity by using specific technical skills. Nurses are largely responsible for monitoring the child's condition using their knowledge of growth and development and pathophysiology, and providing and initiating care which has a firm research rationale. It is interesting that the competencies of the registered children's nurse produced by the UKCC centre mostly on these skills and barely mention other roles. The body of knowledge required to fulfil this role is huge and is, of course, never static. Children's nurses have to know about the physical and psychological growth and development of the child from conception to adolescence. They have to understand all the factors which influence this growth and development and cause disease and disability. They also have to know how to meet the needs of the child with a specific problem.

THE ADVISOR

Counselling is a highly complex activity which has little good research to support its effectiveness (Wilkinson, 1995). There is a growing tendency for lay people to take on the role of counsellor without adequate training or preparation. Health professionals tend to see themselves as counsellors because they listen to families' problems and offer advice. This is not counselling and there is a danger of trivialising true counselling by calling it such. Counselling or personal-centred psychotherapy was founded in the 1940s by Dr Carl Rogers, and is concerned with helping people to understand their personal perceptual world and to use this knowledge to move towards being able to direct their own lives. Most nurses' roles are more concerned with being an advisor and supporter.

In this advisory role the nurse encourages the child and family to share their feelings and thoughts, and helps them to cope with or resolve problems. This involves some of the skills of counselling such as active listening, probing, reflecting, responding with empathy and helping the patient to explore their options. Davis and Fallowfield (1991) agree that nurses are not equipped to counsel patients but talk about nurses using basic counselling skills to improve communication with their patients.

THE ADVOCATE

As an advocate the nurse helps children and their families to make informed choices and act in the child's best interest (Rushton, 1993). Ellis (1995) believes that nurses are best placed to take on this role because their care is more holistic, and they have more opportunity to get to know the individual child and family than other health care professionals.

Some families are assertive and confident enough to act as their own advocates but many will have lost their usual abilities in the stress of the hospital environment (Darbyshire, 1994). In this situation the role of the nurse is to ensure that children and their families are informed and that they have the opportunity to express their opinions. It is a difficult role for nurses to undertake as there may be instances when they do not agree with the family about what action is in the child's best interests. Advocacy is not about overruling families' wishes but respecting and representing their beliefs. Another difficulty is when the child's wishes contradict those of the parents. Again, the nurse as an advocate must give both sides opportunity to express their wishes without imposing personal views.

Activity

Identify occasions in your practice when either you have acted as an advocate or you have observed this role. What skills are needed?

To be an advocate the nurse needs the necessary knowledge to be able to explain all treatment and procedures and the available options in an unbiased manner. This enables the child and family to make informed choices. Advocacy also involves enabling parents of the appropriate way to change existing practice. Assertiveness is often required to speak out on behalf of children and families but care should be taken not to become aggressive and confrontational. On occasions advocacy will involve ethical decision making, so the nurse also needs to have an understanding of ethical theory and principles and skills in moral reasoning.

THE RESOURCE

A major part of any nurse's role is liaison with other members of the multidisciplinary team. The nurse, who tends to have most contact with the child and family, is ideally placed to coordinate the care. The nurse also knows the most appropriate personnel to refer the child and family when their need is outside the nurse's usual practice. This may occur in hospital, for example, when the nurse recognises the family's need for expert counselling, spiritual help or the specialist advice of a paediatric dietician. It may also occur on discharge when the nurse may be able to give families information and contact with community services or self-help groups.

Activity

Create an annotated list for yourself of all the self-help groups with which you have contact during your practice. What benefits do these groups offer?

Basic counselling skills

Make the situation safe
- use an open posture and manner
- avoid interruptions

Use active listening techniques
- let the parent or child talk freely
- use only short prompts or helping statements

Encourage the expression of feelings
- gently encourage emotions to be displayed
- accept displays of emotion calmly

Show empathy and understanding
- reflect back the expressed thoughts and feelings
- avoid giving instant advice
- do not over-emphasise one's own experiences

Help resolve the problem
- aid with setting objectives, determining options

(Nichols, 1993)

Guidelines for teaching parents

Assessment

- what does the family already know?
- have they any immediate concerns?
- how do they learn best?

Planning

- consider what you have to teach
- break content into small steps, possibly into different sessions
- select your teaching method, using as much variety as possible
- choose a suitable time and place

Implementation

- use simple terms, avoid jargon
- introduce the most important issues first
- re-iterate important points
- use verbal praise to reward learning but do not patronise
- have written material for parents to consolidate your learning

Evaluation

- allow time for parents' questions
- check learning has taken place

Cross reference

Role of children's nurses in child health promotion – page 167

Compliance – page 229

Nurses, through previous experience, can also act as a valuable guide to mechanical resources, aids to living, dressings and medication. They are able to give a balanced view of the disadvantages and advantages of using one resource over another.

Acting as a resource involves being able to answer questions about aspects of care or treatment.

THE TEACHER

As well as being able to answer questions, children's nurses also act as a teacher. They are required to teach parents and their children about health, and they are often involved in teaching them about technical care so that the child and parents can continue this care independently.

Every children's nurse acts as a health educator. An increasing part of this role is health prevention which needs a good understanding of the socioeconomic factors in the families' environment which may affect their health. Health prevention in hospital has to be tackled with particular tact as often the accident or illness has already occurred. However, accidents often occur because parents do not recognise the child's abilities and the nurse is in a good position to discuss potential problems and advise preventive measures related to the child's stage of development. Health education posters, information leaflets and displays cannot change motivational or risk-perception factors but they can provide education when used imaginatively in the clinic or ward. This specific part of the teacher's role is discussed in more detail in Module 3 (page 167).

Children's nurses teach children and their families and therefore need the skills to teach both age groups. It is important to assess their willingness to learn and not to make parents feel pressurised into taking on aspects of care. It is useful to teach more than one member of the family so that no one person feels that they carry sole responsibility for the care. Children learn best through play and the nurse can use this strategy to teach knowledge and skills. Teaching parents is often more difficult as they lack confidence because of their anxiety about their child and they often have the competing demands and fatigue caused by other children and other jobs. However, they are usually well motivated and are able to use their past experiences to aid new learning. In comparison to answering questions as a resource person, teaching is not a casual role and should be well planned out beforehand to obtain the best results. Although education is not the sole factor in ensuring compliance, parents who are more knowledgeable about their child's condition are more likely to comply with treatment (Ley and Llewelyn, 1995). The nurse's relationship with parents should help in identifying the most appropriate way of imparting the knowledge; an American study found that 30–50% mothers taught by doctors did not understand terms such as asthma, virus, vitamin or fever (Gablehouse and Gitterman, 1990).

THE LEADER

Nurses may act as leaders in several ways. Although care plans are best negotiated with the child and parents there may be occasions when the nurse is more directive in determining care, e.g. after surgery. Being a primary nurse involves acting as a leader for other colleagues and ensuring continuity and consistency of care. Children's nurses also act as leaders for other nurses or health care professionals who are not used to caring for children. In this role, for instance, they may give specific advice to community staff or nurses in adult intensive care units about the care of children. The nurse in a multidisciplinary team is often the only member of the team with specific knowledge of the child and family and is likely to be the only member with the specific skills to care for children (Fradd, 1994). Nurses must be feel confident and competent in their knowledge and skills to be able to share them in this way.

Activity

Compile a list of the characteristics which you consider an effective leader should have.

Leadership skills
- Time management
- delegation
- accountability
- assertiveness
- communication
- resource management
- inspires and motivates others
- team management

At the 1996 Annual Conference of the Society of Paediatric Nursing, the chief nursing officer for England told delegates that there were great opportunities for children's nurses to lead the way in developing services for children. She was referring to all practising children's nurses because leadership has more to do with personal skills and attributes that one's position in the nursing hierarchy (Sams, 1996). Leadership skills are intrinsic to everyday nursing practice and crucial if nurses are to initiate and implement change rather than have it imposed upon them (Sams, 1996).

THE DEVELOPING PRACTITIONER

Discussion about Peplau's model of nursing (page 607) explains how Peplau believes that the nurse develops from each and every encounter with a patient. She believes that each nurse–patient relationship brings some new learning to the nurse. Benner (1984) recognised that nurses learn their intuitive knowledge by experience but that this experiential learning could not expand and develop unless they began to record what they learn from their experiences. Nurses are now beginning to recognise this valuable source of new knowledge and are using reflection to identify it in a more concrete way.

Guidelines for reflection
- Briefly describe the experience, its context and any influencing factors
- Reflect upon what you did and why
- Examine the reactions of yourself and others
- Consider what influenced your behaviour and actions
- Think whether you could have behaved or acted differently
- Summarise what you have learned from this experience and how it will affect your future practice

Activity

Reflect upon a recent encounter with a child and family and identify what you learn from this occurrence.

Cross references

Research – page 674

Reflective practice – page 619

PREP categories of study – page 622

Reflection need not only be centred on professional practice. Personal incidents such as a bereavement, or a period of time as a patient, may be a valuable learning experience and affect the way in which you practice.

Nursing knowledge can also expand and develop through research. Nurses are now more involved in research but this involvement tends to be confined to those in specialist roles. Clinically based nurses have greater opportunity to observe child and parental behaviour and children's responses to care and treatment, and often use innovative ways to encourage children to comply with treatment. They could be using this experience in an investigative way to challenge accepted practice or introduce new ideas.

The professional bodies in nursing also expect registered nurses to develop their practice. The UKCC Code of Professional Conduct (1992b) states that the nurse has a responsibility to: 'maintain and improve professional knowledge and competence'. In addition, from 1st April 1995 it became mandatory for all registered nurses, midwives and health visitors to provide evidence of their continuing post-registration development in order to re-register every 3 years (UKCC, 1994b). This evidence must include:

- at least 5 days of study in every 3-year period relevant to the individual's role and area of practice, showing how the area of study has enhanced practice;
- a notification of practice form (or a statutory Return to Practice programme after a break of 5 years or more);
- a personal professional profile.

Nurses also develop their practice by gaining increasing technical skills to meet the demand of technological advances. It is important that children's nurses keep abreast of new developments and continue to enhance their own practice if they are to maintain their identity and prove their unique contribution to child health.

Key points ➤

1. Although there is much support for the uniqueness of children's nursing, it is difficult, but necessary to maintain the speciality, to define exactly what this uniqueness means.
2. Children's nursing consists of nine interlinking roles: stranger, surrogate, technical expert, advisor, advocate, resource, teacher, leader, and developing professional.
3. The children's nurse needs to be self-aware to be able to undertake many of these roles.
4. Effective communication is fundamental to all the roles of the children's nurse.

5. Children's nurses need a wide knowledge base to carry out all the roles effectively.

6. Children's nurses owe it to themselves and their profession to develop their role as specialist nurses.

3 MODELS OF NURSING – USELESS THEORY OR AN AID TO PRACTICE

INTRODUCTION

Ever since organised nurse training began, nurses have been theorising about nursing. In Britain, early theories about nursing were communicated by Florence Nightingale in 1859. She described nursing as both an art and a science and her ideas provided the foundation of a knowledge base unique to nursing. After Nightingale, the emphasis moved from nursing to medical knowledge, although this was limited in 1850s, and nursing began to focus on medical phenomena such as signs and symptoms, disease, and medical and surgical procedures.

It was not until almost a hundred years later that there was any effort to develop or define nursing. In the 1950s, with the advent of university education for American nurses, ideas about nursing began to develop which questioned both the nature of nursing and its traditional foundations. These ideas which were called models of nursing have had varied reactions. On the one hand, theory is seen as necessary if nurses desire a professional identity, wish to improve standards of care and consolidate, and want to increase and clarify the knowledge base of nursing. On the other hand, the continued production of multiple models of nursing is seen as elaborate waffle which does not relate to reality and is only indulged in by those academic nurses in teaching who never actually lay hands on a real patient. Thus, at the moment, nurses are divided in their opinions about the usefulness of models; Engstrom (1984) attempted to describe this situation: 'In all a portrait of the profession is one of confusion and lack of consensus'.

To discuss the values of models both from an historical viewpoint and as a means of progressing the discipline of nursing, the following questions need to be considered:

- What are models of nursing?
- Why did models develop?
- Were these reasons valid?
- What do models aim to do?
- Are they achieving their aims?

DEFINITIONS OF MODELS

Models of nursing have been defined in different ways by different authors, but the common theme appears to be that models are expressing the reality of nursing and enabling nurses to be able to work towards common goals. This promotes continuity of care and benefits the nursing team and the patient.

Nursing – what it is and what it is not

' ... Nursing is occupied with the control of the patient's environment so that nature may act upon him or her.'

'It has been said and written scores of times that every woman makes a good nurse. I believe on the contrary that the very elements of nursing are all but unknown.'

Nightingale (1859)

Definitions of models of nursing

' ... a collection of ideas, knowledge and values about nursing which determines the way nurses, as individuals and groups, work with their patients and clients.'

(Wright, 1990)

' ... a descriptive picture of practice which adequately represents the real thing.'

(Pearson and Vaughan, 1986)

' ... Representations of the reality of nursing practice. They represent the factors at work and how they are related.'

(Aggleton and Chambers 1986)

Activity

Discuss with your colleagues how you would define nursing. Look critically at some of the models of nursing you have seen in practice and assess whether you consider your views have been incorporated.

THE EMERGENCE OF MODELS

It appears that models of nursing emerged for several reasons. It is useful to consider if these reasons are actually valid. One of the reasons given for the need to define nursing is nurses' constant bid to achieve professionalism. Professionalism is difficult to define and there appears to be no general consensus on one definition. One of the earliest writers in this field was Abraham Flexner who suggested that the attributes of a profession were (Flexner, 1915, cited by Jolley and Allan, 1989):

- basically intellectual;
- learned in nature, because it is based on a body of knowledge;
- practical rather than theoretical;
- in possession of techniques taught through education;
- well organised internally;
- motivated by altruism.

Several desirable consequences arise from the ability to claim professional status. These include monopoly of service, autonomy, public recognition, prestige, power and authority (Gruending, 1985). The benefits to nursing of professionalism would include relative freedom from supervision outside the discipline as well as monetary and status awards. However, Davies (1996a) suggests that nurses' desire for professionalism is outdated and instead of aiming for power, authority and mastery of a unique body of knowledge, they should be aiming to develop supportive practice, empowerment of patients and knowledge gained by reflection.

Another of the reasons that models of nursing have developed is to provide the body of knowledge that can be applied to its practice – a dominant characteristic of a profession. However, in the obsession with the idea of professionalism, many models have been developed. Do these different theories about nursing, which all to often have not been proven, actually aid in the quest to be seen as a profession?

It may be argued that models of nursing emerged to improve standards of care. All thinking people process views of the world, their work and the subject of their work – in the case of nursing, the patient or clients. In nursing, the care given to patients or clients is influenced by the people who give the care. For example, in a team of nurses, one nurse may align the practice of nursing with that of medicine and aim for the efficient carrying out of medical treatment. Another may see the social activities as important in enabling the patient to function as an individual. One nurse may consistently do things such as washing and dressing for the patient because she sees doing things for people as an essential part of nursing. A second nurse may observe or support someone to do things for himself as she sees helping the patient to be independent as important.

All nurses are as individual as their patients, and, consequently, their past lives and experiences which influence their behaviour and values are unique. Thus it is likely that each nurse has a slightly different image of what nursing is. It is the purpose of models to bring together these images so nurses have shared goals and can improve standards of care, as the alternative is a lack of direction and confusion not only for the patient but for other members of the health care team.

Obviously if models are to improve care by ensuring a consistent approach they need to describe actual nursing as it is and not as some theoretical ideal. Opposers of nursing models suggest that models are unrealistic because:

- British nurses have tended to become dominated by American models. Are these theories realistic as their health care system is so different? Should developments in models of nursing from other countries be studied?

- Terms used are often obscure and incomprehensible. A *Nursing Times* correspondent comments that 'I suspect that many of us cannot understand it ... I am sceptical whether *"consideration of supply of sustenal imperatives to the eliminative subsystem"* will do much to alert the nurse to a particular patient's need for brown bread for breakfast'. Models are more likely to be read and noticed if they are written in a clear, concise language.

- Most models have been developed by nursing theorists who see nursing as it ought to be rather than 'as it is'. Nursing is primarily a care giving discipline so surely any model of nursing must be closely related to this practice?

In spite of such criticisms nursing needs to be able to measure its standards of care and prove its value to patients. A theoretical framework for care could be a useful tool in enabling nurses to manage their own budgets.

Models of nursing have also emerged to meet the need to consolidate, increase and clarify the knowledge of nursing.

> *Practice without theory is like a man who goes to sea without a map, in a ship without a rudder.*
>
> (Leonardo Da Vinci)

The model which traditionally guided nurses was the medical model which concentrated information and decision making in the hands of doctors. As nurses have become more educated they have tried to emphasise the important role that nurses play in health and illness.

The medical model centres around patients' diseases and the physical care needed to cure them. Emphasis is placed on routine and getting the work done. Knowledge is related to the physical sciences and the nurses' role in such a model of care is centred around the achievement of tasks. This model saw the patient as a malfunctioning machine and, as in a factory, different people were given different jobs to correct the malfunction. This has allowed the emergence of nurse specialists (pain, TPN, IV therapy, etc.) which actually do not help the development of nursing models which see the patient as unique and advocate holistic care. Whilst task oriented care can confuse patients who may have several nurses attending to their needs, it may also be reassuring to both parties. Nurses find they do not really know any patient well and this can protect them from becoming emotionally involved. Patients do not feel neglected if their nurse is not available and feel able to turn to other nurses for help.

Activity

Discuss the following issues with your colleagues:
- does task orientation reduce stress?
- do all nurses want to change the traditional handmaiden role?
- do nurses really want to increase nursing knowledge?
- does the specialist nurse practitioner role help individualised care?

While Project 2000 may change traditional views, at the moment any nurse who achieves further knowledge and becomes skilled at bedside care is promoted away from the bedside or develops a speciality as above which prevents the patient being seen as a whole person. Care often ends up being given by the unskilled and untrained. Will this be perpetuated by the emergence of health care assistants? Some nurses are already being managed at ward level by non-nurses – is this because nurses have not been able to clarify what nursing is? Models may add to nursing knowledge but do they really clarify it?

AIMS OF MODELS

Wright (1990) suggests that models may have a value for practice because they aim to define:
- the nature of the person and his/her environment;
- the concept of health;
- the concept of nursing.

In addition, a model also aims to offer guidelines on:
- what kind of research is relevant to nursing;
- how nursing should be managed;

The traditional biomedical model
- Gives the doctor the power for decision making
- Devalues the role of nursing
- Loses sight of the patient as an individual
- Concentrates on the physical diagnosis
- Ignores the holistic view of health and illness
- Emphasises technology to the detriment of caring

Cross reference

Specialist roles for children's nurses – page 639

Figure 3.1

Components of models.

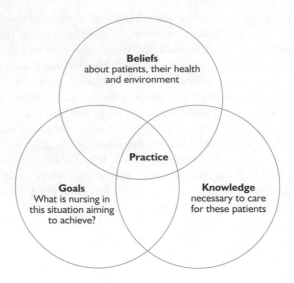

- the content and style of educational programmes;
- the conduct of nursing practice to provide high quality care (Figure 3.1).

Activity

Take a critical look at some of the models you have used in practice. Do they all achieve these aims?

On close inspection, many models of nursing omit large areas of detail, e.g. Newman's model does not attempt to define nursing and even suggests that the model can be used by other health care workers! Much detail is given on the need to change, but there is lack of advice on how to achieve the change. Nursing tends to impose change from above but this is inappropriate if the model is to reflect actual practice. Nurses who are ward based surely need to be helped to choose and develop a model which suits their area of practice otherwise it will be used in theory and not in practice. Wright (1990) agrees with this and advocates that if a model is to be realistically applied to a particular setting, it should be created by those working in that area. Some nurses have created or adapted established models for use in their own setting. An example of this is the Burford model (Johns, 1994).

Cross reference

A reflective model of nursing – page 620

Activity

Opposers of nursing models consider that those models which originate outside the UK cannot accurately reflect nursing in this country. Discuss with some colleagues whether the nature of the patient and the concepts of health and nursing can be defined in universal terms.

Critics of nursing models appear to suggest that the administration of health care in different countries affects the delivery, and thus the definitions, of nursing care. If this is true should nurses in this country be looking for different definitions of nursing now that health care is largely managed by NHS Trusts and fundholding GP practices?

Activity

Talk to nurses of different generations. Do they have very different ideas about nursing?

Activity

Consider if models of nursing should change to reflect changes in society and the Health Service.

If nursing is to remain as a recognised, independent and accepted discipline the development of a unique knowledge base is essential. This knowledge base must be directly related to and useful in nursing practice. Whilst there is still a lack of consensus and frustration about the relevance of models of nursing, consideration of how they can be developed, used and validated for nursing cannot progress.

Activity

Discuss with colleagues their views about models of nursing and consider whether they are worth pursuit in the quest of knowledge about the uniqueness of nursing.

➤ **Key points**

1. Ideas about nursing began to become formalised in the 1950s when models of nursing were first created.

2. At present, nurses are divided in their views about the usefulness of nursing models for practice.

3. Models of nursing aim to define nursing, the nature of the patient and to offer guidelines on the knowledge, attitudes and skills necessary to maintain and develop nursing practice.

4. Opposers of nursing models believe that models are incomprehensible, unrealistic and unrelated to nursing in the UK.

5. Those in favour of nursing models argue that models help to clarify the uniqueness of nursing and enable nursing to be accepted as a profession.

4 MODELS OF CHILDREN'S NURSING

INTRODUCTION

As discussed in the previous section, models of nursing aim to reflect the beliefs and values about nursing in specific settings. They aim to prevent disunity and conflict by clarifying these ideas and promoting a common philosophy of nursing.

In the UK, children's nurses generally share the philosophy of family-centred care; believing that parents should be enabled to participate in the care of their children at all times. This philosophy is supported by the DoH which states that parents should be closely involved in their child's health care (DoH, 1991). In other countries this philosophy has been slow to develop and Hostler (1992) reported that in 30 leading American hospitals there were no examples of nursing models which reflected family-centred care. Up until 1988 there were no specific models of nursing in the UK for the care of children, and children's nurses tended to use either Roper, Logan and Tierney's model of activities of living (Roper *et al.*, 1980), Orem's model of self-care (Orem, 1985) or Peplau's interpersonal relationships model (Peplau, 1952). In 1988, Casey developed the partnership model of nursing specifically for use in child care settings.

This section will summarise the concepts of each of these models, and explore their usefulness and effectiveness for paediatric practice, thus enabling children's nurses to take a critical look at the model used in their area of practice.

ROPER, LOGAN AND TIERNEY'S ACTIVITY OF LIVING MODEL

In the UK, this is probably the best known and most widely used model of nursing. It centres around the philosophy that an important part of living relates to the everyday activities which individuals regularly perform. They call these the 'activities of living'. The model is concerned with the individual's ability to carry out these activities independently, recognising that physical, psychological, environmental, politico-economic and sociocultural factors may all affect an individual's level of independence. It emphasises the individuality of each person's activities of living. The model recognises that fetal development, as well as physical, intellectual, emotional and social development in childhood and adolescence, affects the individual's ability to perform daily activities independently. It also discusses the impact of social relationships and the effect of the family upon the socialisation of children. It is these ideas, which relate to the care of children, which have made the model a popular choice for children's nursing.

The role of the nurse is seen as preventing, comforting and promoting maximum independence. The aim of nursing being to

Activities of living

- Maintaining a safe environment
- Communicating
- Breathing
- Eating and drinking
- Eliminating
- Personal cleansing and dressing
- Controlling body temperature
- Mobilising
- Working and playing
- Expressing sexuality
- Sleeping
- Dying

(Roper *et al.*, 1980)

assess the individuals level of dependence in each of the activities of living and planning how to help that individual move towards independence.

Activity

Read the case study (Figure 4.1 – page 604) describing Roper, Logan and Tierney's model in practice and identify:
*   how Sarah's usual levels of dependence/independence have altered because of her illness;
*   how the roles of the nurse, as described by the model, will be used to help Sarah return to her usual dependence/independence.

The activities of living model has been analysed and criticised by many authors. A popular criticism is that the model is medically biased because the activities of living relate to physiological systems (Aggleton and Chambers, 1986). Lister (1987) denies this claim because at least some of the activities of living have a strong psychological bias. Although many studies have been written about the use of this model they do not examine its appropriateness to nursing practice (Fraser, 1996). Recent evidence appears to show that nurses find the model too simplistic (Parr, 1993) and Fraser (1996) could find no literature to describe its use outside the UK.

In relation to paediatrics, although the model recognises the importance of the family and developmental factors in shaping the individual, it does not consider the role of the family in helping the individual towards independence. This omission would appear to make the model difficult to use in any area where the philosophy was family-centred care.

OREM'S SELF-CARE MODEL

In contrast, Orem's model of nursing centres around the belief that all individuals have self-care needs which they meet themselves whenever possible, but when unable to self-care they require help from others. The individual's ability to self-care depends upon the therapeutic self-care demand which is affected by the individual's maturity, knowledge and life experience as well as their physical and mental health. The essential requirements for life are termed universal self-care requisites and these needs may alter as a result of developmental or life changes. They also alter as a result of ill-health or disability (health deviation self-care requisites). Individuals can often adapt their own care to meet deviations but intervention is required when the individual can no longer make these adaptations. This intervention may be made by friends or family, and it is only when their care becomes inadequate to overcome the deviation that nursing intervention is required. The role

Figure 4.1

*Roper, Logan and Tierney's
model in practice.*

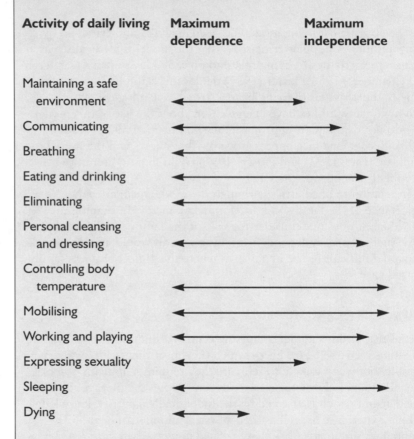

Sarah was a 9 year old who had been admitted to the ward as a newly diagnosed insulin-dependent diabetic. On admission, she was feeling ill due to hyperglycaemia and keto-acidosis.

Once Sarah's immediate medical problems had been treated a nursing assessment was carried out and Sarah's dependence/independence during health and illness was noted. When she was well Sarah was fairly independent at most activities. Her mother did say that she needed reminding to brush her teeth before bed and that she needed help to wash and dry her long hair. Her usual level of dependence/independence was thus assessed as follows:

Activity of daily living	Maximum dependence	Maximum independence
Maintaining a safe environment		
Communicating		
Breathing		
Eating and drinking		
Eliminating		
Personal cleansing and dressing		
Controlling body temperature		
Mobilising		
Working and playing		
Expressing sexuality		
Sleeping		
Dying		

During her first 24 hours in hospital Sarah was very dependent. She felt unwell and had an IV infusion running to overcome her dehydration and was having sliding scale IV insulin. Although I explained all her care, she was not ready to eat and drink normally or to be taught how to test her blood and urine.

of the nurse, which may involve being wholly compensatory, partially compensatory or educative/developmental, is to use various types of helping methods to:

- eliminate any self-care deficits;
- enable the client to decrease the self-care deficit;
- help others to give dependent care;
- meet the self-care needs directly.

Orem defines nursing as being needed when the individual can no longer maintain the necessary self-care to sustain life and health. She recognises that in the care of children, nursing intervention is required when the parent can no longer maintain the appropriate therapeutic amount and quality of care. Thus, this model appears to recognise some important concepts of nursing children. The developmental changes in self-care and the role of parents in meeting their child's needs are recognised. The nurse's role in teaching and helping parents to meet health care deviations is also made explicit.

Orem's language and writing style has been criticised as being very tortuous and jargonistic (Fraser, 1996). Other criticisms include the individual's desire for self-care. Lacey (1993) considers that some individuals have no desire or motivation to be involved in their own care. Lacey also suggests that some nurses, especially those in nursing homes, are happier for patients to remain dependent upon staff for their care. However, in spite of this it is a model which is used world wide in many different fields of nursing. It has been found suitable for mental health (MacDonald, 1991), theatre (Weir, 1993) and oncology nursing (Richardson, 1992) as well as in the care of the elderly (Kitson, 1986).

The suitability of the model for children's nursing is demonstrated by a study performed by Lasky and Eichelburger in 1985. They studied the health beliefs and behaviour of 75 children aged 4–6 years. They discovered that these children understood health promotion and could relate this to their own behaviour. Some health-related activities were carried out independently by the children, some were performed by the parents and some were joint child and parent activities. The study also confirmed the parental influence upon health beliefs and attitudes. Whilst the study was carried out in America and not specifically related to Orem's model, it does illustrate the self-care concepts of the model related to the care of young children.

Activity

Read the case study (Figure 4.2) overleaf using Orem's model in practice and identify:
- examples of how the various helping methods are used;
- the nursing roles used, with examples;
- what knowledge and skills you would need to use this model.

Universal self-care requisites
- Sufficient intake of air, food and water
- Appropriate excretion of waste products
- Optimum balance between activity and rest
- Optimum balance between solitude and social interaction
- Avoidance of hazards to life and well-being
- Conformity with what is currently considered to be a normal lifestyle

(Orem, 1971)

Roles of the nurse
- Wholly compensatory to carry out all care for the patient, e.g. unconscious patient
- Partially compensatory to help the patient carry out care, e.g. helping a small child do up buttons and laces after the child has dressed independently
- Educative/developmental to teach the patient about care, e.g. showing the diabetic child self-injection technique

(Orem, 1971)

Figure 4.2

Orem's model of nursing in practice.

Edwin was a 15 year old with cystic fibrosis. He was admitted to hospital for re-assessment of his deteriorating respiratory function and treatment of a chest infection. Although Edwin was very breathless and had a high temperature, he was anxious to remain as independent as possible. On admission he and I made the following plan to meet his needs in hospital.

Universal self-care requisites

Sufficient intake of air	I would monitor his respiratory function 4 hourly. Edwin would perform his own chest physiotherapy.
Sufficient intake of water	Edwin would choose the time, content and amount of his food and meals according to his breathlessness. He would note down all his intake so that I could advise on calorie intake.
Balance of activity and rest, social activity and solitude	Edwin would determine this and put a note on his door when he required privacy. He had his own TV and computer games.
Elimination	Edwin would report any constipation.
Prevention of hazards	Edwin could meet his own needs. I would monitor his temperature 4 hourly.
Promotion of normal lifestyle	Edwin could go out to eat or meet his friends if he told a nurse first.

Developmental self-care requisites

Life cycle stage. As Edwin was an adolescent I needed to be aware of his need to assert his independence and establish his own personality. He wanted to take responsibility for himself and his illness, and I needed to respect that and allow him to make decisions about his care.

Life changes. Edwin was beginning to recognise that his lifespan could be shortened by his condition. He was concerned about his future and his employment/career prospects. He needed help and support to discuss these issues.

Health deviation self-care requisites

Edwin's chest infection required IV antibiotic treatment which he was keen to learn how to do for himself. I would teach him how to do this.

PEPLAU'S INTERPERSONAL RELATIONSHIPS MODEL

Hildegard Peplau was one of the first nurse theorists and she developed her model of nursing primarily for the field of mental health. Peplau believes that nursing is a significant therapeutic interpersonal relationship and is concerned with working in partnership with the individual to make health possible. The concept of stress is fundamental to this model. Peplau considers that every individual has biological, psychological and social qualities which motivate them to live. When these qualities are impaired tension occurs. These tensions can produce a positive reaction by the individual to overcome the tension and, as a result, to increase their personal growth and development. Alternatively, the individual may react in a negative way and be unable to function effectively. At an extreme level this may cause regression. Using this model, the aim of nursing is to alleviate tensions, and to help the individual to overcome problems in a positive way, thus increasing self-esteem. According to Peplau, the nurse uses six main roles to develop the necessary interpersonal relationship with the individual to be able to help in the resolution of problems. Central to the concepts of this model is the development of the nurse. Peplau believes that the nurse becomes more expert as a result of the knowledge, skills and attitudes gained by the therapeutic relationship with each patient.

Activity

Consider your nursing experience to date. How do you think that you have developed as a result of your interaction with children you have nursed?

Although Peplau does not explicitly explore the use of her model for children's nursing, it is easy to make comparisons with the concepts of the model and the beliefs about nursing children. There is much research evidence to show that children do regress as a result of physical and psychological stress (Grey, 1993), and the role of the nurse is very concerned with minimising this stress and helping the child to cope with it. The nurses relationship with the child and family is very crucial to the success of the treatment and most children's nurses would describe this as working in partnership with the parents. Nursing children is about accepting them as they are with their own home routine and it is also concerned with helping them develop and learn about health care. Whilst some of the roles of the nurse described by Peplau may relate more to the nurse's relationship with parents, they are very appropriate to the care of the older child. The role of surrogate carer has always been suspect when caring for children, as the nurse does not wish to replace the family, but Peplau's definition of this role is that this is a temporary role until the patient is able to be independent again.

Peplau's roles of the nurse

The nurse as a stranger
- accepts and treats the patient as an individual
- initiates the nurse–patient relationship
- orientates the patient to the care setting

The nurse as a surrogate
- helps the patient to become aware of the nurse as an individual
- is self-aware and presents her/himself to the patient
- promotes an interpersonal relationship

The nurse as a resource person
- provides specific answers to questions
- acts as a source of knowledge for improving health
- interprets prescribed care and treatment

The nurse as a teacher
- promotes the patient's interest in learning
- develops innovative teaching to meet individual needs
- uses individual outcomes

The nurse as a counsellor
- helps the patient to understand her/himself
- enables the patient to express feelings
- facilitates patient insight and discovery

The nurse as a leader
- encourages patient participation
- indicates new possibilities
- helps the patient to overcome problems
- develops patient independence

Activity

Read the case study (Figure 4.3) of Peplau's model in practice and identify:
- how Peplau's roles of the nurse are used;
- what knowledge and skills you would need to practise this model.

Figure 4.3

Peplau's model of nursing in action.

Bethany, aged 10 months, was re-admitted to the ward for re-assessment of her multiple physical disabilities. Due to problems caused by a rare genetic defect, she had a tracheostomy to help her breathe and was fed via a gastrostomy. She was also profoundly deaf and wore glasses to help her poor eyesight. Her facial features were very abnormal and she was small for her age.

During my assessment of Bethany using Peplau's model I needed to discover whether the physical stress of her disabilities was causing her mental and physical potential to develop or regress. Lisa, Bethany's mother, was resident during this admission, and I needed to find out if the stress of caring for Bethany's many problems was affecting her physically, psychologically and socially.

To achieve all of the above, I needed to get to know Bethany and Lisa (whom I had never met before) and help them both to gain from their situation by using my previous personal and professional experience. As a result of this relationship I would learn more about them as individuals as well as the stress of such situations. As Bethany's nurse, I also needed to:

- provide care in Lisa's absence
- coordinate the specialist services needed for Bethany's re-assessment
- identify outside agencies and equipment which could help Lisa
- show Lisa nursing techniques to improve her caring skills
- enable Lisa to express any concerns

CASEY'S PARTNERSHIP MODEL

Casey also centres her model around the concept of partnership but, because this model was developed for use in paediatrics, it clearly states that this partnership is one between the parents and the health care professional. This model believes that the patient is both the child and family. It recognises that the child is an individual who is growing and developing physically, psychologically, spiritually and socially. It accepts that each family construction may be different and that in each situation the family must include anyone close to the child. It also believes that the role of the children's nurse is to support and strengthen the family's ability to care for their child. Casey's philosophy of children's nursing states categorically that the best people to care for the child is the family with varying degrees of help from appropriately qualified health care professionals. She believes that this model can be applied in any setting where children are nursed.

To apply this model to practice, it is important to assess the child and family as an individual unit. What is the child's usual behaviour and how has the health problem changed it? Who is important to the child and how do they wish to be involved in the child's care? It is also necessary to discover the child's usual family care so that this can be followed as closely as possible. The child's plan of care can then as far as possible involve the child's usual carers and routine, while the nurse can work in partnership with the family to assess the child's return to health.

Activity

Read the case study (Figure 4.4) overleaf using Casey's model in practice. Identify how the roles of the nurse as described by Casey are used. Consider what knowledge, skills and attitudes are required to practise this model.

The concept of partnership has been the subject of much discussion. The Audit Commission (1993) discovered that many parents were unclear about their role when resident in hospital with their child and felt that their knowledge of their own child was often ignored. In this audit of hospital services for children both parents and children thought that they were not involved in care decisions. Campbell and Glasper (1995) point out that hospitals which provide meals for children but do not cater for resident parents can hardly be said to be enabling partnership. Similarly, families need to be enabled to be the constant factor in the child's life in hospital, as they are at home. Darbyshire (1994) discovered that most children's units have difficulty offering adequate facilities for one parent and do not cater at all for other family members. Other impediments to providing a partnership philosophy of care are staff shortages, skill mix and other health care professionals' attitudes (Campbell and Clarke, 1992). Freidson (1970) argues that partnership is impossible if one member of the partnership has more knowledge and power than the other. Nurses practising the partnership model should take care to share their knowledge with the child and family. However, this does not remove the fact that the nurse is in a more powerful position because of this extra knowledge. Other writers suggest that some nurses avoid partnership with children and families as a means of avoiding the stress that such close relationships can bring (Nichols, 1993).

Activity

Discuss with some colleagues whether nurses can ever truly work in partnership with all children and their parents. Discuss how you can make children and families feel valued and equal in their relationship with the nurse.

Casey's roles of the nurse
- *To provide family care* – when the child or family are no longer able to provide the care which they would normally carry out independently at home. This may be because the child is too ill or when parents cannot be resident
- *To administer nursing care* – the specific health care intervention required by the child
- *To act as a teacher* – by teaching parents to give family care and specific nursing care during their child's illness
- *To provide support* – by helping the family come to terms with their child's illness and treatment and to be available to enable the expression of concerns
- *To be a resource* – by providing specific answers to questions and liaising with other agencies to enable continuing care in the community

Cross reference
Family-centred care – pages 612–617

Figure 4.4

Casey's model in practice.

Toby, aged 5, was admitted to the ward for elective surgery following recurrent severe episodes of vomiting, abdominal pain and diarrhoea. These episodes had been increasing to such a degree that it had now been decided to perform an ileostomy. Sue, Toby's mother, planned to be resident whilst grandparents looked after the rest of the family. It was decided that I would be Toby's named nurse, and when Toby was admitted I spent some time with him and Sue assessing and planning his care. Sue and Toby had been in hospital many times before and Sue knew that, while she wanted to be involved in Toby's care, she was not very good at it as she was frightened of hurting him. She also knew that since his illness Toby had become very clingy and she was anxious about leaving him.

Sue, Toby and I therefore agreed a plan of care which involved Sue but also gave her time alone for meals and to relax. In the pre-operative period I spent time with Sue and Toby getting to know them and their routines and answering questions about the surgery. During the post-operative period when Toby's nursing needs were at their greatest, I provided his specific nursing care and met his hygiene needs with Sue's help. I cared for the ileostomy until Toby started to mobilise when I helped Sue and Toby to learn how to do this. Each day when I arrived on duty, we would all plan the day so that Toby had either Sue or myself present. In the evenings when Dad visited, I would help them settle Toby for the night and then he was happy for them to go out together knowing I was available if he needed me. At the weekends we organised the day to allow Toby plenty of rest so that he could enjoy his late afternoon visits from his grandparents, siblings and the family dog.

Even when Toby and Sue were able to meet Toby's physical needs without me, I made sure I was available to talk, answer questions or just be there while Sue went for a break.

When partnership in care is achieved, its benefit is well documented. Families feel more confident and competent to care for their sick child and thus feel less stressed by the hospital environment. Nurses gain more job satisfaction, and both nurses and families develop more skills in the care of children (Curley and Wallace, 1992).

1. Most UK children's nurses have a philosophy of family-centred care, but this is a concept that is relatively new in other countries.
2. Family-centred care involves the acceptance of individual family's beliefs and values.
3. There are a number of models of nursing which encompass some of the concepts of caring for children but only Casey's partnership model was developed specifically for use in paediatrics.
4. Partnership is a difficult concept to achieve in practice.
5. More research is needed to validate the concepts of nursing models and their appropriateness for children's nursing.

➤ **Key points**

5   FAMILY-CENTRED CARE

INTRODUCTION

Previous chapters have discussed the historical background to involving parents in the care of their sick child and the concept of partnership as expressed by Casey's partnership model of nursing. Now it seems important to discuss the issues involved in practice when enabling parents to be with their sick child in hospital and to be an active participant in their care. This idea of family-centred care, which is supported by the government (DoH, 1991), is part of the philosophy of every paediatric unit and children's nursing course curriculum. However, Darbyshire (1995) warns that without careful consideration of the meaning of family-centred care it could become just an academic, abstract notion which is not actually practised.

There are three main principles of achieving family-centred care. Firstly, that children are admitted to hospital only if the care they require cannot be as well provided at home, in a day clinic or on a day care basis in hospital (DoH, 1991). In this way they can be nursed at home mainly by the family with input from community staff and resources as required. Secondly, that the philosophy is clearly explained to all the staff and family so they can understand and negotiate their roles. Finally, the philosophy has to be implemented in such a way as to take account of all the elements of family care.

CARE AT HOME OR IN HOSPITAL?

The concept of hospital admission only when there is no other suitable option appears to be in the best interests of the child and family. However, is it what parents want? I remember parents of children, referred by their general practitioner to a paediatrician, who have been sent home with medication and advice and who have been clearly unhappy at that decision because they feel unable to cope. All staff working with children need to be aware that not all parents feel able to care for their sick child. This may because of work commitments, other dependent family members or a lack of appropriate skills and knowledge. Remember too, that not all parents feel at ease with sickness and simply feel unable to become involved in nursing care, and the children's community service has yet to develop to such a degree that it can offer a service to all sick children being nursed at home.

In North America, where community children's teams are not available, Care by Parent units have been developed to overcome this deficit. Cleary *et al.* (1986) argued that such units were surplus to requirements in the UK because of the development of children's community teams. On the contrary, such units may form a useful facility

Cross reference

Community nursing – pages 371–377

for parents who are frightened of being left alone at home to care for their child.

There is evidence to show that parents are taking on a greater role in the care of their sick children at home. The Audit Commission (1993) found that children now stay in hospital for a significantly reduced amount of time when compared with 30 years ago. In 1962, children's length of stay in hospital was an average of 13 days. In 1993 this had reduced to an average of 3.5 days. This may not be entirely the result of complying with government guidelines, but a natural reduction caused by better treatments – a similar reduction is seen in the length of stay for adults. This reduced length of stay is helped by the expansion of day care for children but the Audit Commission (1993) noted that this facility is variable and could be developed further. Should this facility be developed further? Is it what parents want and are they offered a choice? Does family-centred care include the selection of a child for day surgery by diagnosis rather than by parental preference? The other reason for the reduced admission time is the development of home care which has been shown to be more cost effective than care in hospital (Chamberlain *et al.*, 1988). There is a danger that economics could take precedence over the family's wishes about home care and it is important to be clear that the choice is the family's. If care is truly family centred the discharge from hospital should be when the family are ready and able to take over the care and not when the hospital is short of beds.

In spite of the reduced length of stay in hospital, shortage of paediatric beds remains a problem. Alongside the decreased in-patient stay is a marked increase in the number of children admitted to hospital. This is unique to paediatrics and seems in opposition to the aims of the service to limit hospital admissions. The increase in admissions which is matched by rising numbers of children being seen in out-patient and A&E departments. These increases may be due to changes in society as well as changing disease patterns, developments in medicine and GP services. In addition, although the shorter stay in hospital has increased paediatric bed availability, this has only caused a lowering of the criteria for admission and a continued bed shortage (Hill, 1989).

Activity

Look at the causes of increased admissions of children to hospital and consider which of these may be pertinent to your area of work.

Gould (1996) suggests that family-centred care is more easily facilitated by the community nurse. The nurse is a guest in the child's home which is a familiar and less threatening environment for the family. In addition, there are no institutional restrictions and regulations usually found in the hospital setting. However, this may be simplifying family-centred care. Unfortunately, community children's nurses have a caseload and have to prioritise their visits, their chosen time may not

---

Causes of increased child admissions to hospital

Sociological changes
- increasing public awareness of health services
- geographical isolation of family members
- less experiential knowledge of home care
- increase in hospital births

Alteration of GP services
- increase in GP deputising service
- consultation only by appointment
- closer liaison with hospital services

Changes in disease patterns
- decrease in acute infectious diseases of childhood (Wyke and Hewison, 1991)
- increase in mental health problems in children (HAS, 1995)
- increases in childhood asthma and diabetes (Audit Commission, 1993)

Increased paediatric bed availability (Hill, 1989)
- day care developments
- shorter lengths of stay
- lower criteria for admission

Developments in medicine
- longer lifespan of children with disabilities and chronic illness
- increased survival rate for low birth weight babies but possibly at the cost of increased health problems during infancy and childhood

Nurses' views about family-centred care

'Kids that are in overnight or two nights, I mean they [the parents] don't make much effort to have contact with us when it's not needed.'

' ... after they've been in for a week, 2 weeks and things are stable then you start expecting the parents to participate in care.'

'I expect them to take care of the non-nursing duties of the child, like, you know, ... the feeding, changing, bathing and things like that, obviously, cos that's what they would do at home.'

'That's why they're there. I mean it's their child, even though they're in hospital. They would have to feed it at home ... '

'We seem to expect that they will, if they're going to stay, help with the care ... that they're not just going to sit there and be bystanders.'

'This woman didn't need our help because the acute stage had passed and she could do all the child's care herself ... I haven't got a relationship with her at all ... and that's because she doesn't need us.'

'I mean the normal things that they would do at home ... the mothering-type things like washing and bathing and feeding ... nothing medical like giving medicines or anything like that.'

'The longer that they're [the parents] in then the more you're able to ... get a more relaxed relationship ... a more friendly relationship with the person, you know, you get to know them and their family involvement.'

'I think that as they become more familiar with the nurses and ... become part of the ward ... I think that the rapport gets better.'

(Darbyshire, 1994)

' ... tactfully encouraged her to try and get some rest, told her there was adequate staff to look after her son whilst in hospital and reassured her we were happy to care for him and did not think badly of her for going.'

' ... talked to parents, constantly reassuring and encouraging them to try and carry out his care as they would at home.'

' ... explained the importance and significance of the mother's continued involvement in the child's care ... '

(Callery and Smith, 1991)

coincide with the family's needs. Families may feel that their home and usual routine is being judged or disrupted by the nurse and they may feel further threatened if a student is present. Strong (1997) found that parents of children with mental health problems trusted health care professionals but were then disappointed by the actual service available, promised visits which did not occur and cancelled appointments.

COMMUNICATING WITH PARENTS

The Audit Commission (1993) found that the root problem in relation to family-centred care was poor communication between staff and parents. Over half of the families involved in their study reported that their involvement in care was never made explicit and 32% felt their role was to substitute for staff shortages. Parents in Darbyshire's study (1995) described their involvement in care as instinctive rather than planned or negotiated. He sensed that many parents felt a moral obligation to care for their child and help the nursing staff rather than an involvement in care.

The Audit Commission (1993) also recognised that nurses play a major role in communicating the concepts of family-centred care. However, for nurses to be able to do this they must have a clear understanding of family-centred care. Evidence suggests that nurses do not have a clear idea of this concept (Callery and Smith, 1991; Gill, 1993; Darbyshire, 1994). Nurses appear to believe that parents have a duty to stay in hospital with their child and carry out the usual parenting care, whilst the more specific nursing care is left to them. There is also the misconception that when parents are actively involved in their child's care that the nurse's role is no longer needed. Indeed, Casey has, in conversation, spoken of the 'dumping' model of nursing which she says occurs when parents are giving all their child's care and are abandoned by the nurses.

These ideas may occur because nurses believe that their role gives them control over the provision of care in hospital and they are loathe to release this control (Callery and Smith, 1991). Coyne (1996) believes that to fully understand the concept nurses should be more aware of parents' physical and psychological needs so that the parents are not put under excessive stress in their role in hospital. Darbyshire (1995) suggests that nurses need to appreciate what it means to be a parent and a parent of a sick child in hospital before they can begin to work with parents to provide real family-centred care. He describes family-centred care as a valuable and meaningful connection with parents based upon genuine mutual respect.

Activity

Discuss the concept of family-centred care with some children's nursing colleagues and parents of children in hospital. Compare their responses with those found in previous studies (see marginal box).

Another strategy for considering the meaning of family-centred care is for nurses to take a critical look at their own understanding of its principles and how they apply these to their practice (Teasdale, 1987).

Activity

Use the discussion questions alongside (adapted from Teasdale's work) to make a critical examination of your own practice.

When considering the principles of family-centred care, the nurse must not presume to be the expert in care or to make accountability the basis for the assumption that parents give up all responsibility for their child because they are in hospital. Teasdale (1987) considers that nurses permit involvement until it poses a problem and then they assert control. Equality should allow the nurse to give advice and only prevent families' wishes when such choices would impair the care of other children and families. The parent is not always right but nor is the nurse, but parents do have the right to choose their level of involvement in care. The difficulty arises when their choice is not the choice of their child, which raises questions about responsible decision making.

The Audit Commission (1993) recommends that information leaflets should be given to parents to explain the main elements of family-centred care. Leaflets have been developed at many centres to provide families with this information but they are mostly designed and written by professionals (Glasper and Burge, 1992). Campbell *et al.* (1993) propose that families should be producing such advice.

Activity

Design a leaflet to explain family-centred care to parents and then discuss its suitability with some parents on the ward.

The lack of information for parents and nurses' misunderstanding of family-centred care may be overcome by improved nurse education which emphasises not only communication and negotiation skills, but family dynamics and psychology (Coyne, 1996). However, this may not help them to fully appreciate the role of the parent and the feelings of guilt, inadequacy, uncertainty, loneliness and anxiety that parents experience when their child is in hospital. One of the mothers in Darbyshire's study expressed this succinctly by saying, 'It's not like being a parent is it? ... You're like a different parent' (Darbyshire, 1994). Nurses, therefore, have to be able to appreciate that parents in hospital can no longer perform as usual; all their intuitive parenting skills have been lost because of a range of emotions resulting from their child's hospitalisation. They need the nurses' help to overcome these feelings before they can return to normal functioning.

Family-centred care?

The principles of family-centred care

- parents cannot be partners in care because they do not have my specialist knowledge and skills and I am accountable for their child's care in hospital
- parents must be informed of what nurses are doing for their child but the final decision rests with the nurse
- each parent has the right to be involved in the nursing care to the extent of their or their child's wishes
- all parents must be given full information and their wishes must be met at all times

The principles in practice

- how much information are parents given on first contact, during any care given to the child and before discharge? What are parents not told? How is handover managed?
- can parents see their child's care plan? Is anything written about the child that parents cannot see? Do other members of the family have access to the care plan?
- how many choices does the parent have during their child's stay in hospital? In which areas do they not have a choice?
- if the care plans disappeared would it make any difference to the care given to that child? (i.e. how much of the care is routine and how much has developed from negotiation with the parents?)

(Adapted from Teasdale, 1987)

The elements of family-centred care

- Appreciation of the family as a constant factor within the child's life as opposed to the variation of health services and professionals with whom they come into contact
- Helping the liaison between parents and health care professionals to occur at all levels within the multidisciplinary team
- Imparting information to parents completely and openly
- Production and implementation of policies and procedures which ensure holistic care for the family as a whole
- Recognising families' individual reactions to, and methods of coping with illness and hospitalisation
- Providing appropriate strategies to meet the developmental needs of siblings
- Enabling and empowering the parent–child relationship
- Designing health care facilities which are appropriate and accessible for families

(Campbell et al., 1993)

IMPLEMENTATION OF FAMILY-CENTRED CARE

Campbell *et al.* (1993) are among many authors who have attempted to define the elements of family-centred care. All these writers agree that the successful implementation of family-centred care involves not only the nursing staff but the entire health care system. The Audit Commission recognised that the implementation of effective policies of child and family-centred care requires a major change in attitudes on the part of managers, doctors, nurses and other staff involved in running the service. Baum *et al.* (1990) suggest that effective policies can only be achieved when parents are seen as essential and equal members of policy-making groups. Whilst these policies would also need to take into account the needs of different cultures, it is also important not to create cultural differences where none exist (Shah, 1994). Surely, individualised care should cater for the individual and recognise any different needs regardless of ethnic background?

Fradd (1996) considers negotiated care plans to be essential for successful family-centred care and believes that families who have been given unbiased and complete information about their child's care are more likely to feel valued and supported. Negotiation is an interactive process and involves the sharing of ideas which helps the nurse to appreciate families' beliefs and values as well as their ways of coping with the stress of having a child in hospital. In this way, the nurse is in a better position to offer appropriate support and to enable parents to provide support for their child in a way which best suits them. The negotiated care must be clearly expressed in the care plan to enable other nurses and members of the multidisciplinary team to continue care when the named nurse is not available. The Audit Commission (1993) recognises this communication of parents' wishes as an important part of the nurse's role in informing and changing others attitudes to family-centred care.

Support for families often includes the care of the sick child's siblings. Siblings are often ignored in the caring process even though their emotional needs are similar to those of their parents (Walker, 1990). Most children's wards struggle to provide adequate facilities for parents and few are able to cater for siblings.

Activity

Explore the facilities for siblings in your hospital on the children's ward(s) and any other area where children are nursed. Talk to some resident parents to discover what facilities they would find useful for their other children.

Even if children are not being cared for as in-patients the families' needs are often not met. Historically, health service facilities for outpatients have always been provided on a 9–5, Monday–Friday basis. This is never a good time for families; parents may have to take time off work and children may miss school, and younger siblings may need alternative care arrangements. Evening and weekend clinics may offer a more appropriate service.

In conclusion, nurses need to have the support of management to be able to implement effective family-centred care. The Audit Commission (1993) recommends that every hospital should have a specific management focus for children's services with appropriate managerial and financial support. Standards for family-centred care should be approved and monitored to ensure quality is maintained.

 Key points

1. Effective family-centred care involves the careful consideration of the criteria for the hospitalisation of children, improved communication between nurses and parents and the strategic implementation of all the elements of family involvement.

2. Parents may not be given sufficient choice about day care or admission to hospital.

3. In spite of changes in children's length of stay in hospital there has been an increase in the number of children admitted.

4. A major reason for the lack of family-centred care is the lack of communication between nurses and parents, mainly due to nurses' misunderstandings about the concept.

5. Parents have problems in functioning as normal parents because of the emotions involved in having a sick child in hospital.

6. Family-centred care relies upon a specific management focus for children's services.

Parental comments about family-centred care

'The only time we saw a nurse was in the morning to make the beds and take the temperatures. If the children who hadn't their mothers there wanted anything, one of the other mothers had to get it for them.'

(Callery and Smith, 1991)

' ... I am not sure of their [the staff] attitude ... they let me do it so that they don't have to do it ... '

(Audit Commission, 1993)

' I dare say it takes a strain away from them [nurses] and they can spend more time with another child.'

'I find I'm feeding her, changing her, putting her down, sitting her up ... all the time, and they're short-staffed sometimes ... can't get a nurse to help you cos they're run off their feet.'

(Darbyshire, 1995)

' ... they tend to expect you to stay. So it was just assumed that I would want to stay.'

'The mums told me where to find things – more help to me than any nurse ... but they're very busy ... '

'They want you to stay and it makes life easier if you do stay, because its better for the nursing staff ... but they don't encourage you to stay because you're not felt welcome or comfortable.'

'It helps me a lot when the staff sorta say do you want to do it? ... and actually standing there watching me not going away and saying get on with it ... '

'If I didn't want to do the care, then they would be there to do the care ... I'm sorta sharing it with them ...

(Coyne, 1996)

'You know they didn't say , Right, change his nappy, and if at any time I don't want to , I can just say, No, I don't want to ... its a wee bit of give and take.'

'They [the nurses] were always friendly, but it's grown into a relationship now ... that's my view anyway ... they really have become friends ... when I was at home I missed them.'

' ... its not a nurse–patient or a nurse–parent [relationship] ... you know, it seems to develop into us, I mean you can talk as if its someone you've known for ages.'

'Some of these nurses, they just click. I don't feel I'm just here and no-one cares about me – I feel I'm part of the whole set up.'

(Darbyshire, 1994)

6 THE NURSE AS A DEVELOPING PROFESSIONAL

INTRODUCTION

Peplau (1952) believed that nurses continue to develop personally and professionally through encounters with different patients. This important aspect of the role of the nurse has only relatively recently been appreciated. Benner (1984) recognised that nurses gained their competence and intuitive grasp of situations from previous experience, and she advocated the use of reflective practice to identify this learning in an explicit way. She believed that while nurses continued to explain their actions as intuitive, the knowledge base for nursing would not expand and develop. Reflective practice is not an easy process as it may discomfort and challenge the reflector. Clinical supervision has developed as a means of guiding and supporting practitioners through the reflective process. The concept of exploring experiences to consider the thoughts, feelings and actions of those involved in the experience, has been recognised by the UKCC as a useful way of providing evidence of continuing professional development.

In 1990 the UKCC recognised the importance of nurses being able to demonstrate the maintenance and development of their professional knowledge and competence and suggested that evidence of such progression was mandatory to maintain registration for practice. This reform was finally agreed and came into force in 1995. One of the post-registration and education (PREP) requirements is to maintain a comprehensive account of all learning and development in a personal profile. These PREP requirements were formal recognition of the need for life-long learning. The idea of life-long learning has developed in the UK as a result of changes in society. In the late 1980s the consequences of demographic changes became apparent. It was realised that the number of young people entering the job market between 1989 and 2011 would decrease by over 2 million (Employment Department, 1992). To counteract this there was a need for all employers to increase opportunities for mature employees. One way of doing this was to provide opportunities for training throughout an employee's working life and to recognise the value of experience. Additionally, the UK needed to be able to respond effectively to increased international competition and technological change by developing the skills of innovation, responsiveness and adaptability of its work force. All employers have had to recognise the need to have a work force capable of adaptation to the constantly changing social environment. The English National Board (ENB, 1994) describes life-long learning as a process which helps nurses to be:

- innovative;

Cross reference

Guidelines for reflection – page 593

Cross reference

PREP requirements – page 594

- responsive to changing demands;
- resourceful;
- change agents;
- adaptable;
- challenging;
- self-reliant;
- able to share good practice.

REFLECTIVE PRACTICE

Whilst deliberate learning takes place in the formal college setting, a large proportion of learning takes place away from educational institutions.

Activity

Consider all the activities you have done since getting out of bed this morning. Think about how you learnt to do these activities.

You will immediately realise that much of your learning has come from experience. For instance, how many of you, as children, made your first cup of tea without first boiling the water? Since then you have quickly learnt through experience, not only how to make a cup of tea, but how to make it exactly as you like it. In the same way you will have learnt through personal and professional experiences how to provide care in different situations. As a student, my class had to practise bed-bathing on each other. I still remember the embarrassment of that experience and how it felt not to be completely dried. This was a valuable learning experience which has affected the way in which I practise. I have learnt so much from the many children and their families for whom I have cared but one outstanding event is that of an abandoned child. This made me realise the importance of security for children, a need which even takes precedence over physiological needs. More recently, the death of my father and my attempts to support my brother through his grieving has highlighted the importance of making it clear to families that it is 'permissible' to share emotions.

The idea that reflection can enhance learning from experience is not new. Coutts-Jarman (1993) states that it was mentioned by Aristotle in his work on judgement and moral action. In the 1930s Dewey discussed reflective thought as a means of reconsidering experiences and linking theory to practice (Dewey, 1933). Although it may be argued that reflection is a sub-conscious activity, Boud *et al.* (1985) consider that it must become a more formal activity for learning to occur and that there is a difference between thoughtful practice and reflective practice. Thinking about an incident does not usually involve the depth of exploration required to learn from the experience.

Qualities required for reflection

- Having an open mind
- Being responsible
- Objectivity
- Ability to assess oneself
- Willingness to explore emotions
- Adaptability to change

Historically, nurses were not expected to question practice or share their emotions and nursing was associated with routine, authority and tradition (Table 6.1). Dewey (1933) describes this as practice which takes the everyday realities for granted. Reflection enables practitioners to question these realities and their reactions to them, 'to think on their feet, improvise, and respond to the uncharted and unpredictable' (Fish and Twinn, 1997). The aim of Project 2000 was to produce nurses who were enquiring, independent, critically self-aware and creative; 'knowledgeable doers' (UKCC, 1986) It would appear that reflection is the ideal tool to help to meet this aim and many universities now use reflection as part of their strategy for the assessment of practice. Johns (1996) believes that reflection in practice helps nurses to concentrate on the caring aspect of nursing and advocates the use of a reflective model of nursing.

Activity

Assess a child and family using the adapted form of Johns' (1994) reflective model of nursing (left). Consider how the use of this model would affect the care of this child and family in comparison with the model you usually use.

It has been argued that reflection has become merely a rhetoric and that there are no accounts to demonstrate its benefit to patients (Newell, 1992). However, there are accounts of its beneficial effects upon child care practice (Wooton, 1997), and Dearmun (1997) argues that this alone should be sufficient rationale for its continuation. Practice which is constantly under critical review is more likely to attract purchasers of health care than practice which is based on ritual and tradition.

CLINICAL SUPERVISION

No one has ever suggested that reflection is easy. It is a process which requires self-examination of attitudes and behaviour which may cause feelings of inadequacy and discomfort. Bond and Holland (1997) suggest that practitioners, managers and educationalists can assist each other to learn in practice. Clinical supervision is one way of providing the time and opportunity for reflection and supporting and developing staff to provide a high standard of practice. Clinical supervision can also

---

A reflective model of nursing

Core question
- what information do I need to nurse this child and family?

Cue questions
- who is this child and family?
- what health event brings this child into hospital or care environment?
- how is this child and family feeling?
- how has this event affected this child and family's usual life patterns and roles?
- how can I help this child and family?
- what is important for this child and family to make the care environment comfortable?
- what support does this child and family have in life?
- how does this child and family view their personal future?

(Adapted from Johns, 1994)

Table 6.1

Traditional versus reflective practice

Traditional	Reflective
Importance of routine	Improvisation
Based on ritual	Research-based
Questioning discouraged	Spirit of inquiry
Didactic teaching	Experiential teaching
Displays of emotions discouraged	Feelings shared and explored
Skills explained by intuition	Knowledge-based skills

provide part of a package of staff development and support. It can be carried out on a one-to-one basis, usually with the line manager, or within a group. It has three main functions, to educate, support and manage. The educative or formative function involves the development of skills, knowledge and attitudes by helping the individual to reflect upon a clinical experience. Provision of support is required to help the individual accept the experience and learn from it instead of becoming overwhelmed by negative emotions – the restorative function. The managerial or normative function, which acts as a quality control, enables the participants to review nursing policy or procedure in relation to the experience and plan for appropriate change (Butterworth and Faugier, 1992).

Activity

Discover how clinical supervision is carried out in your area of practice. How do the participants feel about the process?

Clinical supervision should not feel threatening or become simply a managerial monitoring of progress. It should not become a forum for the discussion of general issues and non-specific complaints. It relies upon clear boundaries to ensure that participants feel valued and supported in their professional development. Clinical supervision and the work arising from it can be used towards meeting the PREP requirements for maintaining registration.

MAINTENANCE OF REGISTRATION

The basic requirements of PREP must be met for maintenance of registration. They include the need to undertake a minimum period of study equivalent to 5 days every 3 years. This study can include:

- attendance at lectures, courses, seminars, workshops;
- distance learning, including the educational supplements in professional journals;
- visits to other areas of practice;
- personal study or research, including reflection of critical incidents.

Any of the above mean little unless the practitioner can identify the objectives and outcome of the study.

The UKCC have firmly placed the responsibility of choosing appropriate study to each individual nurse but Bagnall and Garbett (1996) criticise them for not being more specific about how the equivalent of 5 days' study may be calculated. However, by giving individuals the responsibility for their own development the UKCC can renounce any commitment for funding continuing education. There has probably been more discussion about the funding of the study

Qualities of the clinical supervisor

The clinical supervisor should be able to:

- challenge thinking
- offer higher levels of skills and knowledge than those supervised
- provide a secure environment in which to share confidences
- offer constructive feedback
- motivate individuals to take responsibility for their own development
- assist with critical reflection
- raise clinical confidence and competence
- be supportive

Table 6.2

PREP categories of study applied to children's nursing

Categories of study (UKCC, 1994a, b)	Examples of application
Reducing risk	
Identification of health problems	Noticing incorrect infant feeding
Protection of individuals	Teaching food hygiene to parents
Raising awareness of health risks	'Safety in the sun' poster for children
Health screening	Introducing BP check for all ages
Health promotion	
Care enhancement	
Developments in clinical practice	New treatment regimes
New techniques	Change of role
Innovative approaches to care	Introducing primary nursing
Standard setting	Writing standards for care of parents
Empowering consumers	Involving parents in policy writing
Patient, client and colleague support	
Counselling techniques	Care of bereaved siblings
Leadership in practice	Setting up a paediatric research group
Clinical supervision	Peer review of critical incidents
Practice development	
External/exchange visits	Visit to children's hospice
Personal study/research	Literature review – HIV in children
Clinical audit	Audit hospital safety for children
Changes in policy and procedure	Parental presence at resuscitation
Education development	
Teaching and learning skills	Teaching package for students
Educational audit	Audit of learning environment

requirements than any other aspect of PREP. It could be argued that compulsory study should be locally or nationally funded, especially as it aims to improve and develop practice. Alternatively, perhaps taking responsibility for self-development should include meeting the costs. Whatever the answer, it is clear that, at present, financial help available to nurses for study depends upon their employer and can vary tremendously.

Activity

Find out what study leave and financial help is available to you in your current employment. How does this compare with that available to colleagues working in other health care areas (e.g. education, private sector)? Also find out how it compares to employment outside health care.

The amount of continuing education available also seems to be unfairly distributed. Bagnall and Garbett (1996) believe that the provision for this is biased towards acute hospital trusts and that staff working in community areas have fewer opportunities and less access to further their education. It would appear from this that staff need to be more innovative about their study and could be helped to explore such options by a preceptor. It is clear from the categories of study (Table 6.2) suggested by the UKCC (1994a, b) that there are many ways of developing practice and meeting the requirements which need not bear a financial burden.

DEVELOPING A PORTFOLIO

The standards for maintaining an effective registration include the maintenance of a personal profile or portfolio to demonstrate the maintenance and development of knowledge. Apart from being necessary to re-register, profiling is a useful exercise as it:

- encourages you to reflect on all your past educational and practice experience;
- clarifies those areas which you want to develop;
- enables you to make comprehensive future plans;
- provides you with an up-to-date record of achievements;
- helps the discussion of achievements and developmental needs with current and future employers;
- may help you to gain accreditation for further study.

Activity

Consider a recent achievement of which you are particularly proud. What did you learn from this experience and how can you provide evidence of this learning?

Sometimes providing evidence of learning can seem difficult. However, attendance at a study day or involvement in a new activity does not necessarily mean that learning has taken place. You need to be able to consider ways of demonstrating your learning if you wish to include the activity in your portfolio to show your practice development.

The UKCC (1994a, b) emphasises that your profile is your personal property. It will undertake random audits of profiles but employers cannot demand to see them. If profiles are used as part of performance reviews it is suggested that areas of your profile outside PREP requirements are kept separately (UKCC, 1996).

PRECEPTORSHIP

PREP is not just about maintaining registration although it may be argued that this area has the biggest impact for most nurses. PREP also

---

Developing your portfolio

Factual information
- personal/biographical information
- professional/academic qualifications
- positions held
- other activities/positions outside nursing
- record of your working hours

Self-appraisal of professional performance
- strengths and weaknesses
- achievements
- analysis of critical incidents
- areas of development

Personal aims and action plans
- goals for development
- action plans for achieving goals
- review of action plans
- outcomes from action plans

Record of formal learning*
- study days/seminars/courses/ conferences attended
- visits to other areas
- time spent on other study (e.g. literature searching)

*Each entry in this category should discuss the relevance to your area of practice, your objectives, the outcomes of the activity and how it has contributed to the development of your practice

introduced the idea of preceptorship. A period of support is recommended for newly registered nurses or those returning to practice after a break of 5 years or more. Benner (1984) describes newly registered nurses as advanced beginners who have yet to gain the experience to enable them to link theory and practice to actual clinical situations. Although this is disputed by Johnson (1996), he does not take into account the feelings of uselessness and loss of confidence caused by the change in role which registration brings. This state of confusion is aptly described by Robinson (1996) in her reflection of her first 6 months as a newly registered nurse. Reading this account, one wonders if a preceptor would have eased this transition from student to staff nurse. Maben and Macleod Clark (1996) found that Robinson's experiences were common and that few nurses received a comprehensive programme of support during their first post as a registered nurse.

Activity

Find out what support is available to newly registered children's nurses in your current area of work. Consider what support you would find most helpful.

Preceptors should be first level registered nurses or midwives who have a minimum of 12 months' post-registration experience within the same or associated area of practice. The preceptor should :

- have sufficient knowledge of the preceptee's programme leading to registration (or return to nursing course) to be able to identify current learning needs;
- help the preceptee to orientate to the new area of practice;
- be able to help the preceptee apply theory to practice;
- understand the potential problems associated with the transition from student to registered practitioner and assist the preceptee to overcome these;
- act as a resource to facilitate professional development.

The idea of support is not as simple as having a committed preceptor. The newly registered nurse also needs a supportive environment which provides approachable, forward thinking, up-to-date staff, a good team spirit, trust, responsibility, feedback on progress and teaching. In addition, preceptors need preparation and support from the organisation to enable them to undertake this important role.

LEVELS OF NURSING PRACTICE

The PREP policy also includes standards for programmes of specialist preparation beyond initial registration. These standards are based on developing nurses beyond the fundamental knowledge, skills and attitudes gained in pre-registration programmes. The UKCC believes that after an initial period of practice with support following registration that specialist health care practice requires practitioners to have additional preparation to enable them to demonstrate higher levels of clinical judgement to:

- monitor and improve standards of care;
- undertake nursing audit;
- develop and lead practice;
- contribute to clinical research;
- teach and support colleagues.

Three levels of post-registration practice are identified. Primary practice meets the basic requirements of PREP and it is envisaged that most nurses will practice at this level. Specialist practice involves an additional post-registration specialist practitioner recordable qualification at degree level. Specialist qualifications are available for community and hospital nurses and include specific qualifications for children's nurses.

Activity

Consider your future career plans and find out what specialist programmes are available to help you reach your goals after your period of primary practice.

Advanced practice is recommended for those who are specialist nurses and act as resources for others. This role, which requires a further recordable qualification, is envisaged as one in which the practitioner leads clinical practice either at local or national level, and is a clinically based post which has direct accountability for practice. The PREP document suggests that these advanced practitioner posts are developed as consultant practitioner posts (UKCC, 1994a, b) (see Figure 6.1). Coyne (1997) suggests that experienced specialist nurses, who otherwise may reach the criteria for such a post, need to develop their marketing skills before being able to act as nurse consultants. He also points out that current pay scales for clinical posts do not provide appropriate remuneration for the complexity of advanced practice. However, the development of consultancy posts would finally give clinical nurses a chance to progress without having to move away from patient care. In particular, it would give children's nurses the credibility to influence the development of children's health care services as recommended by the Audit Commission in 1993.

Figure 6.1

UKCC continuum of practice.

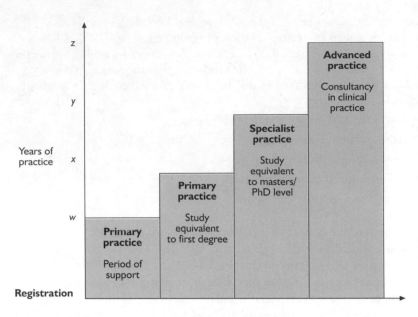

Maintenance and development of professional
knowledge and competence

Key points ➤

1. Peplau (1952) and Benner (1984) believed that nurses' knowledge, attitudes and skills developed through their experiences with different patients and that this enabled them to practise at a higher level.

2. The UKCC recognises the need for practising registered nurses to demonstrate this development of knowledge and skills.

3. Reflective practice is one way in which nurses can learn from their experiences and add to nursing knowledge.

4. Clinical supervision can educate, support and manage nurses' experiential learning.

5. Maintaining a profile can be a systematic way of recording professional development.

6. Preceptorship can support the newly registered nurse to gain confidence and ability in a new role.

CHILDREN'S NURSING IN A MULTI-CULTURAL SOCIETY 7

INTRODUCTION

Effective nursing care of children and their families in any setting is dependent on an appreciation of that family's beliefs and values. In the UK there is an increasing diversity of cultures and there are many differences between the values and beliefs of the average British citizen and those of the minority groups. In Britain, Asians, who comprise 4.5% of the population, are the main minority group, and in some large towns and cities they can form up to 50% of the local population (Baxter *et al.*, 1990). Some of the marked differences among different racial and ethnic groups are related to the attitudes and practices surrounding birth, pain and death and their specific susceptibility to certain diseases.

Generally, health care professionals in the UK and other Western countries have been taught according to the beliefs and values of a White, middle class society, and only in recent years has transcultural education begun to identify that minority groups do not share these beliefs and values. Denial of these differences can create conflict and prevent children's nurses from working in a true partnership with children and families. Children's nurses need to accept that different health concepts and behaviour to their own are not necessarily better or worse – just different.

When discussing the needs of children and families with different concepts of health and related areas, it is important to appreciate the meanings of the terms used to identify why individuals from different backgrounds develop different attitudes and practices. Culture is defined as the unique way of life a group of people have developed in specific physical and social circumstances which acts as a frame of reference for their particular values and beliefs. The lifestyles of most cultures are influenced by religion, a particular system of faith and worship. Ethnicity refers to a specific group of people, usually a minority, who share the same cultural, linguistic or racial background. Race is described as a distinct group of people connected by common descent and identifiable by certain common characteristics such as colour. Individuals' values and beliefs are also influenced by the way in which they 'socialised' and learnt the accepted behaviours of their cultural group as children.

The Children Act (DoH, 1989) states that help provided for the child and family should be appropriate to race, culture, religion and language, and that regard should be paid to the different racial groups to which children and families belong. In addition, the UKCC code of conduct advises nurses that they 'must: recognise and respect the uniqueness and dignity of each patient and client and respond to their need for care irrespective of their ethnic origin'. Whilst there is no doubt that health care professionals have a duty to provide care which takes into account the child and family's specific cultural needs, Shah (1994) warns that cultural awareness training can sometimes reinforce stereotyping and racism. Nurses need to remember that all their patients are individuals regardless of race, ethnicity or culture.

RACE AND ETHNICITY

Race and ethnicity cause specific differences in physical characteristics, predisposition towards certain disorders and susceptibility to disease. David (1990) found that Asian and Black neonates are significantly smaller than white newborns. Black babies seem to overcome this difference quickly to become taller and heavier between the ages of 5 and 14 years than their white comparisons. Oriental children, however, are smaller throughout childhood. It is because of these differences that attention is now being given to the growth charts used to identify children who are outside the normal growth limits. These charts were first compiled in the 1960s, and revised in 1993 to take account of the increased height and weight of people in the UK since the publication of the first charts. However, they still do not take into account the multicultural variation in growth now seen in the UK (Fry, 1993).

Different racial and ethnic groups have a specific predisposition to certain disorders. Cystic fibrosis is one of the commonest inherited disorders in Caucasian people but is rare in Black and oriental families (Dodge *et al.*, 1993). Tay Sachs disease occurs mainly in Jewish children and sickle cell disease is only seen in Black Africans.

Race and ethnicity also affect the resistance to disease. Migrant families usually suffer more illness than the indigenous population. The first major immigrant mortality study in England and Wales was published in 1984 (Marmot, 1984). Mortality rates vary according to the country of origin, but all immigrants showed a higher mortality rate than the average for England and Wales for tuberculosis and accidents. They all had a lower than average mortality rate for chronic chest diseases. These inequalities have remained largely unchanged, as does the high mortality rate for babies of mothers born in Pakistan. It is difficult to know how much this is due to different immune factors or availability of health services.

Health care in the UK is mainly directed towards the needs of the white middle class population (Whitehead, 1992). Immigrant families, particularly those who have just settled in this country, may lack the ability to access the appropriate services. In addition, their health beliefs and traditions do not tend to consider preventive health measures; instead they seek help only at the time of illness. Nurses have a responsibility to help them appreciate the value of preventive health care in a way which relates to their culture.

HEALTH BELIEFS AND PRACTICES (TABLE 7.1)

Individuality is mostly determined by culture. Culture influences most of the way in which people live; their diet, their language, their mode of dress, their beliefs and values, and the accepted mode of behaviour for their cultural group. Variations in the growth and development of children are thought to be largely due to cultural factors.

Activity

Consider your own beliefs and values (using the questions overleaf), and think carefully about how these developed.

As well as family influences, sub-cultures such as ethnicity, religion, peer groups, social class and schooling can all have impact upon the way in which children learn to socialise and affect the way they view health and illness. Nurses need to be aware of their own views and the reasons why these developed before they can truly appreciate others' beliefs. The assessment of cultural beliefs is an important part of the nursing assessment process because compliance with treatment is influenced by the effect that treatment may have upon roles and lifestyles.

Different cultures have different views about health and the causation of illness. They differ in their beliefs about how much control individuals have over their health. Western cultures tend to believe that certain behaviours, such as overwork, stress, lack of exercise or sleep, are causes of illness. Other cultures believe that supernatural forces, 'the will of God' or fate causes disease and that health can only be restored by the same influence. These cultures may rely on wearing amulets or other religious symbols to protect them from disease. Asian, Oriental and Arab cultures believe that illness is caused by an imbalance of hot and cold forces. Health is regained by restoring the balance. For example, respiratory infections are thought to be caused by cold forces and must be treated by food or drugs considered to be 'hot'. For this reason children of these cultures who may have a pyrexia due to a respiratory infection will be overdressed to balance the cold force which caused the problem.

Beliefs about the cause of illness may also lead parents to try alternative medicine or homoeopathy. Provided these do no harm to the child they should be used in conjunction with conventional medicine. Complementary therapies can often reduce the pain and anxiety associated with illness and thus induce a feeling of well-being. Until more research becomes available about the use and efficacy of such therapies it is worth considering their potential.

COMMUNICATION

Communication skills are an important skill in nursing and usually have a prominent part in any nurse education programme but the skills taught

Beliefs and values

- What are your beliefs and values?
- What are your beliefs about death?
- What are your religious views? How important are they for you?
- Do you feel comfortable talking about religion and death?
- How would you describe your own culture?
- Do you think that health and illness is determined by fate, one's own behaviour or some other cause?
- What behaviour in others really upsets you? How do you react if you meet this behaviour?
- Do you believe that touch is important? Do you ever feel uneasy if a child or family gets too close to you (in a non-threatening manner)?
- How do you feel if others disagree with your beliefs and values?

Table 7.1

Cultural and religious influences for nursing practice

Cross reference

Religions, cultural beliefs and diet – page 182

Culture	Childbirth	Diet	General care	Death and dying
Buddhism	An astrologer provides the initial letter of the child's name and date of birth. Birth control and abortion are condemned	Fasting days occur on religious days. No alcohol	Analgesia or sedation may be refused as it may affect the ability to meditate	The dying patient should be visited by a Buddhist monk
Christian Science	Contraceptive pill not generally used. Abortion permitted only in life-threatening situations	No alcohol or tobacco	Surgery, prostheses and drugs may be refused. Prayer is used for healing	Another Christian Scientist is usually welcomed as a support
Established and Free Church (of all denominations)	No special requirements	No special requirements	No special requirements	May require Holy Communion and/or the presence of their priest or minister
Hinduism	Special ceremony after birth. Parents choose name from priest on 10th day	No meat (especially beef), fish, or dairy produce which contains animal fats	Married women cannot have their hair cut or consent for surgery without their husband's permission. Patients prefer treatment from a doctor or nurse of the same gender as themselves	Family (especially eldest son) should be at bedside. Relatives prefer to wash the body
Jehovah's Witness	Baptism not practised. Abortion not acceptable	No tobacco. No meat from animals which have been strangled (e.g. poultry). No blood products (e.g. black sausage)	Transfusion of blood and blood products is not acceptable	Support and prayers of fellow witnesses are appreciated
Jews	Male circumcision at 8 days by a trained circumciser. Men will attend and name the baby at this time	Meat only obtained from ritual slaughter. Shellfish, pork and game forbidden	No drugs derived from the pig (e.g. porcine insulin)	Body should not be left unattended until burial (24 hours after death) and not touched by a non-Jew unless wearing gloves

Mormons	Abortion opposed	No tea, coffee, cola drinks, alcohol or tobacco 24-hour fast 1st Sunday in the month unless undergoing medical treatment	White one or two piece under-clothing not usually removed	Dying should be dignified and pain free Church elder gives blessing for the dying
Muslims	May refuse vaginal examination Baby must be bathed immediately after birth Family prefer to bury placenta 7th day – baby's head shaved (unless unwell), circumcised by family and named Birth control not permitted	Pork and pork products unacceptable All other meat must be ritually slaughtered (Halal) Annual fast during sunrise for 1 month unless menstruating, following recent childbirth, old, weak or ill No alcohol	Prefer to be at home during religious festivals Exposure of body considered unacceptable After toileting, cleansing done with water and left hand Showers preferred to baths Washing of hands, neck, ears and feet, rinsing of mouth necessary before prayer five times a day	Family wash body prior to burial (without coffin) 24 hours after death Post-mortem not acceptable
Plymouth Brethren	Birth control not usually permitted	Eating with non-Brethren not always permissible	Patients may not be seen naked TV and radio may not be watched or listened to	No special requirements
Rastafarianism	Use of birth control unacceptable	No pork, shellfish, milk, coffee or tobacco	Most prefer not to cut hair or beards Blood transfusion from family members only Unacceptable to wear second hand clothing, therefore disposable gowns should be used	Family prefer to be present at bedside
Roman Catholicism	Artificial birth control is unacceptable Natural birth control (e.g. rhythm method) may be practised	Some Catholics do not eat meat on Fridays	No specific requirements	Sacrament of the sick (previously known as the Last Rites) administered by the priest Family may wish to have holy water, rosary, or crucifix by the bed
Sikhs	Abortion not generally acceptable	Vegetarians No alcohol or tobacco	Showers preferred to baths Handwashing and rinsing of mouth before meals Males do not like to remove their turban or Sikh symbols (uncut hair, comb, bangle, sword or shorts) in public Women prefer a female present during examinations	Passages from the holy book read by a Sikh leader Family wash and dress the body before cremation

Adapted from CRACKNELL, R. and COX, J. (1993) *Cultural and Religious Aspects of Caring Professionals*. Luton: University of Luton.

are usually related to the Western culture. Apart from the different language used by many other cultures, Western communication 'rules' may have quite different interpretations for these people.

Communication with families who do not speak English is best carried out by a nurse who speaks their language. When this is not possible an interpreter should be used, ideally from within the family. Even this strategy has its drawbacks. If the interpreter is not familiar with medical terminology, or if there is no corresponding word in their language, confusion or misunderstanding may occur. The family may find it difficult and embarrassing to explore personal issues with an interpreter outside the family group. The nurse may find it difficult to know if the interpreter is relaying the exact information required. I have vivid memories of a crying baby clinic where the doctor was seeing a Turkish mother who was obviously distraught by her baby who cried for about 20 hours a day. The doctor recognised and empathised with the mother's distress and showed great understanding of the mother's situation, wanting to admit the baby to give the mother some respite. However, the husband clearly believed that the mother should cope with the baby and it was difficult to know how much the male Turkish interpreter was able or willing to transmit the feelings of empathy from the doctor to the mother.

Activity

Discuss with others from different cultures whether it is possible to interpret feelings as well as information.

We are all aware that if we do not understand someone or we have not quite heard what they said we just agree. Consequently, it is important that we ensure that families with poor or limited language really do understand when they smile or nod agreement so that they are enabled to give informed consent. The oriental culture believes in avoiding confrontation and these families may agree simply to avoid conflict (Weller, 1994). The lack of questioning by families, does not always imply understanding, as in Asian cultures questioning persons in authority is seen as disrespectful (Orque, 1983).

In Western cultures avoidance of eye contact is seen as disrespectful or a sign of disinterest, boredom or deceitfulness. In other cultures the reverse is sometimes true and some cultures avoid looking directly at the nurse as a sign of respect.

Emotions are also expressed differently in different cultures. In Western cultures public displays of emotion are viewed as embarrassing and inappropriate, but in Jewish and Latin cultures people are expected to share their emotions openly and loudly with others.

Cross reference

Religious, cultural beliefs and diet – page 182

Dietary customs

Food preferences for different ethnic groups tends to originate from the easy availability of such food in their native environment. Most children's wards allow parents to bring food in for their children, and the family may prefer to do so as they can be sure that it is appropriate to their beliefs and the child's appetite. However, hospitals should be able to provide a variety of meals for different cultures and not put added pressure on parents who may feel obliged to bring in suitable foodstuffs.

Activity

Take a critical look at how your own area of practice caters for the dietary needs of different cultures. If changes are necessary what would you recommend?

Nurses should be careful not to impose their dietary values upon other cultures. Baxter *et al*. (1990) found that disabled Asian children in the UK are often taught to eat with cutlery because staff do not realise that eating with fingers is an important part of the Asian culture.

RELIGION

Religion is an important part of most cultures. It determines families' wishes in relation to practices concerning birth and death, and there may be other important rituals to be performed during childhood or illness. It is not enough for the nurse to ask the family's religion on admission. Burnard (1988) discovered that the majority of British people call themselves Christian although they do not formally belong to a church. Bradshaw (1996) warns that the same may be true for other cultures, and that it may be dangerous to assume that Sikhs, Jews and Muslims take their religion seriously. The nurse's assessment should ascertain if there are any special religious practices or needs which are important to the family and not make assumptions from their given religion. Some families, regardless of culture, turn to religion in times of stress for support and may appreciate talking to the hospital chaplain or a member of their own religious group. Others find that severe illness in the family challenges their previous beliefs and find it difficult to gain support in this way.

Whilst everyone may not have religious beliefs, they do have a spirituality (Burnard, 1988). Spirituality has been defined as the meaning, value and purpose of life which may have nothing to do with religion (McSherry, 1996). Bradshaw (1996) argues that meeting families' spiritual needs is an intrinsic part of providing holistic care and should not need to be separated out as a specific topic. It is about helping families to express their feelings and emotions about their child's condition, and how that condition has challenged the meaning, value and belief that a disabled child is punishment for sins from their previous life (Baxter *et al*., 1990). Disability in the family reduces the marriage prospects for the rest of the family in a culture where arranged marriages are the norm and often causes shame, particularly if the disabled child is male. Language problems often make it difficult for Asian families to find out about their child's disability and the community support available. Voluntary support groups for the disabled are usually set up and run by white middle class families and tend not to cater for cultural differences (Shah, 1992). Shah (1992) also found that Asian families found it difficult to accept respite care because they were uncertain that their religious beliefs would be upheld. It is important for children's nurses to appreciate that Asian families coping on their own with a disabled child may not be doing so because they do not want help but simply because they are not aware of the help available.

Key points ➤

1. The UK is a multicultural society with Asians comprising the main ethnic minority group.

2. It is important not to make assumptions about people's beliefs; individuality is more important than race, ethnicity or culture.

3. Health care in the UK is mainly directed towards the needs of the white middle class and is difficult for ethnic minority groups to access.

4. People from different ethnic origins often have different beliefs and practices in relation to health, illness, diet, and religion. They have a different physical appearance and are likely to experience different diseases.

5. Nurses should care for all children and their families in the same way regardless of their ethnic origin, but they should take care to appreciate and respect individual beliefs and values.

6. Nurses need to be aware of their own beliefs and values and the origin of these before they can fully appreciate the beliefs and values of others.

THE FUTURE OF CHILDREN'S NURSING 8

INTRODUCTION

The secret balance of life's current paradox is to allow the past and future to co-exist in the present.

(Handy, 1994)

If Charles Handy's philosophy is to be believed children's nurses need to demonstrate insight and a wider vision to recognise future trends, and to develop children's nursing to meet innovations in practice. Fish and Purr (1991) believe that unless nurses are able to react in this way that they will find the government will impose reforms upon the profession from outside. Nurses cannot be content to let this happen and should be exploring how their current knowledge and skills can be used to influence their future.

In 1988, when Anne Casey was developing her family-centred care model of nursing she questioned over 300 practising children's nurses about their beliefs regarding children's nursing and its future. The most common responses related to the development of:

- recognition of children's nursing as a speciality;
- research-based evidence for paediatric practice;
- specialist roles within children's nursing;
- family-centred care;
- children's community nursing;
- children's nurses' role as health educators;
- technology in children's nursing.

These seem useful headings to use to explore current knowledge and skills and to discuss how their development may affect the future of children's nursing. However, children's nursing is part of the wider field of nursing and its developments cannot be explored without also looking at the future of nursing as a whole.

CHILDREN'S NURSING AS A SPECIALITY

The future of nursing as an independent profession began to be questioned in the 1990s and the possibility of nursing being phased out has to be considered before discussing the development of children's nursing as a speciality. In 1990, managers began to consider that nurses were too expensive to be employed to perform fundamental caring and that less qualified, less expensive health care assistants should be used instead. This idea was steadily accepted by post-NHS reforms and many trusts now employ a large percentage of unqualified support workers. These changes cannot be considered without comparison with previous trends. Before the advent of Project 2000, wards were largely staffed by student nurses and enrolled nurses who were a relatively inexpensive work force. Once student nurses started to become supernumerary and the second level nurse was deemed inappropriate it was too expensive to replace them all with registered nurses. Thus the health care assistant (HCA) came into being. Initially, the HCA role was created to assist the registered nurse in non-nursing duties but shortages of staff have led nurses to allow HCAs to take on more and more of the nursing role until nursing has become difficult to define.

Activity

Take a critical look at the work of unqualified staff in your own area. How much of this would you define as nursing? Why is it not being done by nurses?

Many HCAs consider that qualified staff are unaware of their role and training needs. Uncertainty about this role can lead to HCAs being used inappropriately (Reeve, 1994) and if these unqualified staff are used to give bedside care, it is they who spend more time with patients and develop a relationship with them. Is that what nurses really want? Unfortunately, the reduction in the number of student nurses in the mid-1990s and the consequent drop in numbers of available qualified staff may force managers to employ more unqualified staff. In 1997 the health department increased intakes of student nurses but the benefit of this will not be apparent until 2000 when the skill mix will have already been diluted (Cole, 1997).

In 1996 a report from Manchester University proposed the creation of a generic health care worker. The lowest grade of this post would perform the bedside nursing as an entry gate into specialities such as physiotherapy or occupational therapy. This is effectively stating that nursing is not a specific speciality which needs a particular body of knowledge, skills and attitudes. Glasper (1993) has suggested that a generic nurse may appear a more cost-effective option and that specialist nurses who are unable to gain work in Europe, America and Australia may support this idea. He proposes that, if nursing does return to the generic route, children's nursing becomes a post-graduate qualification. However, this is an expensive option that may only be taken up or available to a few very motivated nurses.

In this climate of uncertainty, what is the future of children's nursing? Campbell (1995) recognises that the speciality could be in danger and warns that if registered children's nurses wish to retain the title children's nurse a concerted effort needs to be made to ensure that the role is uniquely identifiable from that of other health professionals and discreet from other roles. With many children's wards not able to meet government recommendations of a minimum of two registered

Cross reference

Generic nurse – page 587

Cross reference

Number of registered children's nurses – page 350

children's nurses per shift (DoH, 1991, 1996a, b; Clothier, 1994) there is a danger that those providing the care will be attributed with the skills of the registered children's nurse and the specialist nurse will be seen as unnecessary. The problem is worse in areas other than children's wards where children are the minority group.

Activity

Discuss with some colleagues how these dangers can be overcome to enable children's nursing to remain as an important speciality.

Several authors have attempted to address this issue. Campbell (1995) believes it important to be able to define the nature of children's nursing. Colson (1996) advocates greater collaboration between service and education managers to develop flexible yet rigorous post-registration programmes to help those nurses working with children who do not possess a children's nursing qualification.

The future of children's nursing may not be bleak. Children's nurses have evidence to show that children have different needs from adults, and that these needs are both complex and demanding. It has been clearly established that admission to hospital can cause children psychological trauma. There is research to support the importance of maintaining the child and family relationship and the value of working in partnership with parents. This body of evidence helps children's nurses to be able to define the nature of their role. The 1996 Royal College of Nursing Society of Paediatric Nursing presented evidence that children's nurses do make a difference and that children's nurses were aware of the need to assert their role and were reacting to current pressures. If government support for children's nurses is to remain, nurses themselves must continue to prove their worth as specialists and not allow their role to be taken over by unqualified staff.

RESEARCH-BASED EVIDENCE FOR PAEDIATRIC PRACTICE

Nursing research has been aided by the movement of nurse education into higher education. However, because nursing had no research history, the first nurse researchers were forced to rely upon established methodology for health care research. This has not helped nursing research to gain credibility and the 1992 Higher Education Funding Council (HEFC) research assessment placed nursing research at the bottom of their leagues of excellence. In addition, funds for health care research are much in demand and other health care professionals who are more experienced and respected as researchers find it easier to gain this funding. This situation is slowly changing; the 1997 HEFC assessment showed that the quality of nursing research had significantly improved with 10 of the 36 institutions assessed improving their rating since 1992.

In 1992, 30 Nursing Development Units (NDUs) were established by the DoH to provide optimum client care through the development of practice. The number of NDUs is gradually increasing and, led by Campbell in 1993, now includes paediatric units. Nurses within NDUs are encouraged to question practice and use evidence-based knowledge to plan care (Vaughan and Edwards, 1994). These units have firmly ensured that nursing research is linked to practice. Now it is important that nurses react to the research findings. Benner (1984) described the expert nurse as one who 'has an intuitive grasp of the situation', but her work must not become an excuse for experienced children's nurses to continue to use intuition to assess and plan care. Practitioners who cannot express their rationale for care are in danger of perpetuating a ritualistic and unproven approach to children's nursing. As Walsh and Ford (1994) noted, rituals are dangerous because they give a feeling of security and decrease the acceptability of change. Equally dangerous is the enthusiastic implementation of research without questioning its value.

Activity

Take a critical look at the care plan of a child you have nursed. Can you give a research-based rationale for all the care prescribed?

Traditionally nurses have tended to cling to routines and have not been good at reacting to research findings. I still meet nurses who tell me that pressure sores are best prevented by massaging the areas at risk. Changes in practice are often painful because they involve an acceptance that earlier beliefs are now outmoded and devalued, but if children's nursing is to develop, children's nurses must be prepared to question practice and accept change. Whilst all nurses cannot lead change or be researchers it is important that all nurses appreciate research (DoH, 1993). By appreciating the value of research all children's nurses can support the development of practice to ensure that children receive the optimum care. Research appreciation may be defined as a critical questioning approach to one's work, the desire and ability to find out the latest research in that area and the ability to assess its value to the situation and apply it as appropriate (Macleod Clark and Hockey, 1989).

There has been considerable debate on the ethical dilemmas and legal issues surrounding research involving children and their families. Jolley (1995) accepts that paediatric nursing research is not without difficulties but argues that a lack of research may lead to unsafe practice. Research may be defined as a careful search or inquiry which aims to discover new facts. Nurses have always done this in an informal way by evaluating their care and by using their past experience to adapt or create innovative ways of caring for specific children's problems. Unfortunately, nurses have tended not to record or analyse their evaluations and their changes to care remain largely unknown. Reflective practice is now helping nurses to question their practice in a more systematic way but they need to be more active in sharing their findings.

UKCC (1992) guidelines for critiquing research reports

The research question
- are the aims clearly stated?

The rationale for the study
- is the importance of the study made clear?
- is any similar work noted?
- is there a comprehensive literature review?

Methodology
- is this appropriate to the study?
- is it explained fully?
- is the sample unbiased?
- are the reliability and validity of the method proven?

Results
- are these clearly expressed?
- is there discussion of the findings?
- are limitations to the study recognised?
- do they add to nursing knowledge?

Cross reference

Research – page 674

SPECIALIST ROLES FOR CHILDREN'S NURSES

The role of the qualified nurse in the UK has expanded tremendously in the last decade. In many areas the nurse is now recognised as a specialist and is an autonomous practitioner. The UKCC advisory document *Scope of Professional Practice* (1992a) gave nurses guidelines on which to base their decisions about developing their role in response to the changing needs of society. Specialist roles for nurses have also arisen because of the reduction in junior doctors' hours. In 1991 the NHS Management Directive proposed a new deal to improve junior doctors' hours and change their conditions of service. This led to an investigation of the junior doctor role and it was suggested that many duties were inappropriate and could be performed by others, including nurses (Hopkins and Hodgson, 1996). These developments have enabled children's nursing to grow.

Activity

Find out what specialist roles are available to children's nurses. Consider how these roles enhance the care of children.

Nurse specialist posts within children's nursing have developed considerably in recent years. Just a few examples of these specialist posts are listed below:

- infant care/feeding advisor;
- adolescent oncology and haematology;
- asthma care;
- cystic fibrosis;
- HIV and AIDS;
- dermatology;
- pain control;
- plastic surgery.

In addition to specialist posts, individual children's nurses' roles have widened to include specialist skills. One example of the developing scope of practice is the role of the children's nurse practitioner. In children's A&E departments these experienced children's nurses are able to assess, diagnose and treat some specified children without referral to a doctor. In Nottingham there are nurse led clinics for children with asthma and enuresis where nurses assess and monitor the child's condition, giving additional advice and support as necessary (Fradd, 1994). From October 1984 community nurses began to prescribe certain drugs and this initiative has gradually developed to include acute paediatric care. Specialist roles can be seen to be re-creating the task aspect of nursing, but Fradd (1994) believes that such developments add

The scope of professional practice – the principles

- Putting the needs of patients and clients first at all times
- Updating and developing your knowledge, skills and competencies
- Recognising limitations in your personal knowledge and skill and taking action to address these deficiencies
- Ensuring that you do not compromise standards of care by new developments to your practice and taking on new responsibilities
- Acknowledging your own personal professional account- ability
- Refusing tasks for which you are not competent

Cross reference

Emergence of nurse specialists – page 599

credibility and increase respect, trust and confidence in the role of the children's nurse. However, she warns that any role development should in the best interests of children and not evolve merely to make other health care workers' jobs easier.

Will this role development continue? General developments in the NHS appear to favour the expansion of the GP role with perhaps a return to GP hospitals for minor surgery. Children's nurses could play a vital role in such developments especially as children comprise over 30% of a GP's workload and the number of children with complex medical problems are increasing. However, it is worth noting that nurses without a general nurse qualification were only able to access Practice Nursing and Health Visiting from 1995, so there are few children's nurses with these qualifications. It must also be remembered that the Health Service is also very cost conscious at present and very experienced, specialist nurses may be too expensive. There is a need to prove the cost effectiveness of such roles if they are to continue.

FAMILY-CENTRED CARE

There is no doubt that the family will always be an important part of children's nursing and that this philosophy of care will continue to develop. Darbyshire's research in 1994 gave valuable information about the reality of family-centred care for nurses and families but further research is now needed into the:

- nurses' perspectives of parental participation;
- social implications of parental participation;
- definition of 'family';
- nature of being a parent of a sick child;
- implications of participation for parental control and autonomy;
- effects of participation upon parental anxiety levels.

Campbell *et al.* (1993) suggest that family-centred research could represent the way forward for the development of children's nursing. They suggest that family-centred care should be broadened to enable parents to be involved in all decision making about children's nursing including deciding research priorities.

COMMUNITY CHILDREN'S NURSING

With evidence of the increasing number of children at home with chronic and complex disorders, it is likely that the community children's nurse service will continue to develop. From April 1996, GP fundholders were able to purchase specialist nursing services and it is known that many GPs and district nurses admit that they lack the confidence, experience and skills to care for sick children at home (Brocklehurst, 1996). Unfortunately, being a relatively new speciality, community children's nursing is poorly understood by GPs. Community children's nurses need to be able to market their expertise and justify the need for such skills and experience to be certain of their survival.

One area of community children's nursing which could help to justify the need for such a service is in the care of children with mental health problems. In 1995 the Health Advisory Service reported that between 10 and 20% of children required help because of mental health problems and recommended the development of primary health mental health services for children. The DoH has recognised that care of these children should take priority as failure to do so may cause increased demands on the social and educational services as well as leading to continued problems in adulthood. Few psychiatric nurses have qualifications in child and adolescent mental health (McMorrow, 1995) but children's nurses have been taught to appreciate the stresses of childhood and ways of helping children to cope with their problems.

However, there are still very few community children's nurses. Courses to prepare children's nurses to work in the community are hampered by the lack of suitably qualified practitioners to act as teachers, mentors and placement supervisors. At the same time those suitably qualified practitioners have to appreciate families' privacy and confidentiality and not endanger their relationship with them by always being accompanied by students. There is a need for innovative ways of teaching nurses how to care for sick children at home. Perhaps by linking with families and other health care professionals working with children in the community is one way of overcoming this issue.

THE ROLE OF CHILDREN'S NURSES AS HEALTH EDUCATORS

The importance of health education for children is gradually being recognised. Whilst most health education used to be aimed at the adult population, there are now specific strategies for health promotion for children. Attitudes and behaviour are established during childhood so it makes sense to influence these at an early age. There has been much debate about whether health education is the role and responsibility of the parent, the teacher or the health care professional, but many adults have already developed unhealthy behaviour and may be confused about the right information to give children.

Whitehead (1995) points out that health care behaviours are not intrinsically rewarding and environmental influences often make it difficult for children to comply with health education. Children's nurses are taught what health education to give and are aware of children's perceptions of health and illness and can adapt the health message according to the ages of their target group. Initiatives which have provided sexual health education for teenagers have shown a reduction in under 16s registering at family planning clinics (Jackson and Plant, 1996). Other specific health education programmes have been developed to teach primary school children about diet, dental hygiene, smoking and skin cancer.

Cross reference

Mental health in childhood – pages 534–543

Cross references

Role of children's nurses in child health promotion – pages 167–176

Developing strategies for health – page 151

Health education has tended to be based in the community rather than hospital. This is slowly changing and needs to continue to do so in the future. Children's nurses working in any field are in the best position to use their influence and experience with children to provide and reinforce the relevant health education to help children to attain both mental and physical well-being whilst not antagonising parents whose beliefs may be different. This is yet another area where children's nurses should exploit their expertise in family-centred care and make good use of their close relationship with the children and families in their care.

Activity

Choose a specific hospital ward or department and consider what health education programmes would be most suitable for the children and families in this area.

TECHNOLOGY IN CHILDREN'S NURSING

Technology in all branches of nursing has increased tremendously over the last 10–20 years. There has been an increase in the number and types of transplantations performed and this type of surgery is no longer a rare event. Nurses have needed to increase their technological skills to care for these highly dependent children. Extracorporeal Membrane Oxygenation (ECMO) is one example of how technology has developed to care for seriously ill children who previously would have died. ECMO provides pulmonary or cardiopulmonary support for children with reversible respiratory or cardiac failure and ECMO specialists have been appointed to complement the existing staff and provide the specific knowledge and skills to maintain and monitor the ECMO process. These specialists are often children's or neonatal nurses.

Community children's nurses are supporting families of children with special needs who are likely to have quite complicated care at home, such as total parenteral nutrition, tracheostomies, gastrostomies and even ventilation. As the resuscitation of infants becomes more sophisticated, this type of situation can only develop further. It is likely that development in general practice care will increase the amount of technology in the community still further. Alongside this, it is likely that children in acute hospitals will require even more highly dependent care.

In addition the reduction in junior doctors' hours has given nurses responsibility in areas they were not previously familiar with. For instance, children's nurses have now become the experts in the care of implantable IV devices while many doctors may have had little experience of such devices.

Children's nurses will need to react proactively to these changes. They need to be certain of their role and not take on extra responsibilities which may result in the reduced provision of nursing care of children and families. It is worth considering how extra responsibilities affect the concept of partnership in care. Perhaps the philosophy of Great Ormond Street Hospital for Children, 'Children first and always', should be remembered when considering any change in practice

> ➤ **Key points**

1. Children's nurses need to be proactive in their response to change to ensure they maintain their role as specialists in the care of children and their families.

2. If generic nurse education develops, children's nursing may become a post-graduate speciality and children's nurses may be less common.

3. Developments in the HCA role and the inability of many children's wards to meet minimum staffing requirements for qualified children's nurses may lead hospital managers to abandon the attempt to gain these more expensive nurses.

4. To maintain the speciality, children's nurses must be able to:
   - define their role and justify its continued existence;
   - demonstrate an appreciation of research findings;
   - only take on new areas of practice which are in the best interests of the child.

5. More research into family-centred care and involving families is needed to strengthen this concept of care.

6. Future developments to the role of the children's nurse include:
   - health education in hospital care;
   - mental health care of children and adolescents;
   - children's practice nurses;
   - continued initiatives in nurse led clinics, nurse-prescribing and specialist roles.

References

AUDIT COMMISSION (1993) *Children First – A Study of Hospital Services*. London: HMSO.

AGGLETON, P. and CHAMBERS, H. (1986) *Nursing Models and the Nursing Process*. Basingstoke: Macmillan Education.

BAGNALL, P. and GARBETT, R. (1996) Continuing education: how well is PREP working? *Nursing Times*, **92** (7), 34–35.

BARNSTEINER, J. and GILLIS-DONOVAN, J. (1990) Being related and separate: a standard for therapeutic relationships. *Maternal and Child Nursing*, **15** (4), 223–228.

BAUM, D., SISTER FRANCIS DOMINICA and WOODWARD, R. (1990) *Listen, My Child has a Lot of Living to Do*. Oxford: Oxford University Press.

BAXTER, J., *et al.* (1990) *Double Discrimination*. London: King's Fund Centre.

BENNER, P. (1984) *From Novice to Expert: Excellence and Power in Clinical Nursing*. Menlo Park, CA: Addison-Wesley.

BESSER, F. (1977) Great Ormond Street anniversary. *Nursing Mirror*, **144** (6), 31–33.

BOND, M. and HOLLAND, S. (1997) *Skills of Clinical Supervision for Nurses*. Milton Keynes: Open University Press.

BOUD, D., KEOGH, R. and WALKER, D. (1985) *Reflection: Turning Experience into Learning*. New York, Kegan Page.

BOWLBY, J. (1951) *Maternal Care and Mental Health*. Geneva: WHO.

BOWLBY, J. and ROBERTSON, J. (1952) *A Two-year Old Goes to Hospital. Mental Health and Infant Development*. London: Routledge & Kegan Paul.

BRADSHAW, A. (1996) The legacy of Nightingale. *Nursing Times*, **92** (6), 42–43.

BROCKLEHURST, N. (1996) Selling children's community nursing. *Paediatric Nursing*, **8** (9), 6–7.

BURNARD, P. (1988) The spiritual needs of Atheists and Agnostics. *Professional Nurse*, **4** (3), 130–132.

BUTTERWORTH, C. and FAUGIER J. (eds) (1992) *Clinical Supervision and Mentorship in Nursing*. London: Chapman & Hall.

CALLERY, P. and SMITH, L. (1991) A study of role negotiation between nurses and the parents of hospitalised children. *Journal of Advanced Nursing*, **16**, 772–781.

CAMPBELL, S. (1995) What makes a children's nurse? *Child Health*, **2** (5), 117.

CAMPBELL, S. and CLARKE, F. (1992) Ethos and philosophy of paediatric intensive care. In CARTER, B. (ed.), *Manual of Paediatric Intensive Care*. London: Harper Collins.

CAMPBELL, S. and GLASPER, A. (eds) (1995) *Whaley and Wong's Children's Nursing*. St Louis: Mosby.

CAMPBELL, S., KELLY, P. and SUMMERSKILL, P. (1993) Putting the family first. *Child Health*, **1** (2), 59–63.

CASEY, A. (1988) A partnership with child and family. *Senior Nurse*, **8** (4), 8–9.

CHAMBERLAIN, T., *et al.* (1988) Cost analysis of a home intravenous antibiotic programme. *American Journal of Hospital Pharmacy*, **45** (2), 2341–2345.

CLEARY, A. *et al.* (1986) Parental involvement in the lives of children in hospital. *Archives of Disease in Childhood*, **61** (8), 779–780.

CLOTHIER, C. (1994) *The Allitt Inquiry*. London: HMSO.

COLE, A. (1997) The state we're in. *Nursing Times*, **22** (93), 24–27.

COLSON, J. (1996) Creating opportunities for children's nurses. *Paediatric Nursing*, **8** (10), 6–7.

COUTTS-JARMAN, J. (1993) Using reflection and experience in nurse education. *British Journal of Nursing*, **2** (1), 77–80.

COYNE, I. (1996) Parent participation: a concept analysis. *Journal of Advanced Nursing*, **23**, 733–740.

COYNE, P. (1997) Developing nurse consultancy in clinical practice. *Nursing Times*, **92** (33), 34–35.

CRACKNELL, R. and COX, J. (1993) *Cultural and Religious Aspects of Caring Professionals*. Luton: University of Luton.

CURLEY, M. and WALLACE J. (1992) Effects of the mutual cooperation participation model of care on parental stress in the paediatric intensive care unit. *Pediatric Nursing*, **7** (6), 377–385.

DARBYSHIRE, P. (1994) *Living with a Sick Child in Hospital*. London: Chapman & Hall.

DARBYSHIRE, P. (1995) Parents in paediatrics. *Paediatric Nursing*, 7 (1), 8–10.

DAVID, R. (1990) Race, birthweight and mortality rates. *Journal of Pediatrics*, **116** (1), 101–102.

DAVIES, C. (1996a) Cloaked in a tattered illusion. *Nursing Times*, **92** (45), 44–46.

DAVIES, C. (1996b) A new vision of professionalism. *Nursing Times*, **92** (46), 54–56.

DAVIS, H. and FALLOWFIELD, L. (1991) *Counselling and Communication in Health Care*. Chichester: Wiley.

DoH (1976) *Fit for the Future – Child Health Services*. London: HMSO.

DoH (1989) *The Children Act – An Introductory Guide for the NHS*. London: HMSO.

DoH (1991) *Welfare of Children and Young People in Hospital*. London: HMSO.

DoH (1993) *Research for Health*. London: HMSO.

DoH (1994a) *The Allitt Inquiry. Report of the Clothier Committee*. London: HMSO.

DoH (1994b) *The Children's Charter*. London: HMSO.

DoH (1996a) *The Children's Charter*. London HMSO.

DoH (1996b) *Services for Children and Young People*. London: HMSO.

DEARMUN, A. (1997) Using reflection to assess degree students. *Paediatric Nursing*, **9** (1), 25–28.

DE MAUSE, L. (1974) *The History of Childhood*. London: Souvenir Press.

DEWEY, J. (1933) *How We Think*. Boston: D. C. Heath.

DODGE, J., MORRISON, S., LEWIS, P., *et al.* (1993) Cystic fibrosis in the UK 1968–1988: incidence, population and survival. *Paediatric and Perinatal Epidemiology*, 7, 156–166.

ELLIS, P. (1995) The role of the nurse as the patient's advocate. *Professional Nurse*, **11** (3), 206–207.

ENGLISH NATIONAL BOARD (1994) *Creating Lifelong Learners: Partnerships for Care*. London: ENB.

ENGSTROM, J. (1984) Problems in the development, use and testing of nursing theory. *Journal of Nursing Education*, **23** (60), 245–251.

FISH, D. and PURR, B. (1991) *The Evaluation Practice-Based Learning in Continuing Education in Nursing, Midwifery and Health Visiting*. London: ENB.

FISH, D. and TWINN, S. (1997) *Quality Clinical Supervision in the Health Care Professions. Principled Approaches to Practice*. London: Butterworth-Heinemann.

FRADD, E. (1994) A broader scope to practice. *Child Health*, 1 (6), 233–238.

FRADD, E. (1996) The importance of negotiating a care plan. *Paediatric Nursing*, 8 (6), 6–9.

FRASER, M. (1996) *Conceptual Nursing in Practice*, 2nd edn. London: Chapman & Hall.

FREIDSON, E. (1970) *Profession of Medicine*. New York, Dodds, Mead & Co.

FRY, T. (1993) Charting growth. *Child Health*, 1 (3), 104–107.

GABLEHOUSE, B. and GITTERMAN, B. (1990) Maternal understanding of commonly used medical terms in a pediatric setting. *American Journal of Diseases in Children*, **114**, 419–425.

GILL, K. (1993) Health professionals' attitudes toward parent participation in hospitalised children's care. *Children's health Care*, **22**, 257–271.

GLASPER, A. (1993) Back to the future. *Child Health*, 1 (3), 93–95.

GLASPER, A. (1995)The value of children's nursing in the third millennium. *British Journal of Nursing*, **4** (1), 27.

GLASPER, A. and BURGE, D. (1992) Developing family information leaflets. *Nursing Standard*, **6** (15), 24–27.

GREY, M. (1993) Stressors and children's health. *Journal of Pediatric Nursing*, **8** (2), 85.

GRUENDING, D. (1985) Nursing theory: a vehicle for professionalism? *Journal of Advanced Nursing*, **10**, 553–558.

GOULD, C. (1996) Multiple partnerships in the community. *Paediatric Nursing*, **8** (8), 27–31.

HANDY, C. (1994) *The Empty Raincoat*. London: Hutchinson.

HEALTH ADVISORY SERVICE (HAS) (1995) *The Commissioning Role and Management of Child and Adolescent Mental Health Services*. London: HMSO.

HILL, A. (1989) Trends in paediatric medical admissions. *British Medical Journal*, **298** (6686), 1479–1480.

HOPKINS, S. and HODGSON, I. (1996) Junior doctors' hours and the expanding role of the nurse. *Nursing Times*, **92** (14), 35–36.

HOSTLER, S. (1992) Personal communication. In JOHNSON, B., *et al*. (eds), *Caring for Children and Families: Guidelines for Hospital*. Bethesda: Association for the Care of Children's Health.

JACKSON, P. and PLANT, Z. (1996) Youngsters get an introduction to sexual health clinics. *Nursing Times*, **92** (21), 34–36.

JOHNS, C. C. (ed.) (1994) *The Burford NDU Model: Caring in Practice*. Oxford: Blackwell Scientific.

JOHNS, C. C. (1996) The benefits of a reflective model of nursing. *Nursing Times*, **92** (27), 39–41.

JOHNSON, M. (1996) Student nurses: novices or practitioners of brilliant care? *Nursing Times*, **92** (26), 34–37.

JOLLEY, J. (1995) Forging the way ahead. *Child Health*, **2** (5), 202–206.

JOLLEY, M. and ALLAN, P. (1989) *Current Issues in Nursing*. London: Chapman & Hall.

KITSON, A. (1986) Indicators of quality in nursing care – an alternative approach. *Journal of Advanced Nursing*, **11**, 133–144.

LACEY, D. (1993) Using Orem's model in psychiatric nursing. *Nursing Standard*, **7** (29), 28–30.

LASKY, P. and EICHELBURGER, K. (1985) Health related views and self-care behaviours of young children. *Family Relations*, **1**, 13–18.

LEY, P. and LLEWELYN, S. (1995) Improving patients' understanding, recall, satisfaction and compliance. In BROOME, A. and LLEWELYN, S. (eds), *Health Psychology*, 2nd edn. London: Chapman & Hall.

LISTER, P. (1987) The misunderstood model. *Nursing Times*, **83** (41), 40–42.

MacDONALD, G. (1991) Plans for a better future. *Nursing Times*, **87** (31), 42–43.

McMORROW, R. (1995) The role of the community psychiatric nurse in child psychiatry. *Child Health*, **3** (3), 95–98.

McSHERRY, W. (1996) Raising the spirits. *Nursing Times*, **92** (3), 48–49.

MABEN, J. and MACLEOD CLARK, J. (1996) Making the transition from student to staff nurse. *Nursing Times*, **92** (44), 28–31.

MACLEOD CLARK, J. and HOCKEY, L. (1989) *Further Research in Nursing*. London: Scutari Press.

MARMOT, M., ADEELSTEIN, A. and BULUSU, L. (1984) *Immigrant Mortality in England and Wales* (OPCS 47). London: HMSO.

MoH (1959) *Welfare of Children in Hospital (The Platt Report)*. London: HMSO.

NEWELL, R. (1992) Anxiety, accuracy and reflection: the limits of professional development. *Journal of Advanced Nursing*, 17, 1326–1333.

NICHOLS, K. (1993) *Psychological Care in Physical Illness*, 2nd edn. London: Chapman & Hall..

NIGHTINGALE, F. (1859) *Notes on Nursing*. London: Harrison.

OREM, D. (1971) *Nursing: Concepts of Practice*. New York: McGraw-Hill.

OREM, D. (1985) *Nursing: Concepts of Practice*, 3rd edn. New York: McGraw-Hill.

ORQUE, M. (1983) Nursing care of South Vietnamese patients. In ORQUE, M., BLOCH, B. and MONRROY, L. (eds), *Ethnic Nursing Care*. St Louis: Mosby.

PARR, M. (1993) The Neuman Health Care Systems Model: an evaluation. *British Journal of Theatre Nursing*, 3 (8), 20–27.

PEARSON, A. and VAUGHAN, B. (1986) *Nursing Models for Practice*. London: Heinemann.

PEPLAU, H. (1952) *Interpersonal Relationships in Nursing*. New York: Putnam.

PRICE, P. (1993) Parents' perceptions of the meaning of quality nursing care. *Advanced Nursing Science*, 16 (1), 33–41.

REEVE, J. (1994) Nurses' attitudes towards Health Care Assistants. *Nursing Times*, 90 (26), 43–46.

RICHARDSON, A. (1992) Studies exploring self-care for the person coping with cancer: a review. *International Journal of Nursing Studies*, 29 (2), 191–204.

ROBERTSON, J. (1958) *Young Children in Hospital*. London: Tavistock.

ROBINSON, R. (1996) A state of confusion. *Paediatric Nursing*, 8 (7), 6.

ROPER, W., LOGAN, N. and TIERNEY, A. (1980) *The Elements of Nursing*. Edinburgh: Churchill Livingstone.

RUSHTON, C. (1993) Child/family advocacy; ethical issues, practical strategies. *Critical Care Medicine*, 21 (9), 387–388.

SAMS, D. (1996) The development of leadership skills in clinical practice. *Nursing Times*, 92 (28), 37–39.

SHAH, R. (1992) *The Silent Minority*. London: National Children's Bureau.

SHAH, R. (1994) Practice with attitude. *Child Health*, 1 (6), 245–249.

STENBAK, E. (1986) *Care of Children in Hospital*. Geneva: WHO.

STRONG, S. (1997) Peripheral parents. *Nursing Times*, 93 (4), 20–21.

TEASDALE, K. (1987) Partnership with patients? *Professional Nurse*, September, 17–19.

THORNES, R. (1988a) *Hidden Children – An Analysis of Ward Attenders in Children's Wards*. London: Caring for Children in the Health Services Consortium.

THORNES, R. (1988b) *Parents Staying Overnight with their Children*. London: Caring for Children in the Health Services Consortium.

THORNES, R. (1991) *Just for the Day – Children Admitted to Hospital for Treatment*. London: Caring for Children in the Health Services Consortium.

UNITED KINGDOM CENTRAL COUNCIL (UKCC) (1986) *Project 2000 – A New Preparation for Practice*. London: UKCC.

UNITED KINGDOM CENTRAL COUNCIL (UKCC) (1990) *The Report of the Post-registration Education and Practice Project*. London: UKCC.

UNITED KINGDOM CENTRAL COUNCIL (UKCC) (1992a) *The Scope of Professional Practice*. London: UKCC.

UNITED KINGDOM CENTRAL COUNCIL (UKCC) (1992b) *Code of Professional Conduct for Nurses, Midwives and Health Visitors*. London: UKCC.

UNITED KINGDOM CENTRAL COUNCIL (UKCC) (1994a) PREP – Government support for UKCC proposals. *Register*, **14**, 4–5.

UNITED KINGDOM CENTRAL COUNCIL (UKCC) (1994b) *Standards for Post-registration Education and Practice (PREP)*. London: UKCC.

UNITED KINGDOM CENTRAL COUNCIL (UKCC) (1996) PREP – putting the record straight. *Register*, **18**, 6–7.

UNIVERSITY OF MANCHESTER HEALTH SERVICES MANAGEMENT UNIT (1996) *The Future Health-care Work Force*. Manchester: University of Manchester.

VAUGHAN, B. and EDWARDS, M. (1994) *The Research Practice Interface*. London: King's Fund Centre.

WALKER, C. (1990) Siblings of children with cancer. *Oncology Nurses Forum*, **17** (3), 355–360.

WALSH, M. and FORD, P. (1994) *New Rituals for Old: Nursing through the Looking Glass*. Oxford: Butterworth-Heinemann.

WELLER, B. (1994) Cultural aspects of children's health and illness. In LINDSAY, B. (ed.), *The Child and Family: Contemporary Issues in Child Health*. London: Balliere Tindall.

WEIR, L. (1993) Using Orem's model. *British Journal of Theatre Nursing*, **3** (6), 19–22.

WHITEHEAD, M. (1992) *The Health Divide*. Harmondsworth: Penguin.

WHITEHEAD, N. (1995) Behavioural paediatrics. In BROOME, A. and LLEWELYN, S. (eds), *Health Psychology*, 2nd edn. London: Chapman & Hall.

WOOD, C. (1988) *The Training of Nurses for Sick Children*. London: Great Ormond Street Hospital for Sick Children.

WOOTON, S. (1997) The reflective process as a tool for learning: a personal account. *Paediatric Nursing*, **9** (2), 6–8.

WRIGHT, S. (1990) *Building and Using a Model of Nursing*, 2nd edn. London: Edward Arnold.

WYKE, S. and HEWISON, J. (eds) (1991) *Child Health Matters*. Milton Keynes: Open University Press.

LEGAL AND ETHICAL ISSUES

Judith Hendrick

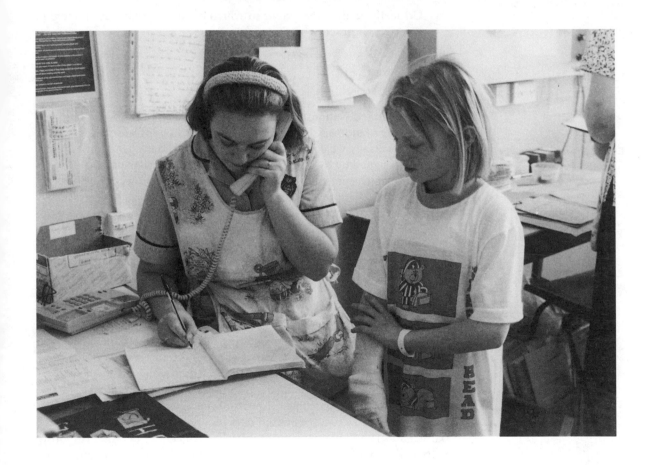

OBJECTIVES

The material contained within this module and the further reading/references should enable you to:

- Understand the legal and ethical principles which underpin children's nursing.
- Critically evaluate the relationship between law and ethics, in particular their interaction in resolving problems which arise in practice.
- Consider the limitations of legal intervention.
- Explore the way in which legal and ethical aspects of children's nursing differ from those of adults.
- Critically analyse the extent to which children's rights are upheld in a variety of practice settings.

Ethical issues terminology

- *Beneficence* – doing that which will produce benefit
- *Non-maleficence* – doing that which will cause no harm
- *Justice* – doing that which respects and acts upon a person's rights. *Fairness*
- *Autonomy* – the quality of having the ability to function independently
- *Deontology* – concerned with *duty*, focusing on the actions rather than their consequences
- *Consequentialism* – concerned with the nature of the outcome of one's actions

INTRODUCTION

The 1989 United Nations Convention on the Rights of the Child has been described as a landmark in the history of childhood not least because it was so universally welcomed. In fact the response to it was so enthusiastic that it was signed up by more countries more rapidly than any other international instrument. Closer to home, the Children Act, which was also passed in 1989, received similar support. Hailed as a children's charter it went further than any other previous legislation in highlighting children's autonomy, acknowledging their independent status and legitimating them as persons rather than objects of concern. Its fundamental principle, however, is the paramountcy of children's welfare and all its provisions in one way or other aim to ensure that children's best interests are always at the forefront. The impact for health professionals of this basic premise cannot be overestimated as it affects every aspect of children's health care and includes both legal and ethical principles.

This module will begin by examining the nature and scope of the law of consent and the extent to which it enhances children's autonomy. It will examine the complex legal and ethical issues which arise when children or those who care for them refuse life-saving treatment. The next section will explore those aspects of the Children Act 1989 which increase children's involvement in decision making, in particular their participation and independence rights. The concept of parental responsibility will also be examined. Other sections in this module look at children and confidentiality, the legal and ethical principles underpinning research, the role of law in allocating resources, and the extent to which it can be used in guaranteeing access to health care. The relationship between law and ethics in regulating and maintaining standards of professional practice is examined. Finally, the issue of children's rights and their implementation in practice is explored.

CONSENT TO TREATMENT 1

The right to consent (or refuse) treatment is one of the most well-established and cherished of 'medical rights' which has long been protected by the law – at least in relation to adults. Recently described as a 'basic human right' it was first expressly recognised in a 1914 American case (*Schloendorff v Society of New York Hospital 105 NE 92 (NY, 1914)*) when the judge said:

> *Every human being of adult years and sound mind has a right to determine what shall be done with his own body; and a surgeon who performs an operation without the patient's consent commits an assault.*

More recently the right to bodily integrity has been acknowledged in DoH guidance and the Patient's Charter. It is also enshrined in almost all medical and research codes of ethics. However, why is the right to consent (which is usually referred to as 'informed consent') regarded as inviolable? Several reasons are usually advanced. One is that it protects health professionals from legal action since touching a patient without consent constitutes the crime of battery and the tort (which is a civil 'wrong') of trespass. Another is its therapeutic benefit, namely that it helps secure the patient's cooperation and trust. A third reason is that it enables individuals to be responsible for their own choices. In short it is the way patients exercise autonomy. As Mason and McCall Smith (1994) state:

> *the seriousness with which the law views any invasion of physical integrity is based on the strong moral conviction that everyone has the right of self-determination with regard to his body.*

Autonomy, which means self-rule or self-government, is highly valued in modern Western society and many of the legal requirements of consent are based on this principle. But autonomy is a complex concept with ancient roots. Our modern understanding of the concept, however, is more recent and dates mainly from the works of two great philosophers – Immanual Kant (a deontologist) and John Stuart Mill (a utilitarian). Its basic idea can none the less be summed up in the phrase '*freedom of thought, will and action*'. Put simply this means that individuals should have the right to be responsible for themselves. In other words control their lives by thinking for themselves, deciding what to do (or not to do) and acting on their decisions.

Few would disagree with the general principle of respect for autonomy given the benefits it is said to confer. These include not just increasing personal well-being by enabling people to lead happier more fulfilling lives, but also by treating people never simply as means to ends

The United Nations Convention on the Rights of the Child recognizes children's right to autonomy under **Article 12** which states that: 'the child who is capable of forming his or own views [has] the right to express those views freely in all matters affecting the child, the views of the child being given due weight in accordance with the age and maturity of the child'.

Cross reference

Deontological versus utilitarian philosophy – page 669

Barriers to listening to children

- *Attitudes* – the greatest obstacles arise from prejudices about children's abilities and beliefs that it is unwise or unkind or a waste of time to listen to children
- *Scarce time and resources* – practical problems such as lack of time, or of a quiet place to talk, lack of pictures or of cards in other languages
- *Lack of confidence* – professionals need to believe that it is possible and valuable to listen to children and that many children can cope with bad news and hard decisions
- *Lack of skill* – failure to hear what young people have to say can result from adult's unwillingness to listen rather than children's inability to form and express their views
- *Language barriers* – Parents may act as two-way interpreters for younger children; explaining the child's terms and views to professionals and translating the technical language into words more familiar to the child
- *Beyond words* – it is helpful to encourage children to express themselves in non-linguistic ways
- *Collusion between adults and children* – professionals tend to communicate mainly with the parents and to young people this may appear like a collusion between adults
- *The need for adults to feel in control* – adults may fear seeming to renege on their responsibility

(Alderson and Montgomery, 1996, page 58)

but as ends in themselves – preventing coercion, exploitation and oppression. However, when applied to children and young people these benefits are commonly questioned, largely because of the myths and assumptions about the nature of childhood (likewise the proper role of parents and health professionals) and misconceptions about children's abilities, needs, and desires for autonomy. It is claimed, for example, that children lack the developed sense of self which an autonomous person requires or they lack the ability to make rational choices or the experience to make wise ones. As such they do not have a will of their own but must rely on others to make decisions for them. Denying children the right to participate fully in decision making far from being inconsistent with their autonomy therefore actually enhances it by enabling them to develop their potential as adults. To do otherwise, that is to burden them with choices which they are incapable of making, is to deprive them of the chance of becoming full human beings.

However, according to Alderson and Montgomery (1996) if children are to exercise autonomy they must be given the opportunity and the permission to do so. As studies have shown (Solberg, 1990) children's independence and competence follow adults' expectations and they increase with mutual respect and trust. This does not mean that all children should be forced to make decisions against their will or always have the final say since respect for autonomy is not an absolute principle but is a matter of degree. Thus, if treatment is complex and carries serious risks, respecting autonomy may involve no more than letting the child express his or her wishes freely. It may even be appropriate to refer the decision to someone else. However, if the treatment is relatively minor a child's wishes could be determinative despite opposition (parental or otherwise).

Activity

Consider the extent to which children ought to be allowed to take responsibility for decisions regarding treatment. Child C, for example, is an average 10 year old. Giving your reasons, identify those medical treatments which you feel he or she should be (a) solely responsible for and (b) never responsible for.

What kinds of things can undermine a person's autonomous choices? And to what extent to they justify paternalism? These are important questions especially in relation to children when paternalistic interference (making a decision for someone else which involves either overriding their expressed wishes or not even consulting them) is not uncommon in practice.

Harris (1985) outlines several factors which undermine a person's capacity for autonomous choice. These are

- *Defects in control.* This may be caused, for example, by mental illness, drug addiction or conditions such as anorexia nervosa, all of which may impair a person's ability to make genuine choices.

- *Defects in reasoning.* To be sufficient to undermine someone's capacity these must arise from, for example, blind acceptance of the views of others or prejudice.
- *Defects in information.* False, incomplete or misleading information, likewise an inability to understand the information, can deprive a person of the chance to make an informed choice.

Other factors which can limit autonomy include the need to balance the autonomy of health professionals with that of the patient. Case law has established, for example, that doctors are not obliged to give treatment which they consider to be contra-indicated. This happened in *Re J [1992] 4 All ER 614* when doctors wanted to withhold life support from a profoundly handicapped baby who was microcephalic, had cerebral palsy, cortical blindness and severe epilepsy. J's mother wanted treatment to be prolonged as long as possible but the court rejected her claim. In so doing it highlighted the potential for tension which exists between autonomy and the principle of beneficence. Beneficence, which basically means doing good for others (Gillon, 1985) requires health professionals and parents to do whatever is necessary to promote and safeguard the welfare of child patients.

Despite this tension there is, none the less, as Bird and White (1995) note, increasing interdependence between the autonomy of health professionals and that of all patients. In relation to consent this focuses in particular on the issue of information disclosure. To make informed choices patients need information – about the risks and benefits of proposed treatment, for example, and alternative options. Health professionals have a key role not only in deciding how much and what information to provide but also in helping patients interpret and evaluate that information. This may mean, if the patient is young, ensuring that the information is given in an age-appropriate way possibly with the help of dolls, story books, drawings and other aids (Alderson and Montgomery, 1996).

Obtaining consent thus involves the application of both legal and ethical principles. As Charles-Edwards (1996, page 67) states

> the debate about children and consent concerns their capacity to understand enough information, and, associated with this, whether they are legally competent and morally autonomous

The concept of competence is thus a central one. And if children's autonomy is to be respected the law must give those who are able to do so the right to give and withhold consent. Yet surprisingly no precise test of capacity (the word capacity and competence are often used interchangeably) has ever been laid down. Typically, though, the following questions are raised when a child's capacity is in issue.

UKCC Exercising Accountability Section D: Consent and Truth states 'informed consent means that the practitioner involved explains the intended test or procedure to the patient without bias and in as much detail (including details of possible reactions, complications, side effects and social or personal ramifications) as the patient requires'.

See **The Gillick case** box on page 657

These are:

- Is the child 'Gillick' competent?
- Who assesses competence?
- If a child is not competent who has the right to make a decision on the child's behalf?
- What if there is a disagreement?

Before looking at these aspects in detail it is important to outline the general legal elements of consent.

GENERAL LEGAL PRINCIPLES

Consent must be effectively obtained

With very few exceptions the law does not prescribe what form consent to medical treatment should take. This means that it can be either express or implied, written or oral. For routine minor procedures consent is usually obtained verbally and may well be implied, such as when patients roll up their sleeves for an injection. More serious procedures especially involving surgery will normally be preceded by written consent using a standard form recommended by the DoH. However, whatever the form of consent it can be withdrawn at any time before or even during the relevant medical procedure. If this happens a fresh consent must be obtained.

Legal definition of treatment

'Surgical medical or dental treatment as well as examination, investigation and diagnostic procedures (and any other procedure which is ancillary to such treatment such as anesthesia).'

(Section 8 Family Law Reform Act 1969)

Activity

- Consider the extent to which the usual forms of consent used for 'minor' procedures in your hospital give autonomy to those involved.
- Consider how the forms of consent which you usually obtain from a child rather than his or her parents respect the child's autonomy.

Legal definition of voluntary consent

'the real question in each case is: Does the patient really mean what he says or is he merely saying it for a quiet life or to satisfy someone else or because the advice and persuasion to which he has been subjected is such that he can no longer think and decide for himself?' In other words 'Is it a decision expressed in form only, not in reality?'

(Lord Donaldson in *Re T [1992] 3, WLR* **782**, page 797)

Consent must be voluntary

To be legally valid consent must be freely given. In other words it must be given without force, undue pressure or influence. This aspect of consent has been described as one of the foundation stones of consent which imposes on professionals a high ethical obligation. In practice whether or not consent is genuine will depend on several factors including the effect of pain, tiredness, drugs and so on. The relationship of the 'persuader' to the patient may also be crucial, especially if he or she is a parent. Note too that the notion of voluntary consent is more subtle than might first appear because although arm twisting and overt threats are not part of medical practice, patients, especially children can be subject to more complicated forms of pressure. They may be over-anxious to please, for example, or easily embarrassed.

Sufficient information must be given

The importance of exercising choice is recognised by the requirements the law imposes in respect of information disclosure. Although no precise legal test has ever been established broad guidelines were set out in *Sidaway v Bethlem Royal Hospital Governors [1985] 1 All ER 643*. Briefly this case basically establishes that patients need only be told what health professionals think they should be told. This means that it is the medical profession itself which decides what should (or should not) be revealed. By adopting this 'professional standard' albeit one which must accord with 'acceptable professional practice' English courts have thus rejected a more patient-friendly approach which would oblige professionals to disclose what 'reasonable' patients would want to know.

Activity

Health Circular HC (90) 22 (DoH, 1990) states that patients are entitled to receive sufficient information in a way that they can understand about the proposed treatments, the possible alternatives and any substantial risks. Consider (a) how this guidance is, in practice, interpreted in relation to child patients, and (b) how information sheets would be helpful to patients.

The combined effect of case law and advice from the DoH is that:

- Patients must be given sufficient information, that is be told in broad terms about the nature and effect of the procedure and its likely risks and harms, in particular those which are substantial and those with 'grave adverse consequences'.

- Patients who ask direct questions, for example, about possible risks should not be lied to. However, they are not entitled to any more information than those patients to whom information has been volunteered. The standard of disclosure is therefore again the professional one and so is determined by responsible professional practice.

- In some circumstances it is lawful to withhold information. This is known as 'therapeutic' privilege and is justified when revealing certain facts might harm the patient, that is damage his or her health or cause psychological damage.

- Information for children should be given in a way which is appropriate for their age and understanding.

Activity

Do you think 'therapeutic' privilege is more likely to be relied on in respect of child patients? If so is it justified? Can you think of examples in your practice?

Patients must be mentally competent

This aspect of the law of consent is still controversial because even though it was assumed that the Gillick case (1986) and the Children Act 1989 had settled once and for all the question of when children could or could not consent to treatment, developments in the law since then have shown that the law's commitment to children's autonomy is far from strong. To explain how the law operates it is necessary to distinguish between children of various age groups and whether they are giving or refusing consent.

16 and 17 year olds

Giving consent

The Family Law Reform Act 1969 (Section 8) applies to this age group. It sets a presumptive standard in that 16 and 17 year olds are presumed (like adults) to be competent unless the contrary is shown. However, even if they are competent the courts (but not parents) retain their protective role and can veto their consent. If young people in this age group are not competent consent can be given by a proxy – usually a parent or someone with 'parental responsibility'.

Refusing consent

Although some might think it illogical to distinguish between a young person's ability to consent to treatment and the ability to refuse in that 'the right to say yes must carry the right to say no' the courts are content to make such a distinction. Thus even though they are competent 16 and 17 year olds can have their 'informed refusal' overridden. This was established in *Re W [1992] 4 All ER 627* in which a 16-year-old girl suffering from anorexia nervosa had her refusal of treatment overridden by the court. Her weight was dangerously low and without treatment her reproductive organs were likely to be damaged. Her life was also in danger. The court held she was not competent because her condition had affected her ability to make a decision about treatment. More controversial, however, were the general principles it laid down about how future cases involving refusal of treatment by young people under 18 should be resolved. Briefly these were that even if they were competent their refusal could be overridden – not just by a court but by parents (or anyone else with parental responsibility) as well. In other words health professionals could rely on the consent of a proxy. The court in Re W also appeared to impose a very stringent test of competency – one which few adults let alone young people could satisfy.

Several reasons are usually advance to justify the courts' paternalistic interference in cases like Re W. A common one is that refusing consent may close down the options (Mason and McCall Smith, 1994). Another is consent 'involves the acceptance of an experience view, refusal rejects that experience – and does so from a position of limited experience'.

But when parents or the court override a competent young person's consent they must act in his or her 'best interests'. This phrase has not yet been precisely defined but it would clearly include therapeutic treatment, i.e. that which is likely to benefit the child after taking into account its risks and harms and likewise the consequences of non-treatment. Whether other treatment, e.g. cosmetic surgery, would be in a child's best interests would depend on the particular circumstances of the case.

Under 16 year olds – 'Gillick' competent

Giving consent

The right of competent under 16 year olds to give consent was established in the Gillick case. This landmark decision acknowledged the independent right of mature young people to control their own health care and introduced the concept of Gillick competence. Within a short time the concept was applied to all medical treatment, not just contraceptive care. The Gillick test sets an evidential standard of competence which means that children are presumed not to be competent unless they satisfy health professionals that they are. However, despite being widely used both in the literature and practice there is still some debate about what the concept actually means and what level of competence the law actually requires children to achieve in individual cases. In short it is a very imprecise and flexible concept.

It is therefore not surprising that the definitions and assessments of Gillick competence vary widely. However, in practice children's competence tends to be underestimated. The age at which children may express a desire to be involved in decision making can also vary, although Alderson (1993) suggests that children of all ages can be helped to participate in decision making. Another study has shown that 14 year olds are as capable of making treatment decisions as adults (Weithorn and Campbell, 1982) according to all the major standards of competency, i.e. evidence of choice, understanding of the facts, reasonable decision making process and reasonable outcome of choice. Given the uncertainty surrounding Gillick competence it is perhaps appropriate to describe it as 'more than a skill; [which] grows and withers within relationships and is perceived subjectively' (Alderson and Montgomery, 1996, page 47).

The Gillick case

In *Gillick v West Norfolk and Wisbech Area Health Authority [1985] 3 All ER 402* the House of Lords held that young people under 16 could give consent to contraceptive advice without their parents' knowledge or consent providing they had 'sufficient maturity and intelligence' to understand the proposed treatment.

Points to note about the Gillick test include:

- it applies to all medical treatment not just contraception
- although there is no automatic age-based cut off, capacity will normally increase with age
- the level of competence required will vary depending on the nature of the proposed treatment
- competence according to *Re R [1991] 4 All ER 117* (a case involving fluctuating capacity), is a developmental concept which must be assessed on a broad long-term basis taking into account a child's whole medical history, background and mental state. As such no child who is only competent on a good day can pass the Gillick test

Activity

Read *Assessment of Mental Capacity: Guidance for Doctors and Lawyers* (BMA and Law Society, 1995), pages 72–76. Critically evaluate the assessment process they recommend in respect of children's capacity.

Deciding when a parents' right to decide should yield to their child's right to make his or her own decisions can thus be very difficult to pinpoint. None the less, respecting a young person's autonomy means at the very least finding out whether a child agrees with his or her parents' wishes. If not, the law requires an assessment of the child's competence. Ethically, too, such an approach is required. As Charles-Edwards (1996) points out a parent's duty to avoid harm and promote good means that as a child matures developing understanding and autonomy, the parents' right to decide on the child's behalf decreases. Finally it is important to note that a court (but not parents) can veto a Gillick competent child's consent.

Refusing consent

It was assumed following the Gillick case that young people under 16 who were competent to give consent were also legally entitled to refuse it. However, recent case law has shown that respecting the autonomy of mature under 16 year olds does not entitle them to refuse treatment – at least not if it is life-saving and offers the child a chance, however slim, of surviving. This means that Gillick competent under 16 year olds can have their informed refusal overridden (until they are 18) by a court or any person with parental responsibility and so may be lawfully treated against their will. In the few cases to reach the courts when parents, their children or health professionals have disagreed about treatment the courts have, nevertheless stressed how important it is to consider the young person's views. Note, too, that as with 16 and 17 year olds, it is only lawful to override refusal of consent if the proposed treatment is in the child's best interests. In *Re E [1993] 1 FLR 386*, for example, a Jehovah's Witness boy aged nearly 16 was refusing (as were his parents) a life-saving blood transfusion urgently needed to treat his leukaemia. The judge imposed a very strict competency test which few adults could have achieved – it required him to consider the manner in which he might die and the extent of his and his family's suffering. Accordingly he was not competent and so he could be treated despite his opposition. Even if he had been considered competent, however, the court (and his parents) could have overruled his refusal because his life was in danger.

Activity

When E became 18 and therefore reached the age when he could refuse treatment he exercised that right and died. Do you think the court was right in denying him the 'right' to die for nearly 2 years? Read the case and decide if you think that E understood what was involved in refusing the blood transfusion. Brief details of Re E can be found in Hendrick (1997, page 190). A fuller report can be found in the law reports.

Children under 16 – not 'Gillick' competent

Permission for treatment for children in this group must come from a proxy – normally a person with parental responsibility or exceptionally someone who is temporarily looking after the child. If there is no such person, or if they are refusing to give consent, an application should be made to court to resolve the issue. The guiding principle is, of course, the child's best interests. In the vast majority of cases this is not problematic. However, what if in the opinion of health professionals they chose an option which is contrary to the child's welfare? This is when a court may be involved as happened in the case of *Re S [1993] 1 FLR 376* when parents of a 4 year old with T cell leukaemia refused consent to a blood transfusion for religious reasons. The court overrode their refusal and authorised the transfusion. This case makes it clear that even when children are too young to make their own decisions parents cannot veto treatment which is thought medically essential. And as the case of Re J (see page 653) shows they cannot demand treatment either.

Consent and the Children Act 1989

When the Children Act 1989 was passed it was hailed as a children's charter not least because several of its provisions enshrined the spirit of Gillick and appeared to give mature young people an absolute right of informed refusal to medical, psychiatric examinations (and exceptionally also treatment). It was not long, however, before the courts intervened (see *South Glamorgan CC v B and W [1993] 1 FLR 574* on page 660) and showed how they were prepared to override the informed refusal of mature young people.

Before concluding this section on consent it is worth noting the position in Scotland, which unlike the UK has yet to litigate the issue of competent young people refusing treatment. It is suggested that certain historical factors and Scottish legislation may give young people greater control over medical decision making.

Provisions in the Children Act 1989 concerning examinations

Children with sufficient understanding to make an informed decision can refuse to submit to medical, psychiatric examinations or other assessments:

- interim care order
- interim supervision order
- full supervision order (this order also covers treatment)
- child assessment order
- emergency protection order

> **Key points**

1. Obtaining consent involves the application of both legal and ethical principles.
2. Assessing children's competence is a complex process which requires consideration of their ability to understand that there are choices and a willingness to make such choices.
3. Definitions and assessments of competence vary widely but good practice requires clear guidance as to the factors which should be considered as relevant or irrelevant to the assessment of legal competence.

The facts of *South Glamorgan CC v B and W [1993]*

A 15-year-old girl with severe behavioural problems had refused to undergo various medical and psychiatric examinations under the Children Act 1989. She had confined herself to the front room of her father's house with the curtains drawn for approximately 11 months and had hardly had any contact with the outside world. If her family refused to obey her instructions she threatened to commit suicide or harm herself. Despite being assessed as competent, her informed refusal was overridden by the court since without being examined it felt that she was likely to suffer serious harm

4. In some circumstances it may be justifiable to override the wishes of a competent child.

5. The ultimate forum for resolving disputes about a child's medical treatment is the court and children should have the opportunity to explain to a judge the reasons for their refusal of consent.

660

CHILDREN ACT 1989 2

There is little doubt that the Children Act 1989 is the most comprehensive and far-reaching reform of child law this century. Designed to bring about a new beginning to the philosophy and practices of the child care system, it radically changes the law relating to children and their families. Its main aims are to:

- promote and safeguard the welfare of children and ensure that their interests are paramount whenever court decisions are made about their upbringing;

- provide new remedies to resolve disputes which were flexible, interchangeable and practical;

- strike a new balance between the protection of children, the integrity of the family and the role of the state;

- emphasise the primacy of the family, i.e. that the best place for children to grow up is with their families;

- identify the independent rights of children and enhance their legal status;

- promote partnership between local authority social service departments and other departments (e.g. health and housing), parents and children.

> **Children Act 1989**
>
> 1. Welfare of the Child
>
> (1) When a court determines any question with respect to
>
> > (a) the upbringing of a child;' or
> >
> > (b) the administration of a child's property or the application of any income arising from it,
>
> the child's welfare shall be the court's paramount consideration
>
> (2) In any proceedings in which any question with respect to the upbringing of a child arises, the court shall have regard to the general principle that any delay in determining the question is likely to prejudice the welfare of the child

The extent to which these aims have been achieved is, nearly a decade later, still uncertain. How far the Act has legitimated children as persons rather than objects of concern is also unclear. This phrase comes from the 1987 Cleveland crisis in which social workers were accused of acting precipitately in removing approximately 100 children unnecessarily from their homes. Events in Cleveland and the inquiry it prompted forced the problem of child sexual abuse into the public domain. They were also major influences on those provisions in the Act which substantially reformed the powers of local authorities to intervene in family life and established a framework within which social work practice could be made more accountable and consistent.

The Children Act was hailed as a children's charter because, unlike previous legislation dealing with children, it relied far less on notions of paternalism which viewed children as defenceless and vulnerable objects of welfare in need of protection. Instead it seemed to be the first statute to take children's rights seriously thereby reconstituting them as persons in their own right (Lyon and Parton, 1995). As such they were no longer possessions over whom power was exercised but individuals to whom duties were owed.

But debate about how far the Act intended to empower children continues. Freeman (1996), for example, considers that because of the paramountcy principle and the primacy it accords to children's welfare, their autonomy must often take a back seat. Others, such as Lyon and Parton (1995), suggest that the way the Act has been interpreted has shown that opportunities for advancing children's wishes and independent action are at best qualified. Alderson and Montgomery (1996) also claim that on the whole the Act's commitment to young people's autonomy is ambiguous.

The main provisions in the Act which have implications for children's autonomy are two-fold, namely those which increase their involvement in decision making (participation rights) and those which recognise their capacity for independent action (independence rights). However, also worth noting in this context is the new concept of 'parental responsibility' largely because it reflects the tension between children's autonomy and their welfare and so also has implications for the exercise of their rights.

PARTICIPATION RIGHTS

Welfare Checklist Section 1(3) Children Act 1989

Ascertainable wishes and feelings of the child (considered in the light of his age and understanding) his physical, emotional and educational needs, the likely effect of any change in circumstances, his age, sex, background and any personal characteristics which the court considers relevant, any harm which he has suffered or is at risk of suffering, how capable each of his parents (or any other person in relation to whom the court considers the question to be relevant) is of meeting his needs, the range of powers available to the court under the Act in the proceedings in question

According to Alderson and Montgomery (1996), participation rights have several advantages. Firstly, they are relatively unconditional in that children do not have to pass any competency test before they express their wishes. Secondly, even very young children can be informed and involved. Thirdly, children can avoid the burden of being blamed for wrong decisions despite having their say. However, participation rights also have their disadvantages, notably being used to deny children the greater status of autonomous individuality. An unequivocal commitment to autonomy could have been assured by making the wishes of mature young people determinative. But, except in relation to medical and psychiatric examinations and assessments (which as was shown in the previous section the courts have since eroded), the Act did not adopt this approach. Instead it gives children the 'right' to be consulted, i.e. to be heard and so have the opportunity to express their wishes and feelings. In practice what this should mean is that there is less chance that children's views will be ignored.

The main vehicle for the child's voice in the Act is the 'welfare checklist'. Introduced to improve and standardise the way court decisions are made the checklist requires the courts to have regard to 'the ascertainable wishes and feelings of the child concerned (considered in the light of his age and understanding)'. This factor is the first in a list of seven. Its prominence suggests it is the most important one but this is misleading since they all carry equal weight. More importantly the child's wishes do not have to be followed even though they can strongly influence the outcome of a case and, in some cases, they may well be decisive providing the court agrees that the child's best interests are thereby promoted.

The Act also significantly increases children's rights to be consulted when they are in the public care system, i.e. being cared for away from home, e.g. by foster parents or a children's home. Hence, local authorities now have to find out their views both before making a decision about their future care and when their case is reviewed. They must also inform children about decisions which affect them.

Whilst these provisions provide no guidance on how a child's wishes should actually be obtained nor what weight should be attached to them – and so can in practice be difficult for children to enforce – they do, as Lyon and Parton (1995) point out, at the very least enhance the legal relevance of their views. Finally, it is worth noting that in court proceedings when a young child's wishes may need to be presented to the court the Act has increased the use of the 'guardian ad litem' whose role is to safeguard the interests of the child and ensure that his or her views are considered.

INDEPENDENCE RIGHTS

Other new provisions appear to acknowledge children's capacity for independent action. As such they arguably 'create the possibility of a more absolute autonomy' (Lyon and Parton, 1995, page 42). Children now have rights to initiate court action. They may, for example, challenge emergency protection orders and ask for a care (and supervision) order to be discharged. Perhaps even more significant is their 'right' to seek the court's permission to apply for a so-called Section 8 order. Of these the most controversial is the residence order which determines with whom the child lives. Often described as the right to 'divorce' parents this order (likewise the other Section 8 orders) can only be sought if the court considers that the child has 'sufficient understanding to make an application'. Designed to filter out inappropriate applications this leave requirement – which has been described by Freeman (1996, page 173) as 'unjustifiable and unnecessary', has been restrictively interpreted. In other words by linking children's empowerment to competence the courts can (by imposing a relatively high degree of understanding) deny young people the right to be treated as autonomous individuals, at least in this context.

> **Section 8 orders (Children Act, 1989)**
>
> - *Contact* – regulates contact between a child and another person, usually a parent with whom the child is not living
> - *Residence* – settles with whom the child lives
> - *Prohibited steps* – prevents something being done without the court's permission
> - *Specific issue* – settles a single issue which has arisen in respect of a child's upbringing

Activity

- Which Section 8 order could be applied for to prevent controversial medical treatment such as sterilisation of a mentally handicapped child?
- Which Section 8 order could be applied for if parents are 'unreasonably' refusing consent to medical treatment for a very young child?
- Find out which Section 8 order health professionals can apply for in respect of a child patient and how they might go about doing this.

PARENTAL RESPONSIBILITY

This term is a central concept in the Act. It describes the legal authority parents have over their children and replaces the phrase 'parental rights' in earlier legislation. The change in terminology was intended to reinforce the idea that the law gives parents authority not as a reward of parenthood but so that they, rather than the state, can raise their child to become a properly developed adult both physically and morally.

The Act does not define parental responsibility in much detail nor does it list the things parents can or cannot do. The absence of written rules means that the scope and nature of the concept remains uncertain. Nevertheless it is usually accepted that those with parental responsibility can take the following decisions:

- *Providing a home*, i.e. deciding how to meet a child's physical needs and emotional needs. It thus includes making major decisions such as where a child lives as well as more mundane ones, e.g. what he or she should eat, etc.
- *Contact*. This is especially important for parents who are not living with their children because it entitles them (subject to any court order to the contrary) to see and spend time with them. In some cases contact can be limited and consist of 'phone calls or letters. It is generally assumed, however, that children benefit from continued contact with both parents.
- *Discipline*. Disciplining a child includes using corporal punishment and other forms of punishment. However, to be lawful discipline must be 'moderate' and 'reasonable', i.e. appropriate to the child's age, health, physique, understanding and strength. Excessive use of corporal punishment which harms a child may result in parents being prosecuted. Note too that corporal punishment is banned in most schools, and whenever children are being looked after by a local authority and living away from their families.
- *Religious upbringing*. Parents have the right to decide what religious faith their child should follow, if any. But, parental choice will not prevail over the strongly held religious views of a mature child.
- *Name*. Although it is usual it is not obligatory for a child of married parents to take the father's surname.
- *Education*. Parents have a wide discretion in deciding how to educate their children although some form of education is compulsory for school-age children (between 5 and 16). Most parents fulfil this obligation by sending their children to school (state or private). However, some opt out of the school system and educate their children themselves at home.
- *Marriage*. A child under 16 cannot get married. Those between 16 and 18 need parental consent.
- *Travel and emigration*. Parental consent is required before a passport will be issued to a child under 18 but those under 16 can be included in their parents' passport.
- *Consent to medical treatment*. Subject to the rights of competent 16 and 17 year olds and 'Gillick' competent under 16 year olds those

with parental responsibility have the right to consent and refuse medical treatment.

LIMITS TO PARENTAL RESPONSIBILITY

Although the scope of parental responsibility is very broad giving parents (likewise anyone else who has acquired it) extensive control over children's lives it is not absolute. It is in practice subject to two major restrictions. The first is the welfare principle. In applying this principle the courts have made it clear that unless parental responsibility is exercised in accordance with that principle it can be challenged and even overridden. The second restriction is that parental responsibility diminishes as children mature and become more capable of making their own decisions. As the courts stressed in the Gillick case:

> the legal right of a parent ends at the 18th birthday, and even up till then it is a dwindling right which the courts will hesitate to enforce against the wishes of the child, the older he is. It starts with a right of control and ends with little more than advice.

OTHER PEOPLE WHO MAY BE INVOLVED IN A CHILD'S CARE

Foster parents

Foster parents look after children but do not have parental responsibility. They may have been appointed by a local authority or be caring for a child as a result of a private arrangement. Foster parents have no legal rights over children but they can make decisions about their day-to-day care by virtue of Section 3(5) of the Children Act 1989.

De facto carers

This group covers a wide range of people who may be temporarily caring for a child, such as childminders, teachers, baby-sitters, relatives and so on. De facto carers do not have parental responsibility, but the Children Act 1989, Section 3(5) applies to them so they too can make day-to-day decisions. These are unlikely to be more than minor ones, however, and would cover such matters as discipline, what the child eats, wears and so on.

Activity

A child of 3 is brought into an A&E department by a nursery teacher and needs stitches on a leg wound. Her parents cannot be contacted. Who can give consent for the medical treatment?

Who has parental responsibility

If a child is legitimate both parents automatically have parental responsibility

If a child's parents are not married only the mother has parental responsibility

An unmarried father can acquire parental responsibility in several ways such as:

- by marrying the mother
- adopting his child
- obtaining a court order
- making a parental responsibility agreement with the mother

How parental responsibility can be obtained by non-parents

Relatives, step-parents and local authorities can acquire parental responsibility through court orders such as residence orders, emergency protection orders and care orders

Section 3(5) Children Act 1989

A person who (a) does not have parental responsibility for a particular child; but (b) has care of the child may (subject to the provisions of this Act) do what is reasonable in all the circumstances of the case for the purpose of safeguarding or promoting the child's welfare

Step-parents

Step-parents do not have parental responsibility even though they have been living with their step-child. However, again by virtue of Section 3(5) they have the legal authority to make day-to-day decisions about a child's care, which given their parental role are likely to more significant than those taken by temporary carers. Step-parents can acquire parental responsibility through a court order (or adoption).

Adoptive parents

Adoptive parents replace a child's biological parents and thus acquire parental responsibility. For legal purposes they are then treated as the child's legal parents and have all their rights and duties.

AGE-RELATED ACTIVITIES

Children acquire certain rights and powers at various different ages. Below are listed some of the most important.

At any age children can:

- initiate proceedings under the Children Act 1989 (if they have sufficient understanding and maturity);
- choose their own religion (unless it is harmful);
- change their name (if they have the maturity to understand the implications of that decision);
- seek advice and counselling (if they are 'Gillick' competent);
- give consent to surgical, dental, medical treatment (if they are 'Gillick' competent);
- apply to see most personal files (whether on computer or held in manual form) provided they understand the nature of their request;
- sue in court (through a 'next friend');
- borrow money;
- inherit property;
- make a complaint about discrimination (on the basis of race, colour, ethnic or national origin, or nationality);
- baby-sit;
- smoke cigarettes (but not buy them until 16);
- enter a bingo club (but not take part in the game);
- have ears pierced.

At 5 children can:

- drink alcohol in private;
- see (or rent) certain films and videos;
- must receive full-time education.

At 10 children can:

- open a bank or building society account;

- be convicted of a criminal offence (if it can be proved they knew what they were doing was wrong);
- in certain circumstances be searched, finger-printed, have samples taken by the police;
- if boys, be capable of committing a sexual offence, including rape (if under 14 the prosecution must prove they knew what they were doing was seriously wrong).

At 12 children can:

- buy a pet;
- be trained to participate in dangerous performances.

At 13 children can:

- work part-time (subject to several restrictions).

At 14 children can:

- be convicted of a criminal offence as if an adult;
- enter a bar on their own, but only buy soft drinks.

At 16 young people can:

- leave school;
- work full-time (subject to certain restrictions);
- leave home;
- marry with parental consent;
- join most trade unions;
- apply for their own passport (but one parent must give written consent);
- buy cigarettes, tobacco, liqueur chocolates, fireworks, premium bonds;
- be street traders;
- sell scrap metal;
- enter or live in a brothel;
- if young men, join the armed forces with parental consent.

At 17 young people can:

- hold a licence to drive certain vehicles (e.g. a car or small goods vehicle);
- if young women, join the armed forces with parental consent.

At 18 young people reach the age of majority and can do most things, such as:

- vote;
- marry;
- serve on a jury;
- make a will;
- own land, buy a house or flat or hold a tenancy;

- buy and drink alcohol in a bar;
- be tattooed;
- donate their bodies or organs;
- pawn goods at a pawn shop;
- enter a betting shop and bet;
- if adopted apply to have their name and address put on the Adoption Contact Register.

At 21 young people can:

- adopt a child;
- stand in a general or local election;
- apply for a licence to sell alcohol;
- hold a licence to drive a lorry or bus.

Key points ➤

1. The key principles underpinning the Children Act 1989 are the paramountcy of the child's welfare, the empowerment of children, and the primacy of the family.

2. The Act's overall objective is to strike a new balance between the protection of children, the integrity of the family and the role of the state.

3. The welfare checklist emphasises the importance of consulting children.

4. The concept of parental responsibility emphasises the duties of parents rather than their rights.

CONFIDENTIALITY 3

To control their health care children need not only the right to consent to (or veto) medical treatment (see above) but also a right of control over personal health information. Laws on confidentiality help secure this control but whilst the principle of confidentiality is one of the oldest in medical ethics and is also widespread in professional codes (likewise the Patient's Charter), research has shown that many teenagers are deterred from seeking professional help around personal and sexual issues because they fear a lack of confidentiality.

The duty to respect confidential information comes from several sources but what is its precise nature and scope? Put very simply the duty of confidentiality means that health professionals must respect their patients' secrets. In other words professionals must not disclose anything learned from a person who has consulted them, or whom they have examined without that person's agreement. Rules of confidentiality are usually justified on two main grounds. One (the utilitarian or consequentialist argument) claims that unless patients feel that they can trust health professionals with potentially embarrassing information and are confident that it will not be divulged they will fail to reveal certain details about themselves (which may be medically very important) or may be deterred from seeking medical care altogether. As a consequence their health may suffer for without full information from patients health professionals cannot 'make accurate diagnoses and prognoses or recommend the best course of treatment' (Beauchamp and Childress, 1994).

The second common justification derives from the deontological school of philosophy. This claims that confidentiality should be respected because it is inherently right to do so. In other words, irrespective of welfare considerations, there are strong moral grounds for keeping information private and secure, notably respect for personal autonomy and fidelity (or promise keeping).

UKCC Code of Professional Conduct (Clause 10)

This requires practitioners to: protect all confidential information concerning patients and clients obtained in the course of professional practice and make disclosures only with consent, where required by court order or where it can be justified in the wider public interest

Consequentialist (or utilitarian) philosophy

This seeks to judge the morality of an act by its consequences. In simple terms this means the right act is that which gives the greatest happiness to the greatest number

Deontological philosophy

This holds that there are rules which govern actions and which tell us whether acts are inherently right or wrong irrespective of the consequences

Activity

Read *UKCC: Confidentiality*: an elaboration of clause 9 of the 2nd edition of the UKCC Code of Professional Conduct 1987 (now clause 10 of the 3rd edition released in 1992).

- Does it make any special reference to children in relation to confidentiality?
- Consider how it defines 'confidential'.

Although the principle of medical confidentiality is universally acknowledged it is not always observed in practice. Some commentators have even suggested that because it is so widely ignored and violated it has become a 'decrepit concept' (Siegler, 1982). However, the duty of confidentiality has never been absolute and almost all codes of practice as well as the law recognise certain exceptions. In relation to children and young people, these exceptions are not always applied consistently and uniformly, largely because of uncertainty about the nature of the legal obligation of confidentiality but also because of confusion as to its relevance to children and young people – in respect of whom disclosure may be considered the only way to protect their welfare.

CHILDREN AND CONFIDENTIALITY

Once an obligation to maintain confidentiality has arisen in law it is owed as much to young people under 18 as it is to any other person providing they are sufficiently mature to form a relationship of confidence. What this means is that irrespective of a child's competence to consent to (or veto) treatment they are none the less in principle legally owed a duty of confidence if they understand what it means to trust someone with secret information. This is, however, subject to any relevant exception (see below). Note too that even if the requested treatment is refused the confidentiality of the consultation should still be respected. Put simply, competence and the duty of confidentiality are not necessarily connected even if in some cases, e.g. very young children they will be, i.e. they will be neither competent nor mature enough to understand what keeping a secret means.

Legal duty of confidentiality

The law recognises a duty of confidentiality when:

- information is not a matter of public knowledge
- information is given in a situation where it is obvious that it is expected to be kept secret
- protecting the information is in the public interest

Activity

Find out:

- Whether under 16 year olds have to visit their own GP for contraceptive advice.
- If an under 16 year old receives contraceptive advice from another GP, whether his or her own GP has to be informed.
- If it is lawful for community nurses, nurses, midwives and health visitors to give contraceptive advice to young people under 16.
- Where young people under 16 can obtain contraceptive advice and supplies.

Useful reading: *What Should I Do? Guidance on Confidentiality and Under 16s* (Brook Advisory Centres, 1996).

EXCEPTIONS TO THE DUTY OF CONFIDENTIALITY

Exceptions to the duty of confidentiality which are most relevant to children and young people are the following.

Consent of the patient

Consent can be expressed or implied but in all cases must be freely given. If patients are too young or too immature consent of a parent is acceptable providing it is in the child's interests. Dimond (1996, page 68) gives the following examples of when parental consent to disclosure may be appropriate, e.g. to the media: a child is being flown overseas for specialist treatment not available in this country; a child is being used as a donor for a sibling who requires bone marrow; a child whose lack of treatment is being used for political purposes to assert deficiencies in the NHS. When a child is 'Gillick' competent then he or she has the independent legal right to consent to disclosure providing he or she understands the consequences of information being revealed.

Disclosing information between health professionals (and others in the multi-agency team) on a need-to-know basis is usually justified on the assumption that patients realise that their welfare depends on relevant information being passed back and forth between all those involved in their care. It is therefore assumed that they have given their implied consent to such disclosure.

Disclosure in the patient's best interests

The ethical principle underpinning such disclosures is paternalism. In other words limiting a person' s autonomy for is or her own sake. In this context it means disclosing information obtained in confidence (to a parent or third party) without consulting the patient (or even despite his or her expressed wishes to the contrary) in order to protect the child's health, safety or welfare. To prevent child abuse, for example, disclosure is likely to be necessary. Hence, a health professional who suspects a child has been abused will, by reporting his or her suspicions to a third party, technically break confidentiality but, by doing so, is almost always going to be acting in the child's interests.

More problematic, however, are cases involving 'Gillick' competent young people who do not want confidential information about their health revealed to a parent. Dimond (1996, page 71) cites several examples when this might be problematic, notably when a young person is:

- having a sexual relationship with an adult;
- suffering from venereal disease, AIDS or is HIV-positive;
- on drugs, smokes, is an alcoholic, pregnant or having an abortion.

In deciding how to balance the duty to respect the young person's confidentiality against his or her interests in disclosing the information a health professional might also have to consider what is in the public's interest (see below). The spread of the HIV virus, for example, has, not surprisingly perhaps, raised many problems relating to confidentiality.

Disclosure in the patient's interest

DoH Guidance on Child Protection: Medical Responsibilities: Addendum to 'Working Together under the Children Act 1989' states in Part 4 that where non-accidental injury or other forms of abuse are concerned, the doctor's responsibility towards the child may appear to be in conflict with his or her ethical duties with regard to confidentiality. There is no dispute that the child's interests are paramount, but the wish to maintain confidentiality may be strong. A doctor may be faced with this dilemma at any stage of the child protection process … At all stages, therefore the doctor needs to make a balanced judgement between the justification for breaching confidence and the distress it may cause, and the withholding of information obtained within the doctor–patient relationship.

Activity

- Critically reflect on examples from your practice, when in relation to a child, you were concerned about disclosing information.

Read the UKCC *Guidelines for Professional Practice* (UKCC, 1996).

- What does it say about confidentiality and children?

Disclosures in the public interest

Legally this exception is the most controversial mainly because its scope is so uncertain – it can be invoked to justify any disclosure which is thought to be for the 'good of society'. Case law suggests that this means when there is a 'real' or 'genuine' risk of danger to the public even though that danger does not have to be imminent. Furthermore the 'risk' must usually be to the public's physical safety, i.e. injury or disease. In one case, *W v Edgell [1990] 1 All ER 836*, an independent psychiatric report commissioned by a patient detained in a hospital secure unit was disclosed (to a hospital and the Home Secretary) despite his opposition. The psychiatrist (Edgell) disclosed his report because the patient had applied to be discharged. However, Edgell considered that he continued to have an abnormal interest in firearms and home-made bombs (10 years previously the patient had been convicted of the manslaughter of five people) and was still a threat to the pubic. The Court of Appeal rejected the patient's claim for breach of confidentiality on the basis that the duty owed to him was outweighed by the overriding public interest in public safety.

The main ethical principles justifying disclosure in this context are non-maleficence and beneficence. Non-maleficence literally means 'do no harm'. It is a negative duty that involves (amongst other things) balancing risks and benefits of a particular action. However, as Charles-Edwards (1996) points out, all medical interventions carry the risk of harm and avoiding harm is not always easy to achieve, especially as the concept of harm is idiosyncratic. In other words people's perception of harm is an integral part of the way they see themselves and their life plan (Gillon, 1985). The principle of beneficence which means 'do good' imposes a positive duty and consists of three elements, notably preventing harm, removing harm and promoting good (Beauchamp and Childress, 1994). However distinct though the principles of non-malficence and beneficence might appear in theory, it is almost impossible to separate them in practice given that health care choices so often involve finely balanced judgements to be made between doing good and avoiding harm. The complex relationship between the two (likewise the difficulties of deciding which principle has moral priority) is well illustrated by vaccination programmes. These may harm a few, i.e. those who suffer serious or even fatal side effects, but are for the greater benefit of many. Charles-Edwards (1996) also warns of the dangers of indiscriminate application of beneficence and how it can involve unjustified paternalism and the disregard of another's autonomy. As she aptly puts it: 'I know what is best for you (best treatment) and you will accept my judgement'.

UKCC definition of public interest

The UKCC advisory paper on confidentiality defines public interest as encompassing such matters as serious crime, child abuse and drug trafficking. It also states that in all cases where the practitioner discloses or withholds information in what he/she believes the public interest he/she must be able to justify that decision

CHILDREN AND RIGHTS OF ACCESS TO HEALTH RECORDS

The relationship of trust and confidence between patients and health professionals is a two-way process. One element is the duty of confidentiality. The other, which is equally important if children and young people are to have effective control over their health care, is the right to know what information has been compiled about them.

Patients' advocates have long been asserted the right to see medical records but it is only fairly recently that rights of access have been recognised by statute. Relevant legislation includes the Data Protection Act 1988 – the first Act to grant access rights which applies to health records kept on computer. Access to non-computerised, i.e. manual health records is governed by the Access to Health Record Act 1990. Both Acts grant children and young people access rights if they have the capacity to understand the nature of their application.

Although both Acts were welcomed as significantly advancing patients' rights neither guarantees access. In other words health professionals are entitled to withhold information which is 'likely to cause serious harm to the physical or mental health of the patient or any other individual or if it identifies a third party'. Note too that parents and others with parental responsibility have rights of access to the records of children if they lack the capacity to make their own application for access or have consented to parental access.

> **Other exceptions to the duty of confidentiality**
> - Statutory justification
> - Court order
> - Medical research
> - Teaching and medical audit

Activity

- Give examples from practice of when it would be appropriate to withhold information from a child patient.
- Read chapter 8 of *Legal Aspects of Child Health Care* (Dimond, 1996). Critically consider how she describes the relationship between access and confidentiality.
- Has a child (or his or her parents) the right to be told that he or she is terminally ill?
- Find out the procedure if a parent or child requests access to their medical notes.

> ➤ **Key points**

1. To control their health care children need a right of control over personal health information.
2. Exceptions to the duty of confidentiality are justified in certain circumstances, in particular when abuse or neglect is suspected.
3. The relationship of trust and confidence between patients and health professionals is a two-way process. One element is the patients' right to know what information has been compiled and the other is the health professionals' duty of confidentiality.

4 RESEARCH

Research on children is now accepted as an important means of promoting child health and well-being. It has also long shaped professional practice. Yet progress, as Taylor (1994, page 78) notes, has often been slow and attitudes reluctant to change. For example, he quotes Myers, writing in 1910 about the treatment of children with tonsillitis who said: 'gargles are of slight use, but painting with glycerine and tannin is more efficacious. The bowels must be kept open'. This 'obsession' between bowels and tonsils continued well into the 1930s with advice in 1938 (Pearce) that: 'rest in bed is essential, an aperient being given at the beginning of the illness, and the bowels kept active'.

Notwithstanding widespread recognition of the need for research, serious doubts still remain about using children as research subjects. These focus mainly on issues of consent, in particular the extent to which the principles which apply to medical treatment provide adequate safeguards – especially when children are too young to make their own decisions. Confidentiality and the risks associated with research are also problematic. Much of the controversy surrounding these issues stems from what Dines (1995) identifies as the inherent dilemma at the centre of research, i.e. the tension between promoting and safeguarding the interests of individual patients and serving the interests of society – both of which are enshrined in the UKCC Code of Professional Conduct. This arises because the research process which aims to advance knowledge (and thus serve the interests of society) may or may not benefit individual patients participating in the research. How then can nurses conducting research claim they are benefiting such patients? As Dines concludes, protecting patients in practice raises difficult questions which are made more difficult by the nurse's dual loyalty to society as well as the patient.

Research can be classified in two ways:

- *Therapeutic research*. This type of research (sometimes called clinical research) aims to benefit a particular group of patients by improving available treatment. It is therefore research which is related to patients' health status and so combines research with their care and treatment.

- *Non-therapeutic research*. This aims only to gain new knowledge and so is unlikely to confer any benefit on participants who may be healthy subjects or existing patients.

Ethical Guidelines on research

The British Paediatric Association (1992) states that research with children is worthwhile if each project:

- has an identifiable prospect of benefit to children
- is well designed and well conducted
- does not simply duplicate earlier work
- is not undertaken primarily for financial or professional advantage
- involves a statistically appropriate number of subjects
- is to be properly reported

Activity

Read chapter 5 in *The Child and Family: Contemporary Nursing Issues in Child Health and Care* (Lindsey, 1994).

- What research on children does he suggest should be undertaken?

- How can children's nurses undertake research?
- Critically assess an example of therapeutic and non-therapeutic research on children in your hospital.

HOW IS RESEARCH ON CHILDREN REGULATED?

Guidance on research derives from several sources. These include advice from the DoH and ethical codes and professional guidelines issues by (amongst others) the Medical Research Council (MRC) and the British Paediatric Association (BPA). All these support research on children in principle but emphasise how it can be justified only if certain principles are observed, i.e.:

- research involving children is important for the benefit of all children and should be supported, encouraged and conducted in an ethical manner;
- relevant information cannot be gained by comparable research on adults;
- legally valid consent must be obtained;
- non-therapeutic research should pose no more than a negligible (or minimal) risk of harm;
- in therapeutic research the benefits should outweigh the possible risks of harm;
- when a choice of age-groups is possible older children should be involved in preference to younger ones.

Activity

Critically evaluate what the Helsinki Declaration says about clinical (therapeutic) research and non-therapeutic research.

In addition to these basic principles, approval should be sought from local research ethics committees (LRECs). Described as 'custodians of good practice' their role is to maintain ethical standards of research, protect subjects of research from harm, preserve the subjects' rights and provide reassurance to the public that this is being done. Note too that research guidelines for LRECs recommend that research should only be carried out on children if it is essential to do so and the information cannot be obtained from adult subjects (DoH, 1991).

Activity

Find out who are the members of the LREC in your hospital. How are they appointed? Critically assess the criteria members must satisfy before they can be appointed.

Declaration of Helsinki

This forms the basis of professional guidelines and lists several basic principles underpinning research, in particular

- research involving human subjects must conform to generally accepted scientific principles and should be based on adequately performed laboratory and animal experimentation and on a thorough knowledge of the scientific tradition
- research cannot legitimately be carried out unless the importance of the objective is in proportion to the inherent risk to the subject
- the right of the research subject to safeguard his or her integrity must always be respected. Every precaution must be taken to respect the privacy of the subject and to minimize the impact of the study on the subject's physical and mental integrity and on the personality of the subject
- in any research on human beings, each potential subject must be adequately informed of the aims, methods, anticipated benefits and potential hazards of the study and the discomfort it may entail
- in the case of legal incompetence, informed consent should be obtained from the legal guardian in accordance with national legislation. Where physical or mental incapacity makes it impossible to obtain informed consent, or when the subject is a minor, permissions from the responsible relative replaces that of the subject in accordance with national legislation

Surprisingly perhaps there is no specific legislation governing research on children. This means that it is regulated mainly by the common law, notably the law of consent and negligence. The principles of consent were outlined in a previous section. However, many claim that these principles should be modified when applied to research, in particular that higher standards of disclosure should be imposed – requiring more information to be revealed than is normally required for medical treatment. Arguably, too, higher levels of understanding and maturity should be reached before children and young people should be considered competent to consent to research.

The legal principles governing research depend both on the age of the research subject, his or her competency and, most importantly, the type of research.

THERAPEUTIC RESEARCH

Young people aged 16 and 17 who are competent, i.e. have the understanding and maturity to understand what the research involves have an independent right to consent. Unless the research only carries minimal risk a relatively high level of competency will usually be required. Note too that for consent to be legally valid it must be freely given and 'informed'. This means that the research subject should be given full information about, e.g. the purpose of the research, its expected benefits and harms, the alternatives and the fact that research is being combined with the patient's treatment. Also crucial is the so-called 'risk/benefit ratio'. The concept of risk is defined in some detail in the BPA guidelines as is that of potential benefit and harm. Thus the assessment of potential benefit includes reviewing several factors, such as how common and severe the problem is which the research aims to alleviate; whether the research is likely to achieve its aims; and its resource implications. Assessment of potential harm raises similar questions, notably how invasive the research is, how severe the harms associated with it are and how likely they are to occur. Also relevant is the recognition that children's responses vary widely, are often unpredictable and alter as they develop (BPA, 1992).

Under 16 year olds can participate in research irrespective of their parent's wishes providing they are 'Gillick' competent. The more invasive and risky the research, however, the more difficult it will be for young people to reach the required level of 'Gillick' competency. And, as with 16 and 17 year olds, consent is invalid unless 'full' information has been disclosed.

Consent to research in respect of incompetent under 16 year olds must be obtained from a proxy – usually a parent. Although not legally required most of the professional guidelines also recommend getting the agreement (or assent as it is sometimes called) of school-age children and in particular to ensure that they do not object. Parental consent is, however, invalid unless the research is in the child's interest, i.e. its benefits outweigh the risks. Information too must be full. Guidance on these issues includes the following advice to researchers, i.e.:

- not to offer any financial inducement to families;
- exert no pressure on families and give them as much time as possible to consider whether to take part;
- encourage families to discuss the project with, for example, relatives;
- encourage parents to stay with their child and assure them that their child's treatment will not be prejudiced by withdrawal from the research;
- respond to families' questions.

NON-THERAPEUTIC RESEARCH

In the past this type of research was widely considered unlawful. Now accepted as justified in certain circumstances it still causes controversy – how can young children who are not competent to make their own decisions be 'volunteered' for procedures which cannot directly benefit them and may carry some risk? That said all the professional guidelines give qualified support for non-therapeutic research providing that the risk to the child is minimal. The concept of minimal risk has been defined above. It has also be defined by the MRC as 'no greater than the risks that reasonable parents commonly expose their children to in everyday life'. The information which must be disclosed must also be full (see above). Indeed some legal commentators suggest that an even higher legal standard of disclosure is required than when the research is therapeutic (which itself is higher than that required for medical treatment).

As regards the age at which children and young people can consent independently to non-therapeutic research, broadly similar rules apply as when the research is therapeutic – subject possibly to the expectation that a higher level of competency be required given that no benefit will be conferred on the research subject. One group, however, namely those who are under 16 and not 'Gillick' competent pose the greatest legal and ethical problems. As Charles-Edwards (1996) notes, since they cannot benefit from the research there is no possible trade-off between the risk and benefit, other than an altruistic reward. However, as she also points out, reliance on altruism in young children to justify them as research subjects is controversial not least because it is difficult to prove.

As far as the law is concerned it seems that parents (and others with parental responsibility) can consent to research on incompetent minors provided it is 'not against their interests'. This criterion is less onerous than the 'best interests' test but its scope has yet to be tested in the courts.

Key points ➤

1. Research on children is justified providing relevant knowledge cannot be gained by research on adults.

2. Research on children is an important means of promoting child health and well-being.

3. When a choice of age-groups is possible older children should be involved in preference to younger ones.

4. Legally valid consent must always be obtained before research is undertaken.

RESOURCES AND RATIONING 5

One of the most poignant cases to reach the courts in recent years was *R v Cambridge Health Authority, Ex Parte B [1995] 2 All ER 129*. It concerned a 10-year-old girl suffering from leukaemia with a life expectancy of 6–8 weeks who was refused a second bone marrow transplant and a third course of chemotherapy costing approximately £75 000 because there was only a small chance of the treatment being successful. In taking the health authority to court B's father hoped to force it to fund the treatment. He failed but the case generated an enormous amount of publicity much of which was critical given the health authority's apparent 'inhumanity' in denying on grounds of cost a child's only chance to live.

Cross reference

The provision of health care – page 711

Activity

Read the case of *R v Cambridge HA, Ex parte B*. Do you think the health authority's refusal of treatment was justified? Give reasons for your answer. Do you think there is a minimal level of care no child patient should be denied? If yes, why? Brief details of *R v Cambridge HA, Ex parte B* can be found in Hendrick (1997, page 24). Fuller details can be found in the law reports.

The controversy was not perhaps surprising given that while health care needs and desires are almost limitless resources are not. This means that priorities have to be set – not just at the 'macro' level but also at the 'micro' level. Sometimes characterised as rationing it is decision making at the micro level which is more likely to directly concern health professionals. This is because rationing inevitably involves making hard decisions, which when the illness is life threatening, can make the difference between the chance of life or death (as in the case of child B, see above). However, who should make the decisions? And what should be the criteria for decision making? These and similar questions raise acute ethical dilemmas which have long been at the centre of health care. However, now, they are increasingly contentious – not because access to health care is much more unequal than it once was (rationing has always taken place but in the past was more secretive) but because the mechanisms of the new NHS make the allocation of resources more visible and open to public scrutiny.

Another factor which affects the rationing debate is that health care expectations – that the state will provide a 'good' heath service and guarantee access to health care – are higher than in the past. As a consequence there is an ever expanding demand for health care. Thus the United Nations Convention on the Rights of the Child expressly recognises children's health care rights. Similarly the European Convention on Human Rights appears to protect everyone's right to

The relationship between microallocation and macroallocation

Macroallocation involves deciding how much of a society's resources should be allocated to health care (which has to compete with housing, education and other social goods) and how it should be distributed. It thus involves determining which categories of illness, injury and so forth should have priority, e.g. heart disease or cancer. Decisions also have to be made about which technologies or procedures should have priority. Microallocation determines who will obtain available resources. It thus involves selecting which patients should be treated (and for what) bearing in mind that resources cannot be provided to everyone who needs them. (See Beauchamp and Childress, 1994) life. However, despite their recognition as basic human rights neither Convention gives any guidance on how these health rights are to be secured and both are silent on the question of the proper responsibility of a health service (Newdick, 1995). While this is perhaps understandable – given that the concepts of 'health' and 'illness' are so broad and flexible that they are almost impossible to define with any precision – it makes the task of setting priorities (both at the micro and macro level) a very complex process.

At the centre of the debate on rationing is the principle of justice. In other words, how to find a 'fair' way of distributing scarce financial and medical resources to satisfy the competing claims of patients. There are several different approaches, e.g.:

- *Needs theory*. Put simply this approach is based on the view that some patients are more 'needy' than others and so should have a special claim on resources. However, what does the term 'need' mean in this context? This is a central question yet the answer is far from clear and to date no consistent principles have emerged nor any criterion agreed by which the notion can be assessed. Furthermore, as Gillon (1985) notes, whilst medical need may well be a necessary criterion for the distribution of resources it does not make choosing between competing candidates (who are agreed to be 'in medical need') any easier.

- *Medical outcome*. This is another value-laden concept (which is sometimes combined with need and referred to as 'medical utility'). Under this approach resources should be allocated according to the probability of medical success. However, as with the needs theory, there are problems in defining what is meant by medical success. How should the concept be measured? As Newdick (1995) points out, there is no objective yardstick by which medical effectiveness can be assessed since it is so influenced by our perceptions of illness and health which vary not only from person to person but also in the same person, from time to time.

- *Maximisation of welfare*. Another way of dealing with the gap between supply and demand for health care has been developed by health economists. It is the theory called 'quality adjusted life years' (QALYS). Often described as 'scientific' it adopts a cost–benefit analysis. As such it measures health care outcomes by evaluating the cost of treatment and the extent to which, and for how long it will improve a patient's quality of life. Not surprisingly the most efficient are those treatments which are the cheapest yet achieve the best quality of life over the longest period of time. The QALYs concept has attracted considerable criticism not least because, as Charles-Edwards (1996) points out, it neglects two fundamental moral principles. One is that everyone's life is of equal value and the other is that life itself, however short, has inherent value.

Protection of the right to life and health care

- *Article 24 United Nations Convention on the Rights of the Child* requires states to recognise the right of the child to the enjoyment of the highest attainable standard of health and to facilities for the treatment of illness and rehabilitation of health and to strive to ensure that no child is deprived of his or her right of access to such health care services
- *Article 2 European Convention of Human Rights* states that everyone's life shall be protected by law. No one shall be deprived of his life intentionally

Activity

- Which approach to rationing do you think is the 'fairest'? Why? Do you think children should be given priority. If your answer is yes, why?
- Do you think individuals should forfeit the 'right' to health if they have a lifestyle or 'habit' such as smoking which adversely affects their health? If so, which kinds of behaviour should 'count' and why?
- What is the 'Oregon' scheme? Do you think it should be adopted?
- What is the relationship between rationing and health targets?

For further reading see Beauchamp and Childress (1994, Chapter 6), FOX and LEICHTER (1991), *The Health of the Nation: A Consultative Document for Health in England*, Cmnd 1523. London: HMSO, and Holliday (1995).

Finally, before concluding this section it is necessary to outline the law's role in allocating health resources. Provision of health care is governed by the National Health Service Act 1977. The Act imposes very comprehensive duties on the Secretary of State for Health, but is unlikely to be of much use to aggrieved patients (whether their claim is based on the allocation of resources at the macro or micro level) who wish to challenge denial (or postponement) of treatment. *In R v Central Birmingham HA, Ex parte Walker [1987] 3 BLMR 32*, for example, a baby needing urgent heart surgery had his operation postponed five times because of staff shortages in a neonatal ward. His mother sought an order from the court that the operation should be performed, claiming inadequate heath resources had been allocated by the health authority. However, the Court of Appeal refused to order the operation saying that it would not substitute its own judgement for the judgement of those responsible for the allocation of resources (unless they had acted unreasonably). In other words the courts would not take what they considered to be essentially clinical decisions.

Other cases – there have only been a handful in the last decade – in which patients have attempted to enforce statutory duties have had similar outcomes. The courts' attitude (which appears to apply whether action is taken against the Secretary of State for Health or individual health authorities) was summed up well Re B when Lord Bingham said:

> *while I have every sympathy with B, I feel bound to regard this as an attempt, wholly understandable but none the less misguided, to involve the court in a field of activity where it is not fitted to make any decision favourable to the patient.*

He then stated how in a perfect world any treatment sought would be provided (if doctors were willing to give it) no matter how much it cost, particularly when a life was potentially at stake. However, the court could not proceed on that basis since it was common knowledge that health authorities were pressed to make ends meet and so had to

National Health Service Act 1977

Section 1(1) imposes a duty on the Secretary of State to continue the promotion in England and Wales of a comprehensive health service designed to secure improvement in:

- the physical and mental health of the people
- the prevention, diagnosis and treatment of illness and for that purpose to provide or secure the effective provision of services in accordance with the Act

Section 3(1) imposes a duty on the Secretary of State to provide throughout England and Wales, to such extent as he considers necessary to meet all reasonable requirements:

- hospital accommodation
- other accommodation for the purpose of any service provided under this Act
- medical, dental, nursing and ambulance services
- such other facilities for the care of expectant and nursing mothers and young children as he considers are appropriate as part of the health service
- such facilities for the prevention of illness, the care of persons suffering from illness and the after-care of persons who have suffered from illness as he considers are appropriate as part of the health service
- such other services as are required for the diagnosis and treatment of illness

make difficult and agonising judgements as to how a limited budget could best be allocated to the maximum advantage of the maximum number of patients.

It is not often that the courts get involved in 'life or death' decisions, but sometimes this is unavoidable especially when urgent decisions have to be made about the withdrawal or withholding of life-sustaining treatment for babies and children. Whilst scarce resources undoubtedly influence decision making other factors are equally relevant. Thus, for example, in the case of *Re J [1990] 3 All ER 930* the court, whilst recognising a strong presumption in favour of prolonging life, none the less allowed treatment to be withheld. This was because it was necessary to perform a 'balancing exercise' – a process which involved judging the quality of life a child would have to endure if given treatment and then deciding whether in all the circumstances such a life would 'be so afflicted as to be intolerable to that child'.

J was born 13 weeks premature weighing 1.1 kg at birth. By the time the case came to court he was 5 months old but had suffered recurrent convulsions and had been ventilated twice for long periods. Despite being able to breath independently his long-term prognosis was very poor: he was unlikely to survive into his teens, and would almost certainly develop serious spastic quadriplegia and be blind and deaf. He would, however, experience the same pain as a normal baby. However, J was not dying nor near the point of death. Nevertheless, the Court of Appeal decided that it would be lawful not to reventilate him if he suffered a further collapse (although he should be treated with antibiotics if he developed a chest infection and hydration should be maintained). In other words the court allowed life-saving treatment to be withheld since this course of action was – given the hazardous and invasive nature of reventilation and the risk of further deterioration – in Js best interests.

Key points ➤

1. Setting health care priorities is a complex process which involves finding a fair way of distributing scarce financial and medical resources.

2. The National Health Service Act 1977 imposes very comprehensive duties on the Secretary of State for Health to provide a comprehensive health service.

3. The reality of scarce resources undoubtedly influences the courts when they are involved in urgent life or death disputes.

4. Demand for health care is increasing but the role of law in guaranteeing access to health is limited.

STANDARDS OF CARE 6

The right to receive a reasonable standard of medical care has, like the right to consent, long been recognised as a legal right. It is also enshrined in several clauses of the UKCC Code of Professional Conduct (the Code).

The 'duties' imposed in the Code do not have legal force. However, given that they aim to establish, maintain and improve standards of professional practice they are expected to be followed. Furthermore, several of them are linked with the law of negligence as they replicate, albeit in broad terms, well-established legal rights. Note too that the implications of the Code are clearly stated in the UKCC Advisory Document which emphasises how it 'provides the backcloth against which any alleged misconduct will be judged'.

But, notwithstanding the similarities between the legal and ethical position on negligence, there are important differences. One of the most significant is that the standards of care contained in the Code are higher than those required by the law. This is perhaps why Rumbold and Lesser (1995) suggest it is possible to identify several levels of care. Firstly, there is the minimum acceptable level which defines legal negligence. Secondly, there is the higher level required by the Code which defines professional negligence. At the top is the 'best possible care' which, ethically, health professionals are obliged to aim at, but are neither blameworthy nor negligent if they do not achieve. In between the second and third of these are the personal standards of individual professionals.

The ethical principles which inform the standards of care set out in the Code are briefly: the principle of non-malficence, i.e. the duty not to harm patients, and that of beneficence, i.e. of positively helping patients by promoting and safeguarding their interests. However, both in practice and in theory there are problems in applying them mainly because all medical treatment involves balancing risks and harms. This of course then raises the question of how they can be reconciled. According to Rumbold and Lesser (1995) the way to achieve this is to (1) ensure that the patient is always informed and consulted and their consent obtained, (2) avoid unnecessary risks and (3) make sure that harm is not inflicted which is clearly greater than the benefit to the patient.

Turning now to legal principles, the standard required by the law is best described as a *minimum* one, i.e. one which is primarily concerned to guarantee a basic level of competence. Practitioners who fall below that standard may be sued and found liable in negligence. The law of negligence (which is another name for medical malpractice) has two broad aims. These are:

- *Compensation*. This seeks to minimise the effect negligence can have on a victim's life. Babies, for example, who are harmed at birth may

---

UKCC Code of Professional Conduct

This states that practitioners are personally accountable for their practice and must:

- act always in such a manner as to promote and safeguard the interests and well-being of patients and clients
- ensure that no action or omission on their part, or within their sphere of responsibility, is detrimental to the interests, condition or safety of patients and clients
- maintain and improve their professional knowledge and competence
- acknowledge any limitations in their knowledge and competence and decline any duties or responsibilities unless able to perform them in a safe and skilled manner

UKCC Advisory Document: Exercising Accountability

This states:

- the exercise of accountability (which is an integral part of professional practice) requires the practitioner to seek to achieve and maintain high standards
- it is recognised that in many situations in which practitioners practice, there may be a tension between the maintenance of standards and the availability or use of resources; it is essential, however, that the profession, both through its regulatory body (the UKCC) and its individual practitioners, adheres to its desires to enhance standards and to achieve high standards rather than simply accept minimal standards

Disciplinary action

Nurses who fail to achieve the professional standards set out in the Code may be the subject of the following action:

- *professional accountability* – proceedings before the professional conduct committee
- *accountability to employer* – in failing to act with care and skill the nurse is likely to have breached her contract of employment

Elements in a negligence action

- *Duty of care* – this means that the health professional was responsible for the patient
- *Breach of duty* – this means that the health professional failed in his or her responsibility
- *Damage* – this means that the health professional's action (or inaction) caused the patient's injuries

The 'neighbour' test

Under this test (which is an objective one) a duty is owed if a health professional can reasonably foresee that a person would be affected by his or her actions or inactions

suffer catastrophic injuries and require long-term nursing care. Damages awarded are thus expected to compensate them for their lost earning potential and higher living expenses.

- *Deterrence.* Here the aim is to reduce the number and seriousness of accidents by making health professionals personally liable. In other words the threat or fear of legal action and potential damage to professional reputations is a powerful incentive to achieve high standards and ensure that greater care is taken.

The three elements which a patient needs to establish to win a negligence case are set out in the margin. All these elements will now be analysed although the focus will be on the second, i.e. breach of duty.

DUTY OF CARE

In almost all health care settings it is easy to establish whether a duty of care exists in that any patient a health professional is currently treating will be owed a duty. So, for example, patients in hospital (whether as in-patients or out-patients), likewise those seeking treatment in A&E departments, are owed a duty of care as are those on GPs' lists. Less clear, however, is the duty owed to colleagues or patients' relatives. In such cases whether or not a legal duty is owed depends on applying the so-called 'neighbour test'.

Note that a duty of care is owed to child patients whether they have sought medical services independently or not. Thus 16 and 17 year olds and young people under 16 who are 'Gillick' competent have the right to apply for inclusion on a GP's list and to seek treatment from other health professionals irrespective of their parents' knowledge or permission. As for children under 16 who are not 'Gillick' competent the request for medical services must come from someone else, usually a parent.

Activity

You are off duty and shopping in a supermarket. A young child has an accident and is bleeding profusely. Are you obliged to offer medical assistance? Is there a difference between your legal and ethical duty? Read Chapter 2 in *Legal Aspects of Child Health Care* (Hendrick, 1997).

BREACH OF DUTY

Proving breach of duty is usually much harder than establishing a duty of care. This is partly due to courts' reluctance to challenge clinical judgement but also the well-established rule for determining the medical standard of care which was set in a famous 1957 case called *Bolam v Friern Barnet Hospital Management Committee [1957] 2 All ER 118*. The case held that doctors are not negligent *'if they have acted in accordance with a practice accepted as proper by a responsible body of medical men skilled in that particular art'.*

The Bolam test (which essentially means that health professionals set their own standards) now applies to all health professionals and basically means that practitioners are judged by their peers, i.e. sisters by sisters, specialist nurses by other specialist nurses, midwives by midwives and so on. In other words legal liability can be avoided if a health professional can show that other reasonably competent (i.e. reasonably skilled and experienced) practitioners would have acted in a similar way. This does not mean they would have done exactly the same but rather their actions were within a range which was acceptable.

Other important issues which the courts have dealt with in establishing what amounts to a breach of duty are given below.

Several schools of thought

No liability arises just because a health professional chose to act in one way rather than another, providing that he or she acted in accordance with accepted practice. Put simply the law recognises medical differences of opinion.

Departing from accepted practice

Deviation from standard practice is by no means conclusive evidence of negligence and may well be acceptable providing the unconventional treatment can be justified, i.e. given the circumstances, innovative or unusual procedures were appropriate.

Activity

Read pages 137–139 of *Medical Negligence Case Law* (Nelson-Jones and Burton, 1995). What types of negligence claims have been taken against nurses? How can these be avoided?
Read *Bolitho v City and Hackney HA [1997] 4 All ER 771*. What is its impact on nurses?

Trainees and inexperience

It is now well settled that the law does not accept a defence of inexperience, lack of ability or knowledge. In short students and other trainees are expected to perform to the same standard as their trained more experienced colleagues. None the less, those 'learning on the job' are expected to know their limitations. They should therefore ask for help (which should be available) rather than undertake a task they are not competent to carry out. In so doing they would normally have a defence to any subsequent negligence claim should a mistake occur. This approach explains the outcome of *Wilsher v Essex AHA [1986] 3 All ER 801* in which a junior doctor who mistakenly inserted a catheter into a vein rather than an artery escaped liability (because he consulted a

The facts of the Bolam case

Mr Bolam claimed that the broken pelvis he sustained during electro-convulsive treatment could have been avoided had he been given relaxant drugs and been properly restrained. He also complained that he was not warned of the risks of treatment. The court rejected his claim because at the time there was evidence that different doctors used different techniques and methods – some used relaxant drugs, other did not. Since both approaches were equally acceptable the doctor was not negligent in choosing one method over another

The facts of the Wilsher case

Martin Wilsher was born prematurely suffering from various illnesses, including oxygen deficiency. His prospects of survival were poor and he was placed in the 24-hour special care unit. He was looked after by a medical team consisting of two consultants, a senior registrar, several junior doctors and trained nurses. He needed extra oxygen to survive and one of the inexperienced doctors monitoring the oxygen in Martin's bloodstream mistakenly inserted a catheter into a vein rather than an artery but then asked the senior registrar to check what he had done. The registrar failed to see the mistake and some hours later, when replacing the catheter, did exactly the same thing himself. In both instances the catheter monitor failed to register correctly the amount of oxygen in Martin's blood, with the result that he was given excess oxygen. Martin claimed that the excess oxygen in his bloodstream caused an incurable condition of the retina resulting in near blindness. But notwithstanding the registrar's negligence Martin failed to win compensation because he could not prove causation (the third element in a negligence claim)

registrar). However, the registrar who repeated the mistake was found liable because he should have known better.

When standards are judged

The law accepts that standards change as current medical knowledge and skills develop. Standards are therefore judged at the time treatment was carried out and not when the case comes to trial (which is typically several years later).

Breaches of the duty of care which are most likely to happen in relation to children are shown in the margin on the next page.

CAUSATION

This is the third hurdle a victim of medical negligence has to overcome and in practice it is one of the hardest. It requires proof that the defendant's conduct caused (or materially contributed to) the victim's injury. In simple terms this means that it was more than 50% probable that the injuries were caused by the negligence. In some cases the link is self-evident such as when a foreign body is left in a patient after surgery. However, in other cases, proving a link is much more difficult – the injuries may have been caused by natural causes or the patient's underlying illness. Sometimes the victim's case collapses because his or her injuries could have been caused by several factors. This is why Martin Wilsher lost his case because even though it was admitted that the registrar had negligently administered excess oxygen (which was well known as a cause of blindness) there were at least five other possible causes of blindness in premature babies. With so many potential competing causes the evidence linking the negligence with Martin's blindness was inconclusive.

Once a victim has proved that the practitioner's conduct caused the injuries he or she will be entitled to compensation (which is normally paid by the health professional's employer). In medical cases damages (the legal term for compensation) consist of several categories including pain and suffering, loss of earnings and earning capacity.

In conclusion it is useful to outline the main difference which Rumbold and Lesser (1995) identify between law and ethics in respect of negligence. These are:

- ethical duties operate whether or not any harm actually follows from the negligence since they apply to actions (and omissions) themselves, and not only to their actual consequences but also to their potential ones;
- the standard of care required by the Code is higher than required by law;
- ethics require a duty of care towards victims of accidents whom a practitioner may come across whilst off duty whereas the law does not require health professionals to be good Samaritans;

- ethics may occasionally require someone actively to prevent an order or policy from being carried out, even though this may conflict with his or her legal duty.

1. The right to receive a reasonable standard of care is a long-established legal right.
2. The UKCC Code of Professional Conduct enshrines both legal and ethical principles of good practice.
3. Failure to reach the required standard of practice can result in legal proceedings.

➤ Key points

Breaches of duty most likely to involve children

Case law and textbooks on medical negligence have shown a clear pattern of when breaches of duty are most likely to occur in relation to children. These are identified by Dimond (1996, page 135) and include:

- *High technology* – developments in medical technology have increased the likelihood of litigation, in particular claims arising from progress in medical treatment, new or quasi-experimental treatment and unproved treatments
- *Failures in communication* – this includes, for example, inadequate instructions to nurses and failure to organise follow-up arrangements. Lack of communication with parents is also a factor
- *Pain relief* – children and parents now have higher expectations in respect of pain relief due to progress which has been made in assessing and measuring pain in children
- *Drug-induced and prescribing errors* – these are commonly due to a breakdown of communication between the practitioner who prescribed the drug and the one who administered it

(See Campbell, 1994)

7 CHILDREN'S RIGHTS
by Tina Moules

> *Most children are not born with rights but with threats.*
>
> (UNICEF, 1989)

RIGHTS

Activity

Before you begin to read, make a list of the rights that you believe you have.

The concept of 'rights' was promoted in the 17th and 18th centuries by philosophers such as Lock and Rousseau. According to Gillon (1985, page 54) rights are 'justified claims that require action or restraint from others ... impose positive or negative duties on others'. The justification for rights lies in either legal or moral principles.

- *Legal rights* – these are rights created by individuals (dictators) or groups of people (parliaments, governments), which are based on what is right and wrong according to law. Legal rights can also be abolished and are therefore subject to change. Bentham (1970) argues that these are the only true rights that exist.

'In order to override a human right one would need to justify the alternative moral device or action, the same way as one would need to justify overriding a prima facie moral obligation.'
(Beauchamp and Childress, 1989)

- *Moral rights* – these rights are based on moral principles and are intrinsically good. They are not therefore subject to change. Gillon (1985) identifies two types of moral right. The first are universal and apply to all humans. Hart (1970) believes that all universal rights stem from one fundamental right which is the equal right of all men to be free, autonomous agents. This then imposes a moral obligation on all people to respect others' autonomy. The second are special rights possessed by some but not by others. These result from prior actions such as reciprocal promises and contracts.

Activity

Look critically at your list of rights. How do you justify them – on legal or moral grounds?

The definition of rights by Gillon (1985) distinguishes between positive rights, i.e. those which impose obligations on others, and negative rights, i.e. those rights which require others not to do things (Beauchamp and Childress, 1989). Brykczynska (1993) proposes that the latter are not easy for children to achieve, e.g. it is as difficult for a child to refuse treatment as it is for them to avoid being smacked for doing wrong.

Activity

Consider critically this latter point with reference to your experience in practice.

THE RIGHTS OF CHILDREN

The notion of children's rights is a relatively recent concept having its roots in the Declaration of Geneva in 1924. The Declaration stated that 'mankind owes to the Child the best it has to give' and emphasised six principles of:

- welfare;
- such means as were necessary for normal development;
- food and medicine;
- relief in times of stress;
- protection against exploitation;
- socialisation to serve others.

The emphasis was on protection of the child with little regard for his right to participate in any decisions or autonomous activities.

This view of children's rights is described by Freeman (1983a) as that of the 'child-savers'. It presumes a paternalistic approach emphasising protection and legalising the intervention of the state. Decision making is controlled by adults who decide what is in the best interests of the child. This protectionist attitude sees adults as defenders of children who often make the assumption that children, particularly young children, are incompetent.

Debate about rights broadened out slightly in the 1950s and the UN Declaration on the Rights of the Child adopted the following principles:

- non-discrimination;
- special protection and opportunities to develop physically, mentally, morally, spiritually and socially in a healthy and normal manner and in conditions of freedom and dignity;
- a right to a name and nationality;
- the right to the benefits of social security (adequate housing, nutrition, recreation and medical services);
- the right of a special needs child to treatment, education and care;
- the need for love and understanding ... in the care and under the responsibility of his parents and in an atmosphere of affection and of moral and material security;
- entitlement to education, free and compulsory, at least in the elementary stages;
- to be among the first to receive protection and relief;

- protection against all forms of neglect, cruelty and exploitation;
- protection from practices which may foster racial, religious and any other forms of discrimination.

Activity

Critically analyse the principles contained within the two declarations above.

Although this declaration was broader, it still did not acknowledge the autonomy of the child nor any concept of empowerment. The emphasis was on welfare and protection. According to Freeman (1983a), this declaration is based on the 'welfare view' of children's rights. The ideas expounded by theorists was similar to that of the child-savers but included acknowledgement of the things that should be afforded to children.

Freeman's third perspective on the approach to children's rights is the liberationist view. Proponents of this view believe children should have equal rights with adults. They believe that British society underestimates the abilities of children and that this becomes a self-fulfilling prophecy as children believe the messages they receive about themselves. The children's liberation movement was particularly active in the 1970s. Holt (1975) suggested that children should be afforded the following rights. The right to:

- equal treatment at the hands of the law;
- vote and take a full part in politics;
- be legally responsible for their lives and acts;
- work for money;
- privacy;
- financial independence and responsibility;
- direct and manage their education;
- travel, live away from home, choose or make their home;
- make and enter into quasi-familial relationships;
- do, in general, what any adult may legally do.

Farson thought along the same lines and saw self-determination as the basis for all other children's rights. He justified his views by saying that (Farson, 1978, page 31):

> We will grant children rights for the same reason we grant rights to adults, not because we are sure that children will then become better people, but more for ideological reasons, because we believe that expanding freedom as a way of life is worthwhile in itself.

Farson (1978) – rights of children

- The right to alternative home environments allowing the child to 'exercise choice in his own living arrangements'
- The right to information that is accessible to adults
- The right to educate oneself (Farson favoured the abolition of compulsory education)
- The right to sexual freedom
- The right to economic power including the right to work
- The right to political power including the right to vote
- The right to responsive design
- The right to freedom from physical punishment
- The right to justice

Activity

Critically analyse the above principles. Compare and contrast the liberationist view with that of the 'child-savers'.

UN CONVENTION ON THE RIGHTS OF THE CHILD

The UN Convention on the Rights of the Child (1989) is the world's first international legal instrument on children's rights, ratified by the UK government in December 1991. Veerman (1992, page 184) sees it as 'an important and easily understood advocacy tool – one that promotes children's welfare as an issue of justice rather than one of charity'.

The Convention is based on three principles:

- Children have special needs which set them apart from adults.
- The best environment for a child's development is within a protective and nurturing family.
- Governments and the adult world in general should be committed to acting in the best interests of the child.

The rights detailed in the Convention can be categorised as follows:

- General rights – the right to life, freedom of expression, the right to information and privacy.
- Protective rights – e.g. from exploitation, abuse.
- Civil rights – relating to nationality, identity and the right to remain with parents unless against the best interests of the child.
- Development and welfare rights.
- Rights relating to children 'in special circumstances'.

Articles 12 and 3 are identified by many as being significant. Freeman (1993) suggests that there is considerable conflict between these. Article 12 emphasises the centrality of the child's views, Article 3 places emphasis on concerns of welfare with the best interests of the child only *a* (not *the*) *primary* consideration.

Whilst the Children Act (1989) goes some way to giving children a right to voice their views in relation to care, Newell (1989) points out there is no obligation on parents to involve children in major decisions at home. In Finland, the Child Custody and Right of Access Act 1983 states that parents who have custody must, before making decisions relating to children, 'where possible, discuss the matter with the child taking into account the child's age and maturity and the nature of the matter. In making the decision the custodian shall give due consideration to the child's feelings, opinions and wishes'. He also highlights that the legislative framework of the education system denies children and young people any formal voice.

Article 12

1. States parties shall assure to the child who is capable of forming his or her own views the right to express those views freely in all matters affecting the child, the views of the child being given due weight in accordance with the age and maturity of the child

2. For this purpose, the child shall in particular be provided the opportunity to be heard in any judicial and administrative proceedings affecting the child, either directly, or through a representative or an appropriate body, in a manner consistent with the procedural rules of national law

Article 3

1. In all actions concerning children, whether undertaken by public or private social welfare institutions, courts of law, administrative authorities or legislative bodies, the best interests of the child shall be a primary consideration

2. States parties undertake to ensure the child such protection and care as is necessary for his or her well-being, taking into account the rights and duties of his or her parents, legal guardians, or other individuals legally responsible for him or her, and, to this end, shall take all appropriate legislative and administrative measures

UN Convention on the Rights of the Child (1989)

Activity

Consider critically the extent to which children are involved in their health care. How might the conflict which Freeman (1993) alludes to be manifest in the care of sick children?

Further reading
FRANKLIN, B. (1986) *The Rights of Children.* Oxford: Basil Blackwell

Franklin (1989) is sceptical about the extent to which the Convention can be implemented. He reviews the Convention critically and comes to the conclusion that in order to achieve rights for children, they must be encouraged to make decisions and act on their own behalf.

Activity

Read Freeman (1993) and Franklin (1989). Consider critically your own views on the Convention with special regard to the care of children in hospital.

In 1992 the Children's Legal Centre published its own 'manifesto for children' in an attempt to translate the concepts contained within the Convention into concrete proposals. They put forward proposals related to:

- the right to be involved in decision making – nationally, within the home, in courts, in schools and other institutions, in meetings and in planning;
- the right to self-determination – giving statutory force to the 'Gillick' principle, adequate social security and youth training;
- the right to services which enable children to develop to their full potential – adequately resourced education, health care and provision for the homeless;
- the right to be adequately safeguarded from injury or abuse – from the environment, legal abuse, bullying, employment;
- the right to equal access to opportunities and to have special needs met – anti-discrimination in relation to nationality, disability, race;
- the right to information about themselves and matters affecting them – access to files and records, accurate sex education.

The extent to which children's rights are upheld depends on the views of the adults around them. Feinberg (cited by Freeman, 1983) argues that the key to differentiating between a claim and a right is the ability of the child to justify the claim in a reasoned manner. However, power relationships between adults and children are such that even a well reasoned argument can be dismissed by an adult. It is therefore the adult who will decide whether there is a justification for awarding a claim the status of a right.

CHILDREN'S RIGHTS AND HEALTH CARE (ARTICLES 6 AND 24)

The previous sections of this module have considered such concepts as autonomy, consent and confidentiality, and have highlighted the often ambiguous position of children within the health care setting. Although children's rights are developing alongside those of other consumers of health care, Freeman (1993) notes that children are often left off the main agenda. A clear example of this was the exclusion of specific reference to children in the Patient's Charter. According to a review of Community Care plans in response to the NHS and Community Care Act, very few included services for children (DH & SSI, 1993). Although the Health of the Nation strategy stresses the importance of infant and child health, it does so on the basis of achieving success in attaining targets for the improved health of adults.

The achievement of health care rights depends on access to opportunities and resources. Although the basic premise of the National Health Act 1946 was that free health services were available to all at the time of use, many would argue that this access is not enjoyed by all. There have been numerous instances of children's vital surgery being postponed due to inadequate resources. According to Carstairs and Morris (1991) children with chronic illness and handicaps tend to be disadvantaged and have poorer access than others to the services they need. Calculations by the Central Statistical Office (1993) show that the amount of health care resources spent on children is disproportionally low. This is particularly so when compared with that spent on the elderly. Children under 16 constitute 20.3% of the population of England and Wales, those 65 and over 15.7%.

The concept of family-centred care has been the basis for care in children's wards for some time. However, the discussion is always of participation by parents, the parents knowing what is best for their child. The power is seen to lie with the nurse and the parent and decisions are often taken on behalf of the child. This attitude is apparent in the government's first report on progress in implementation of the UN Convention. The report (DoH, 1994) states that young children are unable to make decisions, with an emphasis on parents, rather than children, as the consumers of health care.

The role of the children's nurse as the child's advocate is to uphold the rights of the child. However, this can be difficult to do when the views of the parent and the child conflict.

Activity

Consider critically the concept of family-centred care. How can we as children's nurses attempt to ensure that the child is the principal? Consider the concept of child-centred care.

Article 6

1 States parties recognise that every child has the inherent right to life

2 States parties shall ensure to the maximum extent possible the survival and development of the child

Article 24

1 States parties recognise the right of the child to the enjoyment of the highest attainable standard of health and to facilities for the treatment of illness and rehabilitation of health

2 States parties shall strive to ensure that no child is deprived of his or her right of access to such health care services

3 States parties shall pursue full implementation of this right and, in particular, shall take appropriate measures ...

4 States parties shall take all effective and appropriate measures with a view to abolishing traditional practices prejudicial to the health of children

5 States parties undertake to promote and encourage international cooperation with a view to achieving progressively the full realisation of the right recognised in this article ...

UN Convention on the Rights of the Child (1989)

Cross references

Family-centred care – pages 612–617

Advocate's role – page 590

Children's Charter

Copies of the booklet *NHS The Patient's Charter: Services for Children and Young People* can be obtained free of charge from:

Patient's Charter & You
FREEPOST
London SE99 7XU
OR
Health Literature Line 0800 555777

Fulton (1996) suggests three priorities in translating children's rights into practice:

- giving children a voice in the provision of their services;
- upholding children's rights to give or withhold consent to treatment;
- ensuring rigorous attention to children's pain control.

She goes on to propose that children's nurses work on the principle that children are presumed competent unless the adult can demonstrate otherwise.

The Children's Charter published in 1996 sets standards for child health care along the lines of the Patient's Charter and based on the principles of the Platt Report (1959). Although the Charter is welcomed, debates about its effect are numerous. The principles of the Platt Report have been stressed and re-stressed many times over by various bodies and individuals. Why then should this Charter succeed where others have failed?

Activity

Consider the terms of the Children's Charter. Critically appraise the services offered by your Trust or hospital in relation to the standards set on page 16 of the booklet.

The rights of children are clearly acknowledged within the terms of the Charter. The poster which accompanies the booklet is aimed at children and explains that they have certain rights and can expect a certain standard of care (see margin box on page 695).

SUMMARY

Article 42 of the United Nation Convention on the Rights of the Child states that:

> *parties undertake to make the principles and provisions of the Convention widely known, by appropriate and active means, to adults and children alike.*

This is seen by Newell (1991) as being vital because unless people know of its existence and the rights afforded children and guaranteed by the Convention, it will be of little use. Much has been done to spread the word by UNICEF and the Save the Children Fund. However, in the authors' experience very few parents and children know about it. The Children's Rights Development Unit, set up to monitor the Convention in the UK, is attempting to make information available. As a children's nurse you can help to make children's rights an issue and encourage the incorporation of the principles of the Convention into all matters pertaining to children.

Address

Children's Rights
Development Unit
235 Shaftesbury Avenue
London WC2H 8EL

Activity

Debate the issue of children's rights with colleagues. Discuss the Convention with family and friends and most of all with children.

> **Key points**

1. An important question to explore when considering the issue of rights is 'what are they and where do they stem from?'

2. There are three main approaches to children's rights: (i) the paternalistic view of the 'child-savers', (ii) the slightly broader approach of the 'welfare' view and (iii) the liberationist view.

3. The UN Convention on the Rights of the Child seeks to promote children's welfare as an issue of justice rather than one of charity.

4. The extent to which children's rights are upheld depends on the views of the adults around them.

5. A major role of the children's nurse is to promote children's rights in partnership with family and other professionals.

References

ALDERSON, P. and MONTGOMERY, J. (1996) *Health Care Choices: Making Decisions with Children*. London: Institute for Public Policy Research.

BEAUCHAMP, T. L. and CHILDRESS, J. F. (1989) *Principles of Biomedical Ethics*, 3rd edn. Oxford: Oxford University Press.

BEAUCHAMP, T. L. and CHILDRESS, J. F. (1994) *Principles of Biomedical Ethics*, 4th edn. Oxford: Oxford University Press.

BENTHAM, J. (1970) Anarchical fallacies. In MELDEN, A. I. (ed.), *Human Rights*. Belmont: Wadsworth.

BIRD, A. and WHITE, J. (1995) An ethical perspective – patient autonomy. In TINGLE, J. and CRIBB, A. (eds), *Nursing Law and Ethics*. Oxford: Blackwell Science.

BRITISH MEDICAL ASSOCIATION (BMA) and the LAW SOCIETY (1995) *Assessment of Mental Competence: Guidance for Doctors and Lawyers*. BMA: London.

BRITISH PAEDIATRIC ASSOCIATION (BPA) (1992) *Guidelines for the Ethical Conduct of Medical Research Involving Children*. London: BPA.

BROOK ADVISORY CENTRES (1996) *What Should I Do? Guidance on Confidentiality and Under 16s*.

BRYKCZYNSKA, G. (1993) Ethical issues in paediatric nursing. In GLASPER, E. A. and TUCKER, A. (eds), *Advances in Child Health Nursing*. London: Scutari Press.

My rights and what I can expect

I have a right to:

- be registered with a doctor
- have my treatment and care explained to me
- know that what I tell a doctor or a nurse is not passed on to anyone else (unless it is important that someone else knows)
- ask questions or complain if things go wrong or if I'm unhappy with anything about my treatment or care
- continue with my schoolwork

I can expect to:

- be told the names of the nurses and doctors who are looking after me
- be asked my opinion about things, like my treatment and how I feel
- have my questions answered and be talked to so that I understand
- be in hospital only when it is absolutely necessary
- be on a ward for children and young people
- visit the children's ward, before I go, to see what it is like
- be asked, if I am older, if I would prefer to be on a children's ward or adult ward and see both before I decide
- have my privacy and dignity respected
- get a choice of healthy food which tastes good
- have a named nurse
- find the hospital staff make sure I am not in too much pain
- be able to find a quiet place if I want to be alone
- be able to mix with and talk to the other boys and girls on the ward

Children's Charter (1996)

CAMPBELL, A. G. M. (1994) The paediatrician and medical negligence. In POWERS, M. and HARRIS, N. (eds), *Medical Negligence*. London: Butterworth.

CARSTAIRS, V. and MORRIS, R. (1991) *Deprivation and Health in Scotland*. Aberdeen: Aberdeen University Press.

CHARLES-EDWARDS, I. (1996) Moral and ethical perspectives. In CARTER, B. and REARNUM, A. (eds), *Child Health Care Nursing, Concepts, Theories and Practice*. Oxford: Blackwell Science.

CHILDREN'S RIGHTS DEVELOPMENT UNIT (1994) *UK Agenda for Children*. London: CRDU.

CHILDREN'S RIGHTS OFFICE (1995) *Building Small Democracies: Civil Rights of Children in Families*. London: CRO.

CSO (1993) *Social Trends 23*. London: HMSO.

DH & SSI (1993) *Caring for People: Implementing Community Care. A Preliminary Analysis of a Sample of English Community Care Plans*. London: DH & SSI.

DoH (1990) *A Guide to Consent for Examination and Treatment*, HC (90) 22. London: HMSO.

DoH (1991) *Local Research Ethics Committees*, HSG (91) 5. London: HMSO.

DoH (1994) *The United Kingdom's First Report to the United Nations Committee on the Rights of the Child*. London: HMSO.

DIMOND, B. C. (1995) *Legal Aspects of Nursing*, 2nd edn. Hemel Hempstead: Prentice-Hall.

DIMOND, B. C. (1996) *Legal Aspects of Child Health Care*. London: Mosby.

DINES, A. (1995) An ethical perspective. In TINGLE, J. and CRIPP, A. (eds), *Nursing Law and Ethics*. Oxford: Blackwell Scientific Publications.

FARSON, R. (1978) *Birthrights*. Harmondsworth: Penguin.

FLETCHER, N., HOLT, J., BRAZIER, M. and HARRIS, J. (1995) *Ethics, Law and Nursing*. Manchester: Manchester University Press.

FOX, D. M. and LEICHTER (1991) Rationing care in Oregon. The new accountability. *Health Affairs*, **10** (2), 7–27.

FRANKLIN, B. (1989) Children's rights: developments and prospects. *Children and Society*, **3** (1), 50–66.

FREEMAN M. (1983a) *The Rights and Wrongs of Children*. London: Frances Pinter.

FREEMAN M. (1983b) The concept of children's rights. In GEACH, H. and SZWED, E. (eds), *Providing Civil Justice for Children*. London: Edward Arnold.

FREEMAN, M. (1993) Laws, conventions and rights. *Children and Society*, **7** (1), 37–48

FULTON, Y. (1996) Children's rights and the role of the nurse. *Paediatric Nursing*, **8** (10), 29–31.

GILLON, R. (1985) *Philosophical Medical Ethics*. Chichester: Wiley,

HARRIS, J. (1985) *The Value of Life*. London: Routledge.

HART, H. (1970) Are there any natural rights? In MELDEN, A. I. (ed.), *Human Rights*. Wadsworth: Belmont.

HENDRICK, J. (1993) *Child Care Law for Health Professionals*. Oxford: Radcliffe Medical Press.

HENDRICK, J. (1997) *Legal Aspects of Child Health Care.* London: Chapman & Hall.

HOLLIDAY, I. (1995) *The NHS Transformed*, 2nd edn. Manchester: Baseline Books.

HOLT, J. (1975) *Escape from Childhood.* Harmondsworth: Penguin.

KHAN, M. and ROBSON, M. (1997) *Medical Negligence.* London: Cavendish.

LINDSEY, B. (ed.) (1994) *The Child and Family: Contemporary Nursing Issues in Child Health and Care.* London: Bailliere Tindall.

LYON, C. and PARTON, N. (1995) Children's rights and the Children Act 1989. In FRANKLIN, B. (ed.), *The Handbook of Children's Rights.* London: Routledge.

MASON, J. K. and McCALL SMITH, R. A. (1994) *Law and Medical Ethics*, 4th edn. London: Butterworth.

MEDICAL RESEARCH COUNCIL (1992) *The Ethical Conduct of Research on Children.* London: MRC.

NELSON-JONES, R. and BURTON, F. (1995) *Medical Negligence Case Law.* London: Butterworth.

NEWDICK, C. (1995) *Who Should We Treat? Law, Patients and Resources in the NHS.* Oxford: OUP.

NEWELL, P. (1989) *Children are People Too.* London: Bedford Square Press.

NEWELL, P. (1991) *The UN Conventions and Children's Rights in the UK.* London: National Children's Bureau.

NICHOLSON, R. (ed.) (1986) *Medical Research with Children: Ethics, Law and Practice.* Oxford: Oxford University Press.

ROYAL COLLEGE OF NURSING (1993) *Ethics Related to Research in Nursing.* London: Scutari Press.

RUMBOLD, G. C. and LESSER, H. (1995) An ethical perspective – negligence and moral obligations. In TINGLE, J. and CRIBB, A. (ed.), *Nursing Law and Ethics.* Oxford: Blackwell Scientific Publications.

SIEGLER, M. (1982) Confidentiality in medicine: a decrepit concept. *New England Journal of Medicine*, **307**, 1518–1521.

SOLBERG, A. (1990) Negotiating childhood: changing constructions of age for Norwegian children. In JAMES, A. and PROUT, A. (eds), *Constructing and Reconstructing Childhood.* Basingstoke: Falmer Press.

TAYLOR, J. (1994) Research and child care. In LINDSAY, B. (ed.), *The Child and Family: Contemporary Issues in Child Health and Care.* London: Bailliere Tindall.

UNICEF (1989) A new charter for children 3/88. *UNICEF/UK Information Sheet No. 8.*

UNITED KINGDOM CENTRAL COUNCIL (UKCC) (1992) *Code of Professional Conduct for the Nurse, Midwife and Health Visitor*, 3rd edn. London: UKCC.

UNITED KINGDOM CENTRAL COUNCIL (UKCC) (1996) *Guidelines for Professional Practice.* London: UKCC.

VEERMAN, P. (1992) *The Rights of the Child and the Changing Image of Childhood.* Dordrecht: Martinus Nijhoff.

WEITHORN, L. A. and CAMPBELL, S. B. (1982) The competency in children and adolescents to make informed treatment decisions. *Child Development*, **53**, 1589.

Address

Children's Rights Development Unit, 235 Shaftesbury Avenue, London WC2H 8EL.

MANAGING PROFESSIONAL PRACTICE

Joan Ramsay

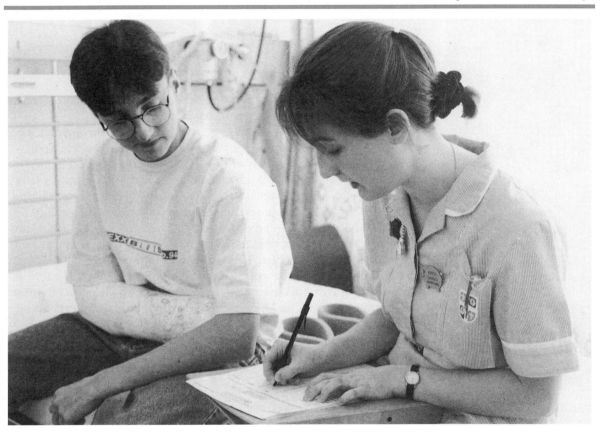

OBJECTIVES

The material contained within this module and the further reading/references should enable you to:

- Examine the discharge planning process.
- Discuss the role of the children's nurse as a leader.
- Explore standard setting and the audit cycle.
- Evaluate the different methods of organising work.
- Consider how to plan staffing levels and determine patient dependency.

INTRODUCTION

One of the most important roles of the children's nurse is that of leader, especially for children's nurses working in a general hospital environment. These nurses need to be able to promote the importance of children's nursing as a speciality and the unique needs of children. This module looks particularly at this leadership role, and explores issues such as skill mix for children's nursing and methods of calculating patient dependency to enable the nurse to justify claims for appropriate staffing levels. It also examines the organisation of work on a children's ward and the advantages and disadvantages of task or patient allocation, and team or primary nursing. In the current market forces of health care the provision of quality care is essential, and this module discusses standard setting and audit as a means of monitoring quality. The importance of cost-effective health care, as well as the need to minimise the length of hospital stay for children who are particularly stressed by being in this strange environment, has meant the need for careful discharge planning has never been so important. The module looks at how this can be best achieved in conjunction with other members of the multidisciplinary team.

DISCHARGE PLANNING   1

INTRODUCTION

Since the Platt Report in 1959 (MoH, 1959) much has been written about the effects of hospitalisation for children. Most of the resulting recommendations suggested that children should only be admitted to hospital if absolutely necessary and this stay should be kept to a minimum. Although the development of community nursing services for children has been slow there has been a significant decrease in the average length of their hospital stay (Audit Commission, 1993). This move towards community care has given impetus to the need for good discharge planning. Good discharge planning not only improves patient care and outcomes of care but minimises re-admission due to inadequate after-care.

Discharge planning must begin with an assessment of the family's wishes, resources and abilities to undertake the care of their child at home. It also involves education of the family and identification of the community and support services available. Because discharge planning is often very complex, government recommendations since 1989 have stated that it should begin as early as possible, ideally during the assessment process at admission, and for booked admissions before the child is even admitted to hospital (DoH, 1989b). Another important guideline was that the family should be at the centre of the planning process.

Tierney *et al*. (1994) found that the majority of families were not consulted about discharge arrangements and that one-fifth of patients had probably been discharged too soon. This latter point was supported by the fact that more than a quarter of the patients were re-admitted within 3 months of their discharge. The psychological benefits and economic advantage of discharging children into the community as soon as possible must be balanced against the risks of discharging highly dependent children into an unsuitable environment with insufficient support mechanisms.

COORDINATION OF DISCHARGE PLANNING

The coordination of discharge is a complex multidisciplinary and multi-agency process. It involves various members of the hospital team, social services, community services and GPs as well as the family. Tierney *et al*. (1994) recommends that a named member of the multidisciplinary team should be given the responsibility of coordinating the discharge arrangements. This named individual should have the responsibility of recording all information relating to the discharge, including the results of any assessments and the services contacted, on a specific discharge plan used by all staff involved in the discharge. A comprehensive

---

Discharge planning – the multidisciplinary team

The family
- education, advice and support

Community nurse/health visitor/GP
- liaison and continuity of care
- ongoing education, advice and support
- clinical input
- maintenance of treatment

Social services
- home/financial assessment

Occupational therapists
- activities of daily living
- home assessment
- equipment

Physiotherapists
- mobility and mobility aids
- respiratory care

Speech and language therapy
- communication skill/aids

Dietician
- enteral feeding
- special dietary needs

School nurse
- continuing care/treatment at school

Discharge planning – points to remember

- Involve the family from the time of admission
- An estimated date of discharge facilitates the support process
- Families may have unrealistic expectations and may not remember all information (see p. 707)
- Discharge is easier to postpone than arrange urgently
- Inform the appropriate therapist on admission when children need to practise skills (e.g. walking with crutches), before discharge
- Ensure family have practised and feel competent in any care they will be giving
- The amount , as well as the frequency, of support should be clearly identified
- If the child needs a key discharge item of equipment (e.g. wheelchair) it should be ordered on admission
- Equipment and/or home alterations may take time and the family should not be given false hopes
- Do not assume that the child's and family's needs on admission will be the same at the time of discharge

discharge planning document, placed either in the child's medical records or at the bedside with the nursing notes, allows all members involved in the discharge, including the family, to be able to see at a glance the progress with the arrangements. This process was supported by the UKCC in 1995 following a report on a survey of current discharge practices in acute hospitals. They recommended that:

- every ward should have a written discharge policy, discharge standards and discharge plans;
- each patient should have a named member of staff designated to take responsibility for the discharge coordination;
- patients and families should know which member of staff is responsible for coordinating their discharge arrangements, be regularly and fully involved in the discharge planning, and be given written information about all arrangements;
- GPs and community nurses should be involved early in the discharge planning process and that community/hospital liaison should be improved;
- improvements were made in the content and speed of delivery of the discharge letter;
- each ward had an audit system for discharge procedures;
- patients should not be discharged at times which were inconvenient for community services;
- wards should receive regular statistical information relevant to discharge planning to enable evaluation of the process.

Activity

Investigate how the discharge planning in your current area of practice meets these recommendations (see Figure 1.1, p. 706).

Coordination and continuity of discharge planning is only as effective as the communication within and between the different agencies and disciplines involved. This is facilitated by a clear understanding of the funding arrangements and the roles of all participants.

NHS FUNDING OF COMMUNITY CARE

In 1995 the government required each health authority to agree eligibility for continuing health care which would be fully funded by the NHS with its local social services department(s).

Activity

Find out the criteria in your own area for fully funded health care.

The eligibility for continuing health care funding does not stand alone. They should be seen as part of the continuum of community care with social services (see Figure 1.2 – page 706). At the lower end of the continuum, chronically ill children may need a minimum amount of health care but a high level of social care. Depending on their financial status, families may be required to contribute to the cost of the social care element. At the opposite end of the continuum, children require a high level of health care and would meet the criteria for fully funded NHS care. At this level the family would not be expected to contribute financially for any part of the care their child receives even if some of this care is provided by social services. At all levels the biggest responsibility for the care of the sick/disabled child falls upon the family and their views about their needs is essential.

The multidisciplinary team is responsible for deciding if a patient is eligible for fully funded NHS continuing health care. The underlying principles for assessing this are that the assessment:

- is part of the care management process;
- involves the child (if appropriate) and family;
- is not initiated until a sufficient period has been allowed for recovery and rehabilitation;
- is multidisciplinary, involving all those providing care or therapy; involves a consultant or GP;
- decision is fully and clearly documented and signed by all those involved.

Most health authorities have additional community funds to pay for a patient's care in the community where this care is not provided under contract with an NHS Trust or other provider. Application for this funding should be part of the multidisciplinary team's assessment.

THE SOCIAL SERVICES PERSPECTIVE

The NHS and Community Care Act (1990) promoted the collaborative working of health, housing, education and social services for the provision of care in the community which included the private and voluntary services. The Act stated that any member of staff could act as the named discharge organiser but in practice this role is often undertaken by the social worker. The named social worker interviews the family to ascertain their wishes and their current resources, including support networks. Other agencies become involved when the amount of care needs are not all within the remit of social services. Any care which involves health needs is put forward to the health authority or GP fundholder to finance. A case conference may need to be arranged when discharge needs are particularly complex.

When a family is not eligible for fully funded NHS care, they may qualify for support from social services. Social services usually assess

---

Example criteria for continuing NHS-funded health care

Families will be eligible for care paid for by the NHS if their child:

- is totally dependent (i.e. where withdrawal or unavailability of help threatens survival) AND has specific additional needs *such as* one of the following:
  – complex methods of feeding
  – care of large pressure sores (grade 4–5)
  – supervision and monitoring of the last stage of cardiac, respiratory, renal or other major organ failure
  – permanent tracheostomy requiring frequent changes and suction
  – skilled lifting and handling needing two or more people
  – unstable or unpredictable medical/psychological conditions requiring specialist clinical intervention
- is terminally ill and needs specialist nursing supervision or support when death is expected within about 3 months
- is in need of ongoing supervision to prevent self-harm or harm to others. (e.g. challenging behaviour with a learning disability or severe behavioural problems arising from a brain injury)
- has needs which individually would not be of sufficient severity to meet the above criteria, but when put together their complexity requires high levels of care
- is in need of phased or intermittent respite care and fall into the above categories
- needs a programme of rehabilitation following an episode of illness or an accident and before long-term needs can be assessed
- will require transport to and from the GP, hospice, health care facilities which is above contracted levels and falls into one of the above categories

(Bedfordshire Health Authority, 1996)

Table 1.1

Social services and health input to different levels of care

	Level of need			
	1	2	3	4
Lead care planning agency	Social services	Social services	Social services	Social services and health care staff
Lead funding agency	Social services	Social services	Social services and NHS	NHS
Social services priority	Medium–high	High	High/more than social service provision	More than social service provision
Example of health input	General medical services (GP, CCN, etc.)	General medical services and specialist nurse	Clinical input above usual PHCT remit	Specialist input from nursing and medicine
Example of social services input	Home care or residential care	Extensive home or residential care	Extensive home and specialist care	Advice to health staff

Assessment of the family and community services for home care

Physical environment
- safe and adequate housing
- telephone in the home
- space for equipment

Psychological status
- firm marital status or alternative support mechanisms
- knowledge of this illness/disability or motivation and ability to learn
- realistic perceptions of the effects of the child's illness/disability upon the family

Available resources
- appropriate equipment available
- appropriate health care personnel available
- home renovation possible
- peer/parent support group available
- appropriate transport available

Cross reference

Community nursing – pages 371–377

the priority of the situation to determine whether families qualify for this support. Only high- and medium-risk priorities are eligible for services (see Table 1.1).

- *High priority* – children in this category require radical intervention to change or ameliorate their situation. They are or may be exposed to significant harm. They may be dependent on others for protection and/or they are not able to be cared for by their own family.
- *Medium priority* – when children need continued support to prevent deterioration of the situation. Their relationship with their family may have broken down and they are unsupported and exposed to risk. This category also includes families with consistent financial problems or substandard accommodation and children in need.
- *Low priority* – When the child's quality of life could be enhanced and/or the risk of deterioration could be significantly reduced.

THE NURSING PERSPECTIVE

On admission to hospital the named nurse and medical team should initiate post-discharge care and determine the approximate length of the child's stay. If parents are actively involved in the child's care planning during hospitalisation it is relatively easy to adapt these care plans for home use. Marland (1994) suggests that sharing nursing care plans with parents in this way not only supports a shared holistic approach to caring for the individual child, but also enables the nurses to assess how parents are coping. The family's named nurse needs to undertake a thorough assessment of the family and the home environment to ensure that the family's emotional and physical resources are able to support the care and responsibility of home care. This assessment should take the child and family's learning needs into account to enable a planned approach to teaching them any new knowledge and skills well in advance of discharge. This gives them opportunity to practise the care before going home, and sometimes it may be appropriate to arrange a trial period at home to ensure they can transfer their skills to the home environment. Ideally, more than one member of the family should be taught so that the burden of this responsibility can be shared. A written plan of teaching which itemises learning goals is helpful for the family and members of the multidisciplinary team to identify progress. This approach is also advocated by Casey and Mobbs (1988) who suggest that it helps clarify the legal implications of parents providing health care.

Written home care instructions should be available not only to remind parents of salient points but to facilitate continuity of care for other professionals involved in the child's home care. These should include a list of useful telephone numbers to enable the family to seek help when needed. Parents should also be advised to discuss their child's home care with their insurance company. If, for instance, their child requires home oxygen, this may alter their fire risk. Local emergency services should also be aware of such home situations to enable them to respond appropriately in case of emergency.

Marland (1994) suggests that good communication between the named hospital nurse and the community children's nurse is the most important factor in transferring care to the home environment. Early liaison with the community nurse also benefits the child and family who can begin to get to know their new nurse before discharge. In Marland's area of practice the community children's nurse met the families of children identified for early discharge on the day of discharge and made the first visit later that same day.

The named nurse should be alert to the fact that home care may not be appropriate in all cases. In addition, even if home care seems initially appropriate, changing circumstances may delay or prevent this option. The nurse may need to help parents come to terms with these changes and make the appropriate alterations to the discharge plan.

THE PHYSIOTHERAPY AND OCCUPATIONAL THERAPY PERSPECTIVE

Discharge planning is essential from the perspective of the physiotherapist and the occupational therapist. The physiotherapist needs time to ensure that the:

- child is fitted with the appropriate equipment;
- child and family know how to use and fit the equipment;
- family know exactly what the child is able to do;
- equipment will be suitable in the home environment.

The occupational therapist (OT) is concerned with promoting independence in the activities of daily living and will identify the appropriate equipment to help with this. Having made the assessment of

Providing resources for discharge

Equipment

Social services
- long-term equipment
- aids and adaptations for the home

Occupational therapy/hospital or community short-term loan stock
- short-term equipment (3 months or less)

Red Cross/self-help groups
- loan equipment for social need only

Prescription items

Dressings, medication, needles and syringes, and feeds provided by the hospital on discharge and then by repeat prescription from the GP

Human resources

Community trust
- community children's nurse
- health visitor
- school nurse
- therapies

Specialist services
- MacMillan nurse
- hospice care

Social services
- home help
- night sitter
- advice about available allowances

Ambulance trust
- transport arrangements

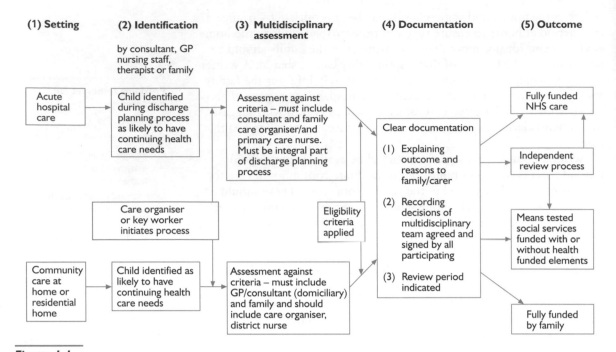

Figure 1.1

Process for deciding whether a family is eligible for continuing health care.

Figure 1.2

The continuum of health and social care.

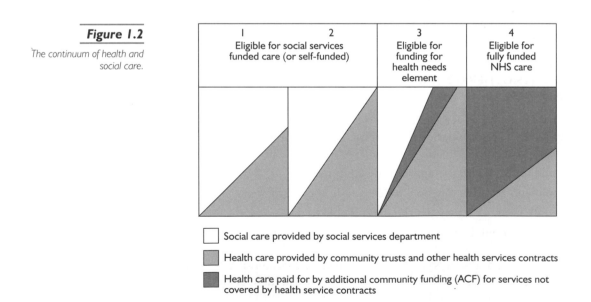

which equipment is required, the OT will then make a referral to social services OTs for delivery of the equipment. The social services usually need substantial notice for any long-term equipment before they can arrange for its delivery.

Activity

Organise a visit to your hospital's OT department and discuss the OT's views on discharge planning and identify the range of equipment available to help children with special needs.

➤ Key points

1. Hospitalisation is traumatic for children and should therefore be kept to a minimum for this group of patients.

2. Effective discharge planning improves patient care and minimises the need for re-admission.

3. Discharge planning should begin before or during the assessment process, on admission to hospital.

4. The family must be at the centre of the discharge planning process which must include all the multidisciplinary team.

5. A named individual should be responsible for coordinating, planning and evaluating discharge for each individual child.

6. Each child's named nurse should be aware of the criteria used to determine eligibility for continuing health care funding and be able to apply for such funding on behalf of the child and family.

Written instructions for home care

Health care needs
- care plan to identify the child's routine of specific health care needs
- list of regular observations required and child's individual norms
- telephone numbers of health care team for advice
- specific information about the child's condition

Equipment
- care of equipment
- problem solving for malfunctions
- telephone numbers of equipment providers in case of failure

Support
- frequency and amount of home support organised
- names and telephone numbers of support agencies involved in home care
- information about self-help groups

Emergency care
- explanation of emergency procedures
- emergency telephone numbers

2 THE NURSE AS A LEADER

INTRODUCTION

As discussed previously, the role of the children's nurse as a leader involves the direction of other nurses or health care professionals who are not used to caring for children. It may also involve influencing those outside the health care field who have some control over health services for children. All children's nurses can act as leaders in this way to ensure the rights of children are maintained and improved.

As families become more aware of children's rights in relation to health, nurses can expect to be involved with the handling of complaints. The acceptance and sensitive handling of complaints about the service can be influential in improving the quality of the service. On occasions the quality of the service can be linked with the available resources to provide that service and all nurses can be instrumental in helping to ensure the best use of the available resources within the budget restraints.

The work of children's nurses can never be context free. It often takes place within health care settings where conditions exist, such as a restricted budget, which influence nurses' actions (Figure 2.1). Nurses clearly need to understand and manage these conditions if they are to achieve effective practice. These contexts of practice can be seen within the immediate environment of health care where nursing takes place and in the wider environment outside this setting. The wider context of practice includes such issues as government policy and how this is interpreted. Salvage (1985) stresses the importance of nurses becoming aware of political issues if they are to act effectively to safeguard areas of influence and promote the interests of individual patients and clients (UKCC, 1992).

POLITICAL INFLUENCES

Activity

Identify the political influences upon the community and hospital care of children.

Children's nursing in the community has changed dramatically over the last 20 years. The move from hospital to community care has been very much influenced by government policy. As a result of a series of reports, the government white paper 'Caring for People' (1989) aimed to provide care in an environment which encouraged a normal lifestyle. This was followed by the NHS and Community Care Act (1990) which gave primary responsibility for the organisation of community care to

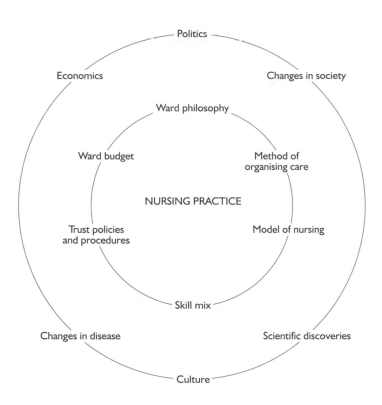

Figure 2.1
Contexts of nursing practice.

the local authorities. This move towards community care has changed the practice of nursing; children in hospital tend to be more acutely ill and community nurses are caring for children who are more dependent and need more resources for their care. Hospital care has also been affected by the NHS and Community Care Act. Hospitals are now NHS Trusts which are autonomous bodies and can introduce their own policies and conditions of service which could drastically alter the way in which nurses work. Some Trusts are already offering financial incentives for children's nurses to overcome a shortage of these specialist practitioners. This may benefit those Trusts with the money to offer such incentives to the detriment of others with less available cash. The government white paper 'Working for Patients' aimed to give more power to the consumers of health care and representation in health care decision making. Additionally, the Children's Charter (DoH, 1996) aimed to make children and parents more aware of their rights in relation to health care. Parents may now be more questioning as a result of this knowledge.

As people become more aware of their rights in relation to health care they begin to demand that their health care needs are met. Unfortunately, this is not always possible, as economic restraints sometimes interfere with the provision of health care. Similarly, nurses,

Cross reference

Children's Charter – pages 694–695

as advocates for children and their families, strive to provide the best resources but are sometimes hindered by economic factors.

MANAGING MATERIAL RESOURCES

The NHS is almost totally funded by the government and must compete for its funds with other government departments, such as Defence and Education. Eighty eight per cent of NHS funds arise from general taxation, which means that the NHS relies upon the country's economic growth. It also means that health authorities have an obligation to function effectively within their budget. Increasing technology and greater demands and expectations of care have set a pattern of financial restrictions and nurses have an important role to play in managing resources and providing high quality care within set budgets. The NHS and Community Care Act (1990) aimed to promote a closer relationship between services and cost by increasing the responsibility for budget management at ward level. It is important for nurses to play a lead role in agreeing these clinical budgets because only they can identify their nursing needs. As nursing becomes more autonomous and involved with technical advances, nurses become concerned with choosing medical stores, supplies and equipment. Although nurses are not usually involved in prescribing drugs their knowledge of the effectiveness and accept-ability of certain medications may influence the doctors' choice.

Activity

Consider ways of encouraging nurses to be more cost conscious in the use and ordering of stores and pharmacy.

Staff cannot be encouraged to budget wisely unless they are aware of the cost of clinical supplies. Marking the prices of items in the store cupboard can raise the staff's awareness of costs but after a time this may be less effective. Monthly information about the usage and expenditure may help staff to appreciate wasteful practices. My own unit was spending so much money on tempadots that these were no longer a cost-effective way of taking temperatures. However, when staff became aware of the high expenditure they identified that they were taking handfuls of tempadots at the beginning of their shift and keeping them in the pockets of their tabards. At the end of their shift any remaining either ended up in the washing machine or had to be discarded as they had changed colour by contact with the nurses' body heat. As a result this practice stopped and the unit made an immediate significant saving.

Savings can also be made by an effective means of stock control. Many areas now use a top-up system so that items in constant use are replaced regularly and the practice of stock-piling is prevented. This system still benefits from nurses' appreciation of costs and the identification of any actual or predicted change in the use of supplies.

Activity

Imagine you are thinking of buying an expensive piece of equipment for yourself (e.g. computer, video recorder, dish washer). The department store has a range of different makes of this equipment. What factors would determine your choice?

The management of material resources is not just concerned with the ordering process. Just as you would do when buying equipment for yourself, the ward manager must consider the following:

- how do the costs of various makes compare?
- does it perform all the functions required?
- how easy will it be to use, how much training would staff require to use it?
- how soon is it likely to be replaced by a better model?
- is it easy to store?
- what are the maintenance costs?
- does it require special equipment to be used with it or can existing equipment be used?

Activity

Take a critical look at the way in which stores and equipment are ordered in your current area of practice. Is it a cost-effective way of managing material resources?

THE PROVISION OF HEALTH CARE

Unfortunately, like resources, the provision of health care, especially in relation to specialist care, is not equally distributed across the UK. The access to certain care is often determined geographically and although this was formally recognised by the government in 1993 in the Tomlinson report, changes have been slow.

Activity

Compare the specialist services available in your nearest major UK city with those in a more rural area known to you.

Rural areas often have limited access to specialist services. Some big cities in the UK have a Helicopter Emergency Medical Service (HEMS)

Cost-effective material resource management

- Stores ordered in a way which prevents stock-piling but ensures a ready supply of items used most frequently
- Authorisation of orders by named staff allows budget control but should not be so restrictive that stores can only be ordered by one person
- A strategy for ensuring a constant turn-over of stock so items do not become unusable because of date or condition
- Clear understanding of the length of time orders take to be dispatched to enable planning of the stock required
- A clear strategy for identifying, reporting and removing obsolete or faulty equipment which is known by all staff
- All staff are aware of the cost and usage of stores and the monthly budget report and know how to report concerns or changes in relation to these

Cross reference

The demand for paediatric intensive care – page 387

Cross reference

Resources and rationing – page 679

Cross reference

Ear surgery – page 459

which significantly improves mortality rates for trauma victims by being able to provide expert care within the first hour (the golden hour) of the incident. Specialist care for children may only be available in selected centres and transfer to these centres inevitably takes time and may affect outcome. In 1996 the tragedy of a child who died whilst being transferred to the only available paediatric intensive care bed highlighted the shortage of such specialist care outside the major UK cities (NHS Executive, 1996).

The alternative argument relates to the success of these specialist centres. Some illnesses of childhood are very rare and the special skills needed to care and treat such children may only be available at major centres where sufficient numbers of these children have been seen. For instance, neonates have a better prognosis if treated in specialist units than if treated by district hospitals (Williams, 1995), and the mortality of children with some types of cancer is lower at tertiary centres (Audit Commission, 1993). Edge *et al.* (1994) identify that the incidence of adverse events are more likely to occur if a child is transported to specialist centres by non-specialist staff and recommend that children are transferred by a dedicated specialist paediatric team.

Children who need costly treatments may be discriminated against by different purchasers of health care. Purchasers, such as fundholder GPs, may be loathe to register children who will use much of their budget on expensive medical treatment. Even relatively inexpensive treatments may not be available to children as NHS Trusts are forced to make financial savings. In some areas routine surgery such as tonsillectomies and insertion of grommets have been curtailed. Whilst this surgery has no proven effect for all children (Black *et al.*, 1990), the Audit Commission (1993) recommended that paediatricians and ENT surgeons jointly determined which children would benefit from surgery. The access to specialised services for children with special needs and mental health problems also varies widely according to geographical area.

As leaders of paediatric practice, nurses who are aware of such discriminatory practices should help families to make an informed choice about the available care and the possible options. Although this may raise questions about the availability of expensive or sophisticated forms of treatment, people are entitled to this knowledge. The NHS can no longer provide for everyone and there is often a partnership between it and the voluntary sector. As the public become aware of this they are often motivated to set up pressure groups and raise money themselves to provide the necessary resources. In 1997, a specialist children's ward was saved from closure because parents organised a series of protests to make sure their concerns were heard (Payne, 1997)

As you can see, nurses and families can influence the provision of care, but fund raising is only one way of doing this.

Activity

Consider other ways in which you, and the families you care for, can influence health care services.

Nurses and families have many different strategies which they can utilise to influence the provision of health care. The effectiveness of such measures will depend upon the continuing motivation of those involved and their access to influential people and organisations. Obviously, nurses have to be careful not to compromise their professional code of conduct and must be able to present their case objectively with valid and reliable evidence to support their argument. Families who are trying to improve services may use the complaints procedure, among other strategies, to highlight a problem.

HANDLING COMPLAINTS

Although praise, thank-you letters and congratulatory notes are offered more freely than complaints (DoH, 1994a), it is only the latter which attract publicity and need investigation. The incidence of complaints, however, does provide an indicator of the quality of care for purchasers of health care who can obtain copies.

Activity

Find out what complaints have been received during the last year in your current area of practice. Who is the complainant in these cases and at what point in the child's care was the complaint received? Consider how you would handle complaints such as these.

Common areas of complaints include:

- inadequate explanations about care;
- misunderstandings about discharge arrangements;
- inedible or unsuitable hospital food;
- care or treatment omitted;
- poor staff attitude.

All these complaints may seem trivial but they are all potentially serious. The first two complaints are related to a lack of communication between health care professionals and families. This is the most common reason for complaints and is usually the easiest to remedy. The omission of care may be due to negligence and have potential legal implications for the Trust and accusations of professional misconduct for the member of staff involved. The complaint about hospital food may reflect upon the quality of care offered by the Trust, especially as evidence shows that nutrition is related to healing and immunity to infection (Westwood, 1997). Families also have a right to expect that appropriate food will be part of children's care in hospital as this aspect is part of the Children's Charter (DoH, 1996). Complaints are often the result of anxieties and feelings of guilt which parents have not been able to express in any other way.

Influencing the provision of health care

Nurses can influence the provision of health care by:

- negotiation with senior managers
- raising local awareness
- appealing to the local league of friends of the Trust
- research to provide clear evidence of the need

Families can influence the provision of health care by:

- drawing up a petition
- obtaining support of the local MP
- writing to the local press
- appealing to the health service commissioner
- involving rotary clubs
- informing the Community Health Council

The value of complaints

- Improving the standards of service
- Providing the encouragement to improve communication
- Emphasising the importance of accurate, timed and dated record keeping
- Reflection upon words and actions
- Ensuring a clear rationale for practice

(Reid, 1996)

Figure 2.2

The NHS complaints procedure.

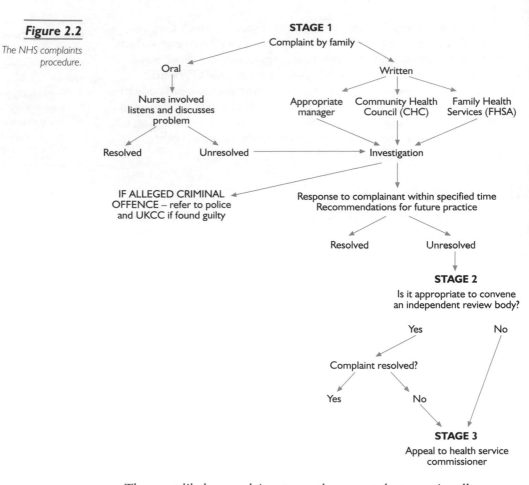

The most likely complainants are the parents but occasionally a relative will complain on their behalf. Most people prefer not to complain while the child is still receiving attention. Many reasons are given for this, such as 'I know you are always busy' or 'I didn't like to bother you', but a more disturbing reason is that of fearing victimisation. Obviously, people who believe this have lost their trust and confidence in the nursing profession. Others may simply want to avoid confrontation. Consequently, most complaints are received after the child has gone home.

The management of complaints will vary according to the type and severity of the complaint but each Trust should have guidelines for handling complaints with which you should make yourself familiar (see Figure 2.2). As stated previously, the commonest cause for complaints is lack of communication, therefore, complainants should initially have an opportunity to discuss their problems and feel that their concerns are being listened to. It is important to acknowledge their concerns and to outline any subsequent action to prevent a reoccurrence of the problem. The Ombudsman has noted that a significant number of complainants do not pursue their complaints when they are satisfied that action has been taken (Blackshaw, 1994). Complaints can be seen as a way of improving services and Reid (1996) suggests that nurses look at complaints rationally and honestly and advises that an explanation and apology can be very reassuring to a concerned parent.

> **Key points**

1. All children's nurses should act as leaders to ensure that the rights of children are heard and acted upon.

2. The political influence on the health care provision for children is great but nurses can also have an effect upon this provision.

3. The provision of health care services for children is unequally distributed across the UK and families may need help to identify the availability of services for their child's needs.

4. Nurses attempting to influence the provision of services for children should do so in a constructive way which will not bring themselves or their profession into disrepute.

5. The management of material resources is one way in which nurses can influence the quality and effectiveness of care.

6. Complaints should be seen as positive as they promote a way of reflecting upon and improving practice.

3 THE ORGANISATION OF PATIENT CARE

INTRODUCTION

There are various ways of organising the care of children in hospital which have evolved over the years to meet the needs of those managing the care and to respond to changes in nursing. These changes have occurred as nurses have become dissatisfied with their image as doctors' handmaidens and have sought ways of raising the profile of nursing. As one result of this dissatisfaction, models of nursing have evolved. These models redefine the traditional nurse–patient relationship and promote the care of patients as individuals. If patients are to be cared for as individuals the system of delivery of care must enable nurses and patients to be able to relate to each other as individuals and be flexible enough to enable nurses to develop innovative ways of meeting individuals' unique needs.

The government supports this notion of individualised care. Standard 8 of the Patient's Charter (DoH, 1994b) states that every patient has the right to receive the care of a named nurse, midwife and health visitor. According to the NHS executive this standard aims to encourage the partnership between the nurse ... and the patient/client which enables the patient/client to be involved in developing a joint care plan. The standard has always been linked with primary nursing but this is not the only way to organise care with a named nurse providing individualised care. As with all methods of organising care, primary nursing has its advantages and disadvantages and nurses need to look carefully at their individual areas of work and identify the method which can offer the best quality of care for their patient group. Shaw (1986) has suggested a framework for measuring quality assurance which enables an impartial discussion of these various organisational methods:

3Es: Efficiency – producing results with minimum effort
      Effectiveness – capable of producing the desired results
      Equity – capable of being impartial
3As: Accessibility – easiness of availability
      Appropriateness – degree of suitability for the job
      Acceptability – endorsement from those involved.

TASK ALLOCATION

In this system the child's care is broken down into a hierarchy of tasks, mostly concerned with physical needs. Traditionally, more senior nurses carried out the more complicated tasks and junior staff did the more fundamental care. This, of course, immediately tends to suggest that the fundamental care is less important. Whilst such care may not be life saving, it is often important for the child and family and often better illustrates the concept of caring than the more technological care. Fundamental care can take some time to deliver and in this organisational system the least experienced staff are with the child and family longer than the qualified staff. Thus these inexperienced staff are in the best position to develop a therapeutic relationship but lack the knowledge and skills to develop and use this partnership. Alternatively, task allocation may mean that the child and family come into contact with a large number of nurses but do not relate to any of them well.

However, task allocation has been shown to be an efficient way of using resources (Huczynski and Buchanan, 1985). With an increasing HCA work force in health care whose NVQ training is task centred, task allocation may be the most cost-effective method of managing care. Cost effectiveness is a powerful argument for NHS Trusts which aim to provide value-for-money quality care. This quality is often measured by standards which reduce care into measurable tasks. However, the question of what constitutes quality in care must be considered. Does the fragmentation of care into tasks provide quality of care?

Huczynski and Buchanan (1985) have also shown that task allocation is effective. It clearly delegates responsibility and is easy to allocate staff whatever the skill mix of those on duty. Task allocation ensures equity by matching highly skilled care to the most experienced staff. It is much less stressful for junior staff who may be anxious about carrying out care in which they lack experience. This argument may be counteracted by the fact that children and families may rely more on them because they are at the bedside for the longest time. Whilst task allocation supports Benner's (1984) ideas about the development of nursing skills, it can hinder personal development if nurses remain only performing tasks in which they have the most practice.

Task allocation gives children and families more access to more staff. This enables them to identify the nurse with whom they feel most comfortable and gives them the choice of the nurse with whom they wish to develop a relationship. Adult patients endorse this method as they find the access to more nurses reassuring and less stressful than relying on one nurse. There is no reason to think that children and families would react differently. Nurses are involved in the care of more children and families and can develop more nursing knowledge as a result of the varied experience available in task allocation. However, it is this increased accessibility which seems to be in direct opposition to the concept of family-centred care. Is it possible for several nurses to create a therapeutic relationship with one child and family? In addition, sociologists have found that this method of work organisation in industry produces boredom, frustration and a sense of alienation and powerlessness amongst workers (Blauner, 1964)

Task allocation appears very acceptable for nursing in the 1990s. Because it matches the increasing unqualified work force, general managers may see it as a way of saving money on qualified, experienced and expensive staff. It may also be attractive to some nurses who find close relationships with children and families too stressful. Its acceptability may be shown by the number of specialist posts in paediatrics which have tended to be task related. For example, a child with Crohn's disease may be cared for by the stoma nurse, the nutrition nurse, the pain control nurse and the nurse providing the day-to-day care.

Activity

Read over the above section on task allocation again and consider the questions posed in the box alongside. Then discuss with some colleagues the future of this method of organising care.

Individualised care – questions to ask

- Does the organisation of care promote an individualised approach to care?
- Does it provide nurses with opportunities to develop relationships with children and their families?
- Does it encourage such opportunities?
- Does it enable the recognition of nurses as individuals?
- Does it give nurses the opportunity to be creative and innovative in meeting individual needs?
- Does it help nurses to gain knowledge and skills about providing individualised care to help future children and patients by enabling (a) an insight into their own feelings and (b) feedback about the care they gave?

PATIENT ALLOCATION

In this organisational method each nurse is allocated a group of patients. This nurse provides all the care for these patients for a specific length of time which can vary from the duration of a shift, or for a week or whenever they are on duty. Patient allocation is efficient because it makes best use of the skills of each nurse to be matched to the patients' needs. However, just because a child and family does not need highly skilled nursing care does not also mean that they do not need a high degree of support or teaching. It is an effective way of delivering care because it clearly defines areas of responsibility and accountability for each shift. It is less effective over a period of time because a number of nurses will have been involved in the care. It is equitable because it assigns patients according to the skills of each nurse on duty and this can be less stressful for junior nurses who may be less confident about caring for acutely ill children.

Patient allocation appears to give children and families optimum access to a number of nurses if it is practised over a period of time. Whilst the families are not dependent on one nurse alone, they do have the continuity of carers by having access to a few named nurses across their period of hospitalisation. This depends on careful planning of off-duty rotas, to match nurses who have just had time off, and are then on duty for several days, with new admissions. If patient allocation is only practised for the duration of a shift, the child and family, as well as the nurse, may not have time to establish a therapeutic relationship. This may suit some nurses who find such relationships stressful. Patient allocation can be very appropriate because it allocates staff according to the appropriateness of their skills. It appears to be an acceptable way of organising care because nurses have the satisfaction of being able to meet all the needs of their children and families who have fewer nurses with whom to relate.

TEAM NURSING

Although patient allocation ideally gives children and families three nurses with whom to relate over a 24-hour period, it can also mean several nurses if the child is in hospital for 7 days or longer. Team allocation tries to overcome this. The ward staff are divided into teams and each team is responsible for the total care of a certain number of patients. The patients are usually grouped in one geographical area of the ward. The team's hours of duty are organised to ensure that at least one nurse from the team is on duty at any time. Kron (1981) suggests that a small group of nurses working together, guided by a nurse leader is more efficient than nurses working alone, but also warns that without good leadership this method of working can lead to fragmentation, a return to task allocation and lack of accountability. It can be an effective way of working as individual nurses can receive help, support and supervision from the rest of the team and therefore feel more confident (Reed, 1988). Thomas *et al.* (1992) found that nurses within a team considered that they had a greater knowledge of their patients and families and that, as a result, they could provide more security for them. This method of working also gives equal status to team members and promotes a democratic view. Children and families have access to a group of named nurses, one of whom will always be on duty. This can provide the child and family with a degree of choice in whom they choose to share their problems whilst maintaining continuity of care. However, team nursing can pose problems with skill mix. If the team member on duty is unqualified the amount of care they can safely provide is limited. However, they can still provide continuity for the child and family even if other nurses may be required to help with specific aspects of care. Good communication and flexible off-duty rotas are key issues in the success of team nursing.

Team nursing is appropriate for an area where the skills and qualifi-cations of staff are different. It also incorporates part-time staff much more easily than other systems of managing care. It enables these staff to recognise their limitations within the security of a supportive team. It is also an appropriate way of meeting the government requirement for a named nurse. The team leader is the experienced and appropriately qualified registered nurse but the family know the other team members when the leader is not present. Thomas *et al.* (1992) found that most staff accepted team nursing well, experiencing greater job satisfaction that with previous organisational methods.

PRIMARY NURSING

Primary nursing was developed by a group of American nurses in the 1970s who were concerned by the fragmentation of care and responsi-bility provided by other systems of patient care organisation (Manthey *et al.*, 1970). A primary nurse is responsible and accountable for the

Primary nursing – nurses' roles

The primary nurse

- is usually a registered children's nurse
- has the responsibility for the total care of a group of children and families from admission to discharge
- acts as an advocate for the child and family
- coordinates and ensures continuity of care
- has accountability and autonomy in decision making
- requires support and help
- acts as an associate nurse for other primary nurses
- acts as a link nurse for student nurses

The associate nurse

- is a first or second level nurse
- works with the primary nurse to carry out agreed care
- provides support and help for the primary nurse
- may also be a primary nurse for other children and families

Primary nursing – changes to the ward sister role

- Devolves autonomy to primary nurses
- Facilitates a supportive environment
- Helps nurses to assess their own practice
- Provides expert advice and teaching
- Organises workloads and shift systems to enable:
  - close nurse/child/family relationships for primary nurses
  - continuity of care
  - even distribution of primary and associate roles
- May act as role model by taking on primary and associate nurse roles
- Helps the multidisciplinary team to understand primary nursing

total care of a group of patients from admission to discharge (and any subsequent re-admissions). The original idea was that this nurse retained responsibility and accountability even when off-duty. When off-duty the care is delegated to an associate nurse who works according to the primary nurse's prescribed care. Any alteration in care, except in emergency situations, is discussed with the primary nurse. Primary nursing is an efficient method of organising care because it makes the optimum use of qualified staff. The appropriately qualified and experienced nurses act as primary nurses with other qualified staff as associate nurses. Unqualified staff take over responsibility for housekeeping duties and are not involved in direct patient care. This is a much more cost-effective use of staff. This system is also effective in producing good results. Gahan (1991) found that continuity of care was facilitated and there was consistency in the approach to care and the information given to families. She found that it enabled a holistic approach to care with the role of the family being better negotiated, clarified and documented than previously. Primary and associate nurses provide support for each other and can experience increased job satisfaction with the increased responsibility and autonomy provided by this way of nursing (Gahan, 1991).

Primary nursing is equitable as it uses the expertise of all staff members. It completely alters the traditional hierarchical roles within nursing and the ward sister develops a clinical specialist and support role. This equity of roles and the destruction of the hierarchy of nursing may have a negative influence unless staff are well prepared and motivated towards primary nursing. Robinson (1991) warns that this type of nursing can lead to the development of an elite core of nurses and this should be prevented by supporting and developing all staff to make the best use of their abilities. Care must be taken in considering the roles of part-time and night staff. Gahan (1991) describes how health care assistants' roles changed from providing direct care to ordering supplies and catering for families' hotel needs. This change gave them a clearer identification of their role and its contribution to the total care of the child and family.

Primary nursing gives the child and family close access to a highly skilled children's nurse. The families are in no doubt which individual nurse is responsible for their child's care. Primary nursing is very suitable for paediatrics, as it provides families the opportunity for partnership in care in a much more structured way than other methods of organising care. It has been shown to be well accepted by nurses (Fradd, 1988) and children and families (Rogers et al., 1992). Binnie (1987) suggests that it is also acceptable to managers as it provides good value for money, and although it usually means a change in staff establishment to increase the number of registered nurses this change improves the quality of nursing care.

Activity

Consider how well each method of care described above promotes individualised care.

Activity

Consider an area in which you have worked and rationalise which method of organising care is most suitable for that specific setting and patient group.

➤ **Key points**

1. There are four main ways of organising patient care, task allocation, patient allocation, team nursing and primary nursing.

2. Whatever method of care organisation is used it should meet Standard 8 of the Patient's Charter and provide the child and family with (a) a named nurse and (b) individualised care.

3. The care organisational method should provide the optimum care for that specific care setting and group of patients.

4. The method of organising care may be evaluated by testing its efficiency, effectiveness, equity, accessibility, appropriateness, and acceptability.

5. Changing care organisational methods requires motivation and commitment from all staff as roles may undergo considerable change.

Potential problems for the implementation of primary nursing

Attitudes of nursing staff
- willing and motivated to undergo change
- able to manage close relationships with children and families
- real knowledge and understanding of primary nursing

Attitudes of medical staff
- willing to accept loss of ward sister as controller
- able to accept in-depth knowledge of the family by the primary nurse

Grades of nursing staff
- need for appropriately qualified and experienced staff

Shift patterns
- need to allow the primary nurse to be on duty for the majority of the child's and family's stay in hospital, or enable the community nurse to be present for the main part of the agreed care

Nature of nurse education
- preparation for the autonomous practitioner
- clinical placements enable the primary nurse role to be appreciated

Unit and hospital policies
- should take into account the autonomy of the primary nurse

4 STANDARD SETTING AND AUDIT

INTRODUCTION

Developing practice using clinical audit is a challenging and complex task. It should be concerned with improving the quality of care provided for children and their parents but it is sometimes viewed with scepticism and suspicion. If it is not performed appropriately it can be seen as a government cost cutting exercise or a regulatory mechanism (Morrell, 1996). Used properly, it provides a tool which contributes to the monitoring of quality, quantity and resources and leads to an improvement in the care provided for patients (see Figure 4.1, page 725).

Changes in the health service in the 1990s have made clinical audit a necessity. The NHS and Community Care Act (1990) required all service providers to define the service their purchasers could expect. Just as you do your main shopping in the store which you believe gives the best quality and value for money, purchasers of health care will opt to place contracts with the service provider who can offer the highest quality, cost-effective care. The development of NHS Trusts has meant that hospitals are in direct competition for the services they offer, so the demonstration of quality is essential.

Nursing and midwifery accounts for nearly half of an acute hospital's pay budget and this proportion rises in non-acute and community services. The NHS Management Executive (1991) argue that this gives nursing the greatest potential for improving the quality of patient services.

Activity

Consider your usual choice of supermarket and jot down your reasons for shopping in this particular store.

Individuals, as consumers of a service, have very firm ideas about what they expect from the people who provide that service. The usual reasons for choosing a specific service are:

- value for money;
- accessibility;
- clean and hygienic surroundings;
- friendly, knowledgeable and helpful staff;
- best quality, up-to-date products.

It is easy to see how these qualities can be applied to health care services. Patients' charters have helped people to realise that they can expect these qualities in the provision of health care as well as in other

Clinical audit

' ... the systematic and critical analysis of the procedures used for diagnosis, care and treatment, the associated use of resources and the effect care has on the outcome and quality of life for the patient.'

(DoH, 1993)

'... a multi-professional, patient-focused audit, leading to cost-effective, high-quality care delivery in clinical teams.'

(Batstone and Edwards, 1994)

'Nursing audit is part of the cycle of quality assurance. It incorporates the systematic and critical analyses by nurses, midwives and health visitors, in conjunction with other staff, of the planning, delivery and evaluation of nursing and midwifery care, in terms of their use of resources and the outcomes for patients/clients, and introduces appropriate change in response to that analysis.'

(NHS Management Executive, 1991)

areas of their lives. Purchasers of health care are given the responsibility of choosing the best health care providers for their customers. Purchasers are either fundholder general practitioners or county community councils.

Activity

Imagine that you are a buyer of clothes for a large chain store. What criteria will you have for purchasing stock?

Purchasers have the responsibility for spending a large amount of money in the wisest way, so their choices are crucial. It is likely that some of the criteria you selected are:

- goods able to be delivered on time;
- quality finish;
- best deal for money in comparison with rivals;
- effective and harmonious communication networks with providers;
- good reputation;
- meets the needs of your customers;
- discount for bulk orders.

These factors can be easily translated into health care, and in the same way that businesses only remain solvent when they maintain a quality service which ensures a regular income and prevents bankruptcy, Health Care Trusts now also have to achieve these aims.

SETTING STANDARDS

Managers of supermarkets and chain stores and chief executives of health care Trusts have to consider how to ensure that their staff are aware of the criteria which indicate the quality of their service. One of the criteria for choosing to shop in a particular store is that staff are approachable and knowledgeable. What does this really mean? If you were asked to demonstrate these qualities would you really know what was expected of you? It is also likely that different people would interpret these qualities differently.

One of the main reasons for setting standards in health care is to let everyone know exactly what is expected of them in order to provide care at the highest level. It also provides an objective way of measuring this high quality care. Nursing standards, which should be written in discussion with all those involved in that aspect of care, are usually written using the following headings:

- *Standard statement* – a broad aim which states the intention to provide an optimum level of care.

The audit process for nursing

- *Objective/standard setting* – a precise definition of what is to be achieved and why which reflects the overall objectives of the service
- *Implementation* – the introduction of clinical, operational and management policies, procedures and guidelines to enable staff to deliver the agreed standards
- *Measuring and recording* – the process of measuring and recording appropriate data in a valid, systematic and objective way
- *Monitoring and identifying an action plan* – the interpretation and use of the data to make any changes in any of the previous stages and/or revise standards as appropriate

Managing the audit process

- *Organisational arrangements* – determine how the audit process operates within the organisation and who will take overall responsibility for acting upon audit findings
- *Leadership* – is required to ensure that staff feel supported and are aware of their role and responsibility
- *Coordination* – to ensure that all those involved in the audit topic are involved and informed
- *Expertise* – in research methodology to make appropriate use of measurement tools
- *Education* – of all staff to provide the appropriate awareness, knowledge and skills to enable them to accept and participate in the audit process
- *Resources* – sufficient funding and/or resources are needed to support the audit process
- *Prioritisation* – of issues to be audited by comparing the desirability and impact of the audit with the feasibility of being able to undertake it and/or act upon the results

(NHS Management Executive, 1991)

- *Structure* – the physical, social and psychological environment and resources necessary for the care to be given.
- *Process* – how the nursing care will actually be performed.
- *Outcome* – the anticipated effect of the care in measurable terms (see Table 4.1).

The DoH (1994b) recommends that standards are a multidisciplinary activity to form a consistent and collaborative approach to improving the quality of patient care. Much of the original work on standard setting was said to be patient centred but patients were not usually involved; in 1995 the NHS Management Executive funded work to develop the involvement of service users. This has resulted in local initiatives where patients have become actively involved in standard setting and monitoring. Once written, standards must be agreed by line managers and made available to all staff.

Activity

Study the standards used in your current area of practice and find out who was involved in writing them. Identify how the involvement of members of the multidisciplinary team and children and their parents could further contribute to these standards.

Standards cannot be set in isolation from the organisation. They should reflect the overall aims of the service which are usually found in the Trust's annual business plan where key objectives are set to provide a framework for the following year. If standards are to be effective and valuable they should also be:

- based on the best available research;
- sub-divided into discrete, observable items of practice;
- capable of being measured;
- realistic and able to be achieved;
- unambiguous and clearly understood by all;
- readily available to all.

IMPLEMENTING STANDARDS

'Standards do not implement themselves' The NHS Management Executive (1991) warns that standards will only improve care if the organisation provides the appropriate policies and resources support the standard. Clinical, operational and management polices, procedures and guidelines and the appropriate human and medical/nursing resources should be in place or introduced to enable the standard to be met and to be audited.

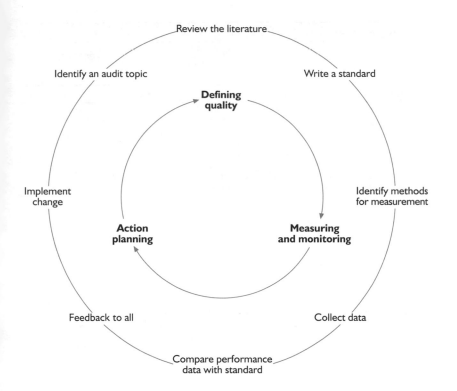

Figure 4.1

The audit cycle.

Activity

Re-read some the standards you studied in the previous activity and identify the policies required to implement them.

MEASURING AND RECORDING STANDARDS

Activity

Study the example standard given in Table 4.1 and consider how you could measure and record the outcomes of this standard.

There are numerous techniques for measuring and recording standards with certain techniques being more appropriate to particular aspects being audited. It is particularly difficult to measure outcomes which relate to feelings and emotions and, for this reason, most standards are best measured using a variety of measuring tools. These tools should follow research rules, procedures and best practices or the audit findings may be invalid (NHS Management Executive, 1991). The Audit Commission's audit of children's services in 1992/3 included an assessment of the quality of care using objectively measured data, the

Table 4.1

Pressure sore risk assessment:
example of a standard

Standard statement		
All patients who are admitted to the Unit shall have a pressure sore assessment chart completed on admission, and reviewed at appropriate intervals, thus providing an individual approach to prevention of skin breakdown in patients.		
Structure	**Process**	**Outcome**
Assessment charts to be available in admission packs	On admission, the allocated nurse will complete the Waterlow risk-assessment chart for each individual patient	Patients will be individually cared for in relation to prevention of skin breakdown
Information on how to use assessment charts available in each clinical area	The admission and subsequent Waterlow scores will be documented on the individual patients' care plans and referred to at report time	Assessment of skin breakdown will be based on current research findings
Nurses who can demonstrate a knowledge of wound assessment	New nurses will be oriented by the ward sister to wound assessment charts	A multidisciplinary involvement in pressure sore risk assessment will enhance communication and understanding in this field
Availability of 'aids' within the clinical areas to prevent skin breakdown	The child's care team will review effectiveness of assessment charts on a monthly basis	Reduction in pressure sores will reduce patient's stay in hospital and overall costs A nursing team committed to and competent in relation to managing individual patients' risk assessment

views of children and parents and staff and observations made by the auditors (Table 4.2).

Questionnaires

There are many patient satisfaction questionnaires which cover a range of issues such as the approachability of staff and the availability and quality of facilities. These questionnaires can be used during or after the patients' stay. Clearly, only older children can use questionnaires and whilst parents can be asked about their satisfaction with their child's care it is difficult to involve younger children in this way.

Questionnaires can also be used to ask staff how standards are being maintained but they cannot be used reliably to evaluate the effectiveness or competence of practitioners. The NHS Management Executive (1991) suggests the use of the Slater Nursing Competency Rating Scale to assess competence. This audit tool uses retrospective ratings on care plans and direct observation of nurse performance.

Observation

An impartial observer from another area, or a health care auditor, can observe the service given and report their findings. Self-recording can be used as an alternative to observers who can be expensive in terms of their time.

Area of care	Objective data	Child/parent view	Staff view	Auditor observation
Named nurse	Identified on care plans?	Do they know who this is?	How does the system work?	Is this made obvious?
Pain relief	Are pain assessment forms in place?	Are they involved in assessment?	How do they assess pain?	Do pain charts show evidence of assessment?
Information	Is a range of information leaflets available?	Have they been given appropriate information?	How do they provide information?	Are leaflets readily available?
Registered children's nurses	Do duty rosters show a minimum of two per shift?		How does the senior nurse maintain the skill mix?	How many RSCN/RN (child) are on duty?
Facilities for parents	What facilities are available?	What do parents think about the facilities?	Can they offer facilities to all parents?	What are the facilities like?

Table 4.2

Auditing the quality of children's services: examples of measurement (Audit Commission, 1993)

Internal monitoring/peer review

Teams of nurses can measure their own standards and this method is probably more reliable than self-monitoring and less threatening than using outsiders. It is still difficult to avoid the subjectiveness of this type of measurement.

Record audit

Spot checks of records provide a way of examining the relevance and quality of nursing practice.

Clinical indicators

Indicators such as measures of health, infection rates or the incidence of pressure sores or accidents provide objective data about clinical care.

MONITORING THE STANDARD AND PLANNING FURTHER ACTION

The monitoring stage of clinical audit processes the information gathered during the measurement of the standard. Once all the information has been collated and reviewed the resulting data should be compared with the standard. Then an action plan can be formulated to identify any further steps which may need to be taken to enhance the area of practice under review. If the standard is shown to have been met it may be appropriate to raise the standard or simply to set the next review date. It is important to remember that a negative outcome may not always mean that the quality of care is poor. At this stage of the audit the validity of the previous steps should be considered:

- was the measurement tool valid and reliable?
- was the sample size sufficient?
- was the implementation of the standard made possible (i.e. was the standard supported by appropriate resources and policies)?
- was the initial standard appropriate?

One outcome of the audit process is a better understanding of appropriate standards (NHS Management Executive, 1991), so if the audit identifies that the standard requires modification the audit should not be considered a failure.

The outcome of the audit process should be clearly summarised to all those involved and any need for change discussed before implementation and remeasurement. The process is repeated as often as necessary to ensure the maintenance and development of clinical excellence (Nursing and Midwifery Audit Information Service, 1996).

Key points ➤

1. The audit process critically examines clinical effectiveness and identifies areas for change.
2. Since the development of NHS Trusts and patient charters, health care policy has placed an increasing emphasis on the quality of care.
3. The first step in the audit process is standard setting. Standards should be evidence based and produced by all those involved in that specific aspect of care.
4. Implementation of standards relies upon the support of appropriate policies and resources.
5. Methods of measuring standards should be valid and reliable.
6. The audit process is cyclical and the comparison of performance data with the standard should identify changes and/or dates for remeasurement.

WORK FORCE ALLOCATION 5

INTRODUCTION

Appropriate staffing levels to meet the care of children depends on many variables such as the dependency of the children, the ward layout, the number of support staff, the shift system and the availability of appropriate staff. Traditionally nurses believed that their areas of work were understaffed but had no objective method of substantiating their claim. The argument used tended to relate to the care the patients received compared with the ideal care which the nurses perceived they should be providing. Unfortunately, this subjective view did little to sway management and has been shown to be a flawed argument (Giovannetti, 1979). Historically, staffing levels tended to be determined in an arbitrary way and nurses have not always had the most appropriate skills for the area in which they worked (Giovannetti, 1984).

This situation eventually prompted nurses to search for an objective planning tool which would enable them to develop a formula to identify the number of staff required to achieve a desired quality of care. Unfortunately, these tools did not help specialist areas such as paediatrics. Most strategies for setting staff establishment levels were designed for acute hospital wards (Hancock, 1980) and do not allow for the uniqueness of nursing children.

SKILL MIX

Skill mix is the term used to ensure that staff with the most appropriate skills are available to meet the needs of the service in the most cost-effective way. It is obviously inappropriate for highly skilled nurses to be performing such jobs as washing up crockery and delivering incontinence pads, yet nurses allow themselves to be used in this way (Hancock, 1992). On the other hand, it is also inappropriate for unqualified staff to be providing unsupervised hands-on care. Research is available to show the cost-effectiveness and improved quality of care provided by qualified staff (Baggust *et al.*, 1992; RCN, 1992). To appreciate the complex role of the qualified nurse it is important to analyse the array of skills used when carrying out any aspect of care.

Activity

Brainstorm and note down typical aspects of nursing care specific to your current area of practice.

Dewar (1992) comments that qualified nurses have difficulty in defining their specific roles. Often nurses first think of manual skills when responding to this activity. In nursing, manual skills are often

---

Calculating staffing

For one nurse on duty at any time :

No. of nurses = (length of each shift × no. of shifts per week) ÷ hours worked per week

For example:

No. of nurses = (8 hours × 3 shifts) × 7 days ÷ 37.5 hours

$$= 24 \times 7 \div 37.5$$
$$= 168 \div 37.5$$
$$= 4.48 \text{ nurses}$$

i.e. to provide one nurse per 8-hour shift each day of the week, 4.48 nurses are required to ensure each nurse only works 37.5 hours per week. This does not allow for sickness, study or maternity leave

---

referred to as basic nursing care or fundamental nursing skills. However, such a response would be supported by the *Collins Dictionary and Thesaurus* which defines a skill as 'something requiring special training or manual dexterity'. This definition implies that these skills require knowledge and understanding. Without an underlying rationale, a skill becomes a meaningless task. In nursing, as in any occupation, it is easy at first to concentrate on the individual components of a skill and forget the subject as a whole. It is only when the nurse becomes proficient at a skill that the actual performance becomes almost automatic and other factors can be considered during the procedure.

Activity

Consider the task of bed-bathing and list what knowledge, skills and attitudes are required to perform this aspect of care proficiently.

When any fundamental nursing task is considered in this way it can be seen that that the nurse uses many different skills apart from that of performing the actual task. When nursing is considered in this way, the notion of manual skills can be broadened to include specialist competencies specific to a particular area of practice. This process of identifying and defining specific skills is important if nurses are to justify their employment. When nurses accept doctors' roles and delegate some parts of their role to unqualified staff they are in danger of eroding the role of the qualified nurse and making it more difficult to define and justify. Budget conscious service managers, who are not always nurses, could decide to employ more unqualified staff for patient care at the expense of qualified staff if their role cannot be clearly identified. Indeed, in 1991, the Audit Commission's report, *The Virtue of Patients*, described cost savings of up to 40 million if health care assistants were used to carry out some of the duties currently performed by qualified staff.

Service managers have the responsibility to ensure a cost-effective skill mix. In other words, each area should employ the right number of qualified and unqualified staff to meet the varying need of each shift during the week. To make decisions about skill mix it is important to know:

- patient dependency levels;
- times of increased workload;
- skills available from each member of staff;
- available hours of duty of staff.

In many areas, information technology has helped to analyse the above information and determine skill mix. Sometimes an emphasis on grading is placed on skill mix, but although this is relevant, it is probably

---

Bathing a bed-ridden child
Task analysis

Knowledge

- areas at risk of pressure sores
- characteristics of healthy skin
- child's disorder and treatment
- prevention of cross infection

Skills

- not causing pain or discomfort during the procedure
- observing: skin colour and condition, temperature and respirations, child's mental state, improvement/deterioration in child's condition
- using play appropriately
- adapting procedure to take account of any medical equipment

Attitudes

- relating to the child appropriately
- talking to the child and family
- explaining/teaching the procedure to the family
- sharing of knowledge in an appropriate way
- negotiating parents' role

more important to look at individuals' different skills and experience. This may be done by an observer who statistically analyses the activities carried out by various nurses in one particular area of practice over a 24-hour period.

Activity

Analyse your own activities for a shift. Construct a spreadsheet to jot down the time spent on each activity during a shift. At the end of the shift you can add up the time spent on each activity and determine the time spent on portering, domestic or secretarial duties.

TIME AND STAFF MANAGEMENT

Part of ensuring an appropriate skill mix is securing round the clock expertise. For this reason, nurse managers have had to consider a more flexible approach to shifts. Most areas now practise internal rotation (when staff rotate from day to night shift) to provide continuity of care and facilitate a team approach. Many areas have also considered variations in shift patterns to reduce the numbers of nurses needed and therefore provide a more cost-effective service.

The numbers of nursing staff required mainly depends on five factors (Roscoe, 1990):

- staffing requirements;
- contracted hours of duty;
- number of shifts per week;
- length of each shift;
- average time absent due to holiday, sickness, study or maternity leave.

Traditionally, nurses have worked two types of daytime shift which overlap in the afternoon. This overlap is often not used to its best advantage and can be seen as a waste of resources to have double the number of required staff for this period of time. Consequently, various initiatives have taken place to counteract this problem.

Shift work inevitably causes problems to humans who have evolved as a diurnal species. Northcott (1995) notes that there is little published work to substantiate the efficacy of any of the various shift patterns available to nurses. Probably the most researched shift is the 12-hour 'long day' which has been introduced in some acute clinical areas. However, Todd *et al*. (1991) suggest that the evidence that these long shifts are beneficial for staff and patients is invalid. In 1995, Barton was commissioned by the DoH to identify the shift system which suited most nurses. She recognised that shift work can affect nurses' psychological health, quality of sleep, cardiovascular and digestive functioning, social

Advantages and disadvantages of 12-hour shifts

Advantages

- 14 shifts/month reduces travel time and expenditure
- increased number of days off per month improves leisure time
- improved continuity of care, especially for short-term patients
- only two hand-over periods per day
- reduced absenteeism (McKillick, 1983)
- improved opportunities for staff education (McColl, 1983)

Disadvantages

- fall off in nurses' performance at the end of the shift (Underwood, 1975)
- overall lower quality of care (Todd *et al*., 1991)
- continuity of care difficult for patients who stay longer than 3–4 days
- possibly contravenes 1974 Health and Safety at Work Act by giving nurses hours which are detrimental to their health and performance
- poor accumulative effect of three to four 12-hour shifts
- reduced communication by ward team members as contact is less

and domestic life and job satisfaction. Barton found that flexible rostering which enabled individuals to cater for their preferences also appeared to reduce some of the health problems and job dissatisfaction associated with shift work. Flexible working is seen as an effective way of recruiting and retaining the work force especially when the workers are predominately women.

Flexibility may also mean allowing a number of staff to work permanently on day or night shifts. Managers tend to prefer internal rotation to night duty believing that it prevents animosity between day and night staff, facilitates professional development for all staff and promotes primary nursing across all shifts. Clinical grading, with senior staff having 24-hour responsibility for their area, has also encouraged the move to internal rotation. The cost effectiveness of internal rotation has not been proven but research has shown that night duty disturbs circadian rhythms and for some individuals this is too stressful to be acceptable (Sadler, 1990).

Northcott (1995) warns that the European Union treaty contains a clause, yet to be agreed, which could enforce all shifts to be a maximum of 8 hours long to minimise the harmful effects of shift work upon staff. For the same reason, this clause would also enforce a maximum 48-hour working week and prescribe a maximum length of time between shifts which may affect the late shift followed by an early shift which is common practice in many rosters. He suggests that nurses should examine their own shift patterns and produce rotas that are safe and acceptable to staff and patients before legalisation forces changes upon them.

Shift patterns

- *Regular* – a fixed roster over a period of time which is repeated when each cycle is completed. Minor variations may occur to meet special requests or to cover annual leave and sickness
- *Irregular* – a duty roster where there is no pattern of shifts and individual preferences are not taken into account; shifts are planned to meet the service need
- *Flexible* – no regular fixed hours or shift patterns. Individuals are consulted about their preferred hours of work and these are matched with the needs of the service

Activity

Look critically at the shift patterns in your own area of work. Are these the most suitable for the staff and the type of work? Is there an even distribution of skills across the 24 hours? Are more staff available for the busiest periods? What suggestions for change could you make?

PATIENT DEPENDENCY

The necessary numbers and skills of staff required in any area is determined by measuring the dependency of the patients in that area. Many scoring systems are available to determine patient dependency but they are often not useful for paediatric areas. For instance, highly dependent, severely ill patients are allocated a high score because they require a lot of highly skilled care, and self-caring patients rate a minimal score. In paediatrics, a toddler without parents present may require almost the same one-to-one nursing care as an acutely ill child. Children with parents present could be rated as self-caring but this would ignore the support and teaching required by the family which may be a highly skilled and time-consuming process.

Another system of determining the necessary resources for specific patients is the case management model. Patients are assigned to a case-type according to their presenting problems and the services they require. Each case-type has a prescribed pathway of care which describes the patient's expected outcomes within a given time scale. The pre-determined care involves all aspects of the patient's care and all personnel involved in that care. As these plans identify the care and resources required for each patient it enables the nurse to spend more time on direct patient care and improves the continuity of care (Mosher *et al.*, 1992). In spite of these advantages it does not seem appropriate for the care of children. With this type of pre-planned care the partnership philosophy of children's nursing may become lost unless the care mapping system is altered to take this into account (Finnegan, 1996). Such systems may also prevent nurses from using their autonomy to plan individualised care.

Activity

Use the patient dependency system on the right to determine the dependency of the children in your current area of work on one specific day. Calculate whether the number and grade of staff are appropriate for these dependency levels. Finally, look critically at your findings. Are they valid? Does the method used take account of all the variables in determining dependency?

Patient dependency studies cannot be considered in isolation from other issues. The available skill mix is important. Some care can be given more quickly by experienced staff than by newly qualified staff but more experienced staff may also have management duties as part of their role. Other staff may require time to teach and assess students.

Activity

Look back to your activity analysis (above) and note the time you spent on non-nursing activities. Multiply this figure by the number of staff on duty during your dependency study (presume that each nurse on duty also used this amount of time for non-nursing). How does this affect your dependency figures?

An example of patient dependency levels

- *Minimal dependency* – 4 hours of nursing care in 24 hours; <10 minutes' direct care/hour (e.g. child having 4 hourly observations, 4 hourly oral/nebulised drugs, ready for discharge, baby with 4 hourly feeds)

- *Low dependency* – 6 hours' care in 24 hours; 10–15 minutes of direct care per hour (e.g. child having 2–4 hourly observations, 4 hourly BM stix, 4 hourly pain assessment, child with parents intermittently resident, baby with 2–3 hourly feeds, routine admission, 48 hours after major surgery)

- *Medium dependency* – 12 hours' care in 24 hours; 15–30 minutes' direct care/hour (e.g. child with IV fluids/analgesia/blood, babies and toddlers with no resident parent, acutely ill admission, child/parents requiring psychological support, children with feeding problems, hourly neurological observations, day 1 following major surgery)

- *High dependency* – 24 hours' care in 24 hours; active and intensive nursing care for 30 minutes/hour (e.g. child with special needs or requiring isolation with no parent resident, child with airway problems (unconscious, croup, severe asthma, tracheostomy), critically ill/multiple injuries child, immediate care after major surgery, care of child and parents following death/emergency transfer to another hospital

Examples of non-nursing activities

- Making empty beds
- Trips to pharmacy, stores, etc.
- Looking for notes or X-rays
- Ordering stores, pharmacy
- Moving beds
- Telephone calls unrelated to patient care

Key points ➤

1. Nurses need to be able to give managers firm evidence of the need for appropriate numbers and skills of staff to meet the needs of the workload.

2. Fundamental nursing activities require specific knowledge, skills and attitudes and cannot be delegated to unqualified staff.

3. Decisions about skill mix depend upon many variables, e.g. workload, availability and experience of staff. Children's nurses need to be able to analyse these variables if they are to convince management of the need for an appropriate nursing establishment.

4. Providing a 24-hour/day service for the care of sick children requires a flexible and innovative approach to shift planning.

5. Patient dependency systems do not always take the uniqueness of children's nursing into account.

References

AUDIT COMMISSION (1991) *The Virtue of Patients: Making the Best Use of Ward Nursing Resources.* London: HMSO.

AUDIT COMMISSION (1993) *Children First. A Study of Hospital Services.* London: HMSO.

BAGGUST, A., SLACK, R. and OAKLEY, J. (1992) *Ward Nursing Quality and Grade Mix.* York: York University, York Health Economics Consortium.

BARTON, J. (1995) Is flexible rostering useful? *Nursing Times,* **91** (7), 32–33.

BATSTONE, G. and EDWARDS, M. (1994) Clinical audit 'how do we proceed? *Southampton Medical Journal,* **10** (1), 13–18.

BEDFORDSHIRE HEALTH AUTHORITY (1996) *Do you Qualify for Continuing Health Care?* Luton: Bedfordshire Health Authority.

BENNER (1984) *From Novice to Expert: Excellence and Power in Clinical Nursing.* Menlo Park, CA: Addison-Wesley.

BINNIE, A. (1987) Structural changes. *Nursing Times,* **83** (39), 36–39.

BINNIE, A., *et al.* (1984) *A Systematic Approach to Nursing Care.* Milton Keynes: Open University Press.

BLACK, N., *et al.* (1990) A randomised controlled trial of surgery for glue ear. *British Medical Journal,* **300**, 1551–1556.

BLACKSHAW, D. (1994) Problems that just refuse to go away. *Nursing Management,* **1** (4), 20–21.

BLAUNER, R. (1964) *Alienation and Freedom: The Factory Worker and his Industry.* Chicago: University of Chicago Press.

CASEY, A. and MOBBS, S. (1988) Partnership in practice. *Nursing Times,* **84** (44), 67–68.

DoH (1989a) *Caring for People.* London: HMSO.

DoH (1989b) *The Children Act: An Introductory Guide for the NHS.* London: HMSO.

DoH (1990) *NHS and Community Care Act.* London: HMSO.

DoH (1993) *Clinical Audit: Meeting and Improving standards in Healthcare.* London: HMSO.

DoH (1994a) *Being Heard. The Report of a Review Committee on NHS Complaints Procedures*. London: HMSO.

DoH (1994b) *The Evolution of Clinical Audit*. London: HMSO.

DoH (1996) *The Children's Charter*. London: HMSO.

DEWAR, B. (1992) Skill muddle? *Nursing Times*, **88** (33), 24–27.

EDGE, W,. KANTER, R., WEIGLE, C. and WALSH, R. (1994) Reduction of morbidity in inter-hospital transport by specialist pediatric staff. *Critical Care Medicine*, **22**, 1186–1191.

FINNEGAN, A. (1996) Managing cost and quality in case management. *Paediatric Nursing*, **8** (8), 25–26.

FRADD, E. (1988) Achieving new roles. *Nursing Times*, **84** (50), 39–41.

GAHAN, B. (1991) Changing roles. *Paediatric Nursing*, **3** (10), 22–24.

GIOVANNETTI, P. (1979) Understanding the patient classification system. *Journal of Nursing Administration*, **9** (2), 4–9.

GIOVANNETTI, P. (1984) Staffing methods – implications for quality. In WILLIS, L. and LINWOOD, M. (eds), *Measuring the Quality of Care*. Edinburgh: Churchill Livingstone.

HANCOCK, C. (1980) Finding the right level. *Nursing Mirror*, **150** (2), 37–38.

HANCOCK, C. (1992) Nurses and skill mix. *Senior Nurse*, **12** (5), 9–12.

HUCZYNSKI, A. and BUCHANAN, A. (1985) *Organisational Behaviour*. London: Prentice Hall.

KRON, T. (1981) *The Management of Patient Care – Putting Leadership Skills to Work*. London: Saunders.

McCOLL, C. (1983) Twelve hour shifts: a way to beat prime time blues. *Canadian Nurse*, **78** (31), 47–50.

McKILLICK, K. (1983) Modifying schedules makes jobs more satisfying. *Nursing Management*, **14** (1), 53–55.

MANTHEY, M., CISKE, K., ROBERTSON, P. and HARRIS, I. (1970) Primary nursing – a return to the concept of my nurse and my patient. *Nursing Forum*, **9** (1), 65–83.

MARLAND, J. (1994) Back where they belong: caring for sick children at home. *Child Health*, **2** (1), 40–42.

MoH (1959) *The Welfare of Children in Hospital (Platt Report)*. London HMSO.

MORRELL, C. (1996) Clinical audit makes progress in care and teamwork. *Nursing Times*, **92** (30), 34–36.

MOSHER, C., *et al.* (1992) Upgrading practice with critical care pathways. *American Journal of Nursing*, **99** (1), 41–44.

NHS EXECUTIVE (1996) *Paediatric Intensive Care Report from the Chief Executive to the Secretary of State*. London: NHS Executive.

NI IS MANAGEMENT EXECUTIVE (1991) *Framework of Audit for Nursing Services*. London: HMSO.

NORTHCOTT, N. and FACEY, S. (1995) Twelve hour shifts: helpful or hazardous to patients? *Nursing Times*, **92** (7), 29–31.

NURSING AND MIDWIFERY AUDIT INFORMATION SERVICE (1996) *Evidence-based Practice and Clinical Effectiveness*. London: NMAIS.

PAYNE, D. (ed.) (1997) This week. *Nursing Times*, **93** (16), 7.

REED, N. (1988) A comparison of nurse-related behaviour, philosophy of care and job satisfaction in team and primary nursing. *Journal of Advanced Nursing*, **13**, 383–395.

REID, W. (1996) Righting wrongs. *Nursing Standard*, **10** (24), 19.

ROBINSON, K. (1991) A primary flaw? *Nursing Times*, **87** (42), 36–38.

ROGERS, M., GAHAN, B., COLE, S. and GOODE, M. (1992) Looking forward. *Paediatric Nursing*, **4** (2), 23–25.

ROSCOE, J. (1990) Planning shift patterns. *Nursing Times*, **86** (38), 31–33.

ROYAL COLLEGE OF NURSING (1992) *The Value of Nursing*. London: RCN.

RUSSELL, I. and WILSON, B. (1992) Audit: the third clinical science? *Quality in Health Care*, **1**, 1–55.

SADLER, C. (1990) Beat the clock. *Nursing Times*, **86** (38), 28–31.

SALVAGE, J. (1985) *The Politics of Nursing*. London: Heinemann.

SHAW, C. (1986) *Introducing Quality Assurance*. London: King's Fund.

THOMAS, D., DUFFY, N. and CAWDRY, S. (1992) Team nursing. *Nursing Times*, **88** (52), 40–43.

TIERNEY, A., CLOSS, S., WORTH, A., KING, S. and MacMILLAN, M. (1994) Older patients' experiences of discharge from hospital. *Nursing Times*, **90** (21), 36–39.

TODD, C., REID, N. and ROBINSON, G. (1991) The impact of 12 hour shifts. *Nursing Times*, **87** (31), 47–50.

UNDERWOOD, A. (1975) What a 12 hour shift offers. *American Journal of Nursing*, **75** (7), 1176–1178.

UNITED KINGDOM CENTRAL COUNCIL (1992) *The Code of Professional Conduct for Nurses, Health Visitors and Midwives*. London: UKCC.

WESTWOOD, O. (1997) Nutrition and immune function. *Nursing Times*, **93** (15), i–vi (supplement).

WILLIAMS, L. (1995) Is the money well spent? *Child Health*, **3** (2), 68–72.

WILLIS, L. and HANCOCK, C. (1980) Finding the right level. *Nursing Mirror*, **150** (2), 37–38.

INDEX

Page references in *italics* indicate tables, those in **bold** indicate figures

Pain (*continued*)
  neonates 550–51
  nurses' perception of 352–3
  post-operative 384
  relief 356–9, *357*, *358*,
    398–400
  sickle cell anaemia 421–2
Pain rating scales 354–5, *354*
Parasuicide 539–40
PARC (Paediatric Aids Resource
  Centre) 495
Parenteral feeding 327–8, 332–4,
  333, 334–5, 549
Parenting *see* Child rearing
Parents
  attitudes 202–3
  and physical illness 205–6
  behaviour and children's
    behaviour 204–5
  and child abuse 242, 244
  and Children Act (1989)
    663–5
  and children's pain 349, 355
  and chronic illness 225, 226,
    227, 228–9
  communication with 277,
    614–15
  and consciousness assessment
    506
  and consent to treatment
    656–7, 658, 659
  and day care 286, 287–8, 288,
    293
  and death 219–20, 222, 223,
    308–11, 396–7, 397–8,
    401, 402
  and disability 232, 234, 235
  disablity or illness of 204
  and drug administration 326
  and education 101–2
  and family-centred care 614,
    614–15, 616, 617
  and home care 364, 373, 374,
    613, 704–5
  hospital facilities 260, **260**
  and hospitalisation 213, 257,
    361, 582–3
    in anaesthetic room 292
    intensive care 389, 390–1
    preparation 264–5, 265,
      266
    in recovery room 292
  separation from 203
  unable to perform usual role
    361
  working patterns 14

  see also Families; Fathers;
    Mothers
Partnership nursing model
  608–10, **610**
Passive smoking 159–60
Patent ductus arterious (PDA)
  437, **439**
Patient care 716
  and confidentiality 671
  patient allocation 718
  primary nursing 719–20, 721
  task allocation 716–18
  team nursing 719
Patient controlled analegsia
  (PCA) 358
Patient dependency 732–3
Patient's Charter 297–8, 693,
  716
Patriarchy 29
PCNs (paediatric community
  nurses) 373, 375, 640–1
  and day care 293
  and disability 235
  and discharge planning 705
  and family-centred care
    613–14
  role of 335, 372, 375–6
  see also Community nursing;
    Nurses and nursing
PDA (patent ductus arterious)
  437
PD (peritoneal dalysis) 483–4,
  484
Peak expiratory flow rate (PEFR)
  518
Pediculosis capitis 527, *532*
Peer education programme 165
Peer relationships 88, *88*
Peplau's nursing model 361, 593,
  607, **608**
Percentile charts 282
Perception, visual 71–3, **72, 73**
Peripherally inserted central
  (PIC) catheter 346
Peritoneal dialysis (PD) 483–4,
  484
Permissive behaviour 21, 38
Personality 83
  development 83–5, *85,* **86**
  and play 98
  and violence 241
Perthes Association 435
Perthes disease *429,* 430
Pertussis 125, *489, 498, 515*
Pethidine *357*
Pharmacological methods 356

Phebitis 343–4, *344*
Phenylketonuria 136, 445, **448,**
  451
Phimosis *478*
Phonology 77
Phototherapy 553–4
Physical abuse 239, *239–40,* 241
Physical assessment 280–5
Physical development 68, *69*
Physical punishment 41, 42
Physiotherapy
  chest 519–20
  and discharge planning 705
Piaget, Jean 74–6
PIC *see* Paediatric intensive care
PIC (peripherally inserted
  central) catheter 346
Placenta 61, 63
Plaster casts 432–3, *432*
Plaster sores *432*
Platt Report (1959) 581, 583,
  694
Play 94–5, 104
  in A&E units 297
  at different ages 95–7
  coping with stress with 264
  for explaining procedures
    268–9
  in hospital 259, 362
  influences on 97–8
  in intensive care 389, 391
  purpose of 98–9, *99*
  views on 98
  whilst confined to bed 365
Plymouth Brethren *631*
PMR (post-neonatal mortality
  rates) 117, **118, 119**
Pneumonia *515*
Poliomyelitis 126, *489, 498*
Politics and health care 349–50,
  708–10
Pollution and health 128–9
Polycystis disease *477*
PONV (post-operative nausea
  and vomiting) 383
Port-a-cath 324, **325,** 347
Portfolios, nurses' 623
Port-wine stain *526*
Positioning of neonates 548–9
Post-neonatal mortality rates
  (PMR) 117, **118, 119**
Post-operative care 378, 382–5,
  442, 443–4
  discharge planning 385
  gastro-intestinal problems
    472